SECOND EDITION

ALEXANDER S. NADAS, M.D., F.A.A.P.

Associate Clinical Professor of Pediatrics, Harvard Medical School;
Cardiologist, The Children's Hospital;   Physician, Sharon Cardiovascular Unit, Children's Hospital Medical Center, Boston

ILLUSTRATED

PEDIATRIC
CARDIOLOGY

W. B. SAUNDERS COMPANY

PHILADELPHIA AND LONDON   1963

To my wife,
Elizabeth McClearen Nadas

FOREWORD

Sixty years ago Dr. Thomas Morgan Rotch, then Professor of Diseases of Children, published the first textbook on Pediatrics from the Harvard Medical School. Even in 1896 there was enough information regarding this relatively new specialty to require a volume of some 1100 pages, but only seven of these were headed Congenital Diseases of the Heart. Obviously there was relatively little to say about this particular pediatric problem and even less stimulus toward further knowledge, for Dr. Rotch wrote that, although "it is usually possible to make a diagnosis of congenital cardiac disease, . . . a diagnosis of the especial lesion is, as a rule, impossible." In any case the exact diagnosis was only of academic interest. In his single paragraph devoted to the management of congenital heart disease Dr. Rotch did mention "the administration of digitalis in small doses and with the utmost caution" as occasionally useful, but concluded that the treatment was "essentially hygienic and symptomatic."

The next textbook of Pediatrics from the Harvard Medical School appeared thirty years later. Professor John Lovett Morse was able to compress what he thought the pediatrician of 1926 needed to know about heart disease into forty pages, less than five of which sufficed for Congenital Heart Disease. Doctor Morse could find one item of progress unknown to Dr. Rotch. But even this was nearly useless, for "the Roentgen ray, which theoretically ought to be of considerable assistance in the diagnosis of special lesions, is practically of little assistance even in the hands of an expert." Yet, "Fortunately the diagnosis of the exact lesion . . . is not of great importance in either prognosis or treatment. . . . There is no curative treatment [and] nothing which will either diminish the deformities or favor the closure of abnormal openings. The treatment, must, therefore, be hygienic and symptomatic."

Now, in 1956 we find ourselves at the end of another thirty-year interval. Judged by the progress before 1926, the mere size of this new book on Pediatric Cardiology from the Harvard Medical School and Children's Hospital of Boston is sufficiently impressive. Even more striking is the preponderance of pages devoted to the diagnosis and treatment of congenital as compared with acquired heart disease. Obviously the sudden increase in knowledge and interest concerning a subject until recently so neglected, is worldwide. Its local history has been traced here only as a convenient example of the size and suddenness of this development. Why should one thirty-year interval (indeed, essentially the last fifteen of those thirty years) have witnessed such striking progress?

A partial explanation is found in the decline of other challenges, such as the feeding methods, formulas and digestive diseases of infancy and childhood. But the real cause was the demonstration by Gross in 1939 and by Blalock and Taussig in 1945 that it was indeed possible to "diminish the deformities or favor the closure of abnormal openings." The essential element was some basis for hopefulness. With hope, interest in diagnosis came suddenly to life; cardiac catheterization became a useful tool rather than a *tour-de-force;* "the Roentgen ray" was belatedly found to be of considerable assistance, indeed, and the "symptomatic and hygienic treatment" took on entirely new meaning and purpose.

The pediatrician—and especially the younger pediatrician—has rightly been unwilling to see all these aspects of diagnosis and treatment handed over to a new subspecialist in cardiology. Fully aware that the surgeon who operates upon the heart of a child requires special skill and training, the pediatrician considers the nonsurgical aspects of cardiac disease in infancy and childhood to be pediatric responsibilities. In rising to meet this new and growing challenge, he will find this volume extremely helpful. Its author once described to me his hope of making this "a do-it-yourself cardiology." I believe he has succeeded.

Dr. Nadas is especially well qualified for this task. His approach as an author parallels that of his own professional life. His residency in Pediatrics at The Children's Hospital in Boston and his year of full-time pediatric responsibility and teaching at the Children's Hospital of Michigan in Detroit were followed by four years of general pediatric practice in a small city some distance from the specialized services of a medical school. With this background of practical experience Dr. Nadas returned to The Children's Hospital in Boston in 1949 to participate in the suddenly and rapidly expanding activities of its Cardiology Division. Now, as Cardiologist to the group of hospitals making up The Children's Medical Center, and Consultant in Pediatric Cardiology to the Boston Lying-in Hospital, the author would, I believe, prefer to be known primarily as a thoughtful and resourceful doctor for infants and children. That Dr. Nadas is also a wise specialist of large experience in cardiology and a teacher of great skill and enthusiasm will be abundantly clear to the reader of the following pages.

CLEMENT A. SMITH, M.D.
Department of Pediatrics
Harvard Medical School

PREFACE TO THE SECOND EDITION

The reasons for publishing a second edition of *Pediatric Cardiology* should be set forth. The first edition, published six years ago, met with an acceptance which, though not extraordinary, surprised the author, his friends, and his publisher. Why, then, tempt fate once more?

The favorable reception of the first edition, and the progress in the discipline during the past seven years, since completion of the manuscript, amply justify revision of the book. Every owner of a copy of the first edition becames a relative, a shareholder in the author's feeble resources. One cannot with equanimity watch respected colleagues, and students, refer to the volume when it clearly contains statements known to the author to be outmoded, even incorrect. The urge to set the record straight and to issue correct information is irresistible. As soon as the revision was begun it became obvious that nearly every page required change—changes based not necessarily on new information in the literature, but more often than not on facts and experience new only to the author and well known for some time to others. Another fact, emerging clearly only at the end of two years' work, is even more painful: portions revised at the outset may already need re-revision at the time of completion of the manuscript. By this time one has gained enough gray hairs to accept this as the human condition.

The reader may note, probably with dismay, that the second edition is appreciably larger than the first. Partly this is due to the growth of knowledge within the field. Secondly the need for more illustrations has become clear. And finally, where in the relatively youthful enthusiasm of 1956 issues appeared in black and white, they now need a more qualified statement. It is hoped that the bringing out of the exception as well as the rule will not make the book less readable and that the relative increase in the erudition of the author, as testified by the larger bibliography, will not make the book more obtuse.

Because of the size of the volume, and the appearance of his separate monograph on the subject, Dr. R. M. Smith and I thought it best to omit

vii

his section on anesthesia from the second edition. Since competition with the magnificent reproductions of angiograms published in recent years by Swedish authors seemed hopeless, no angiograms will be found in this edition. The tables in the present volume are all together at the end of the book to facilitate their use as a ready reference. All the self-imposed limitations announced in the preface to the first edition are still in force. Wherever possible, only first-hand information is discussed. Surgical techniques and physiologic principles will be alluded to only so far as they would assist the clinical pediatric cardiologist. In spite of the "simplicity" of recent open-heart techniques, this volume still shies away from giving instructions as to how to perform cardiac surgery.

The author would again like to express his deep appreciation to his colleagues in the Department, particularly Dr. Anna J. Hauck and Dr. Paul G. Hugenholtz, for their invaluable assistance, direct and indirect, in the compilation of this manuscript. Special thanks are due to Dr. Robert E. Gross, Dr. Edward B. D. Neuhauser and Dr. Martin H. Wittenborg for what they continued to teach me and to Dr. Charles A. Janeway for allowing me the freedom within the Department to write this book.

I also wish to thank Mrs. Marcia Lawson for editing, Mr. Ferdinand R. Harding for the reproductions, and my secretaries, Mrs. Sheila Nelson Franklin and Miss Susan McCartney, for being generally cheerful and helpful through the years. The W. B. Saunders Company have been extremely cooperative and patient throughout the preparation of this volume.

Boston, Massachusetts.   ALEXANDER S. NADAS, M.D.

PREFACE TO THE
FIRST EDITION

This volume is intended to be a handbook for the pediatrician, the general physician and the medical student. It does not claim to be a treatise on the physiology of the heart, though obviously physiological data will be presented in an attempt to explain the clinical picture. I have tried to make every chapter fairly complete by itself; thus a certain amount of repetition is unavoidable.

My intention has been to put proper emphasis on clinical recognition and management of heart diseases in children. Techniques of cardiac catheterization and angiocardiography, for example, have been described; but primary emphasis has been kept on the principles and procedures of clinical management.

I have written almost exclusively about our own experiences at The Children's Medical Center during the past ten years, and I did not intend to write a reference book. Diseases and even important therapeutic procedures such as open heart surgery and hypothermia with which I had little personal contact have been discussed only cursorily. The interested reader may do better to look up these topics in the reference material rather than have me interpret other people's work for him. The list of references, like the book itself, is a subjective one. I did not aim at completeness, but rather included only the books and articles I have found particularly interesting and useful through the years.

The list of people to whom I am indebted—directly or indirectly—in helping me complete this work would easily fill a whole page.

I want to start with my mother and father. The memory of my father, a writer who always wanted to be a doctor, inspired me particularly. I felt that I was paying homage to him by fusing in this volume the profession of the writer with that of the physician. The little emblem at the foot of this preface was the trademark of his magazine published many years ago in Budapest, Hungary.

On the professional side I should like to begin with Dr. Charles A. Janeway, Thomas Morgan Rotch Professor of Pediatrics at Harvard Medical

School, who gave me the opportunity to work in the field of pediatric cardiology. Doctor Clement A. Smith, friend and teacher, has helped me in many ways during the past fifteen years. I want to express my sincere thanks to Drs. Edward B. D. Neuhauser and Martin H. Wittenborg, who taught (and fought) me in radiology, and to Dr. Robert E. Gross for much invaluable teaching and the use of his patient material. Doctors Abraham M. Rudolph and Walter T. Goodale, my associates in the laboratory, assisted me in collecting and interpreting the physiological data presented. Without the help of Drs. Patrick A. Ongley and Donald C. Fyler I am sure the illustrations would not have been completed in time. I would also like to thank Dr. Robert M. Smith for his contribution in writing the section on Anesthesia.

I would like to express my sincere appreciation to Mr. Walter T. Hall, who, through the establishment of a fund for the support of research in pediatric cardiology, helped to defray expenses of publication.

I wish to thank my secretary, Miss Myrtle R. Westhaver, for her efficiency in holding together the cardiology department during the trying period in which this book was written, Mrs. Marcia Lawson for the editing of the manuscript, Mr. Ferdinand R. Harding for the photography, Mrs. Margaret M. Steele for the typing, and Miss Mary E. Delaney for the illustrations.

Finally, I want to thank sincerely the W. B. Saunders Company for the many patient ways by which they helped me prepare this volume and efficiently bridge the Atlantic with their galley proofs.

Groningen, The Netherlands ALEXANDER S. NADAS, M.D.

CONTENTS

xii   **Contents**

Part Three   CONGENITAL HEART DISEASE

THE TOOLS
OF DIAGNOSIS

PART ONE

1

HISTORY, PHYSICAL EXAMINATION AND ROUTINE TESTS

HISTORY

The history in pediatric cardiology should encompass the principal pediatric and cardiac features of heart disease. It should begin with a résumé of the chief complaints. It is extremely important to learn, from the outset, how sick the child really is, and how many of the complaints are entirely "iatrogenic" in origin and secondary only to the discovery of a heart murmur. The entire picture in a child who is sick "because the doctor said so," who is "too active" and whose limitation of exercise is the result of parental restriction will be different from that of another youngster who "will not gain or grow like others," "gets blue" or "breathes heavily."

If the presence of a murmur represents a significant portion of the complaint, it is vital to elicit certain facts about its timing and the circumstances of its discovery. Was it present at birth? If not, how long after birth was it discovered? Was it discovered by a physician who had been taking care of the youngster all along or by a new physician who was seeing him for the first time? How closely had the child's health been supervised before the discovery of the murmur? Were there febrile illnesses, especially sore throats, immediately preceding its appearance, and, if so, what was the time interval between the occurrence of the sore throat and the appearance of the murmur? Precise information related to these points

3

may, on occasion, be the only clue on which to base a differential diagnosis between congenital and acquired heart disease.

Next, the history of the present illness should be elicited. This should be a detailed chronologic account of the child's disease from the first time his health was questioned. It is important that the inquiry about the present illness should not reach back only to the time when heart disease was first diagnosed. In many instances, especially in cases of acquired heart disease, cardiac disorder or its significant antecedents may have been present before there was any clear indication of involvement of the circulatory system.

A careful systemic review is, perhaps, the most important part of the history. As to the gastrointestinal system, the question of appetite should be raised; if the appetite is poor, especially in an infant, one ought to inquire whether the mother believes that this may be due to fatigue or whether it represents a general lack of interest in food. Parents should be questioned carefully about weight gains and losses. A history of abdominal pain may raise the suspicion of rheumatic fever. The genitourinary system should be considered, particularly in respect to a decrease in urinary output, characteristic of congestive failure. In adolescent girls, especially cyanotic ones, the effect of the onset of menses on general well-being and exercise tolerance should be questioned.

Inquiry about the cardiorespiratory system is the most essential part of the systemic review. An excellent idea of the exercise tolerance of these patients may be obtained by careful questioning about the average distance they can walk on level ground or the flights of stairs they can climb without undue fatigue. Inquiries should be made about the influence of weather, or the time of day, on exercise tolerance. One should ask not only about their playing habits and how well they can keep up with their contemporaries, but also how much the average game "takes out" of them. According to their parents, some of these children "never give in," although they obviously look exhausted after playing an hour or two.

In infants and small children who do not walk or run, the effort of taking a bottle, of sitting up for a definite length of time or of crawling around the playpen may represent a rough test of exercise tolerance. One seeks information about dyspnea or wheezing. The child's breathing when he is asleep is a particularly important criterion of respiratory effectiveness; one should note the rapidity of respirations, the use of ancillary muscles (alae nasi) and the presence of grunting. A vivid description of the forcefulness of cardiac action can sometimes be obtained by asking parents whether they themselves could feel the child's heart beating against the chest wall. The time of onset of cyanosis, its permanent or paroxysmal nature, its severity, progression and localization, are all important data. One should inquire about the presence of squatting, and also other favorite positions (such as knee-chest) which the child is likely to assume when tired. Such positions strongly suggest a cyanotic type of congenital heart disease, particularly tetralogy of Fallot.

It should be ascertained whether there have been "anoxic spells" (p. 353); and if so, exact information about their time of appearance, duration, frequency and nature should be obtained. It is also important to note, specifically, whether these spells are accompanied by loss of consciousness or by convulsions. Tendency to excessive perspiration should be noted. Often this is an early sign of congestive heart failure. A persistent cough at night, or after vigorous exercise, may also be a sign of cardiac decompensation.

The number, type and severity of respiratory infections through the years should be established; these are usually increased in patients with large left-to-right shunts, and they may predispose to rheumatic fever. Inquiries should be made about chest pain and hemoptysis, particularly in older children and adolescents. One ought to ascertain the number and severity of sore throats, particularly in patients suspected of having rheumatic heart disease. Nosebleeds may be important because of their frequent occurrence in patients with rheumatic heart disease and pulmonic stenosis.

Investigation of the central nervous system should include inquiries about the child's motor and intellectual development. Although no causal connection between mental retardation and congenital heart disease has been established, unquestionably, a higher percentage of mental retardation occurs among these children, particularly those having cyanosis, than in the average population. This does not negate the also well known observation that some of the most severely handicapped children are among the brightest ones. Furthermore, since in infancy motor development is frequently used as an index of intellectual function, a false impression of mental retardation may be arrived at on the basis of extreme exercise intolerance (e.g., when there is transposition of the great arteries).

The history of a "stroke" should be carefully elicited, since it may alert one to the possibility of endocarditis. More often it signifies severe cyanotic disease. Headaches, personality changes, or somnolence, particularly in an older child with tetralogy of Fallot, could lead to the diagnosis of brain abscess. Symptoms of chorea should be sought for in any child suspected of having rheumatic fever. Discovery of a history of weakness and incoordination may easily lead to the exact classification of a "myocarditis of unknown origin" (Friedreich's ataxia or muscular dystrophy).

The bones, joints, muscles and skin should be subject to inquiry, particularly for the occurrence of rashes, petechiae, rheumatic nodules, "growing pains" and arthritis. The number of joints involved, the duration of involvement, the presence of swelling, heat and tenderness are all important pieces of information.

The family history is of increasing interest as attention is being focused on the etiology of congenital and rheumatic heart disease. Of course the question of consanguinity of the parents should be raised. The number of miscarriages, stillbirths, the familial occurrence of even minor congenital anomalies may be important. The postmortem diagnosis of congenital heart disease in a cousin who died many years ago in early infancy may be a most important clue toward diagnosis in a new patient. Familial occurrence of sudden, unexplained death may direct the physician's attention to familial myocardial disease. A strong history of diabetes may dispose to certain types of congenital heart disease (transposition, hypoplastic left heart syndrome). The tendency of rheumatic fever to appear in several members of one family barely has to be mentioned. The familial occurrence of heredodegenerative diseases of the central nervous system (Friedreich's ataxia) and of the connective tissues (Marfan's syndrome) is well known; both have strong tendencies to involve the heart.

The prenatal history is important, particularly in regard to the first trimester. Inquiries should be made about bleeding, toxemia, febrile illness and exposure to communicable diseases, particularly German measles. Questions about the birth and type of delivery should be made. Particular emphasis should be placed on the occurrence of cyanosis, the use of resuscitative measures, and the administration of oxygen, all signs of fetal distress. Evidence of congenital heart disease is often suggested by a history of delayed discharge from the hospital after birth or of failure to regain birth weight in the expected time.

Feeding, development, immunization and past history require the kind of attention customary in the taking of a good pediatric history.

PHYSICAL EXAMINATION

The physical examination of the child suspected of having heart disease should follow along well established pediatric lines. It is valuable to have a routine sequence which will reduce omissions to a minimum. The following points require particular emphasis.

General Description

Does the child appear ill, or is he happy and playful? Is he in distress of any sort, and if so, what kind? The body build should be expressed by recording the absolute weight and height in terms of percentiles on a well accepted developmental chart. This latter point is particularly important as one follows a patient along through the years and watches his development, the influence of intercurrent illnesses and the effects of surgical intervention. The phrases "well developed" and "well nourished" are particularly irritating and meaningless unless they are supplemented by percentiles of the average. A developmental chart should be part of the record of every child with heart disease.

In addition to expressing the body build in terms of height and weight, note the presence of associated congenital anomalies. Certain combinations of these suggest certain specific congenital heart diseases. It is necessary to refer only briefly to the endocardial cushion defects associated with mongolism, to pulmonic stenosis occurring in children with broad cheek bones, round faces and hypertelorism. The specific lesions seen with Turner's syndrome (coarctation, pulmonic stenosis, atrial septal defect) and the cardiac complications of Marfan's syndrome (aortic and mitral regurgitation, atrial defect and myocardial disease) are well recognized. Wood[748] drew attention to the fact that patients having abnormalities of the forearm tend to have ventricular defects. I have noted that patients having patent ductus arteriosus often have small cavernous hemangiomas. Evans[235] mentioned the association of accessory nipples with pulmonary hypertension. The product of a pregnancy complicated by German measles in the first trimester shows the characteristic association of congenital heart disease, cataracts, deafness and mental retardation. That patent ductus arteriosus is the most common cardiac lesion among these children is well known. I have been impressed by the relative frequency of patent ductus arteriosus associated with pulmonic or aortic stenosis in these patients.[333]

No general description of a child suspected of having congenital

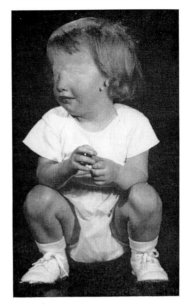

Figure 1. Child squatting.

heart disease should fail to mention his preferred posture, particularly the presence of squatting (Fig. 1). The color should be noted, with particular attention to cyanosis. If cyanosis is present, its depth and distribution pattern are always pertinent. Sometimes patients with minimal arterial unsaturation (such as isolated pulmonary stenosis, Ebstein's disease or pulmonary hypertension) are not frankly cyanotic; their cheeks and lips have a peculiar high color, however, with a slight bluish tinge. Noticing this, the experienced observer will estimate the arterial oxygen saturation to be in the 85 to 90 per cent range. Often this color is misleading, however, and even the trained clinician may mistake the flush of a healthy child entering a warm room for borderline cyanosis.

Jaundice is less common in children with heart disease than in adults. Pallor is, obviously, an important sign; the particular discrepancy of pallor and a relatively adequate hemoglobin level is characteristic of the rheumatic patient. The yellowish pallor (*café-au-lait*) is typical of subacute bacterial endocarditis. The particular combination of cyanosis and pallor in patients with cyanotic heart disease and relative anemia is known as "Picasso blue" in our Clinic.

Head and Neck

The conjunctivae should be inspected with particular care for the presence of anemia or cyanosis. It is surprisingly easy to examine the fundi of most children sufficiently well to note the presence of papilledema and venous engorgement. Carious teeth are, unfortunately, common in patients with cyanotic congenital heart disease, and may be the source of subacute bacterial endocarditis in these patients as well as in those with rheumatic fever. Although the tonsils are not regarded with as much awe today as they were twenty-five years ago, nevertheless the connections between streptococcal sore throat and rheumatic fever on the one hand, and membranous tonsillitis and diphtheritic heart disease on the other, are significant enough to warrant careful evaluation of these organs.

Inspection of the neck can furnish important clues. Vigorous arterial pulsations commonly can be seen in patients with severe aortic disease (coarctation of the aorta, patent ductus arteriosus or aortic regurgitation); they are practically unknown in instances of atrial septal defect. Distention and pulsation of the jugular veins will be discussed later; suffice it to say here that they furnish the best indirect information about the happenings in the right atrium. A thrill palpable at the suprasternal notch is practically pathognomonic of one of four conditions: aortic stenosis, coarctation of the aorta, pulmonic stenosis or patent ductus arteriosus. Evidence of cervical lymph nodes may be extremely helpful in the diagnosis of rheumatic fever, and less commonly of diphtheritic heart disease or even infectious mononucleosis. The rare instance of thyrotoxic heart disease may be suspected if goiter is discovered. A thrill and continuous murmur localized over the neck should raise the suspicion of an arteriovenous fistula. Finally, a continuous murmur of evanescent nature heard over the neck vessels constitutes a venous hum. The differential diagnosis of this will be discussed in some detail in the chapter relating to patent ductus arteriosus (see p. 474).

Heart

Inspection and Palpation. The examiner should start by noting the presence or absence of deformities in the chest. A symmetrical increase in the anteroposterior diameter of the chest, similar to that seen in patients with emphysema, is commonly noted in children with congenital heart disease and pulmonary hypertension. Vigorous pulsation of a significantly enlarged right or left ventricle leads to visible left-sided chest prominence (congenital heart disease with left-to-right shunt or rheumatic valvular disease). Right-sided chest prominence is present occasionally in patients having tricuspid atresia. Visible pulsations, sometimes rocking the entire chest, and characteristic in certain patients with congenital heart disease involving tremendous shunts (patent ductus arteriosus or large ventricular septal defects with aortic regurgitation) and in children with rheumatic aortic regurgitation. Severe mitral regurgitation on a rheumatic or congenital basis may also give rise to a rocking cardiac impulse. On the other hand, a relatively quiet beat may be seen in the face of cardiac enlargement, in patients with Ebstein's deformity, primary myocardial disease and, of course, pericardial effusion.

The presence of thrills and their timing, intensity and localization should be noted. The nature of the cardiac impulse should be observed with great care.[208, 746] A good estimation of the hypertrophy of the right or left ventricle can be achieved by noting the point of maximal impulse of the heart beat. If this is at the xiphoid process or the lower left sternal border, with visible up-and-down pulsations, the chances are that the right ventricle is dominant. Conversely, if the cardiac impulse is maximal at the apex, with visible outward pulsations in this area, the left ventricle is likely to be enlarged. A cardiac impulse palpable at both the xiphoid and the apex strongly suggests combined hypertrophy. It is well worth mentioning that a markedly enlarged right ventricle may occupy the entire anterior surface, as well as the left border, of the heart and, thus, may give rise to pulsations suggesting combined enlargement. In true biventricular enlargement, however, a distinct differentiation is possible between the left ventricular pulsation propulsing forcefully from the back to the apex and the anterior pulsation of the right ventricle. The two are not exactly synchronous, and sometimes an area of relatively diminished pulsations between the two ventricles may be noted. It may also be possible to obtain some clue as to which ventricle underlies which part of the anterior chest wall by looking at the unipolar chest lead in the electrocardiogram. A rightward systolic pulsation of an enlarged right atrium in tricuspid regurgitation may be striking. The nature of the cardiac impulse may be tapping and quick, suggesting a relatively large volume work, or heaving and slow, indicating increased pressure work. Percussion of the entire cardiac silhouette is tiresome, time-consuming and barely justifiable in this age of easy availability of radiograms. At its best this procedure can give the physician only an approximate idea of the size of the heart; at its worst it may be completely misleading.

Auscultation. After inspection and palpation have furnished information about the size of the heart and the intensity and location of its pulsations, the examiner should concentrate on auscultation. To obtain maximal benefit from this most valuable part of the physical examination, the proper instrument must be used. The usual "pediatric stethoscope" with the flat chest-piece edged with rubber is totally useless for reliable auscultation of the heart.[570] Almost equally useless in the examination of infants are the huge adult stethoscopes, especially the ones with only a diaphragm chest-piece; these instruments, when placed on the tiny chest of a baby, cover practically the entire cardiac silhouette. A third kind of stethoscope should be used only when necessary—someone else's stethoscope. The pernicious practice of picking up any stethoscope in a hospital ward is to be deplored. A stethoscope is a personal instrument, much like a fountain pen. Best results can be achieved only by the continuous use of the same ear- and chest-pieces. Not everyone's aural canals are of the same size and shape. The ear-pieces have to fit the canals tightly without discomfort to assure optimal auscultation.[661] It is to be hoped that sartorial considerations will never prohibit the doctor from carrying his own stethoscope in his pocket.

What type of stethoscope should be carried for the examination of children with heart disease? It should be a so-called binaural stethoscope with a combined bell and diaphragm chest-piece. The length of the rubber tubing should probably not be longer than 10 to 12 inches, the bore $\frac{1}{8}$ inch.[572] Within recent years the Sanborn Company began marketing a stethoscope incorporating the ideas of the late Maurice Rappaport, who was their chief engineer, and those of Dr. H. B. Sprague, who has contributed much to the science of auscultation of the heart. This well constructed instrument, with its variable-sized chest- and ear-pieces, is singularly adaptable to auscultation in various-sized patients. If the physician can afford one of these instruments, and in our "affluent" society even some interns manage to own one, he will select the ear-pieces most suited to his auditory canal. Then he will routinely use the size bell and diaphragm which best fit the majority of his patients. The other chest-pieces should be carried in his bag or pocket to be applied to patients smaller or larger than his average. Other excellent stethoscopes, less adaptable but very satisfactory, are those designed by Leatham in England and, recently, by Littman in this country.

One ought to listen not only at the apex and the other conventional points, but also at selected areas over the entire cardiac silhouette. The neck and the chest should be carefully mapped out with the stethoscope, using the bell-piece first, the diaphragm later. Low frequency murmurs are best heard with the bell applied lightly to the chest, whereas the higher frequencies are best perceived with the diaphragm firmly pressed against the precordium. The low frequency first, third and fourth sounds are best heard with a bell, whereas the second sound and high frequency component of clicks are best analyzed with the diaphragm. If possible, the first attempt at listening to any patient's heart should be with the patient lying flat, to be followed by turning him on his left side, and finally by having him sit up. When examining a small infant, one cannot be too demanding, and one should examine the heart in the position most comfortable to the child, irrespective of the gymnastics it may require on the part of the physician. It is remarkable how many children who are completely unmanageable if put on an examining table will be quiet and cooperative when held on the mother's lap.

HEART SOUNDS. On auscultation the first things to be noted are the rate and the rhythm, after which one ought to concentrate on the heart sounds. I have found it useful to try to listen to the sounds one at a time, aiming to determine the following characteristics of each: (1) Where is it heard maximally (apex, second left interspace, and so forth)? (2) What is its absolute intensity? (3) Where is it observed minimally? (4) What is the degree of splitting? This type of analysis of the first, second, third and, possibly, fourth heart sounds should precede the evaluation of murmurs and is of the greatest importance. A loud first sound at the apex occurs commonly in mitral stenosis.[9]

A loud, systolic ejection sound at the pulmonary or aortic area[413] has been observed in conditions associated with dilatation of the ascending aorta or the main pulmonary artery (valvar stenosis, pulmonary hypertension, or idiopathic dilatation of the pulmonary artery). This is referred to as a systolic click. The click originating from the pulmonary artery is best heard at the upper left sternal border and changes its intensity with respirations, whereas the aortic click is usually independent of respirations and is heard best at the lower left sternal border and the apex. The earlier the click, the more severe the stenosis.

A booming second sound at the pulmonary area usually indicates pulmonary hypertension,[578] unless the sound heard in this region actually represents aortic closure. Thus transposition of the great arteries, partial or complete, has to be excluded before definitive conclusions about pulmonary arterial pressure are drawn from the intensity of the second sound at the second left interspace. Careful observance of the two components of the split second sound (see p. 113) may be of considerable help in this regard; almost invariably (except in cases of maximal left ventricular hypertension) the first component represents aortic, and the second, pulmonic closure. Consequently, one may say with assurance that a loud second component of the second sound at the second left interspace means pulmonary hypertension. A loud single second sound may or may not be indicative of such. Absence or diminution of the second sound at the pulmonary area means that the pulmonary arterial pressure is low or that the vessel is in an abnormal position.[2]

In most infants and children an appreciable (0.01 to 0.03 second) splitting of the second sound may be noted on moderate inspiration. Normally, the split widens on inspiration and disappears on expiration. This phenomenon may be observed best at the second left interspace.

A single second sound may indicate either synchronous closure of the two semilunar valves (pulmonary hypertension, ventricular septal defect) or an inaudible pulmonary component (severe pulmonic stenosis with ventricular septal defect). A moderately split second sound (0.03 to 0.05 second), particularly if it does not change with respirations and if the 2 components are of equal intensity, is almost pathognomonic of atrial septal defect.[37] A widely split second sound (0.05 to 0.10 second), with a diminished second component and only slight variation with respirations, indicates severe pulmonic stenosis with an intact ventricular septum. A widely split second sound in which A_2 and P_2 are of equal intensity, with only slight variations, is typical of right bundle branch block. Finally, a moderately split second sound with inspiratory narrowing of the split (paradoxical splitting) indicates left ventricular stress (aortic stenosis, patent ductus arteriosus).

A well defined third heart sound at the apex is common in normal children and adolescents; on the other hand, it may be the precursor of a mid-diastolic rumble. A fourth, or atrial, sound may be specific for conditions with right atrial hypertension (severe pulmonic stenosis, essential pulmonary hypertension, Ebstein's anomaly and total pulmonary venous anomaly). An "opening snap" of the second heart sound may, on occasion, be the only diagnostic clue indicating stenosis of the mitral or even the tricuspid valve.[9]

MURMURS. Analysis of the heart rate, the rhythm, and the nature of the sounds having been accomplished, the murmurs are then identified and described. At least six aspects of every murmur should be recorded: (1) timing: (a) systolic (early, late or pansystolic), (b) diastolic (protodiastolic, mid-diastolic or presystolic, and (c) continuous; (2) nature: (a) systolic (ejection, stenotic, regurgitant, rough, blowing or musical), (b) diastolic (blowing, rumbling, crescendo or decrescendo), and (c) continuous (machinery or to-and-fro); (3) grade of maximal intensity (1 to 6, according to Levine[421]); (4) duration; (5) point of maximal intensity; and (6) degree and localization of transmission (special emphasis to neck and back). On the basis of this type of analysis, information not obtainable by any other method can be secured. The sea-gull type of apical systolic murmur of mitral regurgitation, the presystolic crescendo of mitral stenosis, the diastolic blow of aortic regurgitation (sounding like an echo of the aortic closure), the harsh murmur of a ventricular septal defect, the soft pulmonary systolic blow of an atrial septal defect, the grating, well transmitted stenotic murmur of pulmonary stenosis, the machinery murmur of patent ductus arteriosus—all these become as familiar to the experienced observer as the "barking of a dog or the meowing of a cat."[427] The graphic demonstration and analysis of these phenomena by means of phonocardiography will be discussed in a separate chapter (see p. 106) and illustrated individually within the framework of their respective pathologic conditions.

EXTRACARDIAC SOUNDS. Extracardiac sounds should also be sought. Among these, the most characteristic is obviously the pericardial friction rub, the sound of which can best be imitated by rubbing one's own hair between one's fingers. This is usually heard best at the lower left sternal border, with the stethoscope pressed firmly against the chest. The friction rub is seldom localized to one part of the cardiac cycle. Occasionally it is loudest in systole; once in a while it is present predominantly in diastole. In the latter instance, particularly in patients with rheumatic carditis, a rub may be confused with the faint blow of aortic regurgitation. Extracardiac "clicks," usually noted in systole, probably are caused by pericardial adhesions.

Lungs

The lungs, like the heart, should be examined by inspection, percussion and auscultation of the chest. Inspection gives invaluable information about respiratory rate and the visible effort of breathing. In patients with severe coarctation of the aorta, inspection and palpation of the ribs over the back may reveal thick collateral vessels. Hyperresonance on percussion indicates emphysema or pneumothorax; dullness suggests fluid, atelectasis or consolidation. Ewart's sign is a triangular dullness at the side of the lower spine, pathognomonic of large pericardial effusion, and resulting from compression of the lung. Auscultation not only reveals the wheezes or rales characteristic of infection or congestion, but also gives basic information as to whether too little, sufficient or too much air is being exchanged.

Abdomen

Gentle, often superficial palpation is needed to discover the liver edge in a young infant. In normal infants and children the liver may be palpable as far down as 3 cm. from the right costal margin in the right nipple line. Daily observation as to the size of the liver is one of the most reliable guides in the estimation of congestive failure in children. Frequently one sees a child admitted to the hospital in congestive failure due to paroxysmal atrial tachycardia, with a liver estimated to be 7 cm. below the right costal margin. Adequate treatment of such a patient may result in the absence of a palpable liver within thirty-six hours.

Although many young children normally have a palpable spleen, definite splenomegaly is one of the cornerstones in the diagnosis of bacterial endocarditis. By contrast, an enlarged spleen is seldom caused by congestive failure. Abdominal situs inversus, with or without thoracic situs inversus, may suggest associated congenital heart disease. The obvious importance of acites requires diligent search for abdominal fluid. Palpation of the abdominal aorta is possible in many children and may be used in the accurate localization of a coarctation of the aorta.

Extremities

Cyanosis of the fingers strongly suggests congenital heart disease. In patients in whom a definite difference between the coloring of the upper and lower extremities is noted, a shunt from the pulmonary artery to the aorta through the ductus arteriosus may strongly be suspected. British authors[746] recommend the use of a hot bath to bring out the cyanosis in the legs.

Clubbing of the fingers and toes commonly accompanies cyanosis, but may be seen in patients without arterial unsaturation (p. 352). Clinically, clubbing has at least two components: one is the rounding of the fingers, especially the thumbnails; the other is a thickening and shininess of the terminal phalanges, with disappearance of the normal creases (Fig. 2). In some patients the fingernails show the greatest abnormality; in others the changes in the phalanges dominate. In children in whom a difference in degree of cyanosis between fingers and toes is noticed the same discrepancy in the degree of clubbing will be observed.

Patients with congenital heart disease often have fiery red fingers and toes. We have learned to recognize this phenomenon as a precursor of cyanosis and clubbing; it is fairly characteristic of those whose arterial oxygen saturation is permanently or paroxysmally low normal or slightly abnormal (±90 per cent) (Ebstein's anomaly, isolated pulmonic stenosis with foramen ovale or ventricular septal defect and pulmonary vascular obstruction). The temperature of the extremities should be noted, particularly in regard to differences between hands and feet; the discrepancy may be rather great in coarctation of the aorta. The joints should be inspected carefully; heat, tenderness, redness and swelling are indispensable features in the diagnosis of rheumatic arthritis. Rheumatic joints are painful and tender; they may easily be differentiated from the nonspecific mild joint pains secondary to orthopedic conditions (flat feet and so forth). Rheumatic nodules (Fig. 3) are most commonly found

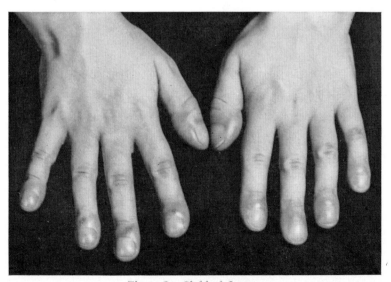

Figure 2. Clubbed fingers.

over the knuckles, the elbows and the knees. Sometimes they can be seen first, and felt only later. They may be recognized better in indirect light as pea-sized, nontender structures attached to fasciae or tendon sheets, which are freely movable with the skin.

Rashes, especially erythema marginatum (Fig. 4), may be seen in patients with active rheumatic fever. Petechiae are characteristic of bacterial endocarditis. Deep, tender, purple spots at the ends of the fingers, representing minute emboli (Osler nodes), are practically pathognomonic of bacterial endocarditis. Pitting edema of the extremities is not common in children; if present, it may indicate right-sided congestive failure.

Palpation of both radial and femoral pulses is of utmost importance. Strong radial pulses with weak and late or absent femorals are diagnostic of coarctation of the aorta. In this and in congenital aortic stenosis a difference between the strength of the left and right radial pulses is also commonly noted. Respiratory variations in pulse volume (pulsus paradoxus) of more than 10 mm. of mercury may indicate pericardial tamponade, though severe respiratory distress (asthma, emphysema or post-thoracotomy states) may give rise to pulsus paradoxus of 20 to 25 mm. of mercury.

Bounding radial or femoral pulses are important clues in the diagnosis of a sizeable runoff from the aorta, either back into the left ventricle (aortic regurgitation), into the pulmonary artery (patent ductus arteriosus), or even exclusively into the peripheral vascular bed (thyrotoxicosis). Lesser degrees of hyperactivity of the carotids may be simply the result of excitement. One important clue to be obtained from the carotids in patients

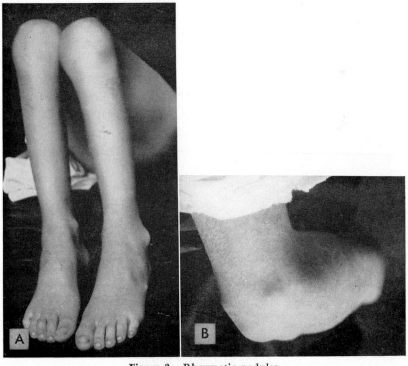

Figure 3. Rheumatic nodules.

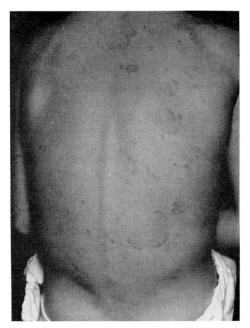

Figure 4. Erythema marginatum.

with aortic stenosis should be mentioned. The patient with critical organic aortic stenosis usually does not have strong carotid pulsations, a fact clearly understandable on the basis of the slow upstroke time of these patients. In contrast, in patients with functional subaortic stenosis, the initial part of the central aortic and carotid tracing has a rapid upstroke. Consequently, these patients may present a picture of critical aortic stenosis with bounding carotids.

Circulatory System

Arterial Pressure. Determination of blood pressure in the arm[315] should be an integral part of every examination. It is important to measure the systolic blood pressure in the arms as well as in the legs in all patients suspected of having congenital heart disease; thus coarctation of the aorta will not be missed by clinical examination.

The auscultatory method, using a mercury sphygmomanometer, is an easy and well accepted procedure in adults and older children. The results can be interpreted without much hesitation.

In children, especially in the younger age groups, the problem is far from simple. To begin with, the patient usually does not cooperate. Second, limbs of different sizes require different cuff sizes. Finally, the results have to be interpreted according to the age of the patient.

To ensure optimal cooperation, it is worth while, if possible, to explain the procedure to the child beforehand. Often an older child may be distracted by watching the up-and-down movements of the mercury column when they are pointed out. Infants often have to be pacified with a bottle of milk while the blood pressure is being taken. Finally, in some instances sedation with barbiturates or morphine may be necessary to ensure some degree of cooperation.

The size of the cuff is extremely important in obtaining results comparable to those of arterial blood pressure determined by direct arterial puncture. As a rough guide, the cuff should cover approximately two thirds of the upper arm or leg. A cuff that is too small gives falsely high readings. For accurate results the pediatrician should have available at least the following cuff sizes: 3-, 5-, 12- and 18-cm. widths. Sometimes a larger cuff, folded over, may be adapted to a smaller limb. The bag should be completely deflated and applied evenly, snugly, without bulging, around the upper arm or leg, and should completely encircle the limb.

Once the cuff of proper size has been applied to the patient, it may be well to obtain a quick reading of the systolic pressure by palpation. The cuff should be inflated to a point well above the disappearance of the radial pulse. Then gradually (2 to 3 mm. of mercury per beat) the pressure should be released until the radial pulse reappears. This point clearly corresponds to the systolic pressure determined by direct measurement.

Once the systolic pressure has been determined by palpation, the systolic and diastolic pressures should be estimated by the usual auscultatory method. According to the latest report of a committee of the American Heart Association, the diastolic pressure corresponds to the level at which the auscultatory sounds completely disappear.[16] Simultaneous measurements of the diastolic pressure by the sphygmomanometer and by an indwelling arterial cannula reveal this not to be the case in every instance. Therefore, if the sounds become obviously muffled at one pressure level and disappear completely at a lower one, both figures should be recorded, since either may represent the true diastolic pressure. As a matter of fact, in our experience, the appearance of the muffled sound more nearly corresponds to measured diastolic pressure. This is particularly obvious in patients in whom Korotkoff sounds may be heard all the way down to zero on the sphygmomanometer, while the diastolic pressure on the intra-arterial tracing never falls to this point.

Though the auscultatory method may not be feasible in a restless infant and the palpatory method may not be adaptable in patients who do not have easily palpated pulses in the lower extremities (coarctation of the aorta), the so-called flush method[315] can be used in both situations. A cuff of appropriate size is placed around the ankle or wrist. The limb is elevated and massaged to produce blanching. The cuff is rapidly inflated to well above the expected systolic level. Then the limb is lowered to approximate heart level, and the cuff is slowly, gradually deflated. The point at which a flush appears below the cuff in the previously blanched limb is taken to correspond to the systolic pressure. The flush pressure is usually lower than the systolic peak pressure obtained by direct arterial puncture or by the auscultatory method. It commonly approximates the level of the mean arterial pressure. Moss and his associates[508] found the flush pressure in normal infants to be lower in the legs than in the arms. This has not been my experience. With these limitations the flush pressure is an extremely useful method of obtaining information about the blood pressure of certain infants when no other method is applicable.

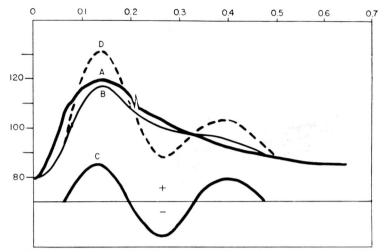

Figure 5. Diagram illustrating the principles of damping and wave summation in the arterial system. *A,* Aortic pressure pulse. *B,* Changes in contour and amplitude due to damping. *C,* Nature of rebound wave. *D,* Summation of curves *B* and *C* (ordinate pressure in mm. of mercury; abscissae line in 0.1 seconds).[729]

Perhaps its prime usefulness is in revealing relative hypertension of the arms, and thus proving the presence of coarctation of the aorta in instances in which this diagnosis could not be made by any other method. Still another method using the principle of oscillometry has been outlined by Keith.[380]

The systolic pressure in the legs is usually significantly higher than in the arms because of a summation effect of the forward pulse wave with the rebound wave (Fig. 5). A reversal of this relation is pathologic and implies the presence of an aortic block. The diastolic pressures in the arms and legs should be identical; a significant difference usually means that the cuff over the leg was relatively small.

The actual height of the systolic pressure has to be interpreted in relation to the patient's age. Various authors have placed the systolic blood pressure level in normal infants at approximately 70 to 90 mm. of mercury between birth and one year of age. Premature infants have correspondingly lower pressures.

Neligan and his associates,[531] recording the systolic pressure of newborn infants, registered an appreciable drop (a mean of 25 mm. of mercury) from the initial value recorded within 5 minutes after delivery to the lowest value reached between one and 4 hours of life (systolic pressure returns to its previous level by the end of the first day). There is a suggestion that newborn infants with the respiratory distress syndrome exhibit a more severe degree of this neonatal hypotension. Between the ages of one and 5 years the average systolic pressure rises to about 100 mm. of mercury; between 5 and 15 years it gradually climbs to 120 mm. of mercury, with a usually transient period of mild hypertension at the time of puberty. The diastolic pressure during the same period changes relatively little, from 55 to 61 mm. Average blood pressures in infants and children, taken from the most reliable sources in the literature, are given in Table 1 (p. 773).

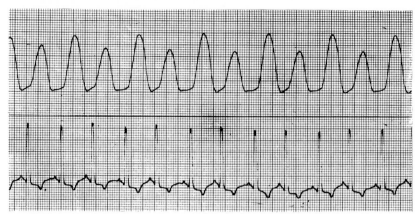

Figure 6. Pulsus alternans in patient with severe aortic stenosis. Note on top line the alternating height of systolic pressure within the left ventricle, and on the bottom the electrocardiogram with QRS complexes of approximately identical height.

The most common causes of persistent and significant elevation of the systolic blood pressure in children, listed in the approximate order of their frequency, are (1) renal disease, (2) coarctation of the aorta, (3) widened pulse pressure (aortic regurgitation, patent ductus arteriosus, thyrotoxicosis), (4) diseases of the central nervous system (poliomyelitis, tumors, encephalitis), (5) poisoning with mercury (acrodynia) and lead, (6) endocrine disorders (pituitary, adrenal tumors, pheochromocytomas), and (7) essential hypertension.

Low blood pressure is most commonly explained by the presence of shock or so-called vasovagal syncope (fainting).

Pulse Pressure. The pulse pressure may be calculated by subtracting the diastolic from the systolic pressure. A widened pulse pressure, detectable by the bounding, water-hammer type of radial pulse, is commonly seen (1) in fever, anemia, thyrotoxicosis, and after vigorous exercise; (2) in aortic regurgitation, patent ductus arteriosus and arteriovenous fistulas; and (3) in complete heart block.

Conversely, narrow pulse pressures may be observed in (1) shock, (2) severe mitral or aortic stenosis, (3) pericardial tamponade or constrictive pericarditis, and (4) certain instances of congestive failure.

Two peculiarities of the pulse may best be detected while determining blood pressure: (1) Pulsus paradoxus, characteristic of the accumulation of an appreciable amount of fluid in the pericardial sac, consists in a decrease of systolic pressure and narrowing of the pulse pressure on deep inspiration. (2) Pulsus alternans, a sign of left ventricular failure, consists in an appreciable drop in systolic pressure in alternate beats (Fig. 6).

Venous Pressure. Determination of venous blood pressure and analysis of the jugular venous pulse waves are extremely useful tools in cardiovascular diagnosis, but are not nearly as widely used as is the determination of the arterial blood pressure. The reason for this neglect may well be the absence of a simple, accurate apparatus, not involving venipuncture, similar to the sphygmomanometer.

In spite of the technical difficulties, a great deal of attention has been paid to the jugular venous pulse in adults by careful cardiologists.

The accurate determination of the venous pressure and detailed analysis of the venous pulse waves are well nigh impossible to obtain in infants because of their lack of cooperation.

In children who cooperate, especially the older ones, simple inspection furnishes reliable information about venous pressure and, indirectly, the right atrial pressure. Perhaps the simplest and most reliable test is inspection of the jugular vein of the patient when he is erect. According to Lewis,[427] the external jugular vein should not be visible above the suprasternal notch unless the venous pressure is elevated. A crude estimation of venous pressure is furnished by measuring the height of the jugular venous column, vertically, in a standing patient, above the suprasternal notch. If the patient is recumbent, the height of the jugular venous column should not rise above an imaginary straight line across the manubrium of the sternum (Fig. 7).

These rough clinical guides usually give satisfactory answers only as to the presence or absence of gross elevation of the mean pressure in the jugular venous system. For purposes of accurate determination, direct measurements by means of venipuncture are necessary. An apparatus for determining venous pressure in this way has been made available commercially.[104] Properly used, this gives accurate and reproducible results.

A simple apparatus which may be made available in the treatment room of any hospital consists of a spinal manometer connected to a **T** tube and mounted on a stand. The zero level of the manometer should be adjustable. One end of the **T** tube is connected to a length of rubber tubing with a glass adapter, to which a number 20 to 22 needle is attached. The other end of the **T** tube is connected with a reservoir by rubber tubing and should have a clamp on it. The reservoir contains saline solution with a drop of heparin.

The patient is propped up at an approximately 45-degree angle, with his arm resting on a pillow. All clothing is loosened, and the patient should be as relaxed as possible. The zero level of the manometer is adjusted to the level of the manubrium of the sternum. If the test is performed with the patient lying flat on an examining table, the zero level should be adjusted at 5.5 cm. above the table top. It is extremely important to record the point at which the zero level of the manometer was placed; only in this way can the results have any comparative value. The manometer is filled with saline solution from the reservoir, and the rubber tubing is clamped. An antecubital vein is entered, and the saline column in the meniscus of the manometer then indicates the height of the venous pressure in millimeters of saline. It is important to watch the rise and fall of the saline column with respirations for a few minutes

Figure 7. Patient lying down at approximately 45 degrees; the pressure (ZL) in the right atrium does not rise above the manubrium line (ML).[427]

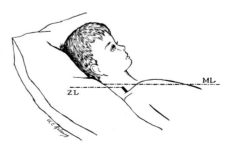

VARIATIONS IN VENOUS PRESSURE IN GROWING CHILD

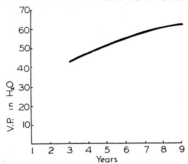

Figure 8.   Venous pressure in children.104

before a definite reading is taken, to see whether it is in free equilibrium with the venous system. The height of the mean venous pressure in children between the ages of 3 and 5 years has been established by Burch[104] as 40 mm. of water, and between the ages of 5 and 10 years, 58 mm. of water (Fig. 8).

Not only is the height of the venous pressure of great importance in the clinical diagnosis of heart disease, but the pattern of the jugular venous pulsation is of considerable interest as well. By careful inspection of the superficial, and preferably the deep jugular, veins a definite pattern of waves and troughs can be observed. A bedside analysis of these is a most important aid in cardiac diagnosis. Normal persons, who do not have elevated venous pressure, should be observed in the recumbent position or at a 45-degree angle. Patients with significantly elevated venous pressure should be in the sitting or standing position when the jugular venous pattern is observed lest the high mean pressure obliterate the individual wave patterns. For the timing of the waves, either simultaneous auscultation of the heart or palpation of the cardiac impulse may be used. With experience, the quick upstroke characteristic of the A wave may be identified by simple inspection and may be differentiated from the slower, later, more undulating V wave. Skillful examination may also reveal the notch corresponding to the C wave on the descending limb of the A. Further inspection may also reveal the depth of the x and y troughs.

For a more accurate analysis of the jugular venous pattern, a suction cup may be placed on the jugular vein and connected to a piezo-electric crystal microphone leading into one of the commercially available amplifiers which register photographically. As a reference tracing, simultaneous registration of the electrocardiogram and possibly the phonocardiogram should be utilized (see Fig. 41, p. 50).

If the jugular venous tracing thus registered is analyzed, three separate waves and two troughs can be distinguished (Fig. 9): (1) The A wave, or presystolic wave, immediately follows the P wave and precedes the Q wave on the electrocardiogram. At the bedside it can be recognized as the wave of the jugular venous pulse which immediately precedes the apical impulse of the heart and is synchronous with or precedes the first heart sound by a fraction of a second. It originates from the reflux in

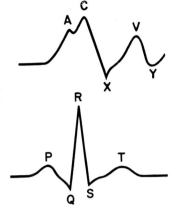

Figure 9. Schematic representation of jugular phlebogram (top), with electrocardiogram as a reference tracing (bottom).

the venae cavae caused by the atrial contraction. (2) The C wave, or early systolic wave, is synchronous with the plateau of the carotid pulse; hence the designation "C." It usually follows one or two seconds beyond the termination of the QRS complex in the electrocardiogram and may be identified clinically as the positive wave immediately following the first heart sound. It is said to originate partly from the isometrically contracting right ventricle pushing back against the closed tricuspid ring and partly from the impulse of the carotid artery itself. (3) The V wave marks the end of ventricular systole. It occurs at the time of, or slightly after, the dicrotic notch at the carotid tracing, usually some distance beyond the T wave of the electrocardiogram, and just beyond the second sound in the phonocardiogram. This V wave is caused by the gradual filling of the right atrium with blood from the systemic venous return. The x depression and the y trough are indicative of the first and second rapid fillings of the ventricles and are identified by their relation to the preceding positive A and V waves, respectively.

Analysis of these elements of the jugular venous pulse reveals a certain characteristic pattern. A large A wave, indicating powerful atrial systole, can be seen characteristically in the phlebogram of conditions causing "P pulmonale," such as pulmonary stenosis with intact ventricular septum, tricuspid stenosis or atresia and Ebstein's anomaly. Obviously, no A waves may be seen in atrial fibrillation. Occasionally a prominent A wave (cannon wave) occurring at irregular intervals interspersed between A waves of average height is seen in patients with complete atrioventricular block. It is caused by an atrial contraction occurring against a closed tricuspid valve (Fig. 10). An exaggerated V wave is seen in tricuspid regurgitation. Tall V waves, preceded by systolic collapse, have been found commonly in patients with large atrial septal defects. Disappearance of the x depression is seen in constrictive pericarditis and right-sided failure. The presence of a well marked, rapid x descent excludes, for all practical purposes, the possibility of significant tricuspid stenosis.

Circulation Time

The bedside determination of the circulation time is of only slight interest in pediatric cardiology today. It is mentioned here mostly for

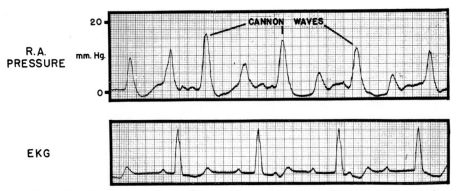

Figure 10.   Cannon waves in the right atrial pressure tracing of a patient with complete heart block. Note the tall A waves (cannon waves) corresponding to the P waves in the cardiogram below. These are the P waves that are not followed by a QRS complex, and thus encounter a closed tricuspid valve. Note, in contrast, the low A waves, corresponding to the conducted P waves.

historical interest. Obviously, circulation time as determined by dye dilution curves is used extensively as part and parcel of the cardiac catheterization procedure and will be discussed at some length in the appropriate chapter (see p. 145).

Clinically estimation of the circulation time is used principally for two purposes: (1) The progress of patients in congestive failure may be estimated by repeated determinations of the circulation time. This is based on the principle that congestive failure is accompanied in most instances by slow circulation time which improves with treatment. By the same token, determination of the circulation time automatically separates the so-called high output failures with rapid circulation time (thyrotoxicosis, anemia or beriberi) from the conventional cases of congestion with slow circulation time. (2) A significantly shortened circulation time in patients with congenital heart disease indicates a right-to-left shunt.

Methods for bedside determination of circulation time are manifold. At the Children's Hospital Medical Center in Boston we have used two methods only. Both give reliable and reproducible results; both measure the arm-to-mouth circulation time. Table 2 (p. 773) contains normal values for the fluorescein method.

In the fluorescein method 0.07 cc. per pound of body weight of a solution containing 5 per cent sodium fluorescein and 5 per cent sodium bicarbonate is injected into the antecubital vein in a dark room. A fluorescent light (a modification of the Wood's lamp) shines on the patient's lips. The end-point is usually sharp when yellowish fluorescein shows up on the patient's mouth. The child should be carefully examined under a Wood's lamp before the test for fluorescent material which may confuse the reading; penicillin and Aureomycin have given trouble in this respect. This test is especially useful with small children when an objective end-point is needed. Doses of more than 5 cc. may cause vomiting.

In the second method Decholin is used in dosages of 2 cc. for children less than 7 years of age and 3 cc. for older children in order to determine the arm-to-mouth circulation time. The material is injected into an antecubital vein, but the end-point here is subjective. The patient should be instructed to indicate immediately by raising his hand when a bitter taste touches his tongue. This test can be used effectively in patients seven or more years old.

ROUTINE LABORATORY TESTS

Routine laboratory tests performed on all children, including those with cardiac disease, will not be described here in detail. Their particular applicability to children with heart disease will, however, be mentioned briefly.

Urinalysis

Patients with congestive failure may have albuminuria, a urine of high specific gravity, and mild hematuria. Hematuria is also found in patients with bacterial endocarditis.

Complete Blood Cell Count

Leukocytosis of moderate degree may be present in congestive failure, bacterial endocarditis and acute rheumatic fever, with or without failure. A high hematocrit value is always found in patients with cyanotic congenital heart disease. In addition to determining the hematocrit level, a careful analysis of the blood indices (mean corpuscular volume, mean corpuscular hemoglobin and mean corpuscular hemoglobin concentration), as well as inspection of the smear, is indicated. Such a careful survey of the hematologic data often reveals the presence of hypochromic anemia requiring iron treatment or a dangerously high hematocrit value (more than 85 per cent). The normochromic or hypochromic anemia noted with bacterial endocarditis and rheumatic fever should be observed.

Acute Phase Reactants

In acute infections, particularly rheumatic fever, certain substances which wax and wane with the progress or subsidence of the disease appear in the blood. These substances are called acute phase reactants. Two tests giving information about these substances should be mentioned.

The erythrocyte sedimentation rate is used universally as a reliable index of rheumatic activity. An elevated erythrocyte sedimentation rate (Westergren, more than 20 mm. per hour; Wintrobe, corrected, more than 15 mm.) is almost invariably present in patients with acute rheumatic fever. One notable exception is the finding of a normal sedimentation rate in some patients with acute rheumatic fever in congestive failure. High sedimentation rate levels are also found in patients having bacterial endocarditis, even in the face of congestive failure, a useful point on differential diagnosis. The phase reactants contributing to the sedimentation rate are probably fibrinogen, alpha$_2$ and gamma globulin.

The C-reactive protein is an acute phase reactant not normally present in the blood. Chemically, the substance is an alpha globulin precipitated with the somatic C-polysaccharide of pneumococci. In the routine laboratory test, rabbit serum is used to precipitate the substance from the patient's serum. It is present with high regularity in almost all patients who have acute rheumatic fever, including those with congestive failure. Patients with certain isolated rheumatic manifestations, however, usually those not accompanied by fever or elevated sedimentation rate (such as chorea, erythema marginatum, or Aschoff bodies in the left atrium), fail, on occasion, to show C-reactive protein in their blood. The principal value of the C-reactive protein determination is that it furnishes excellent laboratory evidence for subsidence of rheumatic activity. Usually the substance disappears from the blood at an appreciable interval after the return of the erythrocyte sedimentation rate to normal.

Bacteriologic and Serologic Examinations

Direct or indirect evidences of a streptococcal infection are found in most patients with acute rheumatic fever. Direct proof is the finding of a group A hemolytic streptococci in nose and throat cultures from patients having acute rheumatic fever. Indirect evidence of a poststreptococcal state is furnished by an elevated antistreptolysin O titer (250 units or more) in the serum. A detectable increase in the antistreptolysin titer starts about two weeks after the onset of streptococcal infecion. The titer usually reaches its maximal level four to six weeks after the onset, and returns to normal within four months. Although, obviously, the diagnosis of rheumatic fever cannot be based on the elevated antistreptolysin titer alone, its absence excludes, for practical purposes, the presence of active rheumatic fever.

A positive blood culture is an integral, though not indispensable, part of the diagnosis of bacterial endocarditis.

2

RADIOLOGY OF THE HEART

No cardiac examination is complete without an adequate radiologic survey of the patient. A complete radiologic examination should include both radiography and fluoroscopy, preferably with appropriate spot films.

FLUOROSCOPY

Cardiac fluoroscopy is the direct examination of the patient's chest and heart under a fluoroscopic screen. Although the proximity of the screen to the chest inevitably results in enlargement and distortion of the cardiac silhouette, fluoroscopy provides certain information not otherwise obtainable.

A word should be included here about the controversy as to whether the radiologist or the cardiologist should perform this relatively simple examination. Ideally, cardiac fluoroscopy should be a cooperative venture. The broad experience of a good radiologist, his ability to survey adequately the entire chest and abdomen under the screen, to recognize the imprint of vascular anomalies on the barium-filled esophagus, to note the adequacy of the diaphragms, all are invaluable in obtaining a good total picture of the patient. On the other hand, the familiarity of the cardiologist with the cardiac silhouette and his mental image of the clinical picture and the electrocardiogram of the patient are indispensable in the darkness of the fluoroscopy room. Optimally, both the radiologist and the cardiologist should be present at fluoroscopy. If, however, there has to be a choice between the two, I believe that, unless the radiologist has made a special study of children with heart disease, the pediatric cardiologist is probably better equipped to perform the fluoroscopic examination.

The disadvantages of cardiac fluoroscopy have been emphasized in recent years. They relate almost exclusively to hazards of radiation. It is a fact that, using conventional, good fluoroscopic equipment, one minute of fluoroscopy time uses approximately 5 r's. Furthermore, even in the most expert hands, one to three minutes of fluoroscopy time is necessary to obtain an adequate survey of the heart and great vessels. On the other hand, a good posteroanterior film of the chest involves the use of only about one hundredth of this value.

These considerations have led to a number of steps modifying the indiscriminate use of the fluoroscope in diagnosing cardiac disorders. To begin with, in many institutions, posteroanterior and oblique films, at a standard 2-meter distance, are used as screening tools for first evaluation. Only if this reveals any abnormality is the patient subjected to fluoroscopy. Of course, time considerations (the child coming from a great distance as an outpatient) may have to modify this policy. Second, gone are the days, in most hospitals, where three, four or more people refluoroscope the same patient "to gain experience." Third, even if initial fluoroscopy is necessary, the follow-up may be done by means of radiograms in most instances. Probably for most patient's, repeat fluoroscopy is not necessary more than once every three to five years. Finally, even this judicious use of cardiac fluoroscopy may be made much safer by the use of the image intensifier, which cuts the amount of radiation to at least one fifth of the original dose.

All these restrictions, and the use of expensive equipment, have diminished considerably the role of fluoroscopy in this entire field. Many cardiologists are nostalgic for the "good old days" when fluoroscopy was performed practically on the kitchen table. Unquestionably, fluoroscopy is becoming more and more a lost art among the younger generation of cardiologists.

On the other hand, what has been lost in this area has been amply compensated for by the more intelligent use of auscultation and electrocardiography in the diagnosis of heart diseases. Furthermore, the films obtained, although more expensive to the patient, furnish much more reliable follow-up data than the little sketches inserted into the records at the time of fluoroscopy.

The most obvious advantage of cardiac fluoroscopy over any other type of roentgenologic technique is that it presents the heart in a dynamic fashion; one may thus obtain a good image of the amplitude of the heart beat. The second advantage is that by rotation of the patient to the oblique and lateral positions the examiner may bring hidden structures into view on the fluoroscopy screen. Third, such extracardiac structures as the thymus can be separated by fluoroscopy from the cardiac silhouette proper. Fourth, by having the patient swallow a barium mixture, one can easily outline the esophagus and thus demonstrate the imprints of adjoining portions of the heart and great vessels. Last, but not least, cardiac fluoroscopy, at a glance, gives a great deal of information about the other intrathoracic organs.

The fluoroscope to be used in pediatric cardiology should be equipped with a tilt table, allowing for the examination of infants lying down and older children standing up. A device for taking spot films is also an important part of the fluoroscope, as is a timing device to remind the examiner of the amount of exposure the patient has had. No more than 5 to 10 minutes of fluoroscopy time at 50 to 70 kilovolts should be used for any one patient. As mentioned previously, in more and more centers, and even in offices, an image intensifier is used for cardiac fluoroscopy. The time used with this instrument is approximately the same as that used with the conventional fluoroscope, but the amount of radiation is reduced to approximately one fifth. A further advantage of this method is that the room does not have to be completely darkened; in spite of this, the sharpness of the image is so great that the presence of pericardial fluid, for instance, may be distinguished from the cardiac silhouette proper.

One cannot emphasize strongly enough the necessity for a dark adaptation period of at least five minutes behind red glasses before starting fluoroscopy if no image intensifier is used. This time can be spent usefully in explaining to the parents and the child what is going to happen. In this way the whole procedure is a great deal less frightening. Also, it gives the child a chance to look around the room and see the people in it. Another point worth emphasizing is that it is almost impossible to use the fluoroscope on a child, especially a small one, without the help of a trained nurse or a technician; her assistance is needed to hold the child and to offer the barium meal in a persuasive fashion.

If the child is cooperative and understands what is required of him, fluoroscopy in the upright position is preferable. Otherwise, much better results can be obtained if he lies on his back with his arms and legs restrained. The first view under the fluoroscope should be of the entire chest. This gives the examiner an opportunity to see the heart size in relation to the entire thoracic cavity and to notice the rate of respiration, the movement of the diaphragms and the site of the stomach bubble. After this general orientation the screen should be narrowed down to the cardiac silhouette and both hili. The child should then be turned from the posteroanterior view to the two obliques (Fig. 11). He should be examined in at least these three views, and preferably in many others. Certain structures, such as the main pulmonary artery, often are seen best somewhere midway between the posteroanterior and the right anterior oblique views.

The individual chambers making up the cardiac silhouette in the different views are schematically presented in Figure 11.

In the posteroanterior view one should try to identify three permanent components of the left border (the left ventricle, the pulmonary artery and the aorta) and search for the outlines of the left atrium. The pulmonary artery may be distinguished from the left ventricle by looking for the rocking beat caused by the contracting left ventricle on the one hand and the expanding main pulmonary artery on the other. Identification of the main pulmonary artery segment from the aortic knob should present no great difficulties; there is usually a definite indentation between the two structures, and the pulsation of the aorta is, as a rule, considerably stronger than that of the pulmonary artery. The aortic knob can also be identified by following the continuous sweep of the aorta from the upper

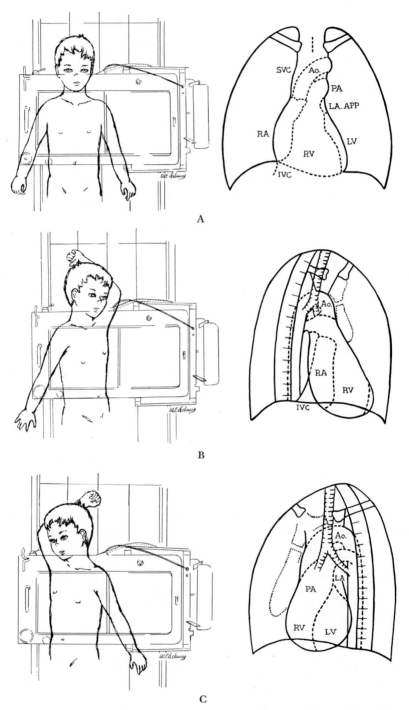

Figure 11.   Schematic representations of (*A*) posteroanterior, (*B*) right anterior oblique and (*C*) left anterior oblique views of the heart at cardiac fluoroscopy.

right border of the heart, up through the sternum, where it juts out on
the left as the knob. If the left atrium projects out on the left border,
it is represented as a double contour, with relatively weak pulsations,
overlapping the powerful contractions of the left ventricle and the main
pulmonary artery. If the left atrium is large enough to project out at the
left border, it usually pushes the barium-filled esophagus to the right in
the posteroanterior view and posteriorly in the right anterior oblique
position. In cases of corrected transposition, the ascending aorta may
occupy, with a broad sweep, the position usually occupied by the pulmonary artery and the left atrium.

The right border of the posteroanterior view, as seen in Figure 11,
is normally made up principally of the right atrium and the superior
vena cava, the ascending aorta contributing to the upper right border.
A large left atrium may also participate in the formation of the right
border, forming a double contour. In this case the other evidences of left
atrial enlargement will also be noted in the posteroanterior and the right
anterior oblique views. The lowest portion of the right border is contributed to by the inferior vena cava. If this vessel empties into the left
atrium, an extremely rare anomaly, a hiatus at the cardiophrenic angle,
may be noted.

The third observation—an extremely important one—to be made in
the posteroanterior view is the size of the hilar vessels. These are best
seen with the fluoroscope concentrated on the vessels $\frac{1}{2}$ to 1 inch away
from the cardiac silhouette. Both the left and right sides should be
surveyed, and the size of the vessels and the presence or absence of
pulsations should be noted. Definite differentiation of intrinsic pulsations
of the hilar vessels ("hilar dance") from activities transmitted from the
main cardiac silhouette requires considerable patience and experience.
Two points help in distinguishing these two kinds of pulsations: the
true intrinsic pulsation is (a) concentric and (b) present at some distance
from the cardiac border.

The final observation to be made in the posteroanterior view is the
contribution of the thymus to the cardiac silhouette. The thymic shadow
may make the heart appear much larger than it actually is, but it can be
separated from the heart relatively easily by noting its "apron-like"
contour and observing its lower tip running up and down with respirations. This distinction is especially necessary in the examination of well
nourished infants, in whom the thymus is usually large. In older children
or emaciated infants the problem should not arise.

The schematic presentation of the two oblique views is found in
Figure 11. The left anterior oblique (LAO) is particularly useful in
determining the relative size of the two ventricles. Incipient left atrial
enlargement may be suspected from the elevation of the left main
bronchus in this view. The size of the ascending aortic arch, as well as
that of the right main pulmonary artery, may be estimated in this view.
The right anterior oblique (RAO) view furnishes a useful measure of
right ventricular enlargement by demonstrating how much of the anterior border is in direct contact with the sternum. The main advantage
of this view, however, is in helping to determine even minimal degrees of
atrial (especially left atrial) enlargement.

Diagnostic Patterns and Their Significance

When cardiac fluoroscopy is carefully performed, certain radiologic patterns emerge. A brief discussion of these will follow.

The cardiac beat may be overactive in anemia, thyrotoxicosis, large left-to-right shunts, aortic or mitral regurgitation, and excitement. An unusually quiet beat is noted in conditions such as congestive failure, myocardial disease and pericardial effusion or constriction. Bradycardia

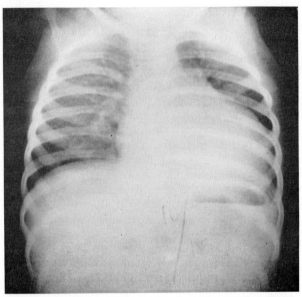

Figure 12. Generalized enlargement of the heart in patient with primary myocardial disease. Note also the pulmonary vascular engorgement.

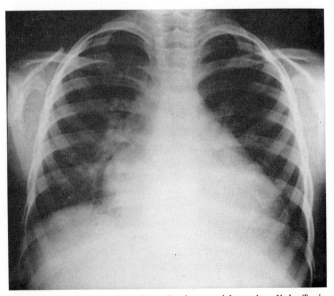

Figure 13. Posteroanterior view of a heart with pericardial effusion.

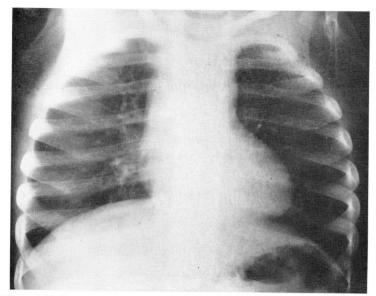

Figure 14. *Coeur en sabot* contour of heart of patient with tetralogy of Fallot.

Figure 15. Posteroanterior view of characteristic figure-of-8 configuration of heart of patient with total anomalous pulmonary venous drainage into the superior vena cava.

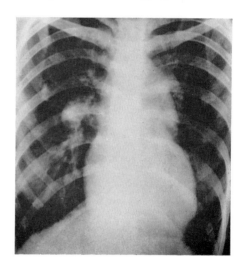

of 50 beats per minute or less usually indicates complete heart block and is well recognizable on the fluoroscopic screen by the relatively rapid atrial and slow ventricular pulsations.

The general contour of the cardiac silhouette may be typical of certain well defined entities. The globular heart, involving enlargement of all chambers, is characteristic of the primary myocardial disease group (Fig. 12). The "water bottle" shape of a large pericardial effusion is easily recognizable (Fig. 13). The "sheep's nose" contour or *coeur en sabot* (Fig. 14) is typical of the tetralogy of Fallot or of some tricuspid atresias. The "figure-8" shape of the heart is seen in total anomalous pulmonary venous drainage into the superior vena cava (Fig. 15). The shoulder-like contour on the left border suggests corrected transposition of the great

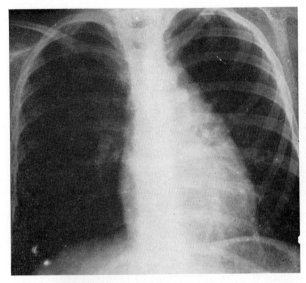

Figure 16. Posteroanterior roentgenogram of patient with corrected transposition of the great arteries. Note the convex sloping shoulder at the left cardiac border representing, in part, the ascending aorta and, in part, the left atrium.

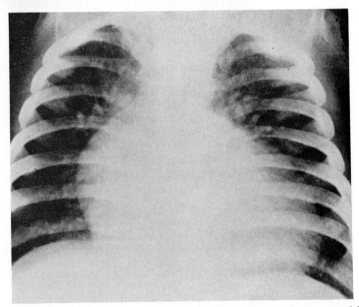

Figure 17. Posteroanterior roentgenogram of patient with complete transposition of the great arteries and intact ventricular septum. Note the egg-shaped cardiac silhouette with the narrow waist and the pulmonary vascular engorgement. This type of roentgenogram in a patient with severe cyanosis is practically diagnostic of the entity.

arteries (Fig. 16). The egg-shaped heart in a child with cyanosis is practically pathognomonic of transposition of the great arteries (Fig. 17). A large heart with gross dilatation of the right atrium and diminished pulmonary vasculature is characteristic of Ebstein's malformation or maximal pulmonic stenosis with intact ventricular septum (Figs. 18, 19).

Minimal enlargement of the left atrium can most easily be detected in the right anterior oblique view by the impression it leaves on the barium-filled esophagus (Fig. 20, *A*). More severe degrees of left atrial enlargement are characterized in the posteroanterior view of the deviation of the barium-filled esophagus to the right (Fig. 20, *B*), and in the left anterior oblique view by the elevation of the left main bronchus. Left atrial enlargement is seen in cases of left ventricular failure, mitral valvular disease, patent ductus arteriosus, ostium primum atrial defect, corrected transposition and, occasionally, in ventricular septal defect. The largest left atria are seen in severe mitral regurgitation; in these cases fluoroscopic examination may disclose a paradoxical pulsation of the left atrium. This observation has been repeatedly confirmed by electrokymography and is a useful sign of mitral regurgitation.

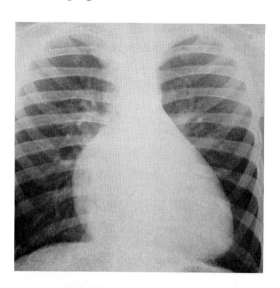

Figure 18. Posteroanterior roentgenogram of patient with Ebstein's malformation. Note the large heart with small pulmonary vessels. The enlargement involves principally the right atrium, bulging out the right border. Characteristically, and in contrast to severe valvar pulmonic stenosis, the main pulmonary artery segment is not prominent.

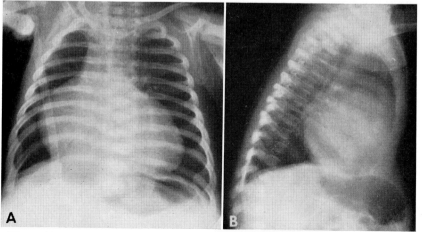

Figure 19. Posteroanterior and right lateral roentgenogram of infant with severe pulmonic stenosis and an intact ventricular septum. Note, to begin with, the close similarity to the roentgenogram of Ebstein's disease, consisting of cardiac enlargement involving principally the right atrium, with diminished pulmonary vasculature. The main pulmonary arterial segment here is not prominent because of the maximal severity of the pulmonic stenosis and the secondary cardiac dilatation. Contrast this with Figure 27.

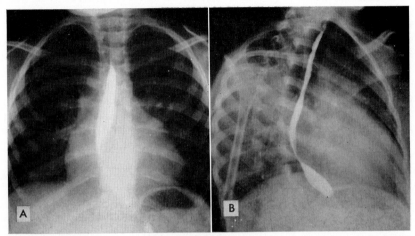

Figure 20. Large left atrium in (*A*) posteroanterior view, displacing the barium-filled esophagus to the right, and (*B*) right anterior oblique view, displacing the barium-filled esophagus posteriorly.

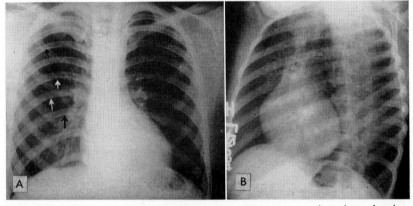

Figure 21. Left ventricular enlargement in (*A*) posteroanterior view, showing the cardiac apex pointing downward (the arrows indicate rib notching in this patient with coarctation of the aorta), and (*B*) left anterior oblique view, showing the cardiac apex pointing downward and posteriorly.

Enlargement of the left ventricle is best visualized in the posteroanterior and the left anterior oblique views (Fig. 21). In both views an enlarged left ventricle manifests itself by producing displacement of the cardiac apex downward and outward. In the posteroanterior view the enlarged left ventricle sometimes causes a rounding of the left ventricular segment. Left ventricular enlargement is characteristic of mitral regurgitation, aortic valvular disease, coarctation of the aorta, patent ductus arteriosus, endocardial cushion defect, certain instances of ventricular septal defect, and tricuspid atresia.

The aorta can best be outlined in the posteroanterior and the left anterior oblique views (Fig. 22). Enlargement of the aortic arch is characteristic of congenital valvular aortic stenosis, aortic regurgitation and patent ductus arteriosus. Hypoplasia of the aorta is generally said to be typical of atrial septal defect (Fig. 23). Vigorous pulsation and collapsing beat of the aorta are seen in aortic regurgitation, patent ductus arteriosus, aortopulmonary fenestration, ruptured sinus of Valsalva, and ventricular defect with aortic regurgitation. The position of the aortic arch can best be demonstrated by asking the patient to swallow a mouthful of barium paste and watching the passage of this radiopaque material down the esophagus. A normal left aortic arch causes slight deviation of the esophagus to the right in the posteroanterior view (Fig. 24, *A*) and posteriorly in the left anterior oblique view. Conversely, if the aortic arch is on the right, the esophagus deviates to the left in the posteroanterior view (Fig. 24, *B*) and anteriorly in the left anterior oblique position. Right aortic arch may be seen without any other cardiovascular anomaly. It is a frequent concomitant of ventricular septal defect with pulmonary stenosis,

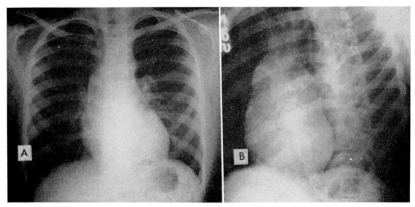

Figure 22.   Large ascending aorta in (*A*) posteroanterior and (*B*) left anterior oblique views.

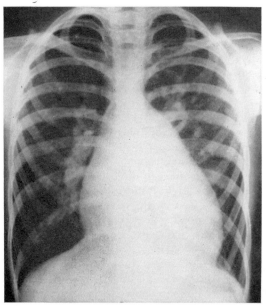

Figure 23.   Hypoplastic aorta in posteroanterior roentgenogram of a patient with a large secundum atrial septal defect.

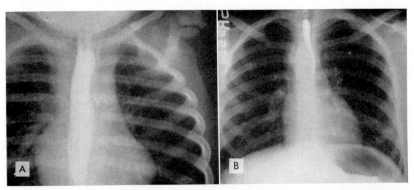

Figure 24. *A,* Normal left aortic arch with depression on the barium-filled esophagus. *B,* Right aortic arch with impression on the esophagus on the right side.

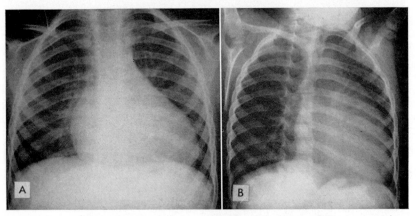

Figure 25. Large right atrium in a patient with Ebstein's disease. *A,* Posteroanterior and, (*B*) right anterior oblique views.

but is practically never seen in conjunction with isolated pulmonic stenosis. The diagnosis of so-called vascular rings by means of a barium swallow is reviewed in some detail on page 571 ff.

The superior vena cava forms the upper right border of the cardiac silhouette in the posteroanterior view. Tremendous dilatation of this structure may be seen in cases of total anomaly of the pulmonary venous drainage. Enlargement to a lesser degree is a fairly constant concomitant of the tetralogy of Fallot syndrome.

Right atrial enlargement can best be demonstrated in the postero-anterior view and in the right anterior oblique view (Fig. 25). An en-larged right atrium is seen with tricuspid disease, Ebstein's anomaly pulmonic stenosis, pulmonary vascular obstruction and atrial septal defect. The largest right atria are seen in tricuspid regurgitation and Ebstein's disease.

Right ventricular enlargement may best be visualized in the postero-anterior view by an upward and outward displacement of the cardiac apex (Fig. 26, *A*). If the right ventricle is large, it may totally displace the retrosternal space in the right anterior oblique view (Fig. 26, *B*). In the left anterior oblique view the generally rounded contour, with an anterior bulge, is characteristic of an enlarged right ventricle (Fig. 26, *C*). Right ventricular enlargement is always present with tricuspid regurgitation, pulmonic stenosis, pulmonary vascular obstruction, mitral stenosis, large ventricular septal defect, and atrial septal defect.

The main pulmonary artery segment is best outlined in the postero-anterior view (Fig. 27) or with the patient turned a few degrees from the posteroanterior toward the right anterior oblique. The right main pulmonary artery is best seen on end in the right anterior oblique position, just below and posterior to the ascending aorta. The left main pulmonary artery is clearly outlined in the left anterior oblique position, below and to the left of the ascending aorta. The pulmonary arteries may be enlarged in pulmonary hypertension, valvular pulmonic stenosis and patent ductus arteriosus. Hypoplastic pulmonary artery or absence of the main pulmonary artery segment is typical of infundibular pulmonic stenosis and transposition of the great vessels. Hyperactive pulsations in the main pulmonary artery segment are characteristic of large left-to-right

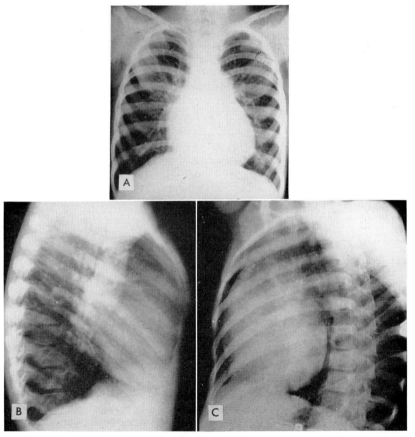

Figure 26. Large right ventricle in a patient with ventricular septal defect and pulmonary vascular obstructive disease. *A*, Posteroanterior, *B*, right anterior oblique and, *C*, left anterior oblique views. Note in *A* the large main pulmonary artery segment, in *B* the heart displacing the retrosternal space, and in *C* the cocked-up apex. The latter two features are characteristic of right ventricular enlargement. The big main pulmonary arterial segment is secondary to pulmonary arterial hypertension.

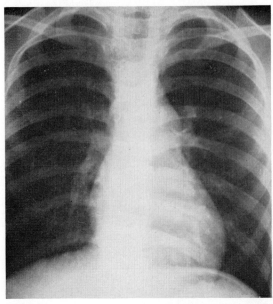

Figure 27. Prominent main pulmonary artery segment in posteroanterior roentgenogram of a patient with pure pulmonic stenosis. Note the similarity of the main pulmonary artery segment in this view to that in Figure 26, *A*. In Figure 26 the dilatation of the pulmonary artery is caused by high pulmonary arterial pressure; in this figure, by poststenotic dilatation.

shunts, pulmonary vascular obstruction and certain cases of mitral valvular disease. In patent ductus arteriosus the amplitude of pulsations in the aorta and the pulmonary artery is frequently identical in intensity and synchronous in timing.

The status of the pulmonary vasculature can best be judged by radiography. Cardiac fluoroscopy gives invaluable information, however, about the presence or absence of intrinsic pulsations, so-called hilar dance. This is noted in all instances of congenital heart disease with a large left-to-right shunt and in cases of pulmonary hypertension. Expansile pulsations are almost never seen with acquired heart disease, even in the presence of pulmonary vascular engorgement.

RADIOGRAPHY

The patient's chest should be in direct contact with the film, and the tube should be 6 feet from the patient. In this fashion, distortion of the cardiac silhouette is kept at a minimum (10 per cent), and the image is reproducible. As a rule, three views are taken: anteroposterior, left anterior oblique, and right anterior oblique, with left or right laterals.

The advantages of radiography over fluoroscopy are that a much higher degree of definition can be achieved, permitting greater recognition of detail, and, of course, the fact that a permanent record is obtained. This record is invaluable in the long-term study of any single patient or disease. The relatively small amount of radiation involved in conventional radiography has been discussed earlier (p. 26).

Cardiac Silhouette

The contour of the normal heart, as seen in the posteroanterior radiogram, depends somewhat on the height of the diaphragm. For this reason, if possible, all films should be taken in either full inspiration or full expiration (Fig. 28).

The age of the patient is also an important consideration in judging the cardiac silhouette. The heart of a normal newborn or young infant has a right ventricular contour corresponding to the dominance of the right ventricle in this age group. This results in a *coeur en sabot* appearance. The pathologic types of right ventricular enlargement, such as tetralogy of Fallot, can be seen only as an exaggeration of the normal configuration. From the age of approximately six months on the heart starts assuming the "normal" left ventricular configuration. This process reaches its culmination in the older age group, in which the patient with hypertensive disease has definite left ventricular enlargement. The

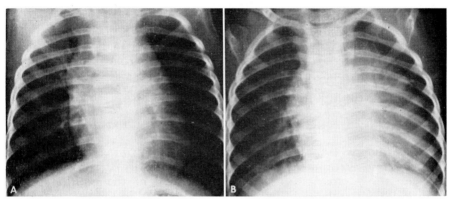

Figure 28. Change in heart size caused by the effect of respiration on the large thymus of a normal baby. *A,* Expiration; *B,* full inspiration.

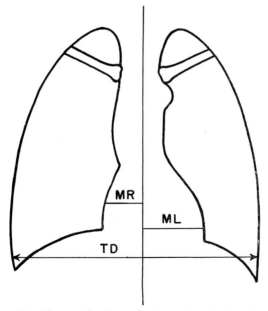

Figure 29. Diagram for determination of cardiothoracic ratio.

left ventricular type of configuration in a newborn or young infant is as distinctly abnormal as is a right ventricular shape in an older child.

Innumerable tables for the determination of the "normal" heart size for any age, height or weight are available. They are cumbersome, difficult to use and far from accurate for children. For practical purposes the use of the cardiothoracic ratio has proved to be as satisfactory as any method, and it is by far the simplest. The ratio consists in the relation of the transverse diameter of the heart to the maximal internal width of the chest (Fig. 29). The transverse diameter is the sum of the midleft and midright diameters; these are determined by drawing a horizontal line from the midline to the farthest left and farthest right borders of the heart. A cardiothoracic ratio of less than 0.5, i.e., a heart which is less than half of the size of the thorax, usually means a heart of average size. This ratio cannot be used with any accuracy in newborn and small infants; here a transverse diameter of 5.5 cm. is taken as the upper limit of normal. All these total measurements are approximations at best. The size of the individual chambers may be more valid than the determination of the size of the heart as a whole. Nevertheless changes in the cardiothoracic ratio through the years in one patient may well reflect the progress of heart disease.

Pulmonary Vasculature

The lung fields may be divided arbitrarily into three vertical sectors: the hilus, and the middle and outer thirds. Normally, the vascular markings are easily observed in both hili. Because of the position of the cardiac silhouette, the right hilus is better visualized in the anteroposterior view than in the left. The vascular elements of the hilar markings consist of the pulmonary arterial and pulmonary venous structures (Fig. 30). Both main pulmonary arteries and the large pulmonary veins converging into the heart may be seen longitudinally. The arteries are sharper and are in the foreground; the outline of the veins is hazier and more in the background. In addition to these large structures seen longitudinally, smaller structures of both the arteries and the veins may be seen on end. Normally, vessels of appreciable caliber are seldom seen in the middle third of the lung field, and never in the outer third (Fig. 30, *A*). Presence of such vessels indicates pulmonary vascular engorgement.

One may assume that the engorgement is active if the enlarged vessels have clear, sharply defined edges (Fig. 30, *D*). Haziness, poor outline and general "filminess" of the lung field are characteristic of passive congestion of pulmonary edema. The differential diagnosis between passive congestion and pulmonary infection is sometimes extremely difficult, even impossible; as a rule, however, passive congestion is best seen in the hilus and the middle third of the lung field, and is uniformly distributed over both sides. Passive congestion, such as seen in mitral stenosis, often results in engorgement of the vessels in the lower, supradiaphragmatic portion, with relative clarity and hyperaeration of the upper half of the lungs (Fig. 30, *C*). So-called Kerley-Fleischner lines, horizontal structures representing engorged lymphatics, together with distention of the interlobar spaces, may also be seen in pulmonary venous congestion. Infectious processes, in contrast, are usually more spotty in distribution and may

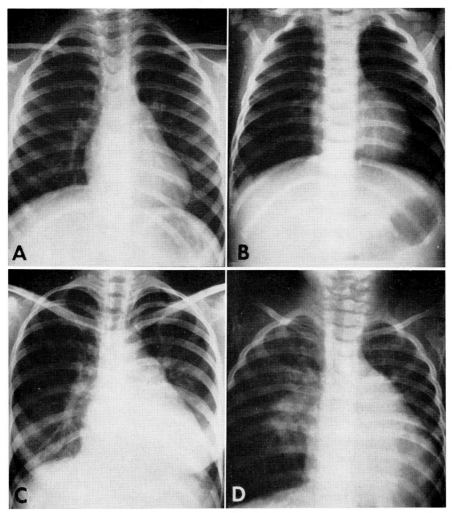

Figure 30. *A,* Normal pulmonary vasculature. *B,* Diminished pulmonary vasculature. *C,* Pulmonary vascular engorgement due to passive congestion. Note the increased translucence of the upper two thirds of the lung fields. *D,* Active engorgement, best noted in the middle third of the right lung field. There is no difference between the upper and lower thirds, and the vessel margins are sharp.

extend throughout the outer third of the lung field without seriously affecting the hilus. A determination of the peripheral pulmonary vasculature also may best be judged by radiography. If the vessels—on end or lengthwise—are small in the middle or outer lung field, we obtain the picture of pulmonary ischemia (Fig. 30, *B*). This, in fact, is the result of normal or diminished amount of blood, with low pressure, in the lungs.

One further peculiarity of the pulmonary vasculature has to be considered here: namely, the collaterals. The question boils down to this: Where do the pulmonary vessels come from? If they originate, as they should, from the left and right main pulmonary arteries, then these principal vessels should be readily visible in the hilus, and the smaller vessels should diminish gradually from the hilus toward the outer third.

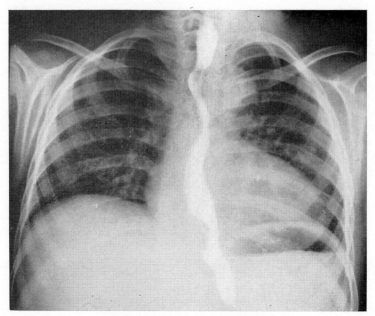

Figure 31. Extensive collateral circulation in patient with pulmonary atresia.

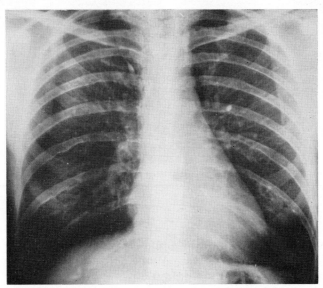

Figure 32. Rib notching in patient with coarctation of aorta.

Conversely, if the pulmonary vasculature is principally made up of bronchial collaterals, such as are seen in pulmonary or tricuspid atresia, the vessels will not originate from a well defined hilar "comma," and their distribution will extend in a lacelike pattern, evenly, throughout the lung fields. Figure 31 shows a predominantly bronchial type of pulmonary vasculature. Unequal distribution of the pulmonary vasculature may be seen in certain congenital anomalies involving atresia of the left or right main pulmonary artery.

Dilated intercostal arteries may exert sufficient pressure on the lower end of the ribs to erode them, giving rise to "rib notching," pathognomonic of coarctation of the aorta (Fig. 32).

ORTHODIAGRAPHY

Orthodiagraphy consists in the tracing of the cardiac silhouette on the fluoroscope screen without distortion, by means of a "single" roentgen beam. The tracing is reproduced on a piece of onion skin paper attached by clips to the screen. This method is accurate and inexpensive, and leaves a permanent record, thus combining the advantages of fluoroscopy and radiography. The principal disadvantages are that it is time-consuming, and occasionally it exposes the patient to more radiation than is desirable. Within recent years I have had no experience with this method. If no equipment for radiography is available, fluoroscopy combined with orthodiagraphy should be used. Excellent descriptions of the technique are available elsewhere.[25] I am afraid that this is another one of the lost arts.

ELECTROCARDIOGRAPHY

Electrocardiography, accurate physical examination, and radiology form the tripod on which rests the clinical diagnosis in pediatric cardiology. Omission of, unfamiliarity with or misinterpretation of any of these three tools spells disaster.

This chapter can perhaps best be introduced by enumerating the things it does not aim to do: (1) It is not a complete treatise on electrocardiography. Excellent textbooks are available for this purpose.[108, 417, 423, 490, 741] (2) It does not make the assumption that the reader knows nothing about electrocardiograms. It is unlikely that an appreciable number of medical school graduates lack this knowledge. (3) It does not describe conditions of no significance in pediatrics. This would be contrary to the purpose of the book.

In a more positive way, the aim is to present a concise and practical discussion of electrocardiograms of children, with emphasis on the normal electrocardiogram as well as on the pathologic recordings.

THEORETICAL CONSIDERATIONS

The Electromyogram

Before the electrocardiogram can properly be understood, certain relatively simple physiologic explanations pertaining to the isolated muscle strip are necessary. The inside of the cell, schematically presented in Figure 33, carries a negative charge, the outer surface a positive one. This potential difference has been measured by micro-electrodes and

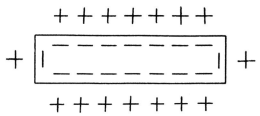

Figure 33.   Resting muscle fiber (schematic drawing) showing the negative charges inside and the positive charges outside the cell.

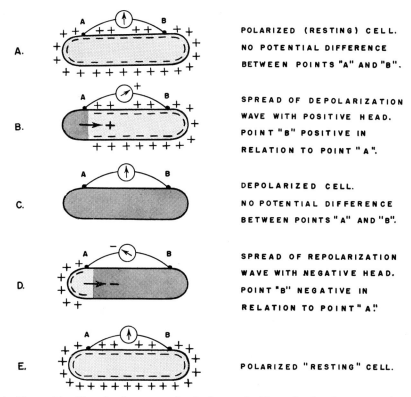

A.   POLARIZED (RESTING) CELL. NO POTENTIAL DIFFERENCE BETWEEN POINTS "A" AND "B".

B.   SPREAD OF DEPOLARIZATION WAVE WITH POSITIVE HEAD. POINT "B" POSITIVE IN RELATION TO POINT "A".

C.   DEPOLARIZED CELL. NO POTENTIAL DIFFERENCE BETWEEN POINTS "A" AND "B".

D.   SPREAD OF REPOLARIZATION WAVE WITH NEGATIVE HEAD. POINT "B" NEGATIVE IN RELATION TO POINT "A."

E.   POLARIZED "RESTING" CELL.

Figure 34.   Electric phenomena in single muscle fiber stimulated at one end.

has been found to be in the neighborhood of 90 millivolts. If a galvanometer is connected to two points on the surface of a resting muscle, no potential difference is registered, since all points on the exterior of the unstimulated cell have the same potential (Fig. 34, *A*). If the strip is stimulated, the potential on the surface of the membrane drops to zero at the stimulated point, because the membrane becomes electrically permeable and the charges on the two sides neutralize each other. As the wave of excitation spreads, the entire surface of the muscle reverses its positive charge. If a galvanometer is connected to two points on the surface of a stimulated muscle, then, in contrast to the resting state, potential differences are registered; the already depolarized portion of the muscle is electrically negative compared to the intact, as yet untouched, portion (Fig. 34, *B*). After the wave of excitation, with a positive head, has completely covered the cell membrane, there remains no potential difference between the inner and outer surfaces of the entire muscle; it is as if the entire electrical energy of the strip had been fired off, or "depolarized" (Fig. 34, *C*). As soon as the depolarization is completed, the muscle strip starts to "refuel," to "repolarize"; during this process the membrane regains its insulating capacity—the outer surface obtains a positive charge, whereas the inside becomes negative. The spread of this "repolarization wave" is in the same direction as the depolarization wave; only, as shown in Figure 34, *D*, the head is now negative instead of positive. With the completion of repolarization the muscle returns to the resting state (Fig. 34, *E*).

If a galvanometer is connected to the end of the muscle strip in such a manner that the positive potentials are registered as an upward deflection and the negative ones as a downward deflection, then the depolarization and repolarization waves are described as a diphasic curve, the so-called electromyogram (Fig. 35).

One final word about the physiologic background. According to recent observations, the changes in membrane potential during depolarization may be defined chemically, to a large extent, by the exodus of potassium ions from the inside of the cell. Conversely, repolarization, according to this theory, may be explained by a re-entry of potassium from the extracellular fluid into the interior of the cell, after which it is sealed in by the membrane.

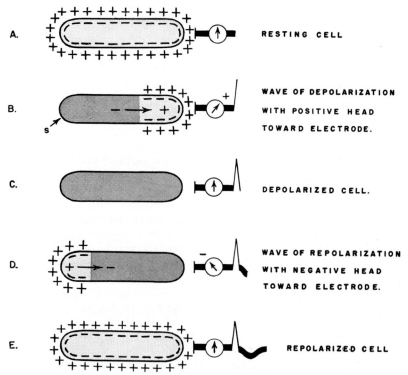

Figure 35.   An electromyogram registered from a galvanometer set up at the end of a single muscle fiber, at the pole opposite the point of stimulation.

The Electrocardiogram

By connecting a galvanometer to the heart, an electrocardiogram may be obtained. This, in contrast to the simple diphasic curve of the myogram, consists of three elements—P, QRS and T—all of which commonly point in the same direction (Fig. 36).

The principal differences between the myogram of a striated muscle and the electrocardiogram probably are due to four main factors: (1) the difference in muscle refractory period, (2) the syncytial nature of the heart muscle, (3) the presence of a rather complicated conduction system, and (4) the problems in placing the galvanometer in the vicinity of the heart.

The refractory period of the heart muscle is considerably longer than that of striated muscle. This fact is responsible for the inability of the cardiac muscle to go into tetanic contraction; it enables the heart to beat rhythmically and to rest between contractions. The striated muscle can go into an "oxygen debt" during prolonged, continuous stimulation, a debt that can be paid during a prolonged resting period. The heart, for obvious reasons, cannot get a prolonged rest; hence the long refractory period furnishes it with time to "refuel" between beats.

The syncytial nature of the heart muscle, doubted recently by electron-microscopists, may be responsible for the fact that the electrocardiogram, in contrast to the myogram, is not a diphasic curve. The wave of depolarization of the ventricles, as represented by the QRS complex, is not followed by a mirror-image repolarization wave, but rather by a lower and wider, most commonly upward wave—the T wave. The deviation of the electrocardiogram from the simple diphasic pattern of the muscle strip is called the ventricular gradient, and, presumably, is due at least in part to the anatomic constellation of the fibers and the resulting differences in duration and intensity of the excitation in different parts of the heart muscle.

The conduction system of the heart is a complicated one (Fig. 37). The impulse is usually formed in the sinoatrial node, in the wall of the right atrium, close to the opening of the superior vena cava. From here it spreads, like a ripple in a pond, through both atria; the anterior portion

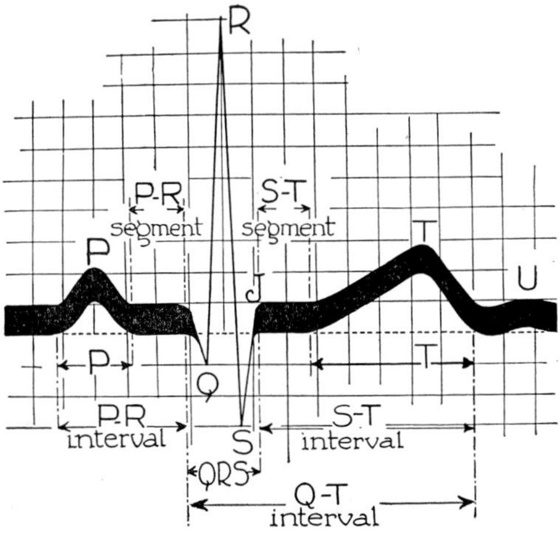

Figure 36. The waves of the normal electrocardiogram.[108]

of the right atrium is activated first, the posterior portion next, the left atrium last. As the wave of excitation spreads through the atria, it reaches the atrioventricular node, in the wall of the right atrium, near the opening of the coronary sinus. From the atrioventricular node the impulse spreads down toward the ventricles through the atrioventricular bundle (His) and its branches. Ordinarily the septum is activated from left to right (Fig. 38). Next, the impulse reaches the narrow wall of the right ventricle for a short time, only to be overpowered by the impulse reaching the thicker left ventricular wall, the final portion of the depolarization process. Remember that the process of depolarization spreads through the ventricular wall from the Purkinje fibers, through the endocardium, out-

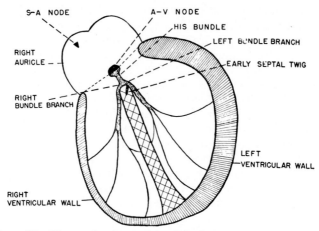

Figure 37.   The conduction system of the heart. (After Wolff.[741])

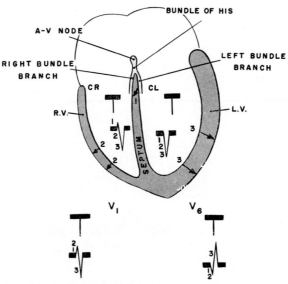

Figure 38.   The spread of the impulse through the normal conduction system as reflected at the right unipolar chest lead (V_1), left unipolar chest lead (V_6), right cavity (CR) and left cavity (CL). For details and explanations of *1, 2* and *3*, see text.

ward toward the subepicardial layers; conversely, repolarization probably begins subepicardially and spreads toward the endocardium.

The position of the electrode is the fourth variant determining the shape of the electrocardiogram. The bipolar leads, described by Einthoven (Fig. 39), originate from the extremities, are assumed to be at infinite distance from the heart, and register potential differences between extremities—the right arm, the left arm and the left foot. Lead I represents potential differences between the right arm and the left arm, lead II between the right arm and the left foot, and lead III between the left arm and the left foot. These are the bipolar extremity leads, or standard limb leads of Einthoven. In contrast, the unipolar leads, the so-called V leads, measure what may be considered actual electrical potentials at some given point in the body. The unipolar limb leads aV_R, aV_L and aV_F[63]

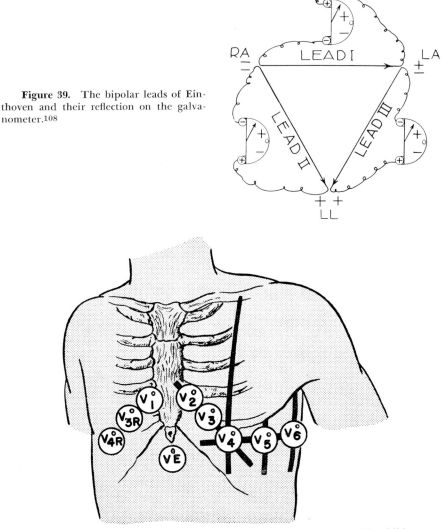

Figure 39. The bipolar leads of Einthoven and their reflection on the galvanometer.[108]

Figure 40. Location of the unipolar chest leads commonly obtained in children.

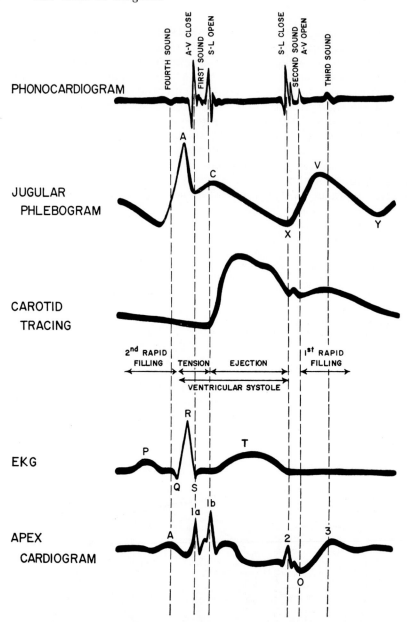

Figure 41. Correlation of the electrocardiogram to the various other external reference tracings and to the cardiac cycle.

(or V_R, V_L and V_F[733]) measure the electrical potentials at one extremity. Lead aV_R measures the potentials at the right arm, aV_L at the left arm, and aV_F at the left foot. The unipolar chest leads measure the electrical potentials of the heart at certain definite points on the chest. By convention, the American Heart Association advocates the use of six chest leads, V_1 to V_6, to which, in pediatrics, three more (V_{3R}, V_{4R} and V_E) often must be added to obtain a clear-cut pattern of progression (Fig. 40).

Various types of curves are obtained, depending on the structure of the heart muscle, the attributes of the conduction system and the position and number of the electrodes. The basic tracing and its correlation with the activities of various portions of the heart are presented in Figure 41.

Certain conventions are observed in the setting of the galvanometer. In the standard limb leads, where potential differences are explored, the galvanometer shows a positive deflection in lead I if the right arm potential is less than that of the left arm, in lead II if the right arm potential is less than that of the left foot, and in lead III if the left arm potential is less than that of the left foot. From these conventions follows the fact that at any one instant in the P-QRS-T complex, the mathematical sum of lead I plus lead III equals lead II. As an example, if the height of R_1 is $+8$ mm. and the height of R_3 is -4 mm., then the height of R_2 must be $+4$ mm.

The conventions ruling the registration of the unipolar leads require that the galvanometer be set in such a way that, when the impulse travels *toward* an electrode, a positive deflection is described, whereas, if the impulse travels *away* from it, the deflection described will be a negative one. Taking the diagram describing the spread of the impulse from the atrioventricular node through the ventricles, it is possible to reconstruct the tracings obtained from various unipolar chest and limb leads (Figs. 38, 42; Table 3, page 774. It may be seen that the initial deflection of V_1, representing a unipolar lead from the right chest, will be a notched positive one made up partly from the activation of the septum from left to right and partly from a short period of right ventricular activation before the thicker left ventricle asserts itself. The final portion of V_1 consists in a deep negative deflection caused by the impulse spreading

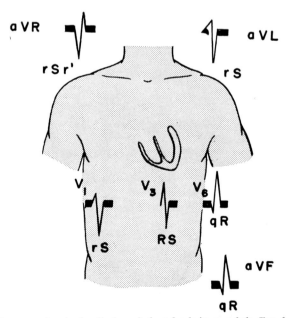

Figure 42. The normal unipolar limb and chest leads in an adult. For details, see text.

through the left ventricle, away from the right ventricular (V_1) electrode. On the other hand, if the electrode is placed on the surface of the lateral wall of the left ventricle, or to V_6, the electrocardiograph characteristically registers a qR pattern. It is demonstrated in Figure 38 that the q is due to the impulse initially traveling away from the left ventricle, activating the septum, and later the right ventricle, from left to right. The tall R ensuing represents the impulse spreading through the bulky left ventricle, toward the electrode at V_6. A third pattern obtainable from the surface of the medial aspects of the left or the right ventricle or from chest lead V_{3-4} is the so-called transitional zone pattern, RS. This is the result of the galvanometer's registering both left and right ventricular potentials with equal deflections. A pattern usually obtained from lead aV_R is the right ventricular cavity pattern, rSr', representing the electrical forces from the back of the heart. Most of the impulses, except those from the very terminal portion of the left ventricle, are directed away from this electrode; hence the predominantly downward deflection. Patterns not ordinarily obtained in the unipolar leads of normal adults are Rs, which represents right ventricular surface potentials and is characteristic of right ventricular hypertrophy, and QS, which is obtainable from inside the left ventricle through intracardiac electrocardiography. A more detailed and logical explanation for the occurrence of these patterns may be found in the section on vectorcardiography (p. 97).

The mean electrical axis, in the frontal plane, may be calculated from a modification of the Bayley triaxial system[46] by adding the unipolar limb leads and forming a hexaxial reference figure (Fig. 43). Lead I connects the left and right arms; thus this is considered a 0 to −180 degree line across the center of the circle. Lead II connects the right arm and left leg and represents the +60 to −120 degree line. Lead III, representing the potential differences between left arm and left leg, makes up the −60 to +120 degree line. The lead axis of aV_F connected with the center of the circle gives the plus and minus 90 degree line, and so on.

Once the system is constructed, the assumption is made that if the mean electrical axis of the heart is exactly perpendicular to one of these

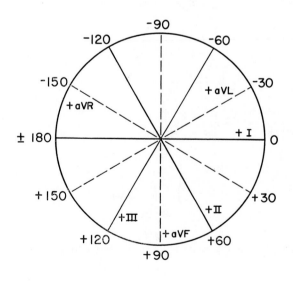

Figure 43. The hexaxial system. For details see text.

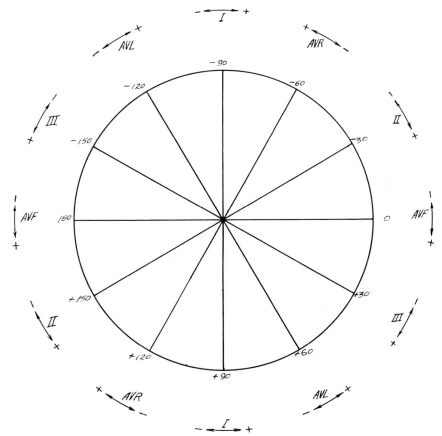

Figure 44. A system of perpendiculars drawn on the standard and unipolar limb leads to be utilized in the estimation of the mean electrical axis.

lead axes, then the complexes in that lead will be equiphasic or conspicuously small. Furthermore, it may be assumed also that if the deflection in one of the six leads is conspicuously bigger than that in any of the others, the mean electrical axis is probably closely parallel to the given lead axis. A second system is constructed, representing the perpendiculars to the limb leads (Fig. 44). In the analysis of any particular cardiogram, lead I is inspected first. If the algebraic sum of lead I (taking area as well as voltage into consideration) is positive, the mean electrical axis will fall to the right of the ± 90 degree line (i.e. the perpendicular to lead I). Next, aV_F is examined. If the algebraic sum of the positive and negative deflections is negative, the mean electrical axis will lie above the 0 to ± 180 degree line (the perpendicular to aV_F). This information, in conjunction with the conclusion reached from lead I, places the mean electrical axis in the quadrant of 0 to -90 degrees. By analyzing in similar fashion the perpendiculars to aV_R and lead II, the mean electrical axis can be determined at a glance within a 15-degree limit.

If all the limb leads are equiphasic complexes, one simply says that the mean electrical axis is indeterminable; i.e. it is perpendicular to the entire frontal plane. If only one lead shows exactly equiphasic complexes, one can assume without further calculations that the mean electrical axis is perpendicular to this particular lead.

One word about area versus voltage. On the whole, it is simplest to use voltage in trying to calculate the mean electrical axis. A lead where R is 10 mm. and s is 3 mm. is considered a positive deflection of 7. This calculation is based on the assumption that the areas under these two deflections will be proportionate to the voltages. In certain situations, particularly in patients with intraventricular conduction disturbances, this assumption may not hold. In such instances, as also in situations in which the positive and negative deflections are of equal height, but one is considerably broader than the other, the positive and negative areas should be considered in calculating whether the entire lead is positive or negative. Exact calculation of the areas would be cumbersome; thus a careful glance, or an "educated guess," taking into consideration voltage as well as area, serves the purpose adequately.

Of course this type of axis calculation may be used not only for the QRS complex, but also for the P and T waves. In our department we calculate mean QRS axes routinely and the P and T axes only if they seem unusual at first glance. Examples of axis calculation are given in Figures 64, 65, 67, 68 and 72.

PRACTICAL ELECTROCARDIOGRAPHY

How to Take an Electrocardiogram on a Child or an Infant

The technique of obtaining an electrocardiogram in an older child should present no particular problem. The techniques described in any handbook by any reputable manufacturer of cardiographs should contain sufficient instructions.

Infants, on the other hand, present considerable, often insurmountable, problems. In my experience, direct writing machines are infinitely more practical than photographic ones in the electrocardiography of infants. The fact that the baby is not likely to hold still for any length of time makes it imperative that the technician see instantaneously whether a few satisfactory complexes, without somatic interference, have been obtained in any one lead. With a photographic machine, even after a great deal of experience, it is often impossible to tell, before developing the film, whether a satisfactory tracing has been obtained. I am well aware of the magnificent records obtained on a two-channel photographic machine by Ziegler[759] of Detroit; I can only express admiration for his ability and, at the same time, express doubts that such tracings could be obtained in large numbers in the majority of institutions.

Only a technician who likes children is likely to obtain clear tracings; the reassurance and kindness emanating from such a person may make a tremendous difference. A bottle of milk or a lollipop may quiet a restless infant; at other times the only way a satisfactory record can be obtained is to have the mother hold the baby in her lap.

In infants the smallest obtainable electrode should be used; a chest piece with a ½-inch diameter usually suffices.

It is important that the electrode paste should touch the chest only at the place where the particular lead is; if the paste is smeared across the chest, a single pattern may be obtained from V_1 to V_6.[36]

Finally, in an infant with a small chest, lead V_3 may be omitted from the series of chest leads. On the other hand, V_E (ensiform process) and V_{4R} or V_{3R} should be taken routinely.

General Evaluation

The general evaluation of the tracing should include adequate evidence of correct standardization; a current of 1 millivolt introduced instantaneously into the machine should produce an excursion of 10 mm. in height, or 10 small squares, and the upstroke time (interval between onset and zenith of the upward deflection) should be less than 0.02 second (Fig. 45, A).

The base line should be free from regular 60-cycle interference (Fig. 45, B) and from irregular somatic tremors (Fig. 45, C). A wandering base line or senseless and irregular deflections are usually due to faulty application of the electrodes.

Determination of Rate and Rhythm

This should begin by identification of the P and QRS complexes, usually in lead II, or in whichever standard limb lead they are outlined

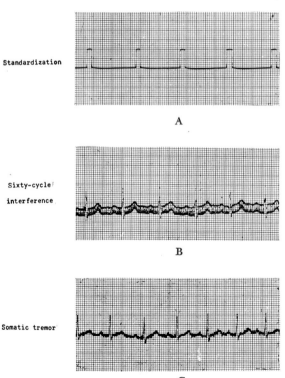

Standardization

A

Sixty-cycle
interference

B

Somatic tremor

C

Figure 45. *A,* Normal standardization for 1 millivolt; *B,* 60-cycle interference; *C,* irregular somatic tremor.

most clearly. Next, the relation between the QRS complex and the P wave must be determined in terms of constancy or variability. If the relation is constant, the ventricular rate per minute is counted; if the relation is variable, both atrial and ventricular rates must be determined. The determination of the rate can most easily be accomplished either by counting the number of small squares between 2 consecutive QRS or P complexes (Table 4, p. 774), or, especially if the rhythm is irregular, by multiplying by 20 the number of cycles between 2 vertical lines (three seconds) on standard electrocardiograms.

Determination of the Mean Electrical Axis

The method for determination of the mean electrical axis was described on page 53. Table 5 (p. 774) gives the normal ranges of P, QRS and T axes for various age groups.

The P-QRS-T-U Complex

The P Wave. The P wave, the first complex in any cardiac cycle, results from the electrical activity of the atria (Fig. 41). There is evi-

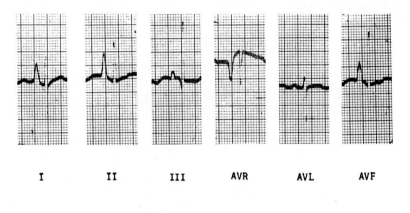

I   II   III   AVR   AVL   AVF

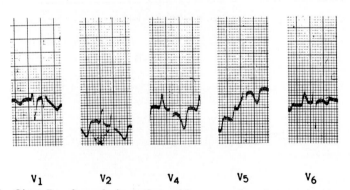

V₁   V₂   V₄   V₅   V₆

Figure 46. Giant P pulmonale in patient with pure pulmonic stenosis. Note tall, thin "Gothic" P wave in lead II and a mirror image of this in aV$_R$; also tall, pointed P in aV$_F$ and V$_4$.

dence that the first part of this wave is the result of the activity of the anterior portion of the right atrium, whereas the final part corresponds to the depolarization of the left atrium and the posterior part of the right atrium. The duration of the P wave in children, measured in standard limb leads, averages 0.06 second (standard deviation equals ±0.02).[32] Its maximum height is less than 2.5 mm. in any lead.[12, 759] The shape of the P wave is usually rounded in the standard limb leads, maximal in lead II, and usually minimal or even inverted (2 per cent of normals) in lead III. The right chest leads usually show diphasic or inverted P waves, the peak appearing early. P in V_5 and V_6, in contrast, is usually upright but low, with a relatively late peak. P in aV_R is normally inverted, in aV_L upright. The mean axis of the P wave in the frontal plane is between +50 and +80 degrees.

It may be said with fair certainty that P waves of more than 2.5 mm. in height or more than 0.08 second in duration are abnormal in children and denote atrial hypertrophy. Some differentiation between right and left atrial hypertrophy is usually, though not invariably, possible. Peaked or "Gothic-shaped," tall, but not prolonged P waves in

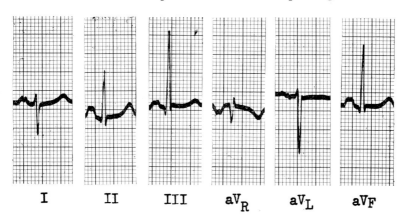

I   II   III aV_R aV_L aVF

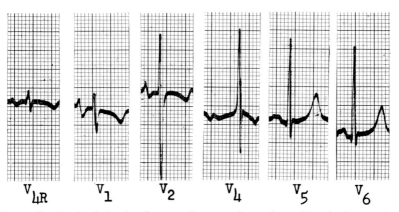

V_{4R} V_1 V_2 V_4 V_5 V_6

Figure 47. P mitrale in the electrocardiogram of a patient with mitral stenosis. Note the wide, notched P waves in all the limb leads and in the left chest leads, V_5 and V_6. Also, notice that the P-PQ ratio is well over 1.6 in aV_F.

leads II and III, coupled with pointed P waves in chest leads V_1 and V_2, with tall initial positivity, usually indicate right atrial hypertrophy (P pulmonale) (Fig. 46). In contrast, flat-topped P waves in leads I and II of normal height, but prolonged duration, with 2 notches at least 0.05 second apart, indicate left atrial hypertrophy (P mitrale) (Fig. 47). The first notch represents activation of the anterior portion of the right atrium; the second notch, most likely, activation of the left atrium, though activity of the posterior portion of the right atrium participates in it as well. Thus it is implied that "P mitrale" represents intra-atrial conduction disturbance. In the chest leads prominent and late P waves may be seen in V_5 and V_6, and the negative component of the P wave is accentuated in V_1 and V_2. British authors[692] maintain that combined atrial hypertrophy may be recognized on the basis of the presence of both tall and broad P waves, the tall, early ones being visible in the right chest leads, the late ones in the left chest leads.

Some South American authors[475] differentiate right from left atrial enlargement by measuring the ratio between P wave and P-Q segment duration (Fig. 48). Normally, this P/PQ ratio is never more than 1.6, and seldom less than 1.0. According to these authors, figures of 1.6 and more indicate left atrial hypertrophy, whereas values of less than 1.0 strongly suggest right atrial hypertrophy.

Absence of P waves in all leads means absence of atrial activity. It is wise, however, to explore the regions above V_1 and V_{4R} with a unipolar electrode, and perhaps even to obtain an esophageal lead before the absence of P waves is diagnosed with certainty. Occasionally, weak atrial activity is not registered in the conventional leads.

Inverted P waves in lead I (Fig. 49) with a P axis of +120 to +150 degrees indicate atrial inversion (right atrium to the left, left atrium to the right), and obviously should be accompanied by an upright P in aV_R and an inverted P wave in aV_L. A P wave of unusual shape with a

P/P-Q   RATIO

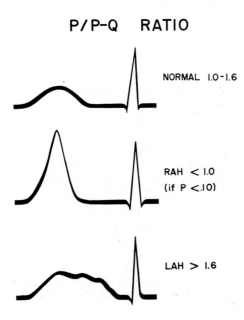

NORMAL 1.0-1.6

RAH < 1.0
(if P <.10)

LAH > 1.6

Figure 48. Schematic representation of the normal P-PQ ratio and the specific deviations from it, indicating right or left atrial hypertrophy.

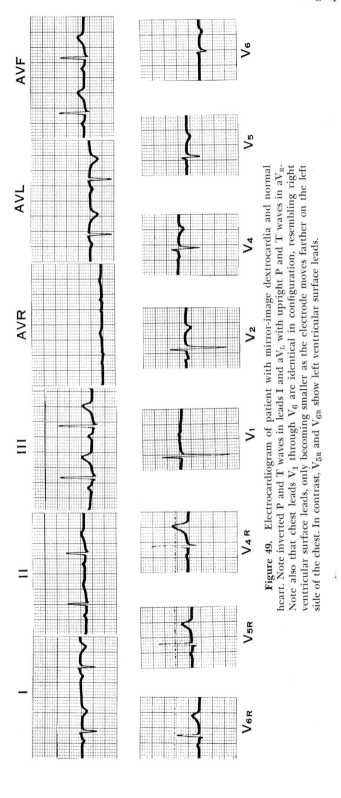

Figure 49. Electrocardiogram of patient with mirror-image dextrocardia and normal heart. Note inverted P and T waves in leads I and aV$_L$ with upright P and T waves in aV$_R$. Note also that chest leads V$_1$ through V$_6$ are identical in configuration, resembling right ventricular surface leads, only becoming smaller as the electrode moves farther on the left side of the chest. In contrast, V$_{5R}$ and V$_{6R}$ show left ventricular surface leads.

I

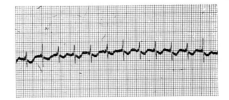

II

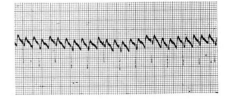

Figure 50. Atrial flutter. Note the regular, triangular-shaped complexes in leads II and III with almost no visible atrial activity in lead I.

III

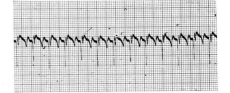

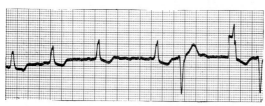

I

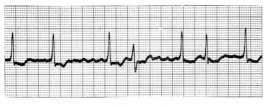

II

Figure 51. Atrial fibrillation. Note the irregularly spaced QRS complexes and the totally irregular atrial activity. Note also the conventionally shaped, and presumably conducted, QRS complexes (1, 2 and 3) in leads I and II, and the irregularly shaped, presumably ectopic, ventricular complexes (4) in lead I and (5) in lead II.

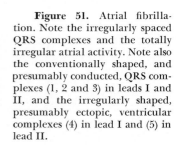

III

P-R interval of less than 0.10 second usually means that the pacemaker is not in the sinoatrial node; hence the designation "ectopic atrial" or "nodal" pacemaker, with a P axis of —60 to —90 degrees.

The normal or nodal P waves may be replaced by bizarre forms of atrial activity known as atrial flutter or fibrillation. In atrial flutter the atrial rate is about 200 to 300 beats per minute; the complexes are regular and triangular in leads II and III, but barely visible in lead I (Fig. 50). The flutter waves are continuous and may be followed through the QRS complexes. Atrial fibrillation, the severest disturbance of atrial activity, with a rate of more than 350 beats per minute, is completely irregular (Fig. 51) and may manifest itself on the tracing as only an irregular baseline.

The P-R Interval. This should be measured from the beginning of the QRS complex, preferably where a clear-cut Q wave is visible. Careful study of a large number of electrocardiograms in adults[534] resulted in the concept that the longest P-R interval found in any limb lead should be taken as the correct value for atrioventricular conduction time.

When determining the P-R interval in children, both the rate and the age have to be considered (Table 6, p. 775), whereas, in the adult, only the rate has to be taken into consideration. By and large, the P-R interval is inversely related to rate and increases with age. But the increase in P-R interval in older children is greater than one would expect from the slowing of the pulse rate alone.

Unusually short P-R intervals (less than 0.10 second) may be seen (1) in infants less than one year of age, (2) if the pacemaker is not the sinoatrial node, or (3) if the atrioventricular conduction is through an aberrant short pathway (Wolff-Parkinson-White syndrome)[740] (Fig. 52). Prolonged P-R intervals may be seen in active carditis, but are not diagnostic of that disorder. Permanently prolonged P-R intervals may be congenital (with or without congenital heart disease) or may be the consequence of past rheumatic infection, without implying rheumatic activity at all.

Regularly variable P-R intervals may be seen in the so-called Wenckebach phenomenon[724] (Fig. 53) and in interference with dissociation (Fig.

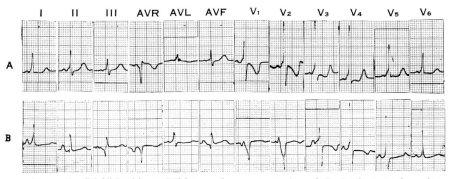

Figure 52. Wolff-Parkinson-White syndrome, types A and B. Both sets of tracings indicate the short P-R interval and the delta waves particularly well seen in V_2 and V_3. The type A complexes on the top line show a dominant R wave in the right chest leads, whereas the type B complexes on the bottom show dominant S waves.

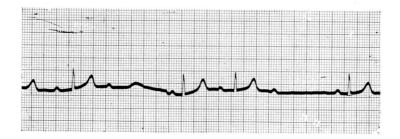

Lead I

Figure 53. Wenckebach phenomenon. Note that the second P wave in the tracing is not followed by a QRS complex. The third and fourth P waves are followed by QRS complexes, but the P-R interval gradually lengthens, and the fifth P wave is again completely blocked.

L   E   A   D   - I -

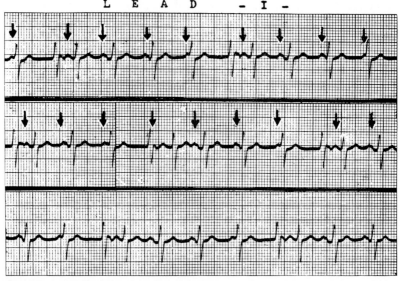

Figure 54. Interference and dissociation. Note the regularly spaced P waves and the regularly spaced QRS complex. The ventricles are beating somewhat faster than the atria; thus the P-R interval consistently shortens. When the P wave falls behind the QRS complex, this stimulates a second QRS complex immediately thereafter. In the top row the P-R interval shortens progressively from the third P wave through the fourth and the fifth. The sixth P wave occurs after the QRS complex, and the next QRS complex comes at a short P-R interval after the seventh P wave.

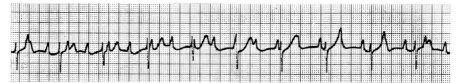

Figure 55. Electrocardiogram showing complete heart block. Note the fast atrial rate (140) and the slow ventricular rate (68). Note the absence of any constant relation between P and QRS complexes. This tracing is from a patient with corrected transposition of the great arteries, Ebstein's malformation and a ventricular septal defect.

54). Completely irregular P-R intervals mean complete atrioventricular block (Fig. 55).

The QRS Complex. The first downward wave beyond the P wave has been designated as the q wave. The first positive deflection beyond the atrial wave is called R, and the negative potential following the first R wave is called S. The term "QS" has been coined for the monophasic negative QRS complex. There may be more than one R or S wave within one ventricular complex. These are designated as R′ or R″ and S′ or S″; their relative sizes may be indicated by using capital letters for the larger deflections and small letters for the smaller ones. This type of detailed description is usually used only in unipolar leads.

The QRS complex is the depolarization wave of the ventricles. Normally its duration is less than 0.10 second; the average duration increases only slightly with age (0.065 second at 24 hours to 0.075 second at 12 years of age),[759] and is influenced relatively little by rate. A QRS complex of 0.10 to 0.12 second in duration is called incomplete bundle branch block; a duration of more than 0.12 second is complete bundle branch block. The measurement should be made in lead II or in one of the chest leads and should be started with the onset of the Q wave and terminated where the electrocardiogram line, returning from S toward the base line, suddenly thickens. The longest QRS in a tracing should be measured. It should also be mentioned here that according to Grant's[298] vectorial analysis of the electrocardiogram, bundle branch block is *not* identical with prolongation of the QRS complex, but rather implies a *change in the normal sequence of excitation*. This may or may not be accompanied by an increased *duration* of the QRS complex.

The range of normal QRS axes in the frontal plane has been tabulated previously; it swings from an almost horizontal position on the right in the newborn period to a somewhat inferior position in infancy, becoming more leftward in childhood, and finally swinging back inferiorly with the linear growth of puberty. In terms of anteroposterior direction, the mean QRS axis changes from a strictly anterior direction in infancy to a more posterior position in adolescence (Fig. 56).

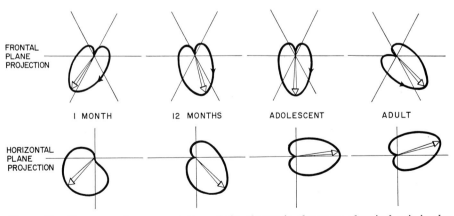

Figure 56. Diagrammatic representation of the change in the mean electrical axis in the frontal and horizontal planes from infancy to adulthood.

The q wave has no great significance in pediatrics. Its vital role in the diagnosis of myocardial infarction in adults is well known. It is not commonly found in lead I, but is frequently present in leads II, III, aV_F and V_5 and V_6. A q followed by R is never found normally in V_{4R} or V_1; on the other hand, a Qr or QS, representing the pattern of the "back of the heart," is common in right chest leads as well as in aV_R. Occasionally in cases of right ventricular hypertrophy a qR is present in V_1; close inspection and special techniques often show this deflection to be not a q, but in fact an rs wave. The duration and the size of the q wave are of no particular importance in children; in normal adults the size should always be less than 25 per cent of the amplitude of the succeeding R wave.

It is well worth mentioning here that, in an infant with the appropriate clinical syndrome, a deep and wide Q in lead I, aV_L or V_5 or V_6 is almost pathognomonic of anomalous origin of the left coronary artery (see p. 262). Furthermore, it should be mentioned that various authors, such as DuShane[209] and Keith[716] (basing their work on that of Cabrera and Monroy[123]), used the presence of deep Q waves, irrespective of width, in the diagnosis of left ventricular hypertrophy in congenital heart disease. As may be seen from Table 8 (p. 776), the *mean* depth of the Q waves in lead V_6 is not more than 1.5 mm. in any age group. Equally clearly, *maximal* Q waves of more than 4 to 5 mm. in depth may be seen in normal persons of all ages beyond infancy, and even within the 90 percentile range, Q waves of more than 2 mm. may be found (Table 8, p. 776). All this means to me that, although the presence of a Q wave may suggest left ventricular hypertrophy, I would hesitate to base the diagnosis on this feature alone. Furthermore, as will be pointed out later, I cannot subscribe to the doctrine that the presence of the Q wave not only indicates left ventricular hypertrophy, but also denotes a specific type, so-called diastolic overloading.

The R wave is the principal positive deflection in the electrocardiogram. It is usually tallest in the standard limb leads, in aV_F and in V_5 or V_6. Certain arbitrary limits of the normal R wave, based on the statistical analyses of large numbers of tracings, have been drawn up.[12, 519, 651, 652, 759] These figures have been useful in diagnosing ventricular hypertrophy, but remember that all such limits are purely arbitrary, and they cannot, with certainty, determine whether or not any individual deflection is of normal amplitude. They can indicate only whether it is likely to be normal or not. With these reservations in mind, the maximal QRS waves in our study of the chest leads of 521 normal infants and children are reproduced in Table 8 (p. 776).

One other measurement of the R wave deserves mention. This is the so-called intrinsicoid deflection designated as "ventricular activation time" (VAT). This is calculated as the time interval between the beginning of the q wave and the peak of the R wave in any one lead. On the basis of certain theoretic considerations, the ventricular activation time was thought to be a measure of the thickness of the portion of the ventricular wall underlying the particular unipolar lead where it was being calculated. Recent information questions the validity of this hypothesis.[625] The normal ventricular activation time for the right ventricle is less than 0.03 second, for the left ventricle less than 0.04 second.

The shape of the R wave gives information about the intraventricular conduction; notching or slurring of the R waves means intraventricular conduction disturbance. Fine notching may not necessarily be abnormal; coarse notchings are almost invariably pathologic. Bizarre and wide (more than 0.12 second) QRS complexes are seen with complete bundle branch block. In the standard limb leads of left bundle branch block (Fig. 57) left axis deviation is present, and R_1 is tall and late and commonly followed by a sharply inverted T wave. In the chest leads of left bundle branch block the terminal forces are directed

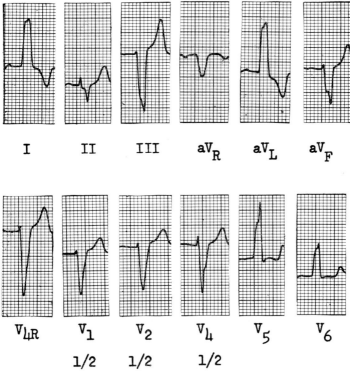

I   II   III   aV$_R$ aV$_L$ aV$_F$

V$_{4R}$ V$_1$ V$_2$ V$_4$ V$_5$ V$_6$

1/2   1/2   1/2

Figure 57.   Electrocardiogram showing left bundle branch block. Note the wide QRS complexes throughout. Note the tall R waves in leads I, aV$_L$, V$_5$ and V$_6$. As expected, there is no Q in the left chest leads.

toward the left. This means that in V$_1$ the terminal portion is negative, whereas in V$_6$ it is positive. Also, the initial forces are altered and point leftward and posteriorly, and there is usually no q wave in V$_6$. Conversely, in right bundle branch block only the terminal forces are altered and, since they originate in the right ventricle, they point rightward and anteriorly. Consequently, the last part of the deflection in V$_1$ is positive and in V$_6$, negative. Obviously, in right bundle branch block, right axis deviation is seen, S$_1$ is wide and deep, and T$_1$ is upright (Fig. 58). The QRS complexes of bundle branch block are identical with those of ventricular premature beats or ventricular tachycardia, but the relation of the P wave to the QRS complex is different in the two conditions. There

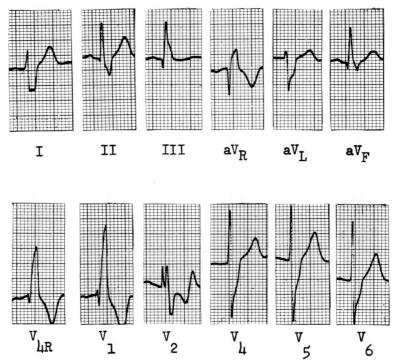

I   II   III   aV$_R$ aV$_L$ aV$_F$

V$_{4R}$ V$_1$ V$_2$ V$_4$ V$_5$ V$_6$

Figure 58. Electrocardiogram showing right bundle branch block. Note the deep and wide S waves in leads I, aV$_L$ and V$_{5-6}$. Note also the tall secondary R waves in the right chest leads. The QRS duration is longer than 0.12 second in all leads.

is a fixed and regular P-QRS relation in bundle branch block, whereas ventricular premature beats or ventricular tachycardia is completely independent of atrial activity.

The appearance of secondary r waves (r′ or R′) in the right chest leads or in aV$_R$ is more the rule than the exception in children. The R′ may represent terminal right ventricular or left ventricular forces, and it is difficult to be sure whether it is normal or abnormal for a given age. The younger the child, the more likely he is to have a secondary r wave to the right. The taller the R, the more likely it is to be abnormal. Often a vectorcardiogram is required to differentiate a normal variation from a grossly abnormal tracing. Whether one refers to the appearance of an r′ in the right chest lead as incomplete right bundle branch block is probably a matter of semantics. We have discarded the expression and, instead, refer to it descriptively as rsr′ or rsR′ to avoid the implication of a conduction disturbance (Fig. 59).

The S wave is usually deepest in leads I, aV$_R$ and V$_1$ and V$_2$. Arbitrary limits of the type mentioned in respect to R waves have also been drawn up for S waves in the chest leads (Table 8). Normal limits of S$_{v-1}$ plus R$_{v5-6}$ have also been calculated.[12, 652] Wide S$_1$ and S$_{v5-6}$ are characteristic of complete or incomplete right bundle branch block. Conversely, wide S$_3$ and S$_{v1-2}$ are seen with left bundle branch block. Deep S$_1$ indicates right axis deviation.

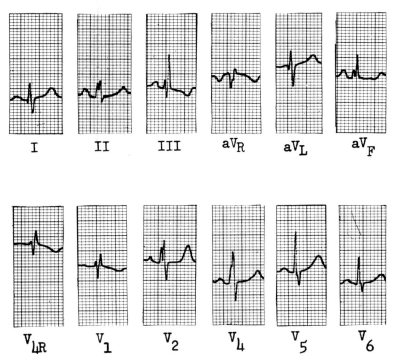

Figure 59. rSR′ pattern in the chest leads of a patient with atrial septal defect, secundum variety. Note the wide S in leads I, aV_L and V_{5-6}. Also note the QRS duration of 0.10 second. This type of tracing is still sometimes called incomplete right bundle branch block.

The RS-T Segment. The RS-T segment is the interval between the end of the QRS complex and the beginning of the T wave. In most instances it is difficult to separate it clearly from the T wave proper, since they are both part of the process of repolarization. The duration of the RS-T segment is almost impossible to determine. Under ordinary circumstances it is at the level of the T-P segment; depressions or elevations of 1.5 mm. or more are probably pathologic and indicate myocardial ischemia or digitalis effect. Prolongation of the S-T segment suggests electrolyte imbalance, specifically hypocalcemia.

The T Wave. The T wave, the terminal portion of ventricular activity, is always positive in lead I. Negative T_2 suggests myocardial damage; negative T_3 is within normal limits. Inverted T_1 suggests either dextrocardia or severe myocardial impairment (ischemia, electrolyte disturbance, and so forth). T in aV_R is always inverted; T in aV_L or aV_F is variable. T_{v5-6} is always upright in normal persons. In contrast, inverted T_{v1-3} is normal in infants and children except during the first few days of life.

Tent-shaped, peaked T waves are characteristic of potassium intoxication (Fig. 60).

The mean T axis in the frontal plane is usually in the same direction as the QRS axis ($+30$ to $+40$ degrees), the angle between the two seldom

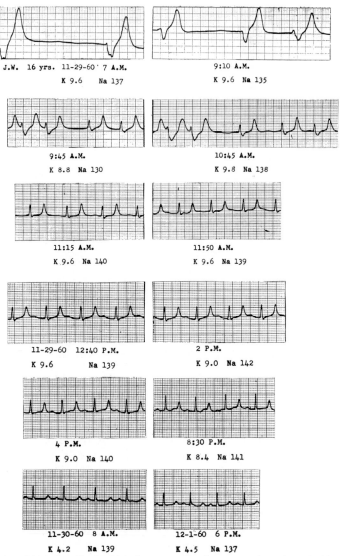

J.W. 16 yrs. 11-29-60 ' 7 A.M.
K 9.6   Na 137

9:10 A.M.
K 9.6   Na 135

9:45 A.M.
K 8.8   Na 130

10:45 A.M.
K 9.8   Na 138

11:15 A.M.
K 9.6   Na 140

11:50 A.M.
K 9.6   Na 139

11-29-60   12:40 P.M.
K 9.6   Na 139

2 P.M.
K 9.0   Na 142

4 P.M.
K 9.0   Na 140

8:30 P.M.
K 8.4   Na 141

11-30-60   8 A.M.
K 4.2   Na 139

12-1-60   6 P.M.
K 4.5   Na 137

Figure 60. Electrocardiographic changes reflecting potassium intoxication from a maximal distortion at 7 A.M. on Nov. 29, 1960, until the return to normal sinus rhythm at 6 P.M. on Dec. 1, 1960. In the interval, note the almost complete absence of the R wave and the tall, tent-shaped T wave in the beginning, with the gradual return of the QRS complexes and eventual lowering of the T waves. Well defined P waves are first seen in the 4 P.M. tracing on Nov. 29.

exceeding 45 degrees. There is little difference in this respect between children and adults. In contrast, the anteroposterior direction of the T axis changes considerably from infancy to childhood, progressing from an entirely posteriorly oriented T wave of the infant to the frontally directed T axis of the child and the anterior T wave of the adult. These changes express themselves in the unipolar chest leads by less and less inversion of the T wave in the right chest leads from infancy to adulthood. The one

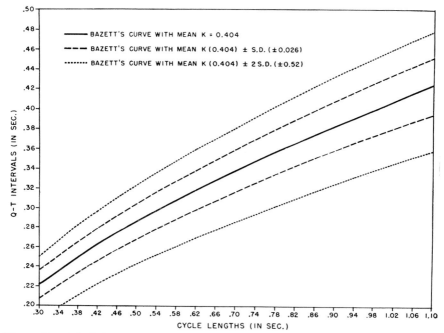

Figure 61. Calculation of the corrected Q-T interval from the actual Q-T measurement and the cycle lengths in seconds.[11]

exception to this, of course, is the upright T_{v1} of the first twenty-four hours of life. *Beyond the first four days of life an upright T wave is surely abnormal in the right chest leads and may indicate right ventricular hypertrophy.*

   The Q-T Interval.   The Q-T interval is the measure of total electrical systole of the ventricles (Fig. 41). Its duration is dependent, much like that of the P-R interval, on age and rate. Much controversy surrounds the measurement and the significance of the Q-T interval.[11, 681] Conventionally, it is measured from the beginning of the QRS complex to the end of the T wave. Lepeschkin[416] conclusively proved that in a certain number of cases the measurement thus performed involves the U wave as well. In any determination of the Q-T interval the averages of at least three complexes, obtained from three different leads, should be measured. The figure thus obtained should then be compared with the table of expected normals for age and rate.[23] Alimurung and his associates,[11] using Bazett's formula $\left(U = \dfrac{Q\text{-}T}{\sqrt{R\text{-}R}} \right)$,[47] constructed a useful graph for the determination of the normal Q-T interval in any given cycle length in children; this graph includes a mean curve and curves to twice the standard deviation, the latter including 95.6 per cent of the normals (Fig. 61). Prolonged Q-T interval is present in a certain number of cases of carditis,[681] in some instances of electrolyte imbalance (potassium or calcium depletion) and after quinidine administration. Shortened Q-T interval may be the result of digitalis administration. According to Taran, it also occurs as the consequence of pericarditis.[681]

The U Wave. The U wave is mentioned only for the sake of completeness. Its practical importance is not known. The U wave is a broad, low wave, discernible in the standard limb leads of about half of the normal electrocardiograms. It may be prominent if the cardiac output is high or if the patient is under the influence of drugs (insulin, digitalis), or it may accompany changes in cell chemistry (potassium, calcium).

Normal Unipolar Precordial and Extremity Leads in Infants and Children

The normal adult left ventricle is thicker than the right ventricle. This anatomic difference is probably the consequence of the pressure differences between the systemic and pulmonary circuits. As a result of these anatomic and physiologic facts, the normal adult electrocardiogram is characterized by left ventricular dominance. This may best be seen in the unipolar chest leads, where, as mentioned before, the typical pattern over the right ventricle is rS, whereas the left ventricular leads show a qR or Rs wave (Table 3; Fig. 42). This is referred to as normal adult R/S progression from V_{1-6}.

In contrast to that of the adult, the circulation of the newborn infant is characterized by anatomic and physiologic dominance of the right ventricle. These facts are clearly mirrored in the unipolar chest leads, where distinct differences between infants and adults are noted. As expected, the unipolar chest leads of the newborn infant show right ventricular dominance or hypertrophy; namely, right chest leads V_{4R} to V_2 show a dominant R wave (Rs) in all instances.[12] The left chest leads show a dominant S (rS), a complete reversal of the adult R/S progression, in 50 per cent of the cases.

Between these two extremes, the heart of the newborn infant and the heart of the adult, the rest of infancy and childhood represents a

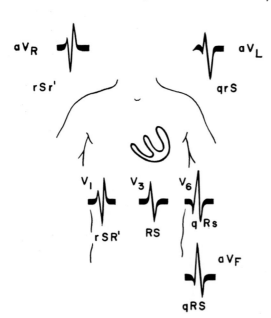

Figure 62. The unipolar limb and chest leads of an infant beyond the newborn age.

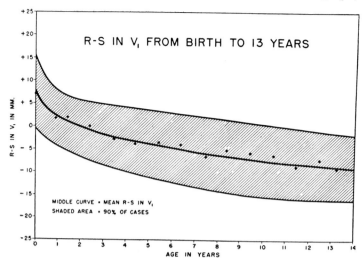

Figure 63.   The algebraic sum of R and S waves in lead V_1 from birth to 13 years.

The infant, not newborn, unipolar electrocardiogram is represented in Figure 62. All that one may state with certainty is that the unipolar chest transitional period from right ventricular to left ventricular dominance. leads of normal newborn infants should represent right ventricular dominance, and those of adults, left ventricular dominance. Whether any particular pattern between these two periods of life is normal or not can be expressed only in terms of probability. The progression from the newborn to the adult pattern is seen in Figure 63, in which the algebraic sum of R and S waves in V_1 is pictured. The sum is a positive one at birth (representing a dominance of R), and gradually becomes a significantly negative one (dominance of S) at thirteen years of age.

Lepeschkin[417] stated the problem in another way by saying, "The ratio of R to S over the right ventricle, the degree of right axis deviation, and the thickness of right ventricular wall in percentage of left show an almost identical course during growth."

A more detailed approach to the same problem is presented in Table 1 (p. 775), in which 521 infants and children are divided into 4 age groups and are analyzed according to the pattern of V_1 in their unipolar chest leads. It may be seen that, whereas 89 per cent of group I show a dominant R, 97.5 per cent of group IV show a dominant S.

The T waves in the right chest leads are upright during the first day of life in at least 75 per cent of normal infants. T_{v6}, on the other hand, is inverted in about 50 per cent of infants within the first 24 hours of life. After the first few days inverted T waves in the right chest leads and upright T waves in the left chest leads are the rule, with practically no exceptions. In infants T wave inversion may extend through V_{2-3}, whereas in older children it is restricted to V_1, and only occasionally extends to V_2 (Table 9, p. 777).

The P waves show almost no change throughout infancy and childhood. They are almost always inverted, or diphasic, in V_{1-2} and, as a rule, are upright in V_{5-6}.

The unipolar limb leads, as discussed previously, give valuable information about the position of the heart. Seventy-five per cent of the infants less than nine months of age have vertical or semivertical hearts. This relation changes but slightly throughout childhood; 66 per cent of patients more than 6 years of age still have vertical or semivertical hearts. The horizontal position of the heart is rare in infants less than nine months old.

One other significant feature of the young infant's heart is the tall R wave encountered in lead aV_R. A dominant R is seen in 28 per cent of infants less than 9 months old (almost exclusively in those less than 2 months old) and in only 2.5 per cent of patients more than 6 years old.

Ventricular Hypertrophy

Perhaps the most important use of electrocardiography in pediatrics is for the determination of the relative thickness of the two ventricles and identification of ventricular hypertrophy.

From what has been said in the section on the unipolar chest leads of infants and children it should be clear that a relatively thick right ventricle, and thus right ventricular dominance, is the rule in infants. Conversely, a relatively thick left ventricle, with left ventricular dominance, is invariably found in normal adults. It clearly follows that a dominant left ventricle in an infant indicates abnormal left ventricular hypertrophy, and a dominant right ventricle in an adult is proof of pathologic right ventricular hypertrophy. Over and above these qualitative differences between infants and adults, quantitative estimates of the degree of ventricular dominance may lead to the diagnosis of left ventricular hypertrophy in some adults, and of right ventricular hypertrophy in some infants.

The diagnosis of ventricular hypertrophy often rests on the height of the QRS complexes alone. If one realizes, however, that the voltages registered by any of the conventional leads depend not only on the thickness of the heart muscle, but also on the thickness of the chest wall, the distance of the heart from the electrode, the position of the ventricle in the chest cavity (displacement by lung or even atria), and the direction of the electrical forces in terms of the particular lead considered, the inevitable fallacies become clear. Also, one has to bear in mind the fact that "normal

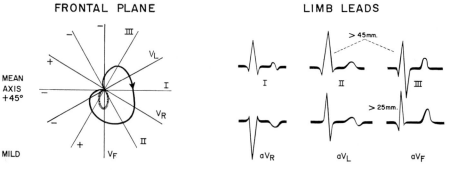

Figure 64. Left ventricular hypertrophy of mild degree as reflected in the frontal plane vector loop and the standard and unipolar limb leads. Note the voltage criteria indicated on the limb leads.

FRONTAL PLANE   LIMB LEADS

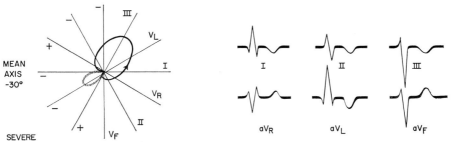

Figure 65. Severe left ventricular hypertrophy represented by the frontal plane vector-cardiogram and the standard and unipolar limb leads.

HORIZONTAL PLANE   CHEST LEADS

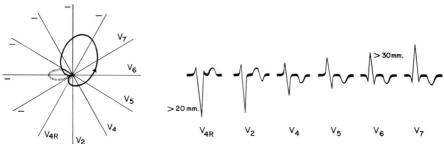

Figure 66. Severe left ventricular hypertrophy as represented in the horizontal plane vector loop and the unipolar chest leads. Note the voltage criteria in the unipolar chest leads. The figure of more than 50 mm. for V_{4R} plus V_6, indicating left ventricular hypertrophy, may be slightly liberal; recent information suggests that it should be closer to 60 mm.

voltages" are based simply on minimums and maximums determined on a large, but not infinite, number of patients. Consequently a warning should be sounded here to the effect that ventricular hypertrophy determined on the basis of voltages alone is not an absolute certainty. It simply means that it is unlikely—statistically improbable—that a normal heart would give rise to voltages beyond a certain magnitude, but it is not impossible in any one case. For this reason, electrocardiographic voltages should be regarded only against the background of other electrocardiographic and clinical criteria of heart disease, and the diagnosis of ventricular hypertrophy should seldom, if ever, be based on voltages alone.

Left Ventricular Hypertrophy. STANDARD LIMB LEADS (Figs. 64, 65). (*a*) The heights of voltages in standard limb leads are useful in the diagnosis of left ventricular hypertrophy. If the sum of the R waves in leads II and III is more than 45 mm., or if the sum of the R wave in lead I and the S wave in lead III is more than 30 mm., the presence of left ventricular hypertrophy should be suspected. (*b*) Left axis deviation (tall R wave in lead I and deep S wave in lead III) of more than —30 degrees indicates left ventricular hypertrophy in 50 per cent of the cases. Intraventricular conduction disturbances, and even horizontal hearts, however, without evidence of left ventricular hypertrophy, may show significant left axis deviation as well.

UNIPOLAR LIMB LEADS (Figs. 64, 65).   These are not pre-eminently useful in diagnosing left ventricular hypertrophy; however, (a) left ventricular potentials, reflected in aV_L or aV_F with R waves of 25 mm. or more may indicate left ventricular hypertrophy, (b) the q waves in aV_F or aV_L (depending on vertical or horizontal position), particularly if coupled with tall symmetrical T waves, suggest, but by themselves are not diagnostic of, left ventricular hypertrophy, and (c) the main deflection in aV_R is always negative in left ventricular hypertrophy.

UNIPOLAR CHEST LEADS (Fig. 66). Unipolar chest leads have been particularly useful in the diagnosis of left ventricular hypertrophy. (a) The height of R in V_{5-6} (more than 30 mm.) and the depth of S in V_{1-2} (more than 25 mm.) may be used as criteria of left ventricular hypertrophy if they clearly fall outside the transitional zone; if V_{1-2} or V_{5-6} still show RS complexes, then positions further to the right or the left must be used as the true potentials of the respective ventricles. If the sum of the R wave in V_5 or V_6 and the S wave in V_1 or V_2 is more than 50 mm. one may be assured that left ventricular hypertrophy exists. (b) S waves in the right chest leads and R waves in the left chest leads, outside the norms given for age in Table 8, are by themselves indicative, *but not diagnostic,* of left ventricular hypertrophy. (c) An intrinsicoid deflection in V_{5-6}, of more than 0.04 second is clear evidence of left ventricular hypertrophy. (d) Depressed S-T and inverted T waves in V_{5-6}, with increased voltages, are conclusive evidence of severe left ventricular hypertrophy with strain. (e) Deep q waves

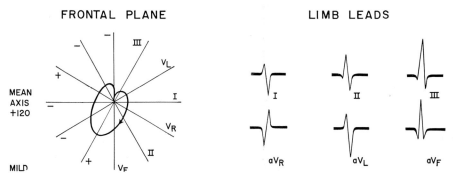

Figure 67. Mild right ventricular hypertrophy represented by the frontal plane vector loop and standard and unipolar limb leads.

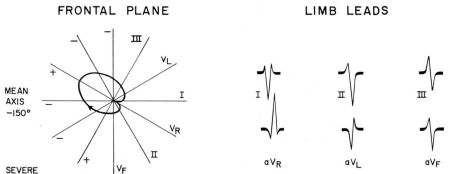

Figure 68. Severe right ventricular hypertrophy as represented by the frontal plane vector loop and standard and unipolar limb leads. Note the clockwise rotation of the frontal plane loop.

(more than 4 mm.) in lead V_{5-6} suggest left ventricular hypertrophy if coupled with tall, symmetrical T waves.

INDIRECT EVIDENCE.   Indirect evidence of left ventricular hypertrophy is furnished by left atrial hypertrophy (Fig. 47) (so-called P mitrale). This is in contrast to the findings in adults, in whom "P mitrale" most often denotes right ventricular hypertrophy secondary to mitral stenosis. In children severe organic mitral stenosis is rare; thus left atrial hypertrophy usually is the result of a failing hypertrophied left ventricle.

In addition to these criteria, as emphasized before, a normal adult type of electrocardiographic record in a young infant indicates left ventricular hypertrophy.

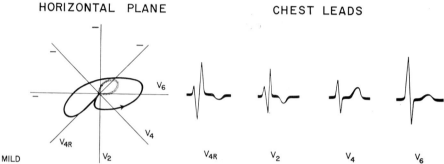

Figure 69.   Mild right ventricular hypertrophy as represented by the horizontal plane vector loop and the unipolar chest leads. Note the counterclockwise inscription of the loop.

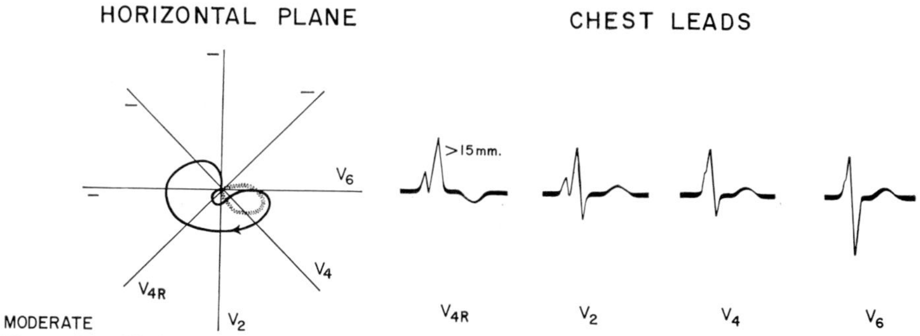

Figure 70.   Moderate right ventricular hypertrophy represented in the horizontal plane by a tall R' in V_{4R} and a wide, deep S in V_6.

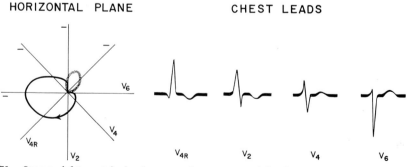

Figure 71.   Severe right ventricular hypertrophy represented in the horizontal plane by a qR in the right chest leads and rS in the left chest leads.

Right Ventricular Hypertrophy. STANDARD LIMB LEADS (Figs. 67, 68). (*a*) Right axis deviation (deep S wave in lead I and tall R wave in lead III) of $+120$ degrees or more is suggestive of right ventricular hypertrophy, with the usual allowances to be given to positional changes. (*b*) A deep S wave in leads I, II and III resulting from a rightward and superiorly oriented mean electrical axis strongly suggests right ventricular hypertrophy.

UNIPOLAR LIMB LEADS (Figs. 67, 68). A dominant R or R' in aV_R is characteristic of right ventricular hypertrophy.

UNIPOLAR CHEST LEADS (Figs. 69 to 71). (*a*) The least certain indication of right ventricular hypertrophy in the chest leads consists in RS deflections from V_1 to V_6, indicating an unusual dominance of the anterior (right ventricular) forces across the entire chest. (*b*) An rsR' pattern in the right chest leads probably indicates right ventricular hypertrophy if the R' is more than 15 mm. in height. The narrower the QRS complex and the taller the R', the more right ventricular hypertrophy is suggested. A late (more than 0.06 second) R' of less than 10 mm. in height probably indicates bundle branch block with not much, if any, right ventricular hypertrophy. (*c*) A tall, unslurred initial R_{v1-2}, with or without a q wave and with small if any S wave, unquestionably indicates right ventricular hypertrophy. (*d*) An intrisicoid deflection of R of 0.04 or more in V_{1-2} is good evidence of right ventricular hypertrophy. (*e*) Inverted T waves in right-sided chest leads, accompanied by depression of the S-T segment, in conjunction with the other changes in the chest leads, indicate severe hypertrophy ("strain pattern"). There seems to be adequate correlation between the severity of the hypertrophy and the extension of the T and S-T changes from V_1 toward V_6. (*f*) Positive T_{v1} in infants beyond the first four days of life suggests right ventricular hypertrophy.

INDIRECT EVIDENCE. Indirect evidence of right ventricular hypertrophy is furnished by peaked and tall P_2, indicating right atrial hypertrophy ("P pumonale") (Fig. 46).

As emphasized before, most of these changes may occur normally in infants, but almost never in normal adults. The use of the tables in the section on normal chest leads should serve as a guide in determining the significance of these findings in older infants or children (Table 8, p. 776). Nevertheless, certain findings always indicate right ventricular hypertrophy, even in the youngest infants. These are (1) the presence of a q wave in V_{4r} or V_1, (2) an R wave in V_4R or V_1 of 20 mm. or more without and S wave, and (3) S-T and T wave changes extending from V_{1-5}. (It is difficult to accept Ziegler's thesis, also stressed by Keith, that a positive T wave in an infant more than twenty-four hours old always means pathologic degrees of right ventricular hypertrophy. My views on the matter can be summed up simply by saying that an upright T_{v1} in normal newborn infants rarely, but surely, occurs. Whether, when it is abnormal it means "systolic overloading of the right ventricle," reciprocal changes from left ventricular hypertrophy or even metabolic abnormalities, may be difficult to determine in the individual case.

The other evidences of right ventricular hypertrophy must be viewed against the background of age and other electrocardiographic and clinical features. For easy review, Table 10 (p. 778) summarizes the criteria of left and right ventricular hypertrophy.

FRONTAL PLANE   LIMB LEADS

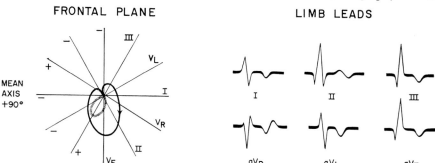

Figure 72. Combined ventricular hypertrophy represented by the frontal plane vector loop and standard and unipolar limb leads.

HORIZONTAL PLANE   CHEST LEADS

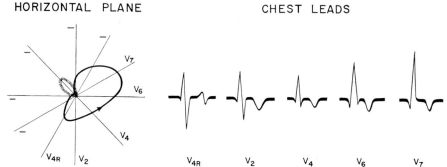

Figure 73. Combined ventricular hypertrophy visualized by horizontal plane vector loop and the unipolar chest leads. Note the dominant R in both the right and the left chest leads.

Combined Ventricular Hypertrophy (Figs. 72, 73). This is usually recognized by one of the following modifications of the left ventricular hypertrophy chest lead pattern: (1) a dominant R wave in V_{1-2}, (2) a shift of the transitional zone to the left, extending often to V_{5-6}, without obviating the tall R of left ventricular hypertrophy, but transferring it to V_7 or V_8, (3) presence of a deep S in lead I, or right axis deviation, and (4) vertical position.

A new concept of ventricular hypertrophy has been suggested by the Mexican School of Cardiology. In a series of papers Cabrera and his associates[123] proposed an electrocardiographic differentiation between increased flow work (diastolic overloading) and increased pressure work (systolic overloading) of the ventricles. They define systolic overloading of the right ventricle as a tall R or qR complex, with or without changes in S-T and T waves, in V_{1-2}. Juxtaposed to this is diastolic overloading of the right ventricle, consisting essentially of an rsR' pattern in V_{1-2}. Systolic overloading of the left ventricle, according to these authors, consists of a tall R wtih flat or negative T waves and S-T depression of the left ventricular leads (aV_F, V_{5-6}), whereas diastolic overloading of the same chamber is recognized by tall R and high, peaked T waves, with an upward-displaced S-T segment in aV_F, V_{5-6}, perhaps coupled with deep Q waves.

This has been an extremely useful and fruitful step in clinical electrocardiography. To begin with, it pointed up the usefulness of the cardio-

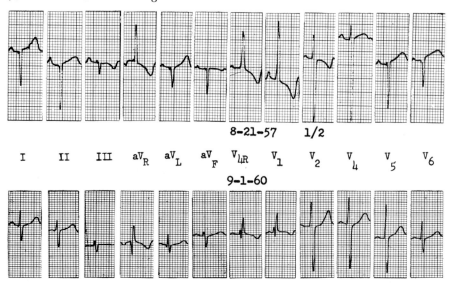

8-21-57   1/2

I   II   III   aV$_R$ aV$_L$ aV$_F$ V$_{4R}$ V$_1$ V$_2$ V$_4$ V$_5$ V$_6$

9-1-60

Figure 74. The change in the electrocardiogram of a patient who has had a successful pulmonic valvotomy. Note the characteristic "systolic overload" in the tracing of Aug., 1957, preoperatively. At this time the right ventricular systolic pressure was more than 150 mm. of mercury. In contrast, note the "diastolic overload" pattern of right ventricular hypertrophy in the patient two and a half years after operation, when the right ventricular systolic pressure was only 50 mm. of mercury.

gram in the diagnosis of congenital heart disease. Second, it departed from the conventional practice of correlating the electrocardiogram with postmortem data, placing these tracings in a dynamic framework by comparing them with physiologic information.

Recognizing the usefulness of the concept, it may be justifiable to point out disagreement with it. I do not believe that the differences in patterns are an expression of systolic versus diastolic overloading. The patterns exist, indeed, but are an expression of quantitative rather than qualitative differences. In other words, what the Mexican group calls diastolic overloading, I call mild right ventricular hypertrophy (which may even be normal in infants and young children). What they call systolic overloading, I refer to as severe right ventricular hypertrophy "with strain." Granted, that the latter degree of right ventricular hypertrophy is usually associated with increased pressure work of the right ventricle (pulmonic stenosis) and that the former is seen most commonly in conditions with increased flow work (atrial septal defect), on the other hand, we have seen unquestionable instances not only of mild pulmonic stenosis showing evidences of rsR' in the right chest leads, but also of a qR pattern of severe pulmonic stenosis being converted, gradually, over a period of months, into rsR' and rsr', after successful surgery (Fig. 74). The same principle holds for the left ventricular patterns, where, through the years, the electrocardiogram of a patient having aortic stenosis changes from one with a tall R and pointed T waves into one with S-T depression and T-wave inversion.

It can well be imagined that both muscle thickness and muscle tension (two important causes of "hypertrophy" in the electrocardiogram) are much greater in patients with aortic stenosis than in those with patent ductus arteriosus. But it is equally clear that one may frequently find a patient with mild aortic stenosis whose left ventricle is no thicker than that of another patient with a sizable patent ductus arteriosus.

Finally, before leaving the electrocardiographic definition of ventricular hypertrophy, it may be worth while to refer to Selzer's excellent summary of the subject as it relates to the cardiogram of adults.[629]

Arrhythmias

Under ordinary circumstances the rate and rhythm of the heart beat are determined by the activity of the sinoatrial node. The average heart rate in resting adults is about 60 to 80 beats per minute. In infants it is considerably higher, approximately 120 beats per minute; in children it is somewhere between these 2 extremes, in the neighborhood of 100 per minute.

To determine the "normal" rate of any person, especially a child, the sleeping pulse rate should be counted. If a child is awake, a number of extraneous factors influence the heart rate to such an extent that it is virtually impossible to obtain a true "resting value."

Rhythms Originating in the Sinus Node.   These are characterized by a P wave of normal and constant configuration and by a P-R interval of at least 0.10 second. Exceptions to the latter point occur in infants less

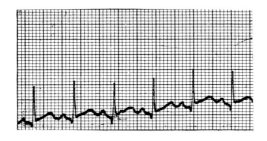

II

Figure 75.   Sinus tachycardia.

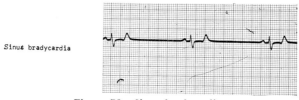

Sinus bradycardia

Figure 76.   Sinus bradycardia.

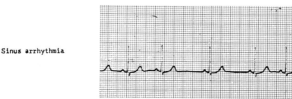

Sinus arrhythmia

Figure 77.   Sinus arrhythmia.

than one year of age and in patients with the Wolff-Parkinson-White syndrome.[740]

Sinus tachycardia is a rapid, regular heart rate ranging to a maximum of 180 to 200 beats per minute, where the normal relation between atrial and ventricular complexes is preserved (Fig. 75). The P wave is almost always easily discernible, although occasionally it may be superimposed on the preceding T wave. Sinus tachycardia may be the result of physiologic conditions (excitement, exercise), pathologic situations not necessarily involving the heart (fever), and, finally, may be the first expression of cardiac embarrassment (carditis, congestive failure). Reflex vagal stimulation (carotid sinus pressure) results only in a gradual decrease of the rate; P waves previously superimposed on the T waves may thus be clearly visible.

Sinus bradycardia (Fig. 76), with rates of less than 100 beats per minute in infants and less than 80 in children, is usually an expression of good cardiac reserve. Occasionally, however, it may be seen in cases of rheumatic carditis. Exercise should raise the rate in sinus bradycardia with ease, in contrast to the relatively fixed rate of complete atrioventricular block.

Sinus arrhythmia (Fig. 77) is a phasic irregularity of the heart beat,

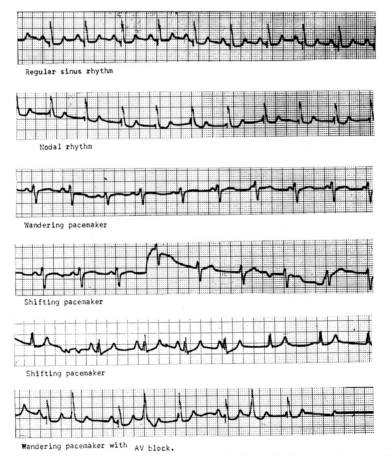

Regular sinus rhythm

Nodal rhythm

Wandering pacemaker

Shifting pacemaker

Shifting pacemaker

Wandering pacemaker with AV block.

Figure 78. Shifting and wandering pacemaker and sinus rhythm in a five-year-old boy with an atrial septal defect.

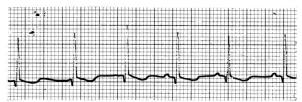

Figure 79.   Sudden shift from nodal to sinus rhythm.

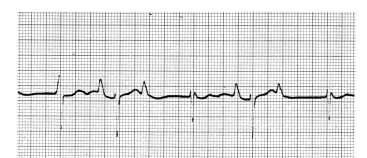

Figure 80.   Sinoatrial block. The second P wave in the tracing is blocked, not followed by a QRS complex. Similarly, the fourth one is blocked as well.

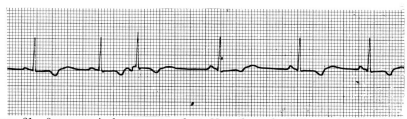

Figure 81.   Supraventricular premature beat. Note the early QRS complex (the third one in the tracing) preceded by an inverted P wave.

speeding up with inspiration and slowing with expiration, but maintaining the conventonal P-QRS relation. Much like sinus bradycardia, it may be an expression of good cardiac function; it is commonly seen in older children and adolescents, seldom in young children, and almost never in infants. Slower rates predispose to it. Sinus arrhythmia is frequently present during convalescence, though patients with rheumatic carditis show little of it, even after recovery from the acute attack.[370]

A wandering pacemaker, another "innocent" arrythmia, represents a gradual shift of impulse formation through several cycles, from one portion of the sinoatrial node to the other. This is pictured (Fig. 78) in the electrocardiogram by a change from a normal upright P wave with an average P-R interval to an abnormal, often inverted P wave with only slight, if any, change in the P-R interval. A shifting pacemaker is a sudden jump from sinus rhythm to nodal pacemaker (Figs. 78, 79). Once the atrioventricular node becomes the pacemaker, the process reverses itself, and the impulse formation gradually reverts to the sinoatrial node. This phenomenon is commonly seen in people without heart disease, but it does occur with rheumatic fever or digitalis intoxication.

Sinoatrial block and sinus arrest are temporary suspensions of the electrical activity of the atria through two or more cycles (Fig. 80). Sino-atrial block is usually episodic and of relatively short duration; the sinus pauses are multiples of the normal sinus rhythm. Sinus arrest is of longer duration, and the length of the pauses bears no mathematical relation to the original cycle length. Both conditions may be secondary to increased vagal tone, anoxia or drugs (digitalis, quinidine).

Rhythms Originating in the Atrium or the Atrioventricular Node. These are called supraventricular rhythms. In contrast to the sinus rhythms, either no P waves are noted, or the atrial waves are unusual in contour, with a P axis of —60 to —90 degrees, and are commonly separated from the QRS complex by less than 0.10 second. With few exceptions, the QRS complexes of supraventricular rhythms are of normal configuration and are less than 0.10 second in duration.

The least significant of the supraventricular arrhythmias is the supra-ventricular premature beat or extrasystole (Fig. 81). This may occur either because an ectopic focus in the atrium becomes unusually active, or because sinus bradycardia or sinus arrthythmia results in a sinus rhythm so slow that the normal threshold of excitation inherent in the atrial wall or the atrioventicular node surpasses it. Supraventricular premature beats are common in healthy youngsters, even in newborn infants, and may have no

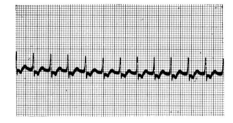

I

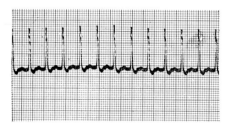

II

Figure 82. Paroxysmal supraventricular tachycardia. Note the rapid rate, the narrow QRS complexes and the absence of well defined P waves.

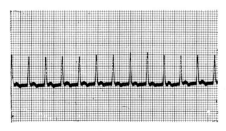

III

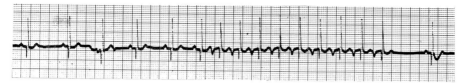

SUPINE

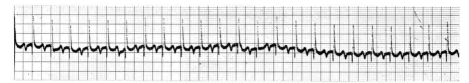

STANDING

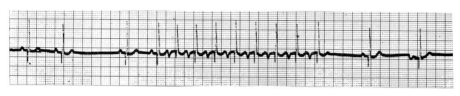

SUPINE

Figure 83. Chronic supraventricular tachycardia. Note the changes accompanying a shift in position. The ectopic focus takes over completely on standing, whereas in the supine position sinus rhythm alternates with bursts of ectopic rhythm.[501]

significance whatsoever. They may also accompany structural heart disease, but the diagnosis must rest on additional evidence. Supraventricular premature beats are characterized by a less than complete compensatory pause; i.e., the length of two cycles, including one with the premature beat, is less than the length of two normal cycles.

A continuous series of supraventricular premature beats, ranging in duration from a few seconds to several years, is called paroxysmal atrial tachycardia (Fig. 82). This, then, represents a complete, temporary usurpation of the function of the sinoatrial node by an atrial or nodal pacemaker. The rate may vary from 160 to 300 beats per minute. The onset, as well as the termination, is sudden in most instances. The rate is completely fixed and unchanging within a fraction of a second. Reflex vagal stimulation either results in the re-establishment of sinus rhythm or has no effect at all. P waves are seldom if ever seen; T waves are usually inverted if the tachycardia has lasted for more than a day. Paroxysmal supraventricular tachycardia often occurs in a child with a normal heart; nevertheless, if it lasts long enough, it may cause congestive failure, and even death. Obviously, this is even more likely to happen if the patient has underlying heart disease.

A transition between paroxysmal atrial tachycardia and supraventricular premature beat is the so-called repetitive tachycardia,[549] a variety of chronic atrial tachycardias in which short bursts of paroxysmal tachycardia alternate with single premature beats from the same focus (Fig. 83). In these short paroxysms the P waves are visible, but abnormal in contour. This should be contrasted with the ordinary type of paroxysmal atrial

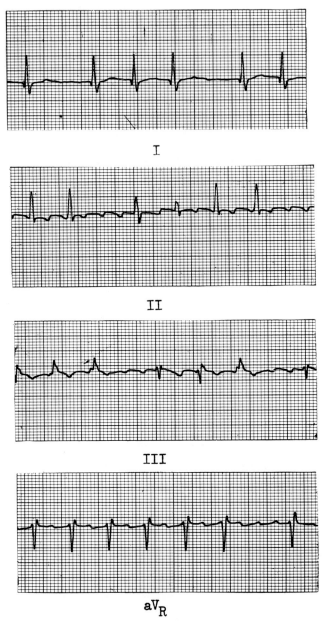

I

II

III

aV$_R$

Figure 84.   Atrial flutter 2:1 to 3:1 response in a patient recovering from an operation for closure of an atrial septal defect.

tachycardia, where no P waves are usually visible. This is usually seen in young people and infants with otherwise normal hearts.

One of the severest supraventricular arrhythmias is atrial flutter. The atria here are in continuous regular activity, ranging from 200 to 350 beats per minute. The ventricles respond with normal QRS complexes in a regular fashion (1:1 to 1:4 ratio), at regular rates of 140 to 300 beats per

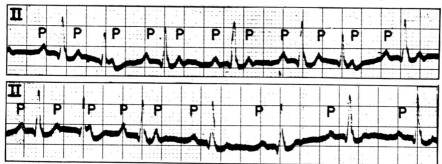

Figure 85.   Paroxysmal atrial tachycardia with block, showing abrupt transition to normal sinus rhythm. (Courtesy Dr. Harold D. Levine.)

minute. Characteristically, in lead I, the flutter waves can barely be noted, whereas in leads II and III they clearly appear in saw-tooth form (Figs. 50, 84). This is a severe arrhythmia and almost always means organic heart disease, especially rheumatic carditis. Occasionally it may be encountered in children with congenital heart disease (corrected transposition) or endocardial fibroelastosis, and it may even occur in normal hearts as paroxysmal supraventricular tachycardia. The effect of atrial flutter on the circulation as a whole depends on the ventricular rate. As long as the ventricles do not respond to more than one third of the atrial impulses, there usually is little difficulty. If the ventricular response is 1:2 or even 1:1, congestive failure will ensue. Reflex vagal stimulation can increase the atrioventricular block and reduce the ratio of ventricular response from 1:2 to 1:3 or even 1:4; often this is the only way by which clear flutter waves, unobstructed by QRS complexes, can be identified.

An arrhythmia encompassing certain features of atrial flutter and certain characteristics of supraventricular tachycardia is the one called paroxysmal atrial tachycardia with block (Fig. 85).[446, 449] This is most commonly the result of digitalis intoxication, but surely may be seen in patients who have never received cardiac glycosides. In this arrhythmia the atria beat at a moderately fast rate, 150 to 250 beats per minute, and the ventricles respond irregularly in 1:1 to 1:3 fashion. The P-R interval is unusually long (0.14 to 0.20 second), and an occasional P wave is completely blocked.

The severest type of supraventricular arrhythmia is atrial fibrillation (Fig. 51). This is a continuous irregular activity of the atria at rates of 400 to 700 beats per minute. The atrial activity may manifest itself electrocardiographically only as a minor irregularity of the base line, so-called fibrillary wave; at other times the atrial waves are coarse and relatively slower, closely resembling flutter waves. These various types of fibrillatory activities may be seen at different times in one and the same tracing. The ventricles respond irregularly, but at a much reduced rate (110 to 150 beats per minute). Both the atrial and the ventricular beats are totally irregular. Atrial fibrillation, for practical purposes, always means severe organic heart disease. It is most common in active rheumatic heart disease, but can be seen in congenital heart disease, especially atrial septal defect, Ebstein's disease, tricuspid atresia or corrected transposition of the great arteries. The effect of atrial fibrillation on the circulation depends for the most part on the ventricular rate. If this is relatively slow, atrial fibrillation

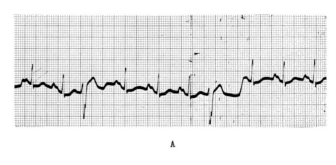

A

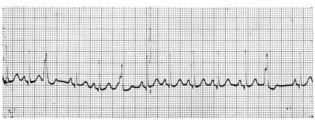

B

Figure 86. Ventricular premature beats, lead I. *A,* Origin of the premature beat in the left ventricle; *B,* in the right ventricle.

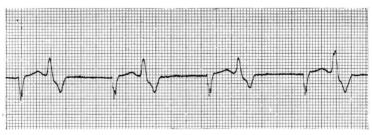

Figure 87. Bigeminy. Ventricular premature beats alternating with supraventricular beats.

may be tolerated for a long time without symptoms. On the other hand, unusually fast ventricular responses often lead to catastrophe. That atrial fibrillation, even with a slow ventricular rate, does not result in optimal circulatory dynamics is demonstrated by the fact that conversion of these slowly beating fibrillatory rhythms to normal sinus rhythm, with the same ventricular rate, is accompanied by great subjective improvement of the patient. Cardiac output studies in patients who have atrial fibrillation show an increase in cardiac output if fibrillation is abolished even without appreciable change in the ventricular rate. Reflex vagal stimulation, if effective at all, results in gradual slowing of the ventricular rate.

Rhythms Originating in the Ventricle.   These rhythms are characterized by a lack of correlation between atrial and ventricular complexes. The P waves are normal in shape. The ventricular complexes, on the other hand, are bizarre in configuration and measure 0.10 second or more; the QRS and T waves often point in opposite directions. Lead I usually gives the clue as to whether the ventricular complex originates from a focus in the right or the left ventricle (Fig. 86). Right ventricular beats resemble left bundle branch block complexes and have a dominant R in lead I, whereas left ventricular beats, similar to right bundle branch block, show a deep S_1.

Ventricular premature beats are the most innocuous among the ventricular arrhythmias. Their significance in pediatrics is only slightly greater than that of supraventricular premature beats. They may occur in perfectly normal youngsters; on the other hand, they may indicate carditis, incipient congestive heart failure, anoxia, or digitalis or quinidine intoxication. Ventricular premature beats alternating with normal beats, so-called bigeminy (Fig. 87), are especially characteristic of digitoxicity. The occurrence of multifocal, multiple-shaped ventricular premature beats has a more serious significance than if the shape of the extrasystoles is always the same within one lead. The characteristic feature of ventricular premature beats, in addition to their shape and their lack of time correlation with atrial activity, is the fact that they are followed by a full compensatory pause. This means that the length of two cycles, including one premature beat, is the exact length of two normal cycles.

A series of ventricular premature beats at a rate of 120 to 180 per minute constitutes ventricular tachycardia (Fig. 88). This phenomenon is rare in children, so much so that, when it does seem to occur, suspicion is immediately aroused as to whether it really represents ventricular tachycardia or supraventricular tachycardia with aberrant intraventricular conduction.

The differentiation between these two conditions is sometimes difficult, but usually is possible on the basis of the following points: (1) Supraventricular tachycardia is influenced by reflex vagal stimulation (carotid sinus or Valsalva maneuver); ventricular tachycardia is not. (2) The P waves in supraventricular tachycardia always show some regularity in relation to the QRS complex, whereas no such connection exists in true ventricular tachycardia. (3) The rates of the P and QRS complexes are similar in supraventricular tachycardia, whereas they are totally different in ventricular

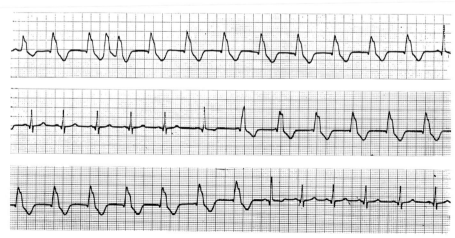

Figure 88. Burst of ventricular premature beats in series, amounting to ventricular tachycardia. The patient had aortic regurgitation and had not received digitalis. The tracing represents a continuous lead I.

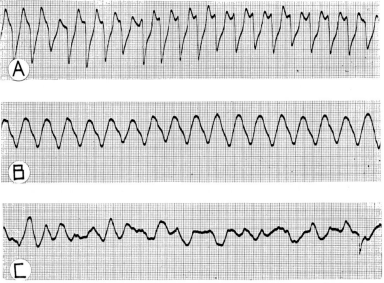

Figure 89. (*A*) Ventricular tachycardia giving rise in (*B*) to ventricular flutter and in (*C*) to ventricular fibrillation. These are consecutive strips of a patient who died after cardiac surgery.

tachycardia. (4) The rate of supraventricular tachycardia is characterized by a clocklike regularity not present in true ventricular tachycardia.

The dangers of ventricular tachycardia are twofold: It may result in congestive failure if the rate is rapid enough and lasts long enough, or it may progress into ventricular flutter or fibrillation. The latter situation is not compatible with effective cardiac output; thus it results in sudden death. Because of this possibility of conversion into ventricular flutter or fibrillation, paroxysmal ventricular tachycardia is regarded much more seriously than is paroxysmal supraventricular tachycardia.

Ventricular flutter and fibrillation are terminal events, and recovery from them is relatively rare. They represent the electrocardiographic substrate of sudden death. The complexes are broad, slurred and notched, and the T waves are fused with the QRS complexes, often resulting in a sine-wavelike pattern. The amplitude varies tremendously within one strip. Many more tracings of this sort have been obtained during and after cardiac operations within the past ten years than were seen in the entire previous history of electrocardiography (Fig. 89).

Effects of Chemical Changes and Drugs on the Electrocardiogram

Potassium. The effect of potassium (Fig. 90) on the electrocardiogram has been amply documented, both in animal experimentation and in man.[51, 230] Whether the electrocardiogram is principally influenced by the potassium level in the serum or within the myocardium itself is the subject of considerable argument. It seems, however, that the proponents of the cellular theory have made a better case.

Potassium intoxication has been produced in animals by infusion or ingestion of large amounts of potassium salts. In man, potassium poisoning is encountered in the later stages of uremia, leukemia and lower nephron

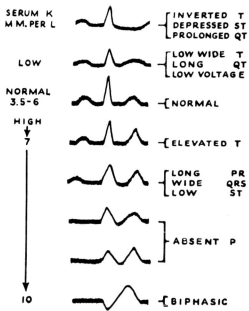

Figure 90. Schematic representation of the changes in P-QRS-T complex in conjunction with potassium levels. (From D. C. Darrow: New England J. Med., Vol. 242.)

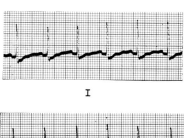

I

Figure 91. Electrocardiogram of a patient with potassium depletion. Note the depressed S-T segment, the prolonged Q-T interval and the prominent U waves.

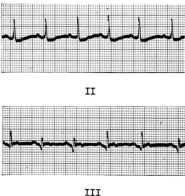

II

III

nephrosis, and after treatment with excessive amounts of potassium. The heart rate usually slows and the P waves become progressively wider and finally disappear, while the P-R interval gradually increases. The QRS complex undergoes changes consisting in widening and diminution of the R waves and increase of the S waves. The T waves become taller and tent-shaped, and eventually surpass the R wave in height (Fig. 60). The disappearance of the P waves may be due to sinoatrial block. The prolongation

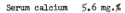

Serum calcium   5.6 mg.%

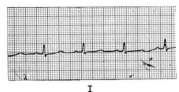

I

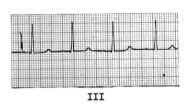

II

Figure 92. Electrocardiogram of patient with calcium depletion. Note the long Q-T interval due to prolongation of the S-T segment with a relatively normal T wave. This contrasts sharply, of course, with the tracing of potassium depletion (Fig. 91).

III

of the P-R interval and the widening of the QRS complex are both evidences of deterioration of conduction throughout all cardiac tissues. No definite correlation exists between serum potassium level and electrocardiographic changes beyond the observation that changes are rarely missed if the serum potassium level is 7 mEq. per liter or more, unless the level of sodium in the blood is unusually low.

Potassium depletion, seen in man in postoperative alkalosis, diabetic coma, long-standing diarrhea, and vomiting, also causes typical changes (Fig. 91), consisting in a prolongation of the Q-T interval with widening and lowering of the T waves, appearance of U waves, and occasional depression of the S-T segment.

Calcium. Calcium depletion, particularly in cases of tetany, also causes prolongation of the Q-T interval (Fig. 92).[51, 230] In contrast to potassium depletion, however, the lengthening of the electrical systole is caused by a prolongation of the S-T segment rather than by a widening of the T wave; the T wave in hypocalcemia is relatively normal, perhaps slightly narrow. The tetanic contraction of the striated muscle is reflected in the somatic tremor noted on the limb leads.

A high level of serum calcium, hypercalcemia, may cause increased irritability of the heart, with premature beats, even paroxysmal ventricular tachycardia.[417] It is also said to shorten the Q-T interval.

Digitalis. The electrocardiogram may be used to determine whether significant amounts of digitalis have been given to a patient and, with some qualifications, whether toxicity is present. The electrocardiogram cannot answer the question: "Has the patient been fully digitalized?" Whether or not full digitalization has been achieved is a question for the clinician to decide; the electrocardiogram only helps to determine whether there is some or too much digitalis in the heart muscle.

The digitalis glycoside, in doses commonly given, does not influence the shape of P waves. But the development of prolonged atrioventricular conduction time or sinoatrial block may be considered a sign of digitalis effect or even mild digitoxicity (Fig. 93). There are no significant changes in the QRS complex with doses usually given to man. Changes in the S-T segment are comparatively common; by changing the ventricular gradient, S-T-segment changes in direction opposite to the QRS complex appear. Possibly by improving the contractility of the myocardium, the repolarization becomes more effective and more near to depolarization; hence the S-T segment is directed opposite from the QRS complex. The same im-

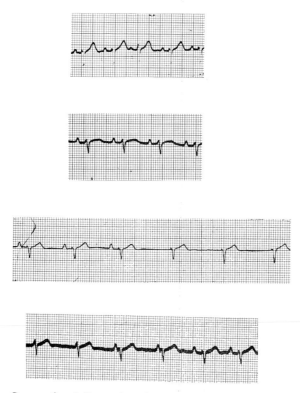

Figure 93. Consecutive daily tracings in patients with digitoxicity. The top tracing shows normal sinus rhythm. The second tracing shows prolonged P-R interval. The third tracing shows changing pacemaker, and the fourth one shows a return of this changing pacemaker to sinus rhythm with progressively prolonged P-R interval.

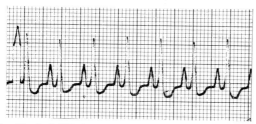

Figure 94. Typical S-T depression in patient with digitalis intoxication.

provement of myocardial contraction may underlie the shortening of the Q-T interval, one of the most consistent effects of digitalis on the cardiogram (Fig. 94). The S-T changes are most obvious in leads with a tall R wave and consist in a straight, angular "step-down" appearance of the S-T segment. S-T changes caused by digitalis administration often cannot be distinguished from those resulting from myocardial damage; however, the straightness and the angularity of the depression, without any convexity, favor a digitalis effect, together with the shortened QT_e. Digitalis affects the T wave only by decreasing its amplitude, not usually changing its direction. Careful analysis of digitalis tracings clearly reveals that most of the change in the direction of the ST-T complex is the result of S-T rather than T changes.

One of the earliest and most favorable results of digitalis administration is a slowing of the heart rate; seldom, if ever, does one see a favorable digitalis effect without a significant drop in rate. This probably represents increased vagotonia, and develops as a result of sinus depression in cases of sinus rhythm, and because of increasing atrioventricular block in cases of atrial flutter or fibrillation. Undue slowing of the rate, to less than 100 beats per minute in infants and less than 80 in older children, is presumptive evidence of digitoxicity.

The development of arrhythmias, in most instances, is evidence of digitoxicity; the one exception is the appearance of a sinus arrhythmia which may simply be the concomitant of the slower rate and increased vagotonia. On the whole, digitalis intoxication results more commonly in atrial arrhythmias in children than in adults, in whom ventricular arrhythmias seem to dominate the picture. Ectopic atrial pacemakers and paroxysmal atrial tachycardias with block are seen relatively frequently as a first expression of digitoxicity. Atrial flutter and fibrillation may also be seen, although much less commonly, and they represent a much more serious degree of intoxication. Ventricular arrhythmias are not seen frequently in children. Ventricular premature beats, if present, are prone to develop in forms of **bigeminy.**

If a patient is receiving digitalis and an arrhythmia develops, the burden of the proof is on the physician who maintains that the change in rhythm, whatever its nature, was not caused by digitalis. The difficulties resulting from this statement are obvious; sometimes it may be extremely hard to decide whether a patient has received too much or too little digitalis. The only reasonable approach to this problem is to try to withhold the drug for a short period, if possible, and to observe the trend of the changes. If the patient is in severe congestive failure, so that withholding the glycoside appears dangerous, then administration of small, frequent doses of a rapidly excreted form of digitalis is recommended, with electrocardiographic control.[446]

The time relation of digitalis administration on the electrocardiogram must be mentioned briefly. In my experience, the earliest effects are the shortening of the Q-T interval and the changes in the T waves. The rapidity of the changes and their duration depend a great deal on the preparation used. Digitalis, even in relatively large doses, affects normal hearts in a minor fashion only, if at all.

Quinidine.   The effects of quinidine on the electrocardiogram consist in slowing of the pacemaker and widening of the QRS complex, the Q-T interval, and the T waves (Fig. 95).

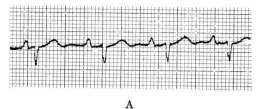

A

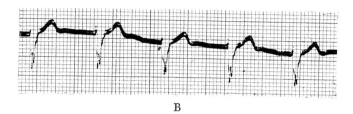

B

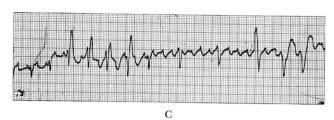

C

Figure 95.   The effect of quinidine on the electrocardiogram. *A,* Normal sinus rhythm. *B,* Nodal rhythm with widening QRS complex. *C,* Tracing from a patient with atrial flutter and quinidine intoxication resulting in multifocal ventricular premature beats.

It has been my practice to consider a widening of the QRS complex by more than 50 per cent as evidence of definite toxicity. Other toxic effects include the appearance of multifocal ventricular premature beats and prolongation of the P-R interval (Fig. 96).

Electrocardiographic changes after a single oral dose of quinidine appear to be maximal in about one hour, and they practically disappear in a matter of four hours.

Pronestyl. The effects of procaine amide are essentially similar to those seen with quinidine administration; doses causing a 50 per cent prolongation of the QRS complex are considered toxic. Occasionally, supraventricular premature beats with aberrant conduction, ventricular tachycardia and even ventricular flutter have been seen as a result of Pronestyl toxicity.

Pericarditis

The electrocardiographic features noted in patients with pericarditis may be the result of two factors. One is pericardial fluid accumulation, or thick scarring (constrictive pericarditis), which results in low voltages

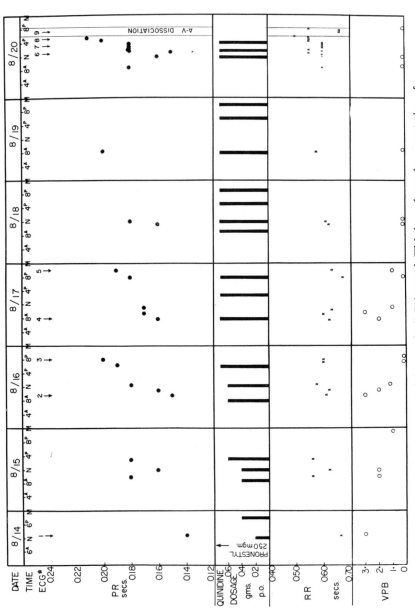

Figure 96. The effect of quinidine on the P-R interval. This is a schematic presentation of the changes. (From J. Menkes, A. S. Nadas and A. Linenthal.)

throughout all leads (Fig. 97). This feature is neither distinctive nor constant; it may be seen in other instances of fluid accumulation, such as the pleural effusion of nephrosis, and it may not be present in severe and advanced cases of pericarditis.

The second type of change—resulting from subepicardial myocardial damage—is more constant and more characteristic. It consists in elevation of the S-T segments throughout all leads, at first. Later the S-T segments return toward normal, and the T waves, particularly in the three standard limb leads, the left chest leads, and aV_F, become negative. Finally, sharp inversion of the T waves is present with perfectly normal S-T segments (Fig. 98). The time relation of these changes is interesting. The S-T elevation occurs early, usually within a week of the appearance of a friction rub. The sharp T wave inversion occurs late (three to four weeks after the onset of the disease), often at a time when all clinical evidences of pericarditis have disappeared. Severe T wave changes may persist one to two months after complete clinical recovery has taken place. Thus, during the time of the most severe clinical changes, the electrocardiogram may be perfectly normal: the S-T segments have already returned to normal, and the T wave inversions have not yet become significant.

A differential point, of almost no importance in pediatrics, should be mentioned briefly. The S-T and T wave changes of pericarditis are similar to those seen in myocardial infarction, with two exceptions: (1) The changes observed in pericarditis are not usually localized to any one

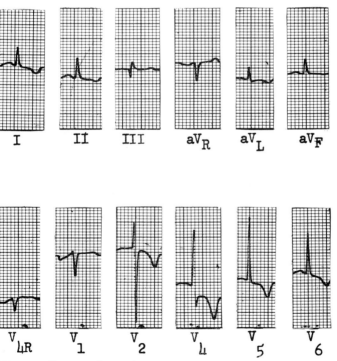

Figure 97. Electrocardiogram of a patient with constrictive pericarditis. Note the diffuse T wave changes throughout and the low voltages in all but the left chest leads.

PURULENT PERICARDITIS

M.B., 7 YEARS, WHITE FEMALE

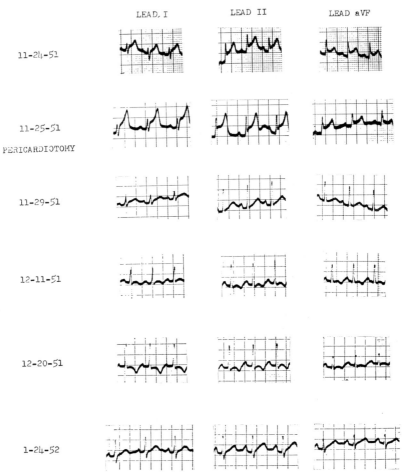

Figure 98. Progressive changes in the electrocardiogram of a patient with purulent pericarditis. Note the appearance of deep S-T and T wave inversions a considerable period after pericardiotomy and clinical cure of the patient. Note the S-T elevation before operation.

area in the chest leads. (2) In pericarditis the changes in the S-T segment are usually absent by the time inversion of the T waves occurs, whereas in myocardial infarction the two changes are more or less synchronous.

P wave changes of the "P mitrale" type are commonly seen in constrictive pericarditis.

4

THE VECTORIAL APPROACH

In the preceding chapters dealing with the electromotive forces of the heart, these phenomena were discussed on the basis of so-called conventional or scalar electrocardiography. This approach analyzes the electrical events of the heart as projected on the various lead axes in the frontal plane. Thus the tridimensional forces (right-to-left, anteroposterior, and superior-inferior) are reduced to positive and negative deflections on a frontal plane reference system.

In contrast, the vectorial approach tries to picture the electromotive forces associated with the cardiac cycle in a tridimensional way. This is accomplished by registering the instantaneous forces serially in their proper magnitude (size of deflection), direction (in the tridimensional space) and sense (positive or negative).

THE VECTORCARDIOGRAM

One method for the registration of the electrical forces of the heart in a tridimensional fashion is by means of a cathode-ray oscilloscope which records the sequence of instantaneous vectors in a loop form. The electrodes are placed at four points on the chest, each presumably equidistant from the others and from the heart. There are various systems of electrode placement (Duchosal's, Wilson's tetrahedron, and Grishman's cube), each claiming superiority over the other. Recently, "corrected lead systems" have been proposed by Schmitt and Frank, utilizing multiple electrodes. The most commonly used ones today in the United States are the Grishman and Frank systems. Our experience so far has been exclusively with the Grishman and Frank systems.

Whichever system is used, and I certainly do not feel qualified to pass judgment upon them, the underlying principle is the same. The electrodes in combinations of twos outline the anteroposterior (Z), right-to-left (X) and superior-inferior (Y) axes. The combination of the anteroposterior and the right-to-left axes outlines the horizontal plane. The right-to-left and superior-inferior axes delineate the frontal plane, and finally the anteroposterior and superior-inferior axes determine the sagittal plane (Fig. 99).

If the electrical impulses from these pairs of leads are connected to an amplifier system, the loop representing the instantaneous electrical forces (vectors) in that particular plane will appear on an oscilloscope connected to the amplifier. Once the loops appear on the oscilloscope screen, they may be photographed by means of a suitable camera to provide permanent records on 35-mm. films (or polaroid positives). By studying the vector loops in all three planes, an excellent tridimensional view of the electrical forces of the heart of any patient may be obtained. Three-dimensional wire models or pipe-cleaner loops may also be constructed to serve as useful teaching guides.

Looking at the spread of the impulse across the ventricles from the atrioventricular node down, the sequence of events described on page 48 is diagrammed in Figure 100, *A*. The initial forces of the QRS complex depolarize the septum in a left-to-right and upward direction (*1*). Next, in rapid sequence, the right ventricular free wall is stimulated (*2* and *3*), and,

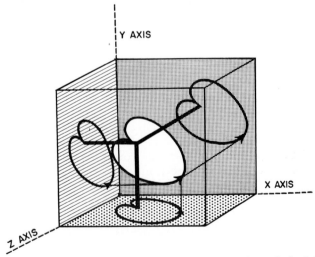

Figure 99. Diagrammatic representation of the vectorial planes derived from the X, Y and Z axes. It may be seen that the frontal plane is derived from the X and Y, the sagittal plane from the Y and Z, and the horizontal plane from the Z and X axes. One may also see the projection of the three-dimensional electrical forces of the heart on these three planes.

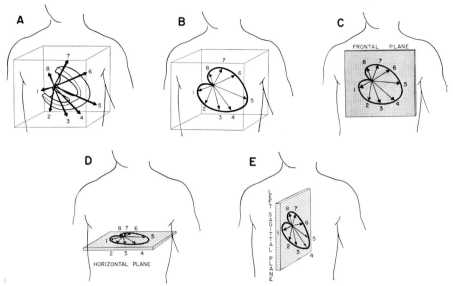

Figure 100. Representations of the instantaneous vectorial forces (*A*), their contribution to the three-dimensional loop (*B*), and the reflection of the loop as well as the instantaneous vectors on the three planes (*C, D* and *E*). For details, see text.

almost simultaneously, the free left ventricular wall begins to depolarize (*4* and *5*). The terminal portion of the QRS complex is almost exclusively made up of left ventricular forces, normally directed leftward and upward (*6* and *7*). In certain healthy persons, particularly in infants and children, and in many patients having pathologic conditions accompanied by right ventricular hypertrophy, the terminal forces are produced by the right ventricular outflow tract and the crista supraventricularis, resulting in a terminal right and anterior force (*8*).

Figure 100, *B*, represents the loop made by connecting the successive mean instantaneous vectors. It cannot be stressed strongly enough that at any one instant a vector represents the summation of *all the forces generated* at that particular time. In other words, point 2 in Figure 100, *B*, represents the vector of the forces generating principally from the right side of the septum and the free right ventricular wall, with only minor contributions from incipient left ventricular depolarization. In contrast, at instant 5 the vector is dominated by left ventricular forces to which the almost completely depolarized right ventricle adds but little.

The time sequence of these resultant forces of ventricular depolarization—vector loops—occurring in a three-dimensional sphere (the heart) may be represented by their projection on the frontal, horizontal and sagittal planes (Fig. 100, *C, D, E*). Figure 101 exemplifies the projection of the tridimensional spatial loop on the horizontal plane. The frontal and sagittal planes may be derived similarly (Fig. 102). Similar loops may be constructed for atrial depolarization (P loop) and ventricular repolarization (T loop).

The normal QRS vectorcardiograms of children and adults in the frontal, horizontal and sagittal planes are described in Figure 103. In gen-

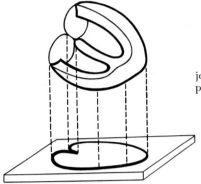

Figure 101. Diagram representing the projection of the vectorial forces on the horizontal plane.

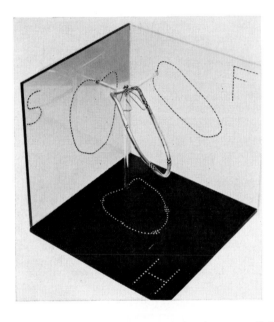

Figure 102. Diagram representing the projection of a model of a vector loop on all three planes.

eral, the P and T loop projection parallels the QRS loops, and the divergence between QRS and T loops should not be more than 40 degrees.

Once the vector loops are obtained, any scalar lead may be constructed from the appropriate planes, or vice versa. For example, the chest leads may be reconstructed from the horizontal plane (Fig. 104) and the standard limb leads from the frontal plane (fig. 105).[304]

THE VECTORELECTROCARDIOGRAM

Several authors, principally Grant,[298] have suggested that vectorial analysis of the electrical forces could be made on the basis of the conventional scalar cardiogram. In contrast to the previously discussed method of vectorcardiography, the term "vectorelectrocardiography" has been suggested. As argument for the superiority of this method, the proponents of vector-

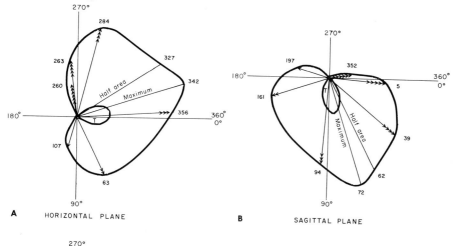

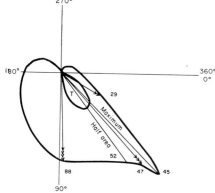

Figure 103. *A, B* and *C* represent normal vector loops in the three conventional planes. The Helm system of annotation from 0 to 360 degrees is used. The QRS loop is drawn in detail. The outlines of the T loop are indicated. The arrows on the individual lines indicate the time sequence. One arrow means 0.01 second, 2 arrows 0.02 second. The figures accompanying this indicate angle.

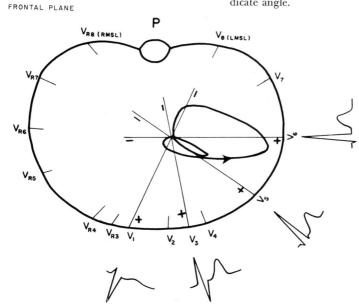

Figure 104. Construction of the unipolar chest leads from the horizontal plane loop.[304]

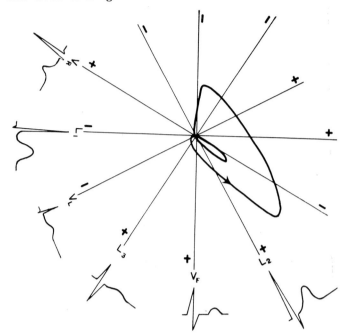

Figure 105. The bipolar and unipolar extremity leads constructed from the frontal plane loop by means of the Bayley hexaxial system.[304]

electrocardiography suggest maintenance of the system that is most suitable for the measurement of the various intervals, that easily pictures separately the P-QRS and T complexes, and of which millions of records throughout the world exist. All they are saying is that the same tracings should be obtained, but that they ought to be looked at differently. Furthermore, no new equipment is needed and no new patterns have to be learned.

It seems to me that a vectorial, three-dimensional view of the conventional electrocardiogram is practically mandatory today. Most teaching institutions use vectorcardiography as well, in selected groups of patients, or for study purposes. Eventually it may come to pass that vectorcardiography, by an improved lead system, with only three loops, or their scalar equivalents, will supplant the present electrocardiogram of at least twelve leads. But until unanimity in regard to electrode placement is achieved on a worldwide basis, and until electronic and photographic equipment becomes simpler and cheaper, the *practicing cardiologist* will continue to use electrocardiography with the standard lead system. He will obtain better understanding of his tracings, however, if he analyzes them by the vectorial method.

The vector loops constructed from the twelve-lead electrocardiograms are closely similar to those obtained by vectorcardiography. Most of the time the only difference is that the vectorcardiogram records every small detail of the loop at every fraction of a second and is easily visualized in three planes, whereas vectorelectrocardiography gives only broad outlines of the frontal plane loop and gives approximation of the horizontal loop. If the difference between the vectorcardiogram and the vectorelectrocardio-

FRONTAL PLANE   STANDARD LIMB LEADS

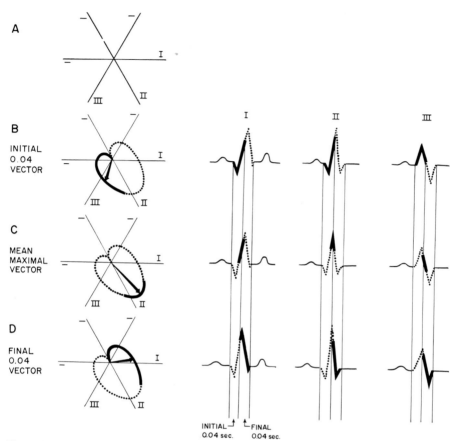

Figure 106.   Details of construction of the frontal plane loop from the standard limb leads by means of the triaxial system. For details, see text.

gram in any one patient shows more significant differences than this, at the present time I am not sure that it may be stated unequivocally which represents a truer picture of the *actual* electrical phenomena.

The frontal plane loop may be roughly and easily constructed from the standard limb leads by means of the triaxial system (Fig. 106, *A*) by determining the direction and magnitude of the initial 0.04, the mean, and the terminal 0.04 vectors, as indicated in Figure 106, *B, C, D*.

A similar use of the standard and unipolar limb leads, by means of the hexaxial reference system (Fig. 43) results in a more detailed, more accurate, but obviously more complex delineation of the frontal plane loop. This method also leads to a more accurate estimation of the inscription of the loop (clockwise or counterclockwise).

The horizontal plane loop may be constructed from the six chest leads by making the assumption that all the chest leads lie in the same plane (Fig. 107). The sagittal plane loop is not usually constructed from the conventional electrocardiogram, though this could be accomplished by utilizing aV_F and V_{4R}.

HORIZONTAL PLANE   UNIPOLAR CHEST LEADS

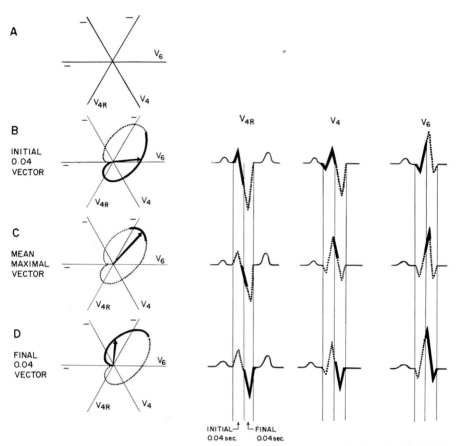

Figure 107.   Construction of the horizontal plane loop from the unipolar chest leads. For details, see text.

CHANGES IN VECTOR LOOPS THROUGHOUT THE PEDIATRIC AGE GROUP

Whichever type of vectorial analysis of the electrocardiogram is used, certain broad generalizations can be arrived at in the development of the vectorcardiogram from infancy, through childhood, into adulthood (Fig. 56).

In effect, there seems to be little, if any, change between the P loops of adults and infants or children. In contrast, the T axis is almost exclusively posterior in orientation in infancy, and becomes anterior in childhood. In young infants (less than three months of age) real and significant differences are noted from the tracings described in the adult.

Newborns

The *frontal plane* QRS loop is usually inscribed clockwise and is directed to the right and inferiorly. The mean vector is between +60 and +110 degrees. The *horizontal plane* is usually inscribed clockwise, and the anterior forces dominate. Sometimes rightward, other times leftward, forces dominate. The *sagittal plane* is mostly clockwise as well, the inferior and anterior forces dominating. The T-QRS angle is less than 40 degrees in all planes.

Variations from these patterns are relatively common. Counterclockwise frontal and sagittal loops are described in normal infants as well as superior, posterior and even leftward orientation of these loops.

Infants

These patterns in newborn infants undergo significant changes within the first few months of life, resulting in less rightward and more inferior, less anterior and more posterior orientation of the spatial QRS vector. Also, the clockwise rotation of the horizontal loop turns into the conventional adult counterclockwise rotation within the first one or two months of life. The exceptions to these conventional patterns are more rare than are exceptions to the patterns of newborns.

Children

In essence, the vectorcardiograms of children are not significantly different from those of adults.

5

PHONOCARDIOGRAPHY

USE AND EQUIPMENT

In view of the emphasis placed on auscultation in the diagnosis of heart disease in children, it seems logical to devote a section of this book to phonocardiography, the graphic registration of heart sounds. This is an excellent tool for the teaching of intelligent interpretation of auscultatory phenomena. It also serves the useful purpose of enabling one to check the accuracy of one's own auscultation, and occasionally plays the role of an unbiased arbiter deciding between two contrary opinions about murmurs and sounds. In this latter respect it is especially helpful for the younger physician or the medical student who, with his own accurate observations now reinforced by the phonocardiogram, can often successfully challenge his elders and teachers. Phonocardiography may thus prove to be a revolutionary instrument in medicine, substituting facts for authority derived from the gray hair of the teacher, enhanced by his academic standing, but sadly limited by the gradually narrowing hearing acuity of age.

Excellent monographs and papers on phonocardiography[412, 423, 453, 468, 476, 543, 570, 571, 678] are available in the literature; hence no complete review of the subject will be attempted here.

The phonocardiograph used up until 1960 at our institution was the Sanborn Twin-Beam. In this recorder two simultaneous tracings are obtained. The top tracing represents the heart sounds and murmurs; the bottom one is used as a reference tracing necessary for timing. The electrocardiogram is used most frequently for reference, but for certain purposes, registration of the jugular venous pulse, the carotid pulse or the apex beat (linear or apex cardiogram) is more suitable.

106

Three kinds of microphones are available with this apparatus. The so-called linear microphone is sensitive to all the vibrations caused by the heart, and, as such, registers primarily the coarse vibrations (less than 100 per second) set up by the cardiac impulse (Fig. 108, *A*), the jugular vein or the carotid artery, and suppresses the finer, higher frequency vibrations, constituting the sounds and murmurs.

The stethoscopic microphone, on the other hand, completely suppresses the coarsest elements and registers only the low frequency sounds, some of them inaudible (between 30 and 200 per second), offered to the ear by the stethoscope (Fig. 108, *B*). The higher frequency murmurs are not brought out well in the stethoscopic tracing. The use of this microphone is principally in the analysis of the heart sounds; it is of less use in demonstrating murmurs.

The logarithmic microphone has the same kind of "bias" as the human auditory cortex. It suppresses not only the lowest vibrations of the cardiac impulse, but also the low frequency murmurs and sounds, and brings out with clarity and logarithmic intensity the highest frequency vibrations (50 to 500 per second) (Fig. 108, *C*). The logarithmic tracing formed the basis of most of our phonocardiographic studies; it was especially useful in the analysis of murmurs.

For the majority of the clinical problems, sound tracings obtained by the logarithmic microphone with electrocardiographic reference are satisfactory. For closer analysis of the heart sounds a stethoscopic and a logarithmic tracing obtained from the apex with jugular venous, linear (apex) cardiographic and carotid arterial reference tracings is desirable.

Three types of chest-pieces are used commonly with the Sanborn Twin-Beam—a medium open bell, a small open bell and a Bowles diaphragm. The first two are used for registering heart sounds and low frequency murmurs; the third is more advantageous for high frequency insufficiency blows and continuous murmurs.

Since 1960 a new 4-channel photographic instrument has been used for phonocardiography in our department. This consists of two Sanborn electrocardiograph amplifiers (for registration of electrocardiograms, carotid and jugular venous tracings, and linear cardiograms) and two Sanborn heart-sound preamplifiers. Two contact microphones and one standard heart sound microphone are used. The recording system of the Sanborn 500M apparatus is used with speeds from 10 to 100 mm. per second. A small oscilloscope is attached to the recording system.

This more complex and considerably more expensive apparatus holds several advantages over the old Twin-Beam. (1) By utilizing four channels simultaneously, exact timing of heart sounds and murmurs is possible. (2) The preamplifier, providing 5 octave-related filter systems with high-pass cutoffs at 25, 50, 100, 200 and 400 cycles per second, furnishes excellent recordings of the various frequencies encountered. Some of the high frequency recordings are among the nicest I have seen. Protodiastolic murmurs of semilunar regurgitation can be demonstrated with surprising clarity. The low-frequency mid-diastolic and protodiastolic rumbles are also registered, though not necessarily any better than with the Twin-Beam. (3) The oscilloscope is extremely helpful in visualizing the tracings to be recorded.

The disadvantages of this machine, aside from its price, are that two

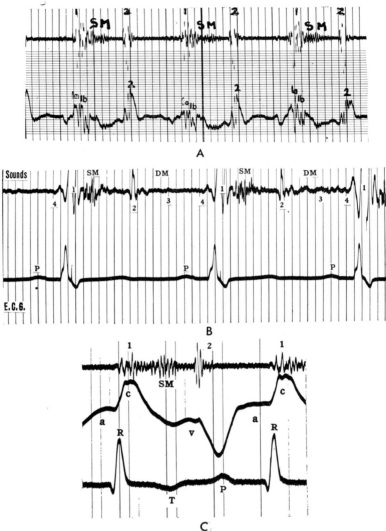

Figure 108. *A,* Upper line, logarithmic phonocardiogram. Lower tracing, linear cardiogram. At the upper tracing note *1* and *2*, indicating first and second heart sounds, and *SM,* indicating systolic murmur. Lower tracing: *1a, 1b* and *2* are waves of the linear cardiogram. For schematic representation of the components of the linear cardiogram (apex cardiogram), see Figure 41.

B, Upper tracing, stethoscopic phonocardiogram. Lower tracing, electrocardiogram. Numbers *1, 2, 3, 4,* indicate first, second, third and fourth heart sounds. SM means systolic murmur; *DM* equals diastolic murmur.

C, Three simultaneous tracings. Upper line, logarithmic phonocardiogram. Middle line, jugular venous pulse. Lower line, electrocardiogram. The phonocardiogram and the electrocardiogram are marked as in (*A*) and (*B*). The jugular venous pulse is marked according to the conventional markings of jugular venous pulse. See Figures 9 and 41.

people are necessary for efficient operation and that the tracings taken from each patient are of necessity longer and bulkier than the older tracings, a fact which eventually may cause a storage problem. Figure 109 represents a few sample tracings obtained with this new apparatus. For most patients these positions, frequencies and reference tracings furnish all the informa-

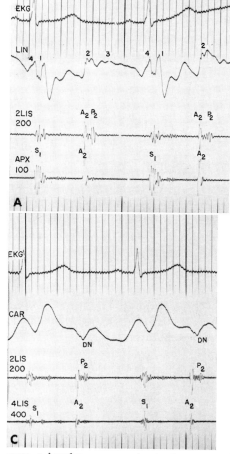

Figure 109. Phonocardiograms obtained with the new four-channel Sanborn phonocardiograph with high-pass filters and appropriate reference tracings. *A* has, as reference tracing on top, the electrocardiogram. The second channel indicates the linear or apex cardiogram with appropriate components. The third channel is a phonocardiogram with the 200-frequency high-pass filter at the second left interspace. The bottom channel is a phonocardiogram at the apex with a 100-frequency high-pass filter. Note the well outlined aortic and pulmonic closure at the second left interspace and the aortic closure identified by the only second sound registered at the apex. *B,* Similar tracings except that, instead of a linear cardiogram, a jugular venous pulse tracing was used for reference, and at the second left interspace the filter is 400 and at the apex, 200. Again, the aortic component of the second sound at the second left interspace may be identified by the second sound registered at the apex. *C,* In this tracing a carotid artery pressure pulse is used for reference in the second channel. Note the presence of the dicrotic notch and its relation to aortic closure.

tion necessary about sounds and murmurs. Of course additional tracings may be taken in individual instances as necessary.

A direct-writing phonocardiograph with six filters has been used to good advantage by Mannheimer and his associates.[397, 476] Unfortunately, I have had no personal experience with this apparatus; hence the reader seeking information on this particular machine is referred to the work of the Swedish authors.

A German direct-writing machine, the Schwarzer apparatus, has gained acceptance in this country within recent years. It has four to six channels and provides an "envelope" type of sound tracing. It has the advantage of simplicity over the photographic machines; at the same time, a certain amount of response fidelity and reproducibility is lost. Also the particular microphone furnished with this recorder is somewhat heavy for use in children. But it is a good machine and gives nice tracings.

Whichever phonocardiograph is used, the problems to be solved are the same, and probably none of the existing apparatus is without shortcomings. The auditory spectrum extends from about 40 to 1000 cycles per second. Through this spectrum the intensity level decreases at the rate of about 6 to 12 decibels per octave. This means that in order to obtain a response which is linear at all frequencies, strong attenuation of the lower frequencies is necessary.

HOW TO TAKE A PHONOCARDIOGRAM

A quiet room is a prerequisite to the taking of a clear phonocardiogram. Soundproofing is useful, but not essential. Telephones and typewriters should not be used at the time a tracing is taken.

The child should rest comfortably on an examining table or should be propped up on a pillow in bed. Only under fortunate circumstances may satisfactory tracings be obtained from children less than three years old, without heavy sedation. The cooperation of an older child may easily be enlisted, even to the extent of having him hold his breath, if the procedure is explained to him.

All tracings should be taken in a definite, consistent sequence, so that when the tracing is developed and analyzed, the identity of each strip will be clear purely on the basis of its position within the series. It is also important, as a further aid in identification, that a permanent notebook be kept containing the patient's name, record number, age, diagnosis and particularly the sequences of each tracing. One should also note the type of microphone, the chest-piece, the amplification, the filter, and the nature of the reference tracing used for every location.

HEART SOUNDS

Four heart sounds are normally registered (Fig. 41). The first sound, or sound complex, is approximately synchronous with the QRS complex in the electrocardiogram and the la and lb of the linear cardiogram; its average duration is 0.10 second (0.05 to 0.15). Its onset can be well timed by the q wave, but its termination cannot be determined electrocardiographically; the C wave of the jugular venous pulse probably serves best as an end-point. The main portion of the first sound results from the closure of the mitral and tricuspid valves (in this order), with some addition from the semilunar opening and possibly atrial and vascular components.

The asynchronism between closure of the mitral and tricuspid valves sometimes may be heard and rather often registered at the lower left sternal border. Normally, this "splitting" of the first sound is not more than 0.03 second, and, as implied earlier, mitral closure precedes tricuspid closure. Luisada and his associates[454] suggested that semilunar valve openings normally contribute to the first sound complex.

A widely split first sound due to the delayed closure of the tricuspid valve and associated with a widely split second sound at the lower left sternal border is characteristic of complete right bundle branch block (Fig. 110). "Incomplete right bundle branch block," i.e., rsR′ pattern in the

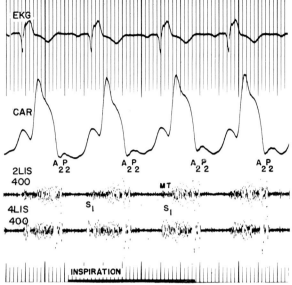

Figure 110. Phonocardiogram of a patient with complete right bundle branch block. Note the splitting of the first sound at the second left interspace phonocardiogram, indicating mitral and tricuspid closure. Also note the well split second sound with little respiratory variation.

electrocardiogram, or left bundle branch block is not associated with splitting of the first sound.

The second component of the widely split first sound should be clearly differentiated from a systolic click or ejection sound. It originates either from the opening of the semilunar valve or from a jet of blood across the valve hitting the wall of the dilated aorta or pulmonary artery.[498] It may be clearly demonstrated with simultaneous pressure tracings that the click occurs well along the upstroke of the carotid or pulmonary artery pressure tracing (Fig. 111, *A*). Pulmonic click is heard at the second left interspace (Fig. 111, *B*), and changes in intensity with respiration. Usually it is separated from the first sound by 0.06 to 0.10 second and consists of high frequency vibrations. Thus these characteristics clearly distinguish a split first sound from a pulmonic click: it is of low frequency, is seldom wider than 0.06 second, does not change with respiration, and is heard at the lower left sternal border. Differentiation of the aortic click, which is heard at the apex, lower left sternal border, or even at the second right interspace, and does not change with respiration, is a little more difficult. Still, the high frequency and the wide separation between first and second components usually serve as distinguishing features (Fig. 112).

Pulmonic click is heard commonly with valvar pulmonic stenosis[413] (usually, but not invariably, mild), idiopathic dilatation of the pulmonary artery, and pulmonary hypertension with dilated main pulmonary artery. Aortic clicks are observed with valvar aortic stenosis,[412] coarctation of the aorta, aortic regurgitation, and in severe cases of tetralogy of Fallot.

A delayed and loud mitral closure sound is typical of mitral stenosis of severe degree (Fig. 113). The distance between the Q wave of the electrocardiogram and S_1 (meaning mitral closure) has been used with some success as a measure of the severity of mitral stenosis.[723] Of course in this case the usual sequence of mitral closure preceding tricuspid closure is reversed.

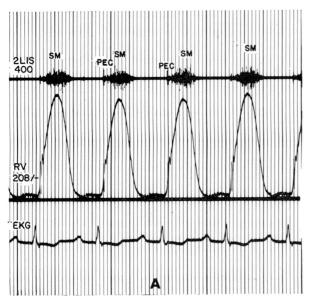

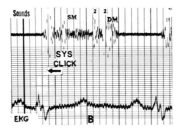

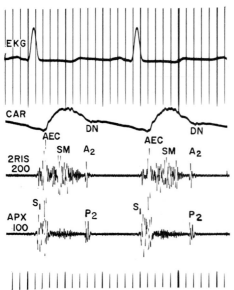

Figure 111. *A,* Tracing obtained in patient with severe valvar pulmonic stenosis and an intact ventricular septum. Note the pulmonic ejection click (*PEC*) corresponding to a notch on the upstroke on the right ventricular pressure pulse. *B,* Systolic click in a patient with pulmonary arterial hypertension and an atrial septal defect. Note the well split second sound and the murmur of pulmonic incompetence (*DM*).

Figure 112. Aortic ejection click in valvar aortic stenosis (*AEC*). Note the relationship of the click to the carotid artery tracing. Also note the narrowly split second sound at the apex. P$_2$ is the second component of the second sound and may be seen only on the apical tracing.

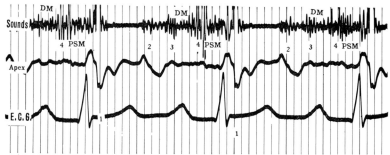

Figure 113. Late first sound in patient with mitral stenosis. Note the diastolic and pre-systolic murmurs.

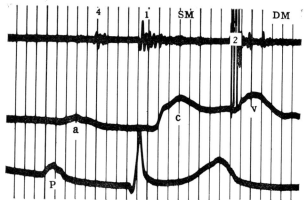

Figure 114. Upper tracing, phonocardiogram. Middle tracing, jugular venous pulse. Lower tracing, electrocardiogram. Note the low-intensity first sound in the phonocardiogram.

A short P-R interval results in a loud first sound,[199, 423] and, conversely, a long P-R interval (shock, myocardial failure or pericardial effusion), results in a faint first sound (Fig. 114). Complete heart block, with variable P-R intervals, is accompanied by a first sound of varying intensity (Fig. 115).

The second sound, or sound complex, although usually occurring beyond the T wave, does not show a close correlation with the electrocardiogram. More accurate timing is possible by using the dicrotic notch of the carotid or pulmonary artery tracing as a reference. Furthermore, the second sound begins with the 2 wave and ends with the 0 point of the linear cardiogram (Fig. 41). Its average duration is 0.08 second (0.03 to 0.12).

The closure of the semilunar valves contributes the main portion of the second sound, with possibly some muscular and vascular elements added. The degree of splitting between the semilunar elements of the second sound should be carefully noted. The two sets of semilunar valves—aortic and pulmonary—close practically simultaneously in the normal adult; the vibrations caused by the closure of these valves are thus superimposed on each other, and no splitting occurs. In contrast, in children, under normal circumstances, the semilunar valves close asynchronously,[37] the aortic first, the pulmonary second. Consequently the trained ear may easily discover a slight splitting, accentuated on deep inspiration, within the second sound of normal children. If measured phonocardiographically,

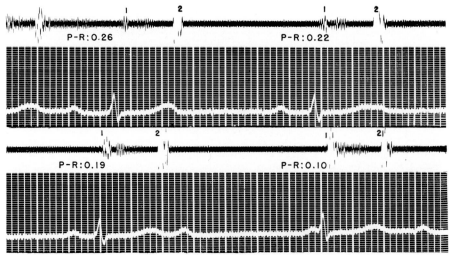

Figure 115. Variable intensity first sound (1) in a patient with complete heart block. Note the low-intensity first sound if the P-R interval is long (0.26) and compare the high-intensity first sound with a short P-R interval (0.10).

the 2 peaks constituting the splitting normally are seldom more than 0.04 second apart on held expiration. In deep inspiration, on the other hand, the distance between aortic and pulmonic closure sounds may widen to 0.07 or 0.08 second normally.

The identification of aortic from pulmonic closure is not always simple. As stated before, under normal circumstances, left-sided events precede right-sided events. Thus, if two high-frequency components of the second sound can be seen, it may be assumed that the aortic comes first. A second way of differentiation is that, barring transposition of the great arteries, the portion of the second sound registered best at the second left interspace probably originates in the pulmonary artery, whereas the aortic component is best visualized at the apex, lower left sternal border or second right interspace. This difference may be brought out particularly well with a phonocardiograph, allowing for two phonoamplifiers with identical filters, registering at the second left and the fourth left interspace or the apex, simultaneously (Fig. 116).

Finally, and most accurately, the origin of a particular component of the second sound may best be determined by identifying the aortic component with a simultaneous carotid artery tracing and the pulmonic closure with a simultaneous pulmonary artery tracing (though because of the nature of the pulmonary artery tracing, the latter is much more difficult). It may be assumed under these circumstances that the portion of the second sound preceding by 0.02 to 0.04 second the dicrotic notch of the carotid artery tracing corresponds to aortic closure. (The time lag between sound and pressure phenomena is due to the length of time it takes the blood to travel from the aortic valve to the carotid artery.)

The final component of the second sound is the so-called opening sound of the mitral valve. This is the terminal portion of the second sound complex, is identified by the 0 point of the linear cardiogram, and consists normally of vibrations too low to be audible or visible in the logarithmic tracing. It can be seen, however, in the low frequency tracings obtained from the apex. No sound effects due to the opening of the tricuspid valve may be seen normally.

It may be assumed that a loud second sound at the second left interspace usually indicates pulmonary hypertension. If the phonocardiogram reveals two distinct components of the second sound with a loud second component, and if reference tracings identify this as corresponding to pulmonic closure, pulmonary hypertension is a virtual certainty.

If the loud second sound at the pulmonic area is not split, it may represent aortic closure alone or synchronous closure of the aortic and pulmonic valves (Fig. 117). The differentiation between these two situations may be difficult at times and may have to be resolved by considering evidences outside the scope of the second heart sound (murmurs, x-rays, and so forth). A loud second sound in the aortic region may well indicate

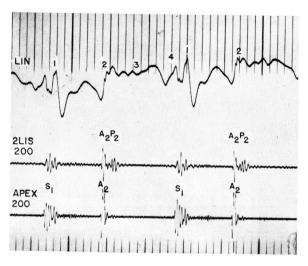

Figure 116. Identification of the split second sound at the second left interspace by using an apical phonocardiogram as a reference tracing.

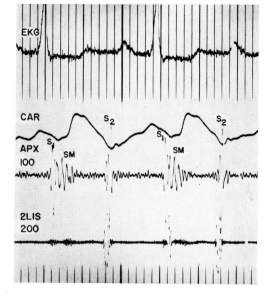

Figure 117. Single loud second sound, encompassing both aortic and pulmonic closure, at the second left interspace and the apex. The tracing was obtained from a patient having a ventricular septal defect and pulmonary vascular obstruction with maximal pulmonary hypertension.

systemic hypertension, particularly if the high-intensity component can be identified as representing aortic closure.

A low-intensity second sound at the aortic area is of no particular significance in children.

The abnormalities of splitting should also be discussed. As mentioned earlier, aortic closure normally precedes pulmonic closure by about 0.03 to 0.04 second in children breathing quietly. In atrial septal defect the split widens to 0.05 second or more on expiration, the aortic and pulmonary components being of the same intensity (Fig. 118). Complete right bundle branch block has the same effect (Fig. 110). Fairly wide splitting of the second sounds (0.05 to 0.06 second) may be noted in patients having small ventricular septal defect (Fig. 119) and particularly in children with ventricular septal defect, pulmonic stenosis and a left-to-right shunt. That the rsR' electrocardiographic pattern is not the cause of wide splitting in patients with atrial septal defect is conclusively proved by the fact that surgical correction of atrial defects abolishes wide splitting without influencing significantly the width of the QRS complex. It is thought that the widely split second sound in these patients is due to the increased volume work of the right ventricle inherent in the physiology of atrial septal defect. A widely split second sound is also noted in patients with pure pulmonic stenosis (Fig. 120), but here, as mentioned previously, the second sound is of low intensity, and the prolongation of right ventricular systole is due to increased pressure, rather than volume, work. Leatham[412] suggested that the degree of splitting is in linear relation to the severity of the stenosis (see Fig. 431). The widely split second sound of severe pulmonic stenosis with intact ventricular septum contrasts sharply with the single second sound, corresponding to aortic closure on the external phonocardiogram, noted in patients with severe tetralogy of Fallot (Fig. 121).

The splitting of the second sound in a normal child widens with inspiration, presumably on account of the increase in systemic venous inflow. In a patient with a large atrial septal defect in whom both atria act like a single filling chamber, the increased venous inflow due to inspiration

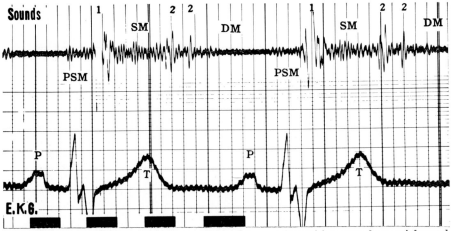

Figure 118. Widely split fixed second sound in a patient with a secundum atrial septal defect. Note the low-frequency systolic ejection murmur and the low-frequency presystolic and early diastolic murmurs.

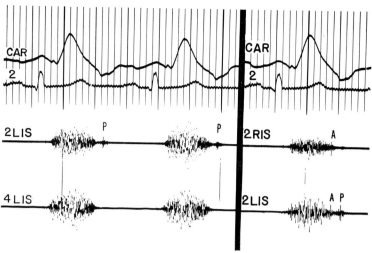

Figure 119. Pansystolic murmur of patient with a small ventricular septal defect. Note the well split second sound at the second left interspace.[705]

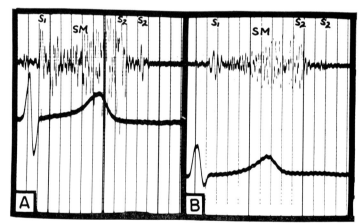

Figure 120. Phonocardiograms from two patients with pulmonic stenosis and intact ventricular septum. *A,* A moderately split second sound with an appreciable pulmonic component, indicating mild stenosis. *B,* Widely split second sound with a low-intensity pulmonic component characteristic of severe stenosis. Note the late apex of the diamond in both instances.

influences the left and right ventricles in similar fashion, and thus there is no change in the degree of splitting between inspiration and expiration (fixed split). By the same token, in patients with severe pulmonic stenosis and maximally prolonged right ventricular systole, inspiratory increase in venous inflow also fails to prolong right ventricular systole further. This "fixed split" is not noted in patients with mild to moderate pulmonic stenosis, in those having atrial defects with a less than 2:1 pulmonary-systemic flow ratio or in right bundle branch block.

A reversal of the normal sequence of semilunar closure, i.e. pulmonic closure preceding aortic closure, results in so-called paradoxical splitting (Fig. 122). This means that on inspiration, when right ventricular systole

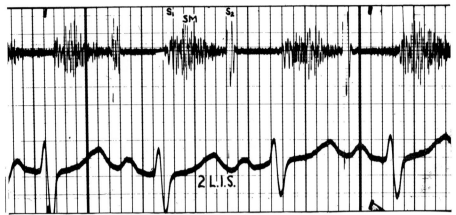

Figure 121. Phonocardiogram of a patient with tetralogy of Fallot. Note the single second sound and the diamond-shaped murmur with the early peak.

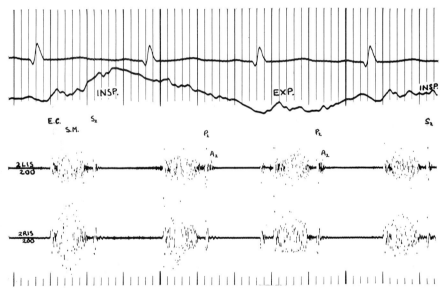

Figure 122. "Paradoxical" splitting in a patient with severe aortic stenosis. Note that P_2 precedes A_2 in the tracing taken at the second left interspace. Left ventricular pressure in this patient was 220/10 mm. of mercury.

is prolonged and pulmonic closure is delayed, the split narrows, and on expiration it widens. "Paradoxical splitting" is a logical concomitant of conditions accompanied by prolonged left ventricular systole, i.e., complete left bundle branch block, severe aortic stenosis, and an increase in pulmonic diastolic pressure (patent ductus arteriosus).

A distinctly audible and clearly registerable terminal component of the second sound complex, synchronous with the O point of the apex cardiogram, and caused by the opening of the mitral valve, is seen almost universally in patients with mitral stenosis (Fig. 123). The distance between the aortic component of the second sound and this opening snap is almost never less than 0.04 second and never more than 0.12 second (average 0.07).

The time interval between aortic closure and opening snap has also been used to gauge the severity of mitral stenosis; the shorter this interval, the higher the left atrial pressure, and thus the more severe the degree of mitral stenosis.[45] Occasionally, in a patient with tricuspid stenosis, Ebstein's anomaly or even atrial septal defect, an opening snap of the tricuspid valve may be seen and even heard. Sometimes it may be difficult to differentiate between an opening snap and a third sound. But the snap is usually of higher frequency, is rarely further than 0.12 second from the aortic component of the second sound, and is registered at the lower left sternal border rather than the apex. More importantly, it is synchronous with the O point of the linear cardiogram rather than the 3 wave. Differentiation of the opening snap from pulmonic closure may also be difficult at auscultation, but should not be hard with a good phonocardiogram and adequate reference tracings.

The third heart sound is identifiable by the 3 wave in the linear cardiogram, and corresponds to the first rapid inflow of blood from the atria to the ventricles. Usually this is clearly audible in children, less commonly in adults. It is well registered, particularly in a low-frequency tracing. The fourth heart sound, or atrial sound, corresponds to the second rapid filling period of the ventricles and is identifiable by the fact that it follows the P wave and precedes the q wave in the electrocardiogram. This sound consists of low frequency vibrations and is usually not heard in normal people, but may be registerable in the phonocardiogram.

Unusually high amplitude or high frequency third (protodiastolic) and fourth (presystolic) heart sounds with tachycardia are recognized with a stethoscope as gallop rhythm (Fig. 124). In most instances this means cardiac failure, particularly if the third or the fourth sound is palpable. In children an unusually loud third sound indicates a hyperdynamic heart, i.e. excitement, anemia, or most commonly a large left-to-right shunt. Mounsey[510] stated that in adults the loudest third sound is heard in constrictive pericarditis (pericardial knock). It is worth noting that, though a

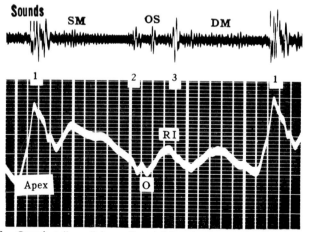

Figure 123. Opening "snap" in patient with mitral stenosis. Upper tracing, phonocardiogram; lower tracing, apex or linear cardiogram. Note *O* at opening snap corresponding to O point in the linear cardiogram.[542]

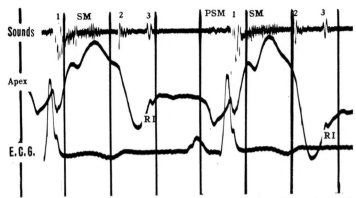

Figure 124. Gallop rhythm consisting of first sound, second sound and loud third sound. Upper tracing, logarithmic phonocardiogram. Middle tracing, apex cardiogram. Lower tracing, electrocardiogram.

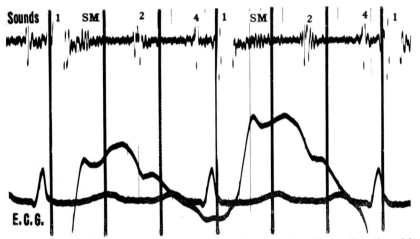

Figure 125. Loud atrial or fourth sound in logarithmic tracing. Upper line, logarithmic phonocardiogram. Middle line, jugular venous pulse. Lower line, electrocardiogram.

loud third sound may be the precursor of mitral stenosis in adults, its presence usually is not compatible with critical mitral stenosis.

A loud fourth sound (atrial sound) (Fig. 125) in children usually originates from the right atrium and may be heard in patients having disorders associated with high right atrial pressure (primary pulmonary hypertension, pure pulmonic stenosis, Ebstein's disease, tricuspid atresia and total pulmonary venous anomaly) and complete heart block. A left ventricular fourth sound is heard in patients with severe left ventricular disease (aortic stenosis, coarctation of aorta).

MURMURS

Vibrations, with frequencies of 50 to 1000 per second, registered between heart sounds, are called murmurs. They are conventionally thought to result from turbulences developing in the laminar flow of blood, although in recent years other physical explanations have been invoked to explain their origin. Occasionally it may be difficult to distinguish a short murmur from a prolonged heart sound. In most instances, however, murmurs have a duration long enough to make differentiation relatively easy.

Occasionally a more serious problem is presented by the occurrence of artefacts (respiratory sounds, noises in the room, defects in the machinery, and so forth). The best way to avoid these is to be scrupulously certain that the phonocardiogram is taken in a quiet room and that the base line between sounds is kept as straight as possible. Furthermore, one ought to suspect all vibrations extending with equal intensity and frequency throughout systole and diastole, especially if appearing periodically rather than constantly, of being artefacts of respiratory origin (Fig. 126).

Once the vibrations of appropriate frequency and timing have been identified in the phonocardiogram as murmurs, their significance has to be decided upon. This brings one to the question of "organic" versus "functional" murmur, a terminology I have tended to discard in favor of "significant" and "not significant" murmur. The auscultatory phenomena associated with permanent anatomic deformities of the heart are commonly called "organic" murmurs and have fairly severe implications. Logically, one would include in this group conditions with such varying significance as mitral stenosis, the mildest form of pulmonic stenosis, aortic regurgitation and small Roger type ventricular septal defect. By contrast, in the "functional" category, with a usually benign connotation, would be included conditions without permanent abnormalities, such as anemia, rheumatic carditis without valvular deformities, fever or thyrotoxicosis.

This differentiation, based on pathologic data, is meaningless today in view of the physiologic information available. It may readily be seen that mild pulmonic stenosis (defined physiologically as a systolic gradient between right ventricle and pulmonary artery of 15 to 20 mm. of mercury, giving rise to a loud systolic murmur) may never be demonstrable at postmortem examination. Will such a murmur be called "organic"? Similarly,

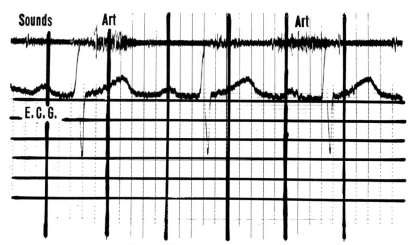

Figure 126.   Respiratory artefact.

shall we classify as "organic" or "functional" the loud murmur of a small ventricular septal defect when there is no demonstrable increase in oxygen saturation at the ventricular level, but when the defect is definitely present at postmortem examination, and even visible at cine-angiography? The terms "organic" and "functional" are clearly wrong in their prognostic implications. A small ventricular defect, though "organic," may be compatible with a long and active life, whereas the "functional" murmur of severe anemia or thyrotoxicosis may be associated with severe cardiac failure.

Finally, if one reviews the available literature to learn which murmurs most authors call "functional" and which "organic," one concludes that all loud systolic murmurs, and everything that occurs in diastole, are called "organic," whereas everything that is faint in systole is called "functional." The fallacy of this reasoning has been proved repeatedly by the finding of a loud early diastolic murmur in the pulmonary area of a patient with an anatomically normal heart (idiopathic pulmonary regurgitation) and by the presence of only a faint systolic murmur in patients with pulmonary atresia or the severest type of mitral stenosis.

In view of these difficulties, then, the murmurs should be properly described in respect to timing, intensity, duration and nature, and then should be correlated with the other necessary and available clinical and laboratory information and designated as being "significant" or "not significant" at that particular time.

Murmurs associated with cardiac symptoms, x-ray evidences of cardiac enlargement or abnormal electrocardiograms should certainly be considered "significant." Even without these ancillary findings, a murmur is likely to be "significant" if it is of high intensity (more than grade 3, according to Levine) and appreciable duration, if it transmits well throughout the precordium, the neck and the back, and if it is not influenced by the phases of respiration or change in position. Diastolic murmurs, on the whole, are more likely to be "significant" than systolic ones.

The "insignificant" or innocent murmur is never accompanied by cardiac symptoms and laboratory evidences of heart disease. Usually it is a murmur of low intensity, low frequency and of short duration, occupying midsystole. It may be heard maximally at the left sternal border or the apex, it transmits poorly, and it shows considerable variations from cycle to cycle with respiration, change in position or for no obvious reasons. A particular type of "insignificant" murmur, commonly heard in healthy adolescents, is strongly localized to the left lower sternal border and sounds much like the plucking of a string (Fig. 127).

Another type of "innocent" murmur, to be described later, is the so-called physiologic ejection murmur at the second left interspace, which is closely similar (practically identical) to the murmur of secundum atrial septal defect. Obviously the second sound, however, is normal. Finally, of course, should be mentioned as a characteristically "innocent" murmur the continuous nonmachinery type of jugular venous hum (Fig 128). Any one of these three types may be designated as an *"innocent murmur"* and meaning *"no significant heart disease."* In the same category of "no significant heart disease" I would include the patient who has the murmur and the clinical and physiologic picture of mild pulmonic stenosis, minimal aortic stenosis, or small ventricular or atrial septal defect. The murmur

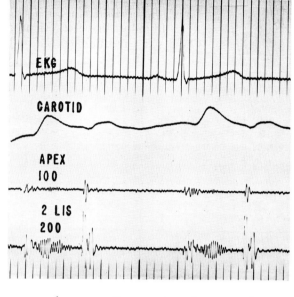

Figure 127. An innocent murmur at the second left interspace. Note the even, harmonic quality of a stringlike murmur. On auscultation this has a musical sound.

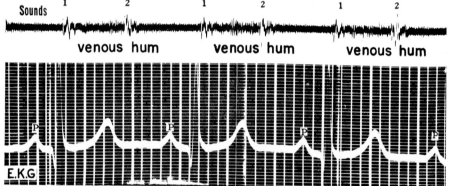

Figure 128. Venous hum under the right clavicle. Note the split first sound, the split second sound with a loud aortic component, and the plateau-shaped, medium-frequency, low-intensity continuous murmur covering the second two thirds of systole and the first half of diastole.[542]

here conforms to a clear-cut "organic" pattern, but the implications of the total picture are those of "no significant heart disease." Finally, the murmur associated with severe anemia, thyrotoxicosis or acute carditis, although "functional," I would not call "innocent," but would indicate that it means *significant* heart disease—just as significant as though it represented organic mitral stenosis.

A word may be said here about the occurrence, nature and significance of murmurs in infants and children. Richards,[586] reporting on more than 5000 newborns, found a systolic murmur at birth in 1.7 per cent, a figure in close agreement with that published several years ago by Lyon and his associates.[463] These studies confirm the impression of most pediatricians that murmurs in the newborn are relatively rare.

But more recent studies, particularly those of Burnard,[113] Halliday

Smith,[322] and others, indicate that if the heart of the newborn is examined carefully and at hourly intervals from birth on, more than 50 per cent of the infants will be found to have transient murmurs within the first 24 to 48 hours. These same murmurs occasionally may be demonstrated in fetal phonocardiograms. It should be mentioned that premature infants are more likely to have murmurs in the neonatal period than are full-term infants, and those with the "respiratory distress syndrome" have them even more commonly. The significance of these observations in relation to the hyaline membrane syndrome will be discussed later. The nature of these neonatal murmurs is hard to determine. A portion of them, unquestionably, originate from a left-to-right shunt across a partially constricted patent ductus arteriosus. These have either a typical continuous, machinery nature or only a late systolic crescendo. Other murmurs have a classic "stenotic" nature; still others sound like those of a typical ventricular septal defect. The majority of them, however, are not classifiable at present. They may be due to temporary mitral incompetence, secondary to increased flow and pressure work that the left ventricle is suddenly called upon to perform. Others may represent an opening in the ventricular septum that closes later. As mentioned, still others represent a patent ductus arteriosus. But *probably no murmurs are associated with the patency of the foramen ovale.*

The probability that a systolic murmur heard at a casual single auscultation within twenty-four to forty-eight hours after birth indicates congenital heart disease is 1 in 7 if the nature and intensity are disregarded. No figures are available as to the ultimate fate of newborns with loud murmurs; my impression is that no more than half of these prove eventually to have congenital heart disease. I have personally observed the disappearance of grade 3 to 4 harsh, left sternal border systolic murmurs within the first one or two months of life. Whereas systolic murmurs are rarely encountered at birth (unless a special study is made in this regard), by one year of age the incidence rises to 7 per cent.[585] Figures quoted by various authors, pertaining to normal children and adolescents, vary between 30 and 50 per cent. The vast majority of these correspond to the group previously labeled "insignificant."

The following principles in regard to murmurs are proposed:

Systolic Murmurs (Occurring between the First and Second Sounds)

1. With appropriate amplification, faint systolic murmurs may be registered in most, if not all, normal persons at the upper and midleft sternal border.[305] The site of origin of these "physiologic murmurs," not audible with a conventional stethoscope, is probably the pulmonary orifice.

2. An exaggeration of this "physiologic murmur" is the soft "pulmonary ejection murmur" consisting of low-intensity and medium-frequency vibrations, with a suggestion of midsystolic crescendo. This is audible with a stethoscope in persons who have generalized high cardiac output (exercise, anemia, pregnancy, excitement) or a high right ventricular output (atrial septal defect) (Fig. 129).

3. A further exaggeration of the same phenomenon, but associated with a pressure gradient across the aortic or the pulmonic valve, is the so-called stenotic murmur (Fig. 130). This is much louder than the first two murmurs

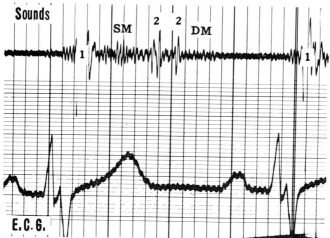

Figure 129. Irregular low-intensity systolic murmur in patient with atrial septal defect. Note also the widely split second sound and low-frequency early diastolic murmur.

mentioned; it is commonly associated with a thrill and is transmitted well to the neck and back, and even to the neck vessels. Phonocardiographically, this is a clearly diamond-shaped murmur of high intensity and high frequency. It is separated from the first sound by an appreciable interval (corresponding to the time needed for the opening of the corresponding semilunar valve) and reaches its zenith sometime in mid or late systole, its decrescendo phase terminating with aortic or pulmonic closure. It should be emphasized that the presence of a "stenotic" murmur does not necessarily mean anatomic stenosis, but rather a physiologic pressure gradient. It should be empasized further that a murmur of similar phonocardiographic characteristics, but having much poorer transmission qualities (since the blood and the muscular wall of the right ventricle dampen it), may be caused by a small ventricular septal defect.

4. In contrast to the previous three systolic murmurs, the murmur of atrioventricular valve regurgitation begins immediately with the first sound and either continues throughout systole (pansystolic) (Fig. 131) or assumes a decrescendo configuration. It is important to emphasize the blowing and musical sound of this murmur and its localization to the lower left sternal border and the apex, with good transmission to the axilla and back. Tricuspid murmurs often increase with inspiration, whereas those of mitral regurgitation are not affected by it (Fig. 132).

5. Another *regurgitant* murmur is the one registered at the upper and lower left sternal border in a patient with ventricular defect. This begins immediately with the first sound, but almost invariably lasts throughout systole, with a plateau shape (pansystolic) (Fig. 133). It has a different quality from the murmur of atrioventricular regurgitation. In frequency and intensity it is more nearly like the murmur of semilunar stenosis, lacking the musical, blowing sound and being rough and grating. On the other hand, it is only rarely diamond-shaped in configuration, and it transmits considerably less well to the neck and back.

6. The *uneven* systolic murmur of a patent ductus arteriosus, which may or may not be followed by a diastolic component, is heard best at the

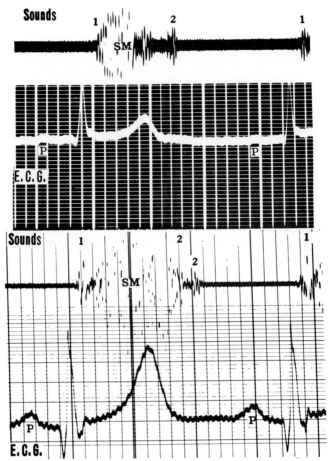

Figure 130. *A,* Diamond-shaped systolic murmur of aortic stenosis. Note the early apex of the diamond a considerable distance before the second sound. *B,* Diamond-shaped systolic murmur in patient with pulmonic stenosis. Note the relatively late apex of the diamond close to the second sound.

upper or midleft sternal border (Fig. 134). It consists of vibrations of varying frequencies and intensities, but like the murmurs discussed in paragraphs 4 and 5, it begins immediately with the first sound; thus it may have the general characteristics of a "regurgitant" murmur. The unevenness of the murmur may be the result of the peculiar physiologic situation in which one powerful stream of blood coming from the aorta through the ductus encounters the other stream ejected from the right ventricle into the pulmonary artery.[530]

Leatham[412] in his excellent article on heart sounds and murmurs classified the murmurs described in paragraphs 1, 2 and 3 as ejection murmurs and those mentioned in paragraphs 4, 5 and 6 as regurgitant murmurs. Although this is a useful concept, indeed, I believe that further specifications, as attempted here, are necessary. In other words, the murmur of a small ventricular septal defect, according to Leatham, is a "regurgitant" murmur, whereas, in fact, it may be indistinguishable from an ejection murmur. Presumably the reason for this is the high resistance to flow

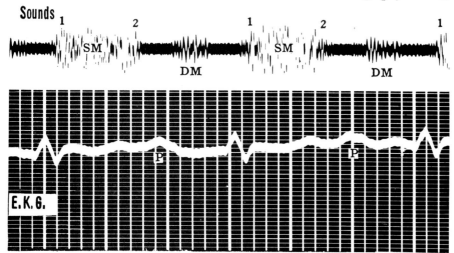

Figure 131.   Plateau-shaped murmur of mitral regurgitation with a low-frequency mid-diastolic murmur at the apex. Note the long P-R interval, placing the P wave before the mid-diastolic murmur. Presystole, however, is free.

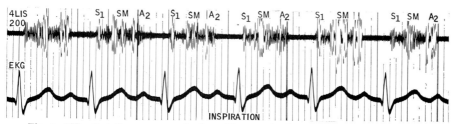

Figure 132.   Systolic murmur of tricuspid regurgitation at the fourth left interspace. Note the increased intensity of the murmur on inspiration, indicated at the bottom of the tracing. Note also the variable intensity first sound and the well split second sound.

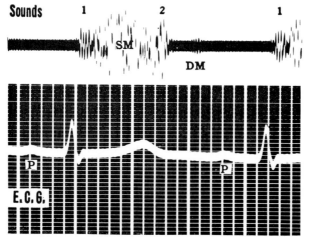

Figure 133.   Plateau-shaped systolic murmur of ventricular septal defect.

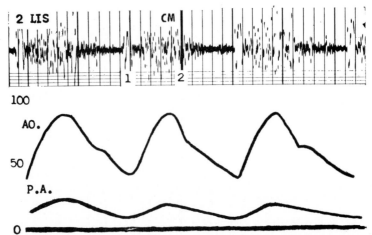

Figure 134. Continuous murmur of patent ductus arteriosus at the second left inter-space. Note the late systolic crescendo, with the apex of the murmur coinciding with the second sound and with the peak of aortic systolic pressure. It is at this point in the cycle that the pressure difference, the gradient, between aorta and pulmonary artery is maximal.

offered by the small defect, which is not much different, hemodynamically, from that offered by the pulmonary valve in pulmonic stenosis. Similarly, although both mitral regurgitation and ventricular septal defect are accompanied by "regurgitant" murmurs in principle, still the frequencies and transmissions of the two are sufficiently different that I think they should be thought of separately.

Diastolic Murmurs (Occurring between Second and First Sounds)

These may be divided into protodiastolic, mid-diastolic, and presystolic murmurs.

1. The murmurs of semilunar regurgitation (Fig. 135) are easily recognized by their high-frequency vibrations occupying protodiastole in a crescendo-decrescendo fashion. Their origin may be an incompetent aortic or pulmonic valve. Accordingly, they may be registered best at the upper right or lower left sternal border (aortic), or at the upper and midleft sternal border (pulmonic). Many are best registered with high-frequency filters and best heard with the diaphragm stethoscope.

2. Most murmurs of atrioventricular stenosis (Fig. 136) originate in the mitral valve, rarely at the tricuspid valve. These are low-frequency, rumbling, low-amplitude vibrations starting with mid-diastole and continuing beyond the fourth sound, often in a crescendo fashion (presystolic crescendo). These murmurs are heard best with the patient in the left lateral position, through a bell stethoscope, and are registered best with low-frequency filters. This murmur is preceded, at an appreciable interval, by an opening snap, and is followed by a late, loud first sound, making this one of the most characteristic auscultatory phenomena (fouttatarou). The third sound is usually faint or absent if the stenosis is of any severity. Murmurs characteristic of mitral stenosis may also be heard in patients having ventricular septal defect or patent ductus arteriosus who have no

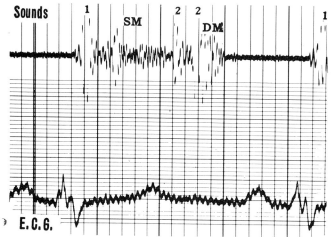

Figure 135. Early diastolic murmur of semilunar incompetence in patient with pulmonary vascular obstruction syndrome. Note also widely split second sound and systolic murmur.

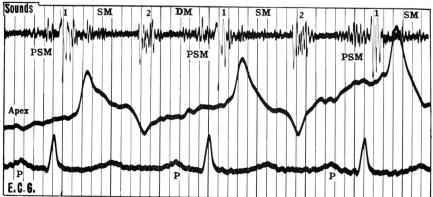

Figure 136. Typical presystolic crescendic murmur in a patient with rheumatic heart disease and mitral valve involvement. Tracing recorded at cardiac apex. Note: (1) prominent first heart sound, *1;* (2) moderately split second heart sound, *2;* (3) decrescendic medium-frequency moderate-intensity systolic murmur, *SM;* (4) mid-diastolic murmur, *DM;* (5) pre-systolic crescendic murmur, *PSM.*

organic stenosis, but rather a tremendous flow through the mitral valve secondary to the left-to-right shunt.

3. Diastolic-flow murmurs (Fig. 137) also originate at the atrioventricular valves; there is no actual narrowing, however, but rather an increased flow through a normal-sized orifice. These are also low-frequency vibrations of even lower intensity than those mentioned in paragraph 2. They are almost exclusively associated with a loud third sound, are heard in early or mid-diastole, extending, rarely, into presystole, and are almost never crescendic in configuration. There is no opening snap, and the first sound may or may not be loud. Diastolic-flow murmurs are heard in all large left-to-right shunts, in acute rheumatic carditis with mitral regurgitation (Carey Coombs murmur) and with aortic regurgitation (Austin Flint murmur). Tricuspid diastolic murmurs sometimes increase in intensity

with inspiration. It may be interesting to note that the diastolic-flow murmurs originating at the tricuspid valve, as in atrial septal defect, are early murmurs and follow closely the pulmonic component of the second sound. In contrast, the flow murmurs of ventricular defect and patent ductus arteriosus, originating in the mitral valve, are more likely to occur in mid-diastole (Fig. 138). These diastolic-flow murmurs are low in frequency and may be heard much better in children than in adults, with the bell stethoscope barely touching the skin.

Leatham[412] divided diastolic murmurs into (1) ventricular filling murmurs, including mitral stenosis, the Carey Coombs murmur, and left-

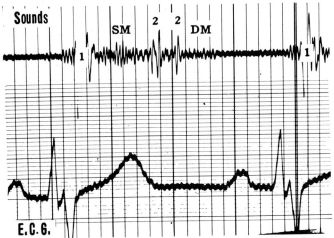

Figure 137. Murmurs of patient with atrial septal defect. Note the low-frequency, low-intensity diamond-shaped ejection murmur, the widely split second sound, and the early, protodiastolic, low-frequency rumble.

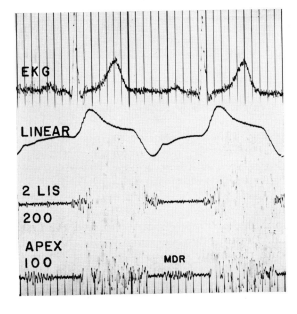

Figure 138. Low-frequency mid-diastolic rumble at the apex in patient with ventricular septal defect.

to-right shunts; (2) atrial systolic murmurs (presystolic) of mitral stenosis and tricuspid stenosis; and (3) diastolic murmurs caused by aortic and pulmonic regurgitation.

Continuous Murmurs

Continuous murmurs extend without interruption throughout the second sound, and must be differentiated first from the to-and-fro murmurs of aortic stenosis and aortic regurgitation. A continuous murmur does not mean that there is a murmur during every period of the cardiac cycle. This may be the case, but does not necessarily have to be so. It is commonly understood, however, that the murmur continues from systole into diastole through the second sound, though it may disappear entirely in presystole and may not start until some time after the first sound.

1. The machinery murmur is heard in patent ductus arteriosus (Fig. 134), aortopulmonary septal defect, coronary arteriovenous fistula, after shunt operation, and in certain cases of persistent truncus arteriosus (type IV). All these murmurs are continuous, according to the definition given, with a late systolic crescendo. They are moderately loud, are constant, and are not influenced by position or respiration. Their point of maximal intensity depends, of course, on their origin. The relative intensity of the systolic and diastolic components depends on the physiologic situation, particularly on the point at which the maximal pressure gradient occurs between the systemic and the pulmonary circuits. For instance, if a patient has a congenital coronary arteriovenous fistula which empties into the left ventrical, clearly the pressure gradient will be maximal during diastole; hence a loud diastolic murmur will be the dominant feature. Conversely, if a similar anatomic structure opens into the pulmonary artery, the systolic and diastolic components will be of equal intensity. These murmurs may be heard best with a diaphragm stethoscope, and may be registered best with high-frequency filters.

2. Venous hum (Fig. 128) may originate from the jugular vein (in normal persons), the pulmonary vein (in patients having pulmonary arteriovenous fistula or anomalous pulmonary venous drainage) or the pulmonary artery (in cases of peripheral pulmonic stenosis). All these murmurs continue in a plateau shape through the second sound, without late systolic crescendo, and are, on the whole, faint and influenced by positional changes and respiration. Their point of maximal intensity depends on the site of origin of the murmur.

6

CARDIAC
CATHETERIZATION

The introduction of cardiac catheterization, a little more than fifteen years ago, as a research tool and diagnostic test revolutionized the entire field of cardiology. Concepts that had been familiar only to physiologists became common knowledge to medical students as well as to practitioners of medicine. The use of the intracardiac catheter made it possible to determine accurately the cardiac output in man by applying the Fick principle. It enabled physiologists to compare the output of the systemic with the pulmonary ventricle; thus shunts from left to right and right to left could be quantitative with reasonable accuracy. By determining the oxygen content of the blood in various areas of the right side of the circulation, the site of left-to-right shunts could definitely be localized in most instances. By accurate analysis of the pressure tracings, stenotic lesions of the right side of the heart were discovered, and pulmonary hypertension was established as a rather common disease. By paying particular attention to the pressure tracing in the pulmonary tree, important conclusions were drawn in relation to diseases affecting the left side of the heart.

Since the first edition of this book was published, six years ago, further advances have been made in this field. Catheterization of the left side of the heart has become almost as widely practiced as that of the right side. Consequently, good, direct information about left-sided events has become available.

Instead of the cumbersome, old gasometric analysis of oxygen content in the blood, newer, quicker, spectrophotometric methods have come into use, allowing multiple samplings with small amounts of blood. Dye dilution curves with Evans blue became extremely popular for a while. They were to be the fountain of knowledge, and all phenomena related to the cardiac cycle were to be calculated from these mysterious curves.[743] Although this extreme view has been discarded by most workers in the field, dye dilution curves with Evans blue and, at the present time, indocyanine green have become useful agents of the cardiac catheterization procedure and are used with increasing skill in the detection of shunts and calculation of cardiac output and regurgitant flows. The presence of shunts may also be detected by the use of other indicator techniques, using hydrogen,[150] cold saline, radioactive krypton or radiopaque dye.[444]

Angiocardiography, in our institution, and in many other centers, has ceased to be a separate procedure, but, by means of multiple selective cine-angiograms, has become another indicator to be performed as *part of* the total catheterization technique. This has been made possible by the radiologic advances inherent in the perfection of the image-intensifier principle.

The magnificent pictures furnished by the Elema and Schonander biplane serial angiocardiograms are still used to great advantage in many places. The clarity of detail and the tridimensional view they furnish are still unsurpassed. In this day of increased consciousness of radiation hazard, however, one begins to wonder whether this procedure is worth the price of the large amount of radiation involved. Certainly, this kind of detailed information may prove to be vital in some instances, but in many cases I believe that a thorough catheterization procedure with cine-angiograms gives just as good or better information with appreciably less radiation.[601, 656]

The widespread use of the strain gauge manometer instead of the old capacitance, or even saline, manometer has contributed appreciably to the convenience and accuracy of pressure measurement.

Finally, intracardiac phonocardiography and electrocardiography have been made part of the catheterization procedure in selected cases.

From all this it may be seen that cardiac catheterization has ceased to be the simple procedure of ten years ago. It is no longer enough to pass a catheter into the pulmonary artery, take one or two blood samples from each of the right heart chambers, and to measure pressures with a saline manometer. The age of innocence is over. The advances in instrumentation and techniques have become so formidable that only personnel highly trained and occupying themselves practically full-time with this method should be allowed to be in charge of a cardiac catheterization laboratory.

As a result of all the information pouring out of the diagnostic and research laboratories of the world, physiologic thinking in the field of cardiology has become even more prevalent within the past five years. Clinical cardiology has moved even closer to the basic science laboratory, but one wonders whether both of them have not moved away from the man who sees patients in the home and in the office. It is hoped that all the new knowledge can be translated into terms of patient care to be of use to physicians taking care of sick people. It should be possible to interpret the clinical data available at the bedside and in the office in the light of physiologic information, in order to improve medical care. This is the principal purpose of this book.

Basic information related to the principles of cardiac catheterization may be found in the classic papers of Cournand,[171] Bing[57] and Dexter.[192] A résumé of the new techniques alluded to in the last few paragraphs may be found in selected references.[398, 601, 743, 763]

WHO SHOULD PERFORM CARDIAC CATHETERIZATION, AND WHY?

Of course, all this is not an unmixed blessing. The question of who should be responsible for the operation of a cardiac laboratory became a real problem. The physician many years and many textbooks away from the physiology courses at medical school had to "relearn" all that he might never even have understood previously. The practitioner—especially the pediatrician, who in the past had felt intellectually rather superior if he could distinguish the P wave from the T wave in the electrocardiogram—was suddenly given the task of analyzing the difference between the left atrial and the pulmonary capillary pressure tracings. The medical man, studiously avoiding the use of the scalpel since he had finished that rotating internship he had never wanted to take to begin with, had to learn how to cut down on veins and poke around the tricuspid valve with a long rubber tube. The surgeon, whose distaste for the stethoscope fully matched the horror of the scalpel experienced by his colleagues in internal medicine, had to rediscover mathematical equations and the use of a slide rule, and even to relearn Ohm's law. One solution to the problem was to turn the whole procedure over to a physician trained primarily in the basic sciences, or even to a Doctor of Philosophy who could make good use of his technical skill acquired in the experimental laboratory and his intellectual superiority carefully cultivated by the various meetings of learned societies. This sounded fine to everyone but the patient, who still wanted to see a doctor, primarily trained in the care of people, with interest in him as a person and not only as a composite of pressures and flows.

Fifteen years after the introduction of the cardiac catheterization technique, this problem has not been solved with finality. Different centers throughout the country have utilized people with different types of training for the operation of the cardiac catheterization laboratory. It seems clear, to me at least, that the best results have been obtained in those centers where various types of personnel are available to utilize fully the benefits derived from the procedure. A physician well trained in physiology has to be in immediate and complete charge of the laboratory; he should be responsible for the analysis of the data and their interpretation and significance in relation to the particular study. A cardiologist should be in charge of the patient. He should decide, subject to the approval of the laboratory head, who should undergo the procedure. He should integrate the physiologic picture and the clinical observations, and should interpret the whole thing to the patient and the family. Finally, taking the entire situation into careful consideration, he should decide about the therapeutic implications, subject, of course, to the approval of the surgeon. In addition, the active participation of members of the Anesthesia Service and the Radiology Department is indispensable. It cannot be emphasized strongly enough that all these people should be in close cooperation and consultation with each other for best results.

INDICATIONS AND RISKS

There is no unanimity of opinion as to the indications for cardiac catheterization. A great deal depends on the experience and temperament of the physician making the decision.

Before embarking on the indications, it must be realized that *this is a major procedure which may terminate in the death of the patient*. This may not be a statistically significant fact; nevertheless it should be made crystal clear to every patient or parent. If death occurs as a consequence of a therapeutic procedure, the relatives usually accept it much more readily than if the catastrophe is encountered as the outcome of a diagnostic procedure. I do not believe that we can quote statistically valid mortality figures, since much depends not only on the skill of the operating team, but also on the material with which they are working. If the physician is conservative and reserves catheterization for sick people only, his mortality figures will be higher than those of his colleague who catheterizes everybody with an apical systolic murmur. But—and this point can scarcely be over-emphasized—some of the latter group, the ones with no significant disease at all, can be seriously harmed and may even die during the procedure. The risk quoted to parents in our department is that about 499 out of 500 of these procedures go perfectly well, but once in about 500 times, trouble arises. Higher risks than these are quoted when patients with pulmonary vascular obstruction or Ebstein's disease are considered for study.

Always remembering these dangers, we recommend cardiac catheterization for the following groups: (1) patients who, on the basis of clinical evidence, do not have operable heart disease, but whose condition is clearly severe, and in whom an operable situation cannot be excluded with reasonable certainty; (2) patients with a clinical picture of operable heart disease in whom the severity of the lesion and the exact anatomic and physiologic details represent part of the operative indications (atrial septal defect, pulmonic stenosis, mitral stenosis, tetralogy of Fallot, ventricular septal defect and aortic stenosis); and (3) patients with a clinical picture of operable heart disease in whom a complicating factor, possibly contraindicating operation, is suspected (patent ductus arteriosus or coarctation of the aorta with right ventricular hypertrophy), and (4) for the postoperative evaluation of patients who have undergone cardiac surgery.

We do not usually recommend catheterization for patients who clearly have operable heart disease with definite indications for operation (severe mitral stenosis, patent ductus arteriosus, coarctation of the aorta, classic instances of severe pulmonic stenosis, aortic stenosis or large atrial septal defect). We are also reluctant to use the procedure in patients without significant heart disease.

The preferred age for cardiac catheterization is three years or older. But successful right heart catheterization has been accomplished in many babies from the newborn period onward, when clear indications existed.

The difficulties encountered consist principally in the development of arrhythmias. For obvious reasons, atrial premature beats or even paroxysmal atrial tachycardia is not nearly as worrisome as are ventricular premature beats, ventricular tachycardia or, of course, ventricular flutter or fibrillation.

In addition to the arrhythmias, we have also seen transient hemiplegias, presumably due to air embolism, develop after catheterization. Hypotension has been reported to occur in severely ill cyanotic patients and those with pulmonary vascular obstruction. In our laboratory this has not been a prevalent cause for concern. Another complication we witnessed was the looping of the catheter in the right atrium with the formation of a knot; cardiotomy had to be performed in order to withdraw the catheter from this patient. Other complications to be mentioned are (1) blood loss due to excessive withdrawal, which may have to be corrected by postoperative blood transfusion, (2) development of transient, but in one case fatal, complete atrioventricular block, (3) cardiac tamponade after percutaneous left ventricular puncture, (4) development of severe anoxia when the catheter is passed through a maximally stenosed pulmonary valve,[552] and (5) perforation of the atrial or ventricular wall by the catheter itself, infiltration of the ventricular musculature, or even rupture of the thin-walled pulmonary artery by the injection of dye under high pressure.

We have never seen proved bacterial endocarditis develop after venous catheterization, although in one instance of left ventricular puncture fatal endocarditis occurred two months after the procedure. A febrile reaction, lasting twelve to eighteen hours, occurs occasionally.

TECHNIQUES

The Technique of Right Heart Catheterization

The technique of catheterization of the right side of the heart consists in the introduction, under sterile conditions, of a long, thin, plastic-coated, woven nylon catheter through a systemic vein into the right side of the heart and the pulmonary arteries.

At right heart catheterization an antecubital vein of the right arm is usually selected and exposed, although the saphenous vein is preferable in infants and young children. In newborns the superficial, or even the deep femoral, vein may be the only one large enough to accept the proper-sized catheter. Although the approach through the right median cubital or basilic vein is the preferred one in older children, the saphenous approach should be used if exploration of the left atrium through the atrial septum is contemplated. It should be mentioned, however, that it is somewhat more difficult to pass the catheter into the pulmonary artery from a vein in the leg than from a vein in the arm. In certain instances it may be necessary to make an approach from the arm to explore the pulmonary artery and a saphenous approach to get across the atrial septum in the same patient.

Soft, pliable catheters, ranging in size from number 4 to 7 and in length from 50 to 125 cm., are used routinely (Fig. 139). Larger catheters with six side openings are used for rapid injection of radiopaque dye; they prevent the uncontrolled recoil imparted to open-ended catheters by the ejected jet of dye. Special catheters are used for intracardiac phonocardiography and electrocardiography.

A saline solution containing heparin is used to fill the catheter, which is then connected to the manometer before insertion into the isolated vein. In this way, pressure at the tip can be monitored throughout the procedure. Then, under fluoroscopic control, the tip is advanced through the superior or inferior vena cava (depending on the arm or leg approach) into the right atrium, right ventricle, pulmonary artery, and as far out to the lung fields as possible. Most of the time, with gentle twisting, turning and pushing, the tip may be advanced with ease; occasionally, however, even with considerable maneuvering, the catheter cannot be advanced in the required fashion, in which case changing the catheter or reintroducing it into another vein may accomplish the desired result. While the tube is being advanced, the patient is connected to an electrocardiograph, and one member of the team watches the tracing on the oscilloscope for the appearance of arrhythmias.

When the catheter reaches the superior vena cava (Fig. 140, A), blood is collected in a heparinized syringe for oxygen analysis. This is handed to a technician, who places it in an ice bath. The catheter is flushed with the saline solution, as it is whenever blood is withdrawn through it. Next, the catheter is advanced into the right atrium, where another blood sample is obtained (Fig. 140, B) and a right atrial pressure tracing is recorded. Then the catheter, connected to the manometer and under fluoroscopic control, is advanced from the right atrium to the right ventricle, which is identified both by the appearance of a ventricular type of pressure tracing on the oscilloscope and by the position of the tip of the catheter under the fluoroscope (Fig. 140, C). A blood sample and a pressure tracing are

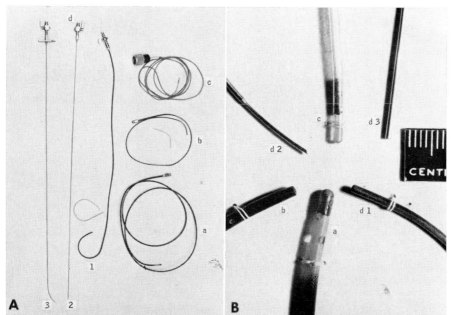

Figure 139. Various catheters used in our laboratory at this time. *A* illustrates the catheters in their entire length, and *B* focuses on the tips. (*a*) National Institute of Health angiocatheter. (*b*) Lehman catheter, 50 cm. (*c*) Phonocatheter with barium titanate tip. (*d*) Components of transseptal catheter. (*d 1*) Catheter as it looks on the outside. (*d 2*) Stylus. (*d 3*) Transseptal needle.

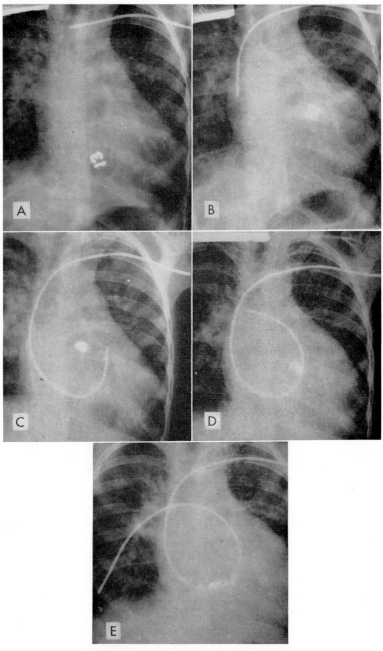

Figure 140. *A,* Cardiac catheter, approaching from the left arm and reaching the border between innominate vein and superior vena cava. *B,* Cardiac catheter in the mid-lateral portion of the right atrium. *C,* Catheter advancing through the tricuspid valve into the right ventricle. *D,* Catheter entering pulmonary artery from the right ventricle. *E,* Catheter in the "pulmonary capillary" position wedged out into the lung fields.

obtained from the ventricle; then, under fluoroscopic and manometric control, the tip is advanced into the pulmonary artery (Fig. 140, *D*). A blood sample having been obtained here, the catheter is again advanced, as before, and "wedged" as far out to the lung fields as possible, into a so-called pulmonary wedge position, where samples and pressures are again obtained (Fig. 140, *E*). When all this is completed, the catheter is pulled back into the pulmonary artery and left there. Now the artery at the site of the "cut down" is exposed and cannulated with a number 18 to 22 needle. With the needle in the systemic artery and the catheter in the pulmonary artery, expired air is collected in a Douglass bag while arterial and venous samples are obtained. This will be used for calculation of cardiac output and determination of oxygen capacity. Pressure tracings from systemic and pulmonary arteries having been obtained, the catheter is withdrawn from the pulmonary artery through the right ventricle into the right atrium. Simultaneous pressure tracings from these sites and from the systemic artery are obtained. Blood samples are collected again from selected areas on the way out. The catheter and the needle are removed, and the "cut down" is sutured.

The entire procedure from "cut down" to suture closure usually takes one to three hours. During this time fifteen to twenty blood samples and many feet of pressure tracings are collected. In our experience a general anesthetic is almost never required.

Sedation is achieved with a combination of 25 mg. of Demerol, 6.25 mg. of Phenergan and 6.25 mg. of chlorpromazine in each milliliter of solution. One milliliter is administered for each 30 pounds of body weight, with a maximum of 2 ml. for children. The drug is administered intramuscularly one hour before the procedure. This serves the purpose adequately in most instances. Exposure to image-intensifier viewing should last no more than thirty minutes.

This is the simplest kind of routine catheterization of the right side of the heart. As implied before, in most instances the procedure is considerably more involved. The technical aspects of the ancillary procedures used in the appropriate situation will be outlined briefly later.

The Techniques of Left Heart Catheterization

Left heart catheterization is not nearly as well standardized as that outlined for the right side. Various methods are preferred in various centers. The following approaches have been proposed.

Approach to the Left Atrium. APPROACH THROUGH FORAMEN OVALE OR ATRIAL SEPTAL DEFECT. This is the simplest method and is probably the procedure of choice in all infants and small children, in whom the foramen ovale is likely to be at least probe-patent. It is also the preferred approach in patients with known atrial septal defect. The technique is identical with that described in relation to right heart catheterization, except that a leg vein (saphenous or superficial femoral) is the obligatory choice for the "cut down." As the catheter approaches the heart through the inferior vena cava, it is usually easy to manipulate it through the foramen ovale (Fig. 141). As a matter of fact, often this seems to be the preferred route for the catheter rather than the sharp angle necessary to traverse the tricuspid valve.

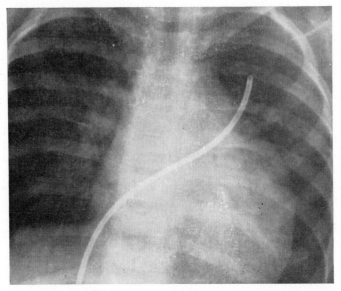

Figure 141. Passage of catheter through the inferior cava, right atrium, foramen ovale, into the left atrium, and out into a pulmonary vein.

Once the left atrium has been entered, pressure tracings and blood samples are obtained. Next, the left ventricle is explored. Because of the acute angle the catheter must take in order to enter the left ventricle, exploration is accomplished from this approach in only about 50 per cent of the patients. Of course this percentage varies tremendously, according to the experience and skill of the operator. Even if the left ventricle can be entered in this fashion, the catheter can seldom be passed through the aortic valve. Determination of the systemic arterial pressure must then be made by entering a peripheral artery directly.

This approach to the left side of the heart is almost routinely attempted in all our patients undergoing cardiac catheterization. It is a safe and easy technique. It furnishes an opportunity for performing ancillary procedures in a number of situations not primarily affecting the left side of the heart. Our interest in this type of information led us to use the saphenous approach routinely in a large proportion of our infants and small children.

APPROACH BY PUNCTURING INTACT ATRIAL SEPTUM. Exploration of the left atrium by means of puncturing the intact atrial septum was described by Ross, Braunwald and Morrow in 1960.[593] The technique is similar to that described for passage through the foramen ovale except that the atrial septum first must be punctured. To this effect, a relatively large catheter is introduced into the right saphenous vein (number 7 or 9), passed through the inferior vena cava, and lodged against the atrial septum. Then a long transseptal needle (number 17 to 19) is guided through this catheter, through the atrial septum, and into the left atrium. Next, a polyethylene catheter is passed through the needle in the left atrium, and samples and pressure tracings are obtained from the left atrium, the left ventricle and, if possible, from the aorta.

Our experience with this method is relatively limited, since a large

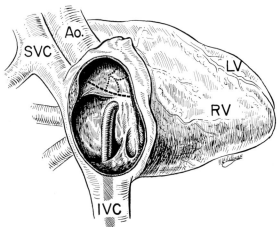

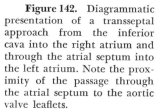

Figure 142. Diagrammatic presentation of a transseptal approach from the inferior cava into the right atrium and through the atrial septum into the left atrium. Note the proximity of the passage through the atrial septum to the aortic valve leaflets.

portion of our patients are small infants, in whom the introduction of the large catheter necessary for this procedure may be somewhat more cumbersome than it is in older children and adults. According to physicians from the National Heart Institute, this procedure has been performed without ill effects in more than 100 instances. A potential danger seems to be perforation of the base of the aorta, located less than 1 cm. from the point where the needle crosses the septum (Fig. 142). Since the problems in pediatric cardiology are associated mostly with the aortic and not the mitral valve, we hesitate to use routinely a potentially dangerous method which does not guarantee direct information about the aortic valve.

Approach through the Right Main Bronchus. We have never used this technique in our department. It was described by Faquet[237] in 1952 and Allison and Linden in 1953.[13] The method consists in the passage of a long needle through a bronchoscope. The anteromedial wall of the right main bronchus is punctured, and the needle is passed into the left atrium. A polyethylene catheter is passed under the guidance of the needle into the left atrium and left ventricle. This is a safe procedure which has been performed to great advantage several hundred times at the National Heart Institute and at other centers where there is a predominantly adult patient load. Because of the trauma inherent in bronchoscopy in small children and because of the relatively small left atria encountered in pediatric cardiology, it is not to be recommended for routine use in pediatric departments.

Approach through the Back. Introduced by Bjork[59] in 1953, the right paravertebral method (Fig. 143) has been used several hundred times in adults with mitral valve disease. We have used the technique, with assistance from our surgical colleagues, in a handful of adolescents in whom our attention has been focused primarily on the function of the mitral valve. One further use for this technique, in infants or children of any age, has been in the diagnosis of cor triatriatum.

The patient lies in the prone position. The skin over the back is sterilized and draped. A skin puncture site is then selected, about 4 to 5 cm. to the right of the spinous processes, at the level most directly opposite to the center of the cardiac silhouette, as determined fluoroscopically. With the patient under local procaine anesthesia, the needle is passed in a left-

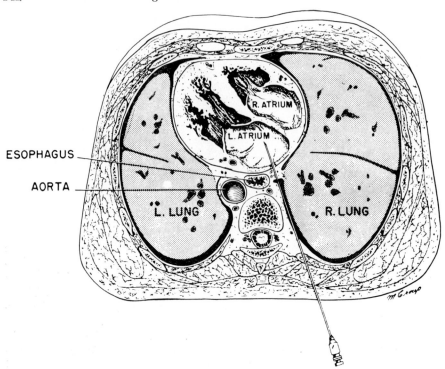

ESOPHAGUS

AORTA

Figure 143.   Approach to the left atrium through the back. Diagrammatic representation.[763]

ward direction toward the center of the heart, into the left atrium. A polyethylene catheter is inserted under the guidance of the needle and passed
from the left atrium to the left ventricle and the aorta. Pressures and
samples are obtained. An excellent detailed description of the technique
may be found in Fisher's article on the subject.[252]

The disadvantages of the technique in infants and children in regard
to the size of the atrium are the same as those cited in regard to the
transbronchial approach. In addition, hemoptysis, pneumothorax, hemo-
thorax and hemopericardium have been reported among the complications.
Fisher referred to a fatality due to puncture of an aortic aneurysm.[251]

Approach to the Left Ventricle.   PERCUTANEOUS PUNCTURE.   This procedure was described by Brock[99] in 1956. With the help of our surgical
service, we have used it for the evaluation of aortic valve disease in more
than 100 cases.

A number 16 or 18 needle is introduced into the ventricle at the point
of maximal left ventricular impulse. The skin is nicked first to facilitate
introduction of the needle. The patient is under general anesthesia. The
needle, attached to a syringe, is directed upward and posteriorly toward
the second right costochondral junction (Fig. 144). Entry into the left
ventricle is verified by withdrawal of bright red blood. A blood sample
is obtained and pressure is measured through the needle. An attempt is
then made to enter the aorta with a thin polyethylene catheter passed
through the needle. This maneuver is successful in more than 75 per cent
of the patients and allows determination of the nature of the aortic ob-

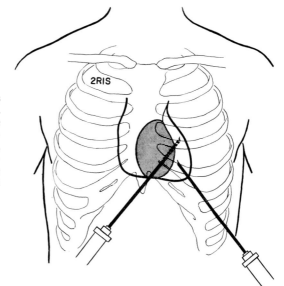

Figure 144. Percutaneous approach to the left ventricle. Note the approach through the apex into the left ventricle directly, and through the xiphoid, in which case the catheter approaches the left ventricle through the right ventricle, via the interventricular septum.

struction (valvar or subvalvar). If the aorta cannot be entered, the brachial artery is cannulated and the pressure in the peripheral artery is used for determination of the aortic valve gradient.

In our department this has been a safe and uniformly successful technique for determining the severity of aortic stenosis. No fatalities have been encountered so far with this method in our institution. The one definite case of tamponade and the bacterial endocarditis questionably caused by left ventricular puncture have already been mentioned. An occasional small pneumothorax has proved always to be transient and without great significance. Brock's group reported 2 deaths among 184 cases, both in older patients with maximal calcified stenosis. So far, direct left ventricular puncture has always been performed by a member of the surgical staff in our institution. This, I presume, is more of a tradition than a necessity.

RETROGRADE CATHETERIZATION THROUGH A PERIPHERAL ARTERY. Although this route of left ventricular exploration was first proposed in 1950,[764] it was not until 1960 that the approach from the femoral or the right brachial artery gained wide acceptance.[504] By skillful manipulation of the catheter introduced into a peripheral artery into which heparin has been introduced distally, the left ventricle may be entered in all patients except those having maximal aortic stenosis. Severe aortic stenosis, even with gradients as high as 100 to 150 mm. between left ventricle and ascending aorta, does not necessarily represent an insurmountable obstacle to passage of the catheter through the aortic valve.

In our laboratory at present, all patients undergo catheterization of the right side of the heart first. Then, if exploration of the left side is deemed necessary, we usually try to pass the catheter through the foramen ovale. If this is not successful, retrograde passage through the aortic valve is attempted. If neither of these approaches is successful, direct left ventricular puncture or the transseptal needle is used. The only disadvantage, or complication, of retrograde catheterization of the left ventricle has been

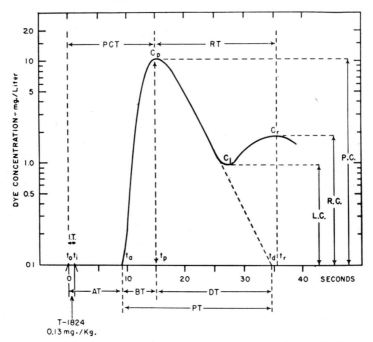

Figure 145. Time and concentration components of an indicator dilution curve in a normal subject. The logarithm of the concentration on the ordinate is plotted against time on the abscissa, and the declining slope of concentration has been extrapolated to the base line, according to the method of Hamilton, to eliminate the effect of recirculated indicator.

All instants on the time base are designated by a lower case t, followed by a suitable subscript. All intervals on the time base are designated in capitals or, for convenience for use in mathematical equations, by a capital T with a suitable subscript.

I.T., Injection time. The interval between the instant of the beginning and the instant of completion of injection of the indicator; $T_I = (t_i - t_o)$.

AT, Appearance time. The interval from the instant of the beginning of the injection to the instant of its first detection at the sampling site; $T_a = (t_a - t_o)$.

PCT, Peak concentration time. The interval from the instant of the beginning of injection to the instant of maximal concentration at the sampling site resulting from indicator traversing the normal circulatory pathway; $T_{PC} = (t_{pc} - t_c)$.

BT, Build-up time. The interval from the instant of first detection of indicator at the sampling site to the instant of maximal concentration resulting from indicator traversing the normal circulatory pathway; $T_B = (t_{pc} - t_a O)$.

RT, Recirculation time. The interval from the instant of maximal concentration of indicator to the instant of next definable peak concentration of the indicator (if any) due principally to indicator which has passed the systemic capillaries; $T_R = (t_r - t_{pc})$.

PT, Passage time. The interval from the instant of first decision of indicator at the sampling site to the instant when the declining concentration of indicator reaches a minimally detectable value eliminating the estimated effect of recirculated indicator; $T_p = (t_d - t_a)$.

DT, Disappearance time. The interval from the instant of maximal concentration to the instant at which the declining concentration of indicator reaches a minimally detectable value, eliminating the estimated effect of recirculated indicator; $T_D = (t_d - t_{pc})$.

MTT, Mean transit time. The average interval required for indicator particles to travel from injection site to sampling site, eliminating the estimated effect of recirculated indicator; $T_M = \bar{t} - t_o)$.

Values for concentration are designated by large capitals or, for convenience for use in mathematical equations, by a capital C with a suitable subscript.

P.C., Peak concentration. The maximal concentration of indicator particles occurring at the sampling site due to indicator that has traversed the normal circulatory pathway (C_p).

(*Continued on page 145*)

some interference with the circulation of the arm in a few cases. This has resulted in loss or weakness of radial pulses and, in one case only, of coldness of the hand. Yet, I have heard of instances in which thrombosis of the brachial artery occurred after this procedure. Well over 200 retrograde arterial catheterizations have been performed in our laboratory without any serious complications.

Ancillary Procedures

Measurement of Oxygen Consumption.   In order to calculate the cardiac output accurately, by means of the Fick principle, the oxygen consumption per minute must be determined. In older children a closed-circuit method with collection of expired air through a mouthpiece into a Douglass bag is readily applicable.

In infants the closed technique has been applied recently by means of a nasal adaptor.[287] An open technique with the use of a mask has also been used to good advantage in this age group.[144]

Indicator Dilution Techniques.   Although the use of Evans blue dye as a diagnostic tool was recommended by Nicholson, Burchell and Wood ten years ago,[535] it has been only within the past five years that this technique has been used to any extent at our institution.

The principle of the technique is essentially one of determining the circulation time and quantity of dye at various sites in the circulation, by various methods.

Indicator substances most commonly used include Evans blue (high spectral absorption in the red region of 640 millimicrons) and cardiogreen (indocyanine green, high spectral absorption in the infra-red region of 800 millimicrons). Evans blue dye cannot be used accurately in patients with arterial unsaturation, whereas cardiogreen is reliable for fully saturated as well as unsaturated blood. Other substances used for dilution curves are radioactive indicators (I^{131} human albumin), methylene blue, Coumassie Blue, or indigo carmine, cold saline solution or hypertonic saline solution. The principle in the use of all these is the same, even though the detector is different.

Indicator dilution curves are used for detection of left-to-right shunts and of right-to-left shunts, and for estimation of valvular regurgitation and of cardiac output.

In its simplest application a measured amount of dye substance is injected into the right atrium. Blood samples are withdrawn from a

---

AC., Average concentration. The mean concentration of indicator particles at the sampling site during their first circulation (passage time) eliminating the estimated effect of recirculated indicator ($\bar{C}$).

R. C., Maximal recirculation concentration. The secondary peak of concentration of indicator occurring at the sampling site, resulting principally from particles which have passed systemic capillaries and recirculated by way of the normal circulatory pathway(C_r).

L.C., Least concentration. The minimal concentration of indicator occurring at the sampling site between the times of maximal concentration and maximal recirculation concentration (C_l).

EC, Equilibrium concentration. The concentration of indicator at the sampling site occurring at a specified interval after injection when uniform mixing of indicator and blood in the circulatory system is assumed to have occurred (C_e).[763]

peripheral artery through a needle into an apparatus capable of quanti- tatively detecting the appearance of dye by spectrophotometric methods (oximeter, densitometer, and so forth). The appearance of the dye in the artery may be registered as a bell-shaped curve. Several points on this curve may be noted (Fig. 145): (1) appearance time, when the very first dye particle reaches the detector; (2) build-up time, the interval over which concentration increases to a peak; and (3) disappearance time, indicating the disappearance of the dye and a return of the curve to the base line.

The site of injection as well as of detection varies tremendously and includes any heart chamber or great vessel amenable to the catheter (Fig. 146).

Foreign Gas Technique. Inhalation of nitrous oxide,[504, 505] radioactive krypton (Kr[85]) and even simple hydrogen gas[150] has been used for accurate detection of even small left-to-right shunts. The gas is inhaled through a mask, and samples are obtained from a systemic artery and the right heart chambers (Fig. 147).

An extension of this technique by dissolving the gases in saline solu- tion has enabled investigators to use the same material for detection of right-to-left shunts by injecting the solution into the right heart chambers and taking samples from a systemic artery.

Intracardiac Phonocardiography. A number of microphones have been introduced into the human heart by means of the cardiac catheter.[424] Our experience has been almost exclusively with the barium titanate microphone designed by Wallace and Brown and put to clinical use by Lewis and Deitz.[424] This microphone is incorporated into a rather soft number 5 plastic catheter. Attached to a suitable preamplifier, it gives good sound tracings. When it is mounted with an open-end catheter, the diame-

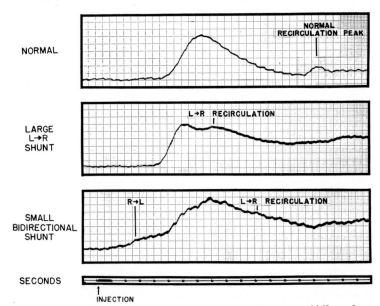

Figure 146. Examples of dye curves. *Top,* A normal curve; *middle,* a large left-to- right shunt; *bottom,* a small right-to-left and a sizable left-to-right shunt. Note the slow return to the baseline, characteristic of a left-to-right shunt, and the early hump, indicating a right-to-left shunt.

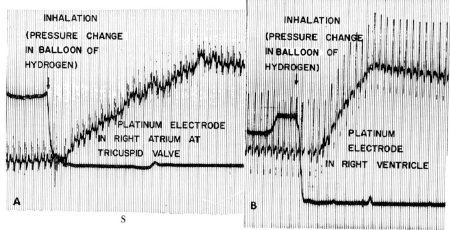

INHALATION

(PRESSURE CHANGE

IN BALLOON OF

HYDROGEN)

INHALATION

(PRESSURE CHANGE

IN BALLOON OF

HYDROGEN)

PLATINUM ELECTRODE

IN RIGHT ATRIUM AT

TRICUSPID VALVE

PLATINUM

ELECTRODE

IN RIGHT VENTRICLE

A

B

S

Figure 147. Example of a hydrogen curve. Note the early appearance time indicating a left-to-right shunt in *A* at the atrial and in *B* at the ventricular level. Each thick time line equals 1 second. The appearance time in *A* is about 1.6 seconds, in *B* 2.4 seconds.

ter is equivalent to number 9 French. The Soulie catheter contains a microphone and a micromanometer at its tip. It, too, is large (number 8 French).

At present this is principally a research tool, though in certain selected situations it may furnish information of much diagnostic significance. One area of usefulness is in the detection of ventricular septal defects too small to give rise to changes in oxygen saturation (Fig. 148). Similarly, it has been useful in the identification of a patent ductus arteriosus associated with a ventricular septal defect.

Intracardiac Electrocardiography. This is also a research tool with practical diagnostic importance only in the identification of Ebstein's anomaly. In this condition an atrial pressure tracing is registered simultaneously with a right ventricular cavity electrocardiogram pattern (rS).[678]

The information made available by intracardiac electrocardiography is of considerable theoretical importance to the understanding of scalar electrocardiograms as well as vectorcardiograms (Fig. 149).

Selective Angiocardiography and Cine-angiography. Since the introduction of angiocardiography as a diagnostic technique by Castellanos[141] in 1937, many strides have been made in this area. First, from the original one exposure per second we have advanced to ten to fifteen per second with the rapid cassette changers and up to thirty to sixty frames per second with cine-angiography. Second, from a simple one-plane angiocardiogram, biplane instruments have been developed for use in angiocardiography as well as cine-angiography. Third, the use of the image intensifier, by increasing the brilliance of the fluoroscopic screen several hundred and even thousand times, reduces radiation to a point at which it is possible to inject dye into several sites in rapid succession without exposing the patient or the physician to excessive amounts of radiation. Fourth, the introduction of new dye substances without any appreciable toxicity has eliminated the risk of multiple injections almost completely (Hypaque, Ditriokon, Renovist). Finally, the development of mechanical or even

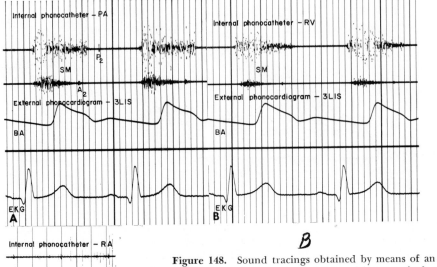

Figure 148. Sound tracings obtained by means of an intracardiac phonocatheter in a patient with a ventricular septal defect. Withdrawal from pulmonary artery (*A*) indicating the high-frequency high-intensity decrescendo systolic murmur and the well noted second pulmonic sound. In the external phonocardiogram obtained at the third left interspace, in the second panel, aortic closure may be seen in addition to the systolic murmur. The third and fourth panels are brachial artery tracing and electrocardiogram, respectively. *B* shows the systolic murmur to be louder in the right ventricle than it was in the pulmonary artery, and pulmonic closure cannot be visualized. The other panels are as before. *C* shows no murmur in the right atrium. An atrial sound may be seen at the beginning and the end of the top panel, corresponding to the P wave in the electrocardiogram on the bottom.

automatic injectors and special catheters allows delivery of the dye with high velocity into specific areas.

As a result of this technical progress, angiocardiography has ceased to be a separate procedure; it is part and parcel of the cardiac catheterization technique. No general anesthesia is used. In our laboratory, cine-angiography is used from selected sites in the left or right side of the heart, depending on the diagnostic problem presented. Thus invaluable information is obtained about shunts, valvar regurgitation and anatomic details. The cine-angiogram is as integral a part of the physiologic study as pressure measurements or oxygen analysis.

Personnel

At least four, preferably five, people are necessary for the efficient performance of the various procedures involved. One handles the catheter; the second one is in charge of the multichannel recorder and watches the electrocardiogram constantly on the oscilloscope. A third person has to handle the Douglass bag for the oxygen collection, the densitometer or

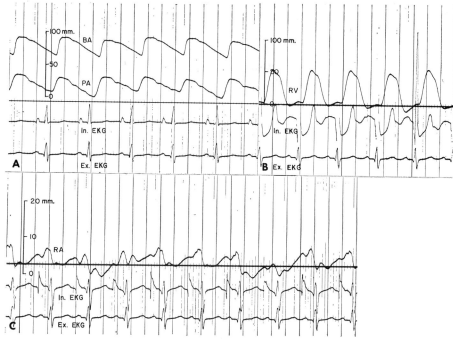

Figure 149. Intracardiac electrocardiogram. *A,* The electrode in the pulmonary artery. Note the P wave and the dominantly upright QRS complex. *B,* The right ventricular tracing. Note the deep Q and tall R in the last complex. *C,* From the right atrium. Note the big P waves and the biphasic QRS complex.

oximeter for dye dilution curves, and the fluoroscopic screen. A fourth person, a technician, handles the blood samples. Finally, a nurse should sit by the child's head, talk to him, quiet him and reassure him.

If it is impossible to obtain the services of five persons for one procedure, the technician handling the blood samples may also be available for managing the screen, the densitometer and the oxygen collection.

Equipment

A good-sized (about 400 square feet) air-conditioned room is necessary for adequate catheterization. The atmosphere should have the characteristics of a well run operating theater; it must be clean, quiet and efficient. Adjoining the catheterization room should be a chemistry laboratory with one or two technicians so that the results of the chemical analyses can be communicated immediately to the catheterization team.

The Fluoroscopic Apparatus. The radiologic equipment necessary for a modern catheterization laboratory should allow for fluoroscopic visualization of the passage of the catheter, permanent recording of catheter positions by means of a spot film device, and cine-angiography or angiocardiography. Demonstration of the catheter position to students and visitors by means of a television screen is optional.

Although all these operations except the last may be accomplished by a conventional fluoroscope and an angiocardiograph with rapid cassette changer, we believe that the use of an image intensifier is practically mandatory today. The principal argument in favor of this equipment is economy of radiation. By effective use of the photomultiplier tube the amount of radiation may be cut to as much as one tenth of that involved with the conventional fluoroscope. This is an important saving, not only for the patient, but also for the physician. A second advantage of the image intensifier is particularly pertinent to children; the use of a semidarkened room eliminates some of the fear inherent in the procedure. Finally, the television screen is an excellent teaching medium which is not available through the conventional fluoroscope.

An image intensifier with a 9-inch tube has been used in our laboratory. In connection with a closed-circuit television unit and a motor-driven camera, it has worked satisfactorily from both the fluoroscopic and the cine-angiographic viewpoints.

The Recorder.   A multichannel photographic recorder has been in use in our laboratory for the past several years. In connection with an oscilloscope it furnishes instantaneous visualization as well as permanent records of the following phenomena, singly or simultaneously: electrocardiograms, pressure pulses, indicator dilution curves, sound tracings, and respirations.

Manometers.   At least two, but preferably more, strain-gauge pressure transducers should be on hand at all times.

Oximeters.   The photometric method of oxygen analysis has all but displaced the cumbersome, gasometric, Van Slyke machine. The speed, precision and accuracy inherent in the photoelectric method have encouraged most workers in the field to rely almost entirely on photoelectric cells for their oxygen determination. The Van Slyke method is used only for an

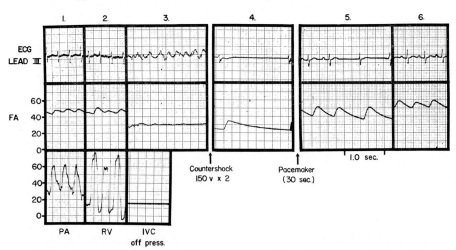

Figure 150.   Development of ventricular fibrillation during catheterization. Note the appearance of ventricular tachycardia in the electrocardiogram when the catheter is in the pulmonary artery and continuing as the catheter is withdrawn through the right ventricle into the inferior vena cava. At this point pressures were not monitored. Between panels 3 and 4 two countershocks were applied. Between panels 4 and 5 the patient's heart was driven by the pacemaker. In panels 5 and 6 normal sinus rhythm has returned, with good femoral arterial pressures.

occasional check on the photometric method and for determination of dissolved as well as hemoglobin-bound oxygen.

In this country light transmission is the most frequently used photometric principle.[742] In Europe the reflection principle, introduced by Brinkman and by Ziljstra,[762] is also widely used for this purpose.

Oximetry may be used for analysis of blood samples obtained in a syringe and transferred to the laboratory or, instantaneously, at catheterization by withdrawing blood into a cuvette oximeter and reinjecting it into the patient. The latter method is quicker and entails little blood loss for multiple samplings. On the other hand, the accuracy is not quite comparable to the syringe technique, and the withdrawal of blood through some of the cuvettes may be time-consuming.

A further modification of the photoelectric technique is one in which the optical density of the blood is measured at appropriate wave lengths. Such a "densitometer," after appropriate calibration, is a most accurate and sensitive detector for dye dilution curves.

Douglass bags, a Pauling oxygen analyzer, and appropriate gauges and mouthpieces are necessary for determination of oxygen consumption.

Surgical Instruments, Catheters, Solutions. Catheterization packs containing hemostats, forceps, knives, blades, syringes, needles, suture materials, sponges, drapes, towels and glassware should be made up daily and autoclaved in one unit.

Lehmann catheters in sizes 4 to 8, varying in length from 50 to 125 cm., should be available in ample supply. Special catheters for angiocardiography, with side holes, and double-lumen catheters for simultaneous sampling from two sites should be on hand for special occasions.

A manual or automatic injector for radiopaque dye is necessary for adequate angiocardiography.

Solutions of isotonic saline, heparin and the commonly used drugs should always be in ample supply.

Emergency Equipment. In addition to oxygen and drugs (digitalis, Pronestyl, quinidine, and pressor agents), a thoracotomy kit and an external defibrillator and pacemaker are indispensable parts of the equipment. It cannot be stressed often enough that not only should these supplies be present, but also their working efficiency should be checked periodically. It is well to arrange an emergency drill every three to six months so that everybody in the laboratory knows exactly what to do, where to go, and what to get in case of an emergency. The three-minute interval between cardiac arrest and irreversible brain damage is very short, and countermeasures must be promptly organized (Fig. 150).

Information Obtained

Basically, cardiac catheterization furnishes information about blood flows and pressures in various segments of the circulation.

Blood Flow. CARDIAC OUTPUT. *Fick principle.* One of the most important results of cardiac catheterization in man is the accurate determination of the cardiac output. One way to calculate this is based on the Fick principle, which states that if we know how much oxygen the organism uses within a measured period (minute oxygen consumption), and if we can also ascertain the amount of oxygen extracted from each liter of circulating arterial blood during the same interval (arteriovenous oxygen difference), then we can calculate how many liters of blood have to go around every minute in order to use up the number of milliliters of oxygen determined by the oxygen consumption test. This line of thought may be expressed in an equation:

$$\text{(1) Cardiac output, L./min.} = \frac{\text{O}_2 \text{ consumption, ml./min.}}{\text{A-V difference, ml./L.}}$$

Preferably, oxygen consumption is *determined* according to one of the methods discussed, or it is *assumed* on the basis of a table of averages collected from our data (Table 11, p. 779). The arteriovenous oxygen difference is calculated by subtracting from the *determined* arterial oxygen content (brachial or femoral artery) the *determined* oxygen content of mixed venous blood. The latter sample, if no left-to-right shunt is present, should be from the pulmonary artery or the right ventricle; samples from the right atrium or the superior vena cava are much less well mixed and much less representative of mixed venous blood. Samples from the inferior vena cava are almost totally useless for this purpose.

An example will clearly illustrate the calculations.

$$\text{(2) Cardiac output} = \frac{\text{O}_2}{\text{A-V difference}} \text{ (see Fig. 151)}$$

If oxygen consumption is 160 ml. per minute, oxygen content of the arterial blood is 190 ml. per liter, and oxygen content of mixed venous blood (PA) is 150 ml. per liter. Then

$$\text{C.O.} = \frac{160 \text{ ml./min.}}{190 \text{ ml./L.} - 150 \text{ ml./L.}} = \frac{160 \text{ ml./min.}}{40 \text{ ml./L.}} = 4 \text{ L./min.}$$

Obviously, comparison of the cardiac output of patients of various sizes can be made only by relating the actual volume to that of a standard-sized person. By convention, a patient having a body surface of 1 square meter is the standard means of comparison. The cardiac output expressed in liters per minute per square meter of body surface is called the cardiac index. The cardiac index is determined by relating the cardiac output to the patient's calculated surface area.

The next equation gives a clear example of this.

$$\text{(3) C.O.} = \frac{150}{190 - 140} = 3 \text{ L./min.}$$

If body surface area is 1.5 square meters, cardiac index is 2 liters per minute per square meter.

The cardiac output determined by the Fick principle is usually accurate and reproducible within a 10 per cent error. The principal source of error is, of course, the determination of the oxygen consumption. A second cause for error may be that the venous blood sample was not truly a "mixed" sample.

With all these sources of error, it is really surprising that the cardiac index usually falls consistently between 3 and 5 liters per minute per square meter at any age. If the output is appreciably higher than this, the patient probably was not in a basal state. Patients in hyperdynamic situations

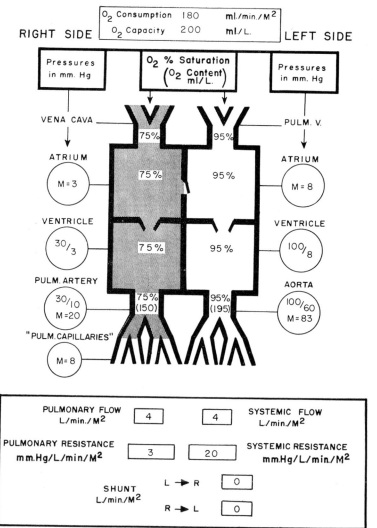

Figure 151.   Diagram of normal circulatory dynamics with pressures, oxygen contents and per cent of saturations.

(thyrotoxicosis, anxiety, anemia, arteriovenous aneurysms) have consistently high outputs. Interestingly enough, patients with compensated severe congenital aortic stenosis may have high normal cardiac outputs also. Low cardiac outputs, if real, are characteristic of hypothyroidism and congestive heart failure. A further reason for low output may be that the determination of the oxygen consumption was wrong and that the mouthpiece was leaking, giving lower than real consumption figures.

Of course, severe exercise invariably increases oxygen consumption to three to eight times the resting value. In normal persons this is accompanied by a corresponding increase in cardiac output. In patients with diminished cardiac reserve (some normal children and, strangely enough, athletes in training) the arteriovenous difference may widen considerably with the result that the cardiac output does not increase appreciably on exercise.

This kind of exercise response suggests, but is not conclusive evidence of, congestive heart failure. In the supine position most of the increase in cardiac output is accomplished by an increase in rate, with relatively little increase in stroke volume. In the upright position an increase in stroke volume occurs within the first few seconds or minutes of the exercise until the stroke volume is increased to its maximum, which equals the supine value; thereafter the rate increase becomes effective again.

Dye dilution method. A second method for determination of the cardiac output utilizes indicator dilution curves. This may be done by the instantaneous injection method, using the Stewart-Hamilton formula or one of its modifications.[743]

$$\text{(4) Cardiac output} = \frac{\text{indicator (mg.)} \times 60 \text{ (sec.)}}{\text{transit time (sec.)} \times \text{mean concentration (mg./L.)}}$$

In this equation, indicator means the dye injected in milligrams, and transit time ($Td-ta$) is the time interval between the extrapolated disappearance time and the appearance time; the mean concentration is calculated by measuring the area underneath the linearly replotted curve and relating it to time.

We have been using this method to determine the cardiac output in patients during left ventricular puncture, when general anesthesia makes it impossible to apply the Fick principle. The dye is injected into a peripheral vein, and a systemic artery is used for sampling.

Another method for determination of the cardiac output by dye dilution curves is the constant-rate injection method, using the following equation:

$$\text{(5) Cardiac output} = \frac{Q}{C_E}$$

Q equals the quantity of dye injected per minute, and C_E is the equilibrium concentration of the dye at the site of sampling. I have had no experience with this method, but others[638] have found it to be satisfactory and of comparable accuracy to the other methods described.

CALCULATION OF SHUNTS. *The oxygen method.* Since no significant change in the oxygen content, or percentage of saturation, of the blood occurs between the various chambers of the right side of the heart under normal circumstances, an appreciable increase in the oxygen saturation in one cavity over that of a proximal one usually means admixture of arterial blood, i.e. a left-to-right shunt. Since the mixing of venous blood is least complete in the right atrium (which receives blood of three different saturations—from the superior vena cava, the inferior vena cava, and the coronary sinus, respectively, in order of diminishing saturation), the amount of change in oxygen saturation in this chamber, compared to that in the superior vena cava, must be rather large to be significant. Samples from the inferior vena cava are so unstable that they should never be used for comparison. The blood in the right ventricle is usually considerably more homogeneous; thus a smaller difference between the oxygen content of this cavity and that of the right atrium is of diagnostic significance. Finally, even minute differences between the oxygen content of the pulmonary artery and that of the right ventricle are important.

Thus it seems clear that the larger the difference between the two chambers and the more distal in the right side of the heart it occurs, the more significant it is. Furthermore, one set of samples showing an increase in saturation is less significant than several sets of samples showing the same general trend. Finally, the level of oxygen saturation at which the change occurs should be taken into consideration, particularly if it is related to the pulmonary venous saturation. For instance, if the oxygen saturation is 85 per cent in the right ventricle, an increase to 90 per cent in the pulmonary artery, if the pulmonary venous blood is 94 per cent saturated, indicates a much larger shunt than an increase from 65 to 70 per cent with an arterial, or pulmonary venous, saturation of 98 per cent.

Taking all these factors into consideration, I believe that a 1.5 volumes per cent change between the superior vena cava and the right atrium, a 1 volume per cent change between the right atrium and the right ventricle, and a 0.5 volume per cent change between the right ventricle and the pulmonary artery are surely of diagnostic significance.

By expressing the same information in percentage of saturation and relating it to the number of sets of samples obtained, smaller differences may be made to count. An increase in oxygen saturation of 15 per cent in one set of samples, between the superior vena cava and the right atrium, or of 10 per cent in at least 2 sets of samples, is deemed significant. Similarly, an increase of 10 per cent in one set of samples and 5 per cent in at least 2 sets of samples is a significant difference between the right atrium and the right ventricle. Finally, an increase of 5 per cent between the right ventricular outflow tract and the pulmonary artery is indicative of a left-to-right shunt into the pulmonary artery.

Also, by expressing the values in this fashion (in per cent of saturation), the influence of oxygen capacity on shunt calculations can be eliminated. Table 12 (p. 780) indicates the magnitude of change in oxygen content caused by changes in capacity. It also demonstrates the different changes in volumes per cent caused by the same change in per cent of saturation at different levels of capacity. Table 12 (p. 780) indicates the effects of pulmonary venous and systemic venous saturation on the size of a left-to-right shunt. A practical application of these figures may be shown by lowering the mixed venous saturation by exercise, and thus demonstrating a significant shunt which was not obvious at the high, resting, venous saturation level. The latter maneuver is best carried out by using two catheters for simultaneous sampling during exercise, one in the right atrium and the other in the pulmonary artery. The fact that it is difficult to appreciate the significance of an increase in per cent of oxygen saturation at high mixed venous saturation levels makes it hard to demonstrate the presence of a ventricular septal defect if an atrial defect is also present. Similarly, a hemodynamically significant shunt at the ductal level may barely be noticed if a coexisting ventricular septal defect raises the saturation significantly within the right ventricle.

All these facts, in addition to the possibility of regurgitation (pulmonary and tricuspid) and the effects of streaming, make the reliance on a single set of samples analyzed for oxygen a dubious basis for calculating left-to-right shunts. Utmost caution is necessary for interpretation of data. Repeated observations and correlations with other physiologic and clinical data are essential for correct interpretation of data on oxygen saturation.

The significance of low systemic arterial saturation is relatively easy to appreciate. The only significant pitfall to avoid is the misinterpretation of pulmonary venous unsaturation. It is comparatively common, particularly in patients under anesthesia or in small infants with pulmonary disease, to find that arterial saturation of less than 91 per cent is due not to a right-to-left shunt, but to pulmonary venous unsaturation secondary to ventilatory trouble. The surest way to differentiate pulmonary cyanosis from that caused by a right-to-left shunt is to determine the pulmonary venous saturation by passing the catheter into the left atrium and the pulmonary vein. If this is not technically feasible, an oxygen study should be undertaken. The patient inhales 100 per cent oxygen for 5 to 10 minutes. At the end of this period an arterial sample is obtained, while the patient is still breathing pure oxygen. If the arterial unsaturation is due to pulmonary factors, the arterial saturation as well as the dissolved oxygen (1.5 to 2.0 volumes per cent by the Van Slyke method) will become normal. If, on the other hand, the arterial unsaturation is due to an intracardiac right-to-left shunt, the arterial oxygen saturation may indeed rise significantly, but the dissolved oxygen will stay low.

Taking all these precautions into consideration, one may now propose the Fick equations for calculation of right-to-left and left-to-right shunts.

$$\text{(6) C.O. systemic } (Q_s) = \frac{O_2 \text{ consumption}}{\text{Systemic A-V difference}}$$
(systemic arterial O_2 content minus mixed venous O_2 content)

$$\text{(7) C.O. pulmonary } (Q_p) = \frac{O_2 \text{ consumption}}{\text{Pulmonary A-V difference}}$$
(pulmonary venous O_2 content minus pulmonary arterial O_2 content)

If Q_p is more than Q_s, there is a left-to-right shunt. If Q_p is less than Q_s, there is a right-to-left shunt.

Two examples readily illustrate the situation.

(8) O_2 consumption = 150 ml./min. Hence: C.O. (systemic) $= \dfrac{150}{190-140} = 3$ L./min.

BA O_2 content = 190 ml./L.

C.O. (pulmonary) $= \dfrac{150}{190-160} = 5$ L.

RV O_2 content = 140 ml./L.
PA O_2 content = 160 ml./L.

Shunt from left to right = 2 L./min. at the pulmonary arterial level.

O_2 capacity   = 200 ml./L.
PV O_2 content = 190 ml./L.
    (assumed)

(9) O_2 consumption = 150 ml./min. Hence: C.O. (systemic) $= \dfrac{150}{170-120} = 3$ L.

BA O_2 content = 170 ml./L.

C.O. (pulmonary) $= \dfrac{150}{190-120} = 2.1$ L./min.

PA O_2 content = 120 ml./L.
O_2 capacity   = 200 ml./L.

Shunt from right to left = 0.9 L./min., level not determined.

PV O_2 content = 190 ml./L.
    (assumed)

It may be seen in example 8 that the systemic output is smaller than the pulmonary; hence the shunt is from left to right, and its magnitude is two thirds that of the systemic output. It is also clear from this example that the shunt occurs at the pulmonary arterial level; hence it indicates the presence of a patent ductus arteriosus.

In contrast, in example 9 the systemic output is about 50 per cent more than the pulmonary output, implying a right-to-left shunt, the site of which cannot be determined from these particular data. It may be seen that in order to calculate the systemic flow in a patient with right-to-left shunt, the assumption has to be made that the pulmonary vein is 95 per cent saturated.

If bidirectional shunting occurs, the "effective pulmonary flow" must be determined first.

(10) Effective $Q_p = \dfrac{O_2 \text{ consumption}}{\text{pulmonary venous } O_2 \text{ content minus mixed venous } O_2 \text{ content}}$

(11) Then the left-to-right shunt $= Q_p$ minus effective Q_p, and the right-to-left shunt $= Q_s$ minus effective Q_p.

Dye dilution method. If dye injected into the venous circuit appears in the systemic artery in an abnormally short time, a right-to-left shunt is indicated. If the first hump on the ascending limb may be sharply separated from the main portion of the curve, a quantitative estimation of the right-to-left shunt is feasible, with certain qualifications. By selective injection of the dye into various right heart chambers, the site of the right-to-left shunt may be determined with relative ease (Fig. 152). For instance, if injection into the right atrium results in an early appearance of dye in the systemic artery, whereas injection into the right ventricle fails to produce an early hump, it may be assumed that the right-to-left shunt occurs at the atrial level.

The presence of a recirculation curve, a late hump on the descending limb, indicates that a left-to-right shunt occurs (Fig. 146). The appearance time and build-up time are normal, but the peak deflection is reduced,

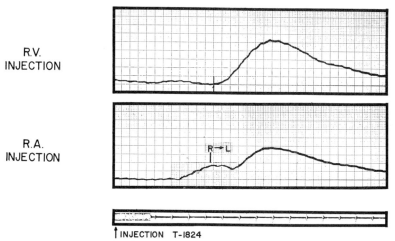

↑INJECTION T-1824

Figure 152. Localization of a right-to-left shunt site by indicator dilution curve. Note the early appearance of dye in the systemic artery with injection in the right atrium and a late appearance if injection is in the right ventricle. This indicates that the right-to-left shunt occurs between the right and left atria.

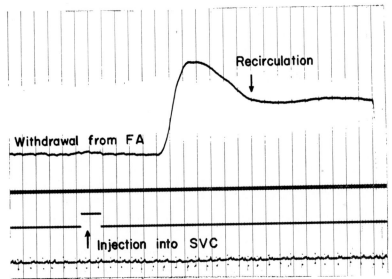

Figure 153. Dye dilution curve indicating aortic regurgitation. Note that the same type of recirculation curve is seen as is commonly noted with a left-to-right shunt.

and the disappearance time is prolonged. Similar tracings may be obtained, for similar reasons, in patients with valvar regurgitation (Fig. 153).

The degree of distortion in the dilution curve is proportionate to the size of the left-to-right shunt; methods for quantitative estimation have been described.

The localization of left-to-right shunts by the dye dilution method necessitates injection into the left side of the heart through one catheter and sampling from various chambers of the right side of the heart through a second catheter. Injection into the left side may be accomplished either by the retrograde approach, through the aortic valve, or by injection into the peripheral pulmonary artery. In the latter instance the dye being injected is assumed to have the same effect as though it had been placed directly in the left atrium.

The difference in appearance time between dye injected into the left and that injected into the right pulmonary artery may be utilized for differentiation of an anomalous pulmonary vein from an atrial septal defect.

Foreign gas method. During the inhalation of an inert gas, such as nitrous oxide or radioactive krypton, its concentration in the right side of the heart and the pulmonary artery is negligible. In the presence of an appreciable left-to-right shunt, significant amounts of the inert gas leak into the right heart chambers and are demonstrable in the blood samples obtained through the cardiac catheter. The ratio of the gas content in systemic arterial and pulmonary arterial blood after ten seconds of inhalation is proportionate to the size of the left-to-right shunt. The site of the shunt may be deduced from the site of the sampling. Right-to-left shunts may be detected by injecting radioactive krypton (dissolved in saline solution) into various right heart chambers and sampling from the systemic artery. Since clearance of the gas in the lung capillaries is almost complete, its appearance in the systemic arterial blood is indicative of a right-to-left shunt. The site of the shunt may be detected by varying the sites of injection within the right side of the heart.

Within the last year, inhalation of hydrogen and sampling with a platinum electrode from the right side of the heart gave promise of an easy method for detection of a left-to-right shunt of even small magnitude.

Cine-angiography and angiocardiography. By selective injection of radiopaque dye through the cardiac catheter into various left and right heart chambers, good visualization of the course of the dye may be obtained. This, of course, is not a quantitative method, but may be an excellent qualitative approach to the left-to-right and right-to-left shunt problems.

CALCULATION OF REGURGITANT FLOWS. I believe that it is fair to say that all methods proposed so far for accurate quantitation of regurgitant flows leave much to be desired. Satisfactory qualitative approaches to the problem are numerous. The simplest and in many ways the most effective way to demonstrate valvar regurgitation is to inject radiopaque dye distal to the regurgitant valve and to document its appearance in the proximal chamber by means of cine-angiography. Injection into the ascending aorta results in filling of the left ventricle in cases of aortic regurgitation. Left ventricular injection opacifies the left atrium if there is mitral insufficiency. Severe valvar regurgitation distorts the dye dilution curves in a fashion similar to that caused by a sizable left-to-right shunt. By selective injection of the dye into the left ventricle and sampling from the left atrium, localization of the regurgitant flow is possible. Korner and Shillingford[400] suggested empirical regression equations for calculation of mitral regurgitation. The method did not stand close scrutiny. Another quantitative method for estimation of aortic regurgitation involved injection of radiopaque dye through a retrogradely introduced arterial catheter. The farther from the aortic valve left ventricular filling occurred, the greater was the degree of aortic regurgitation.

Pressure Measurements. Perhaps the most important, and in many ways the most accurate, information obtained by the cardiac catheterization procedure is the measurement of pressures in the various heart chambers.

The recording of pressure pulses, through a long, fluid-filled catheter, through various connecting tubes, by means of a pressure transducer containing air or liquid, introduces some inevitable distortions. These may be exaggerated by the "fling" of the catheter in high velocity portions of the circulatory system (Fig. 154). Damping may be introduced by air bubbles or clots (Figs. 155, 156). Nevertheless, by skillful use of a critically damped system, adequate and reproducible tracings may be obtained. The catheters, the recording device and the manometers used in our laboratory have been described.

Phasic tracings are recorded in all chambers. Mean pressures are obtained by electrical integration in all but the ventricular cavities. Various pressure attenuations are used in various chambers under varying circumstances. In addition to the invaluable information about hemodynamics furnished by adequate pressure tracings, they also serve as a monitor in localizing the position of the catheter. Table 13 (p. 780) indicates the range of normal pressures obtained in patients in our laboratory. Zero point is at midchest.

The following facts are obvious even on cursory inspection of normal pressure pulses: (1) Atrial mean pressures and ventricular end-diastolic pressures are closely similar. There is even closer similarity, in fact practical

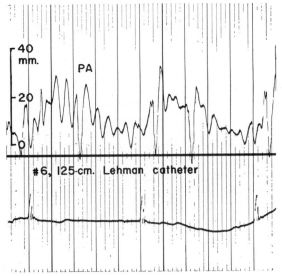

Figure 154. Undamped pulmonary arterial tracing indicating "fling."

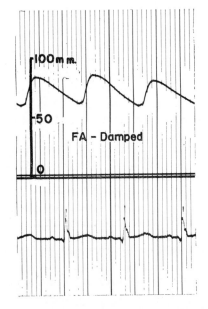

Figure 155. Femoral arterial tracing before flushing of the catheter.

identity, between the A wave and the end-diastolic pressure in the ventricle. (2) A definite rise in systolic pressure occurs between atria and ventricles. (3) A definite rise in diastolic pressure occurs between ventricles and great arteries. (4) There is no systolic gradient across the pulmonic or aortic valves. (5) Systolic pressures on the left side are appreciably higher than those in the corresponding chamber on the right. The normal range of pressures in the various heart chambers is listed in Table 13.

ATRIAL TRACINGS. In effect, *right atrial* pressure pulses are identical to the jugular venous pulse tracings (Fig. 157). Of the three waves, the A and the V with their respective x and y depressions can be seen well, but

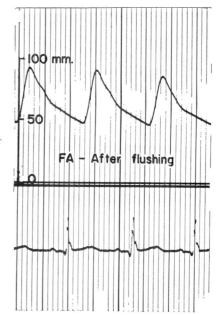

100 mm.

50

FA – After flushing

0

Figure 156.   Femoral arterial tracing after flushing of the catheter.

the C wave is often missing. Presumably, this is due to the lack of the reflection of the carotid pulse. Even during quiet respirations the atrial pressure varies appreciably with the intrathoracic pressure. In dyspneic infants the fluctuation may amount to 10 to 15 mm. of mercury (Fig. 158). *Left atrial* tracings are similar to right atrial tracings, but are not identical to or synchronous with them. The mean pressure, as seen in the table, is higher, as are the A wave and the V wave. The reason for this probably lies in the different volume-pressure characteristics of the left ventricle. Left atrial systole begins consistently within a fraction of a second after right atrial systole. Whereas placing the cathether in a midlateral position in the right atrium is fairly easy, in the small left atrial cavity artefacts are more likely to be introduced, either because of pressure of the catheter against the wall or because the catheter is too near the mitral valve. If the catheter is withdrawn continuously on "mean" pressure through a foramen ovale, a drop in pressure clearly indicates the point at which the catheter enters the right atrium from the left atrium (Fig. 159). Close similarity or identity of left and right atrial mean pressures is characteristic of atrial septal defect (Fig. 160).

Tall A waves on the right side may mean pulmonic stenosis, pulmonary vascular obstruction, tricuspid atresia or stenosis, or Ebstein's disease. Tall A waves in the left atrium may indicate left ventricular hypertension (either essential, or that caused by aortic stenosis or coarctation), mitral stenosis or atresia, ventricular septal defect or patent ductus arteriosus. The A wave is not present in atrial fibrillation, in which a fusion of the x and y descent occurs.

Tall V waves in either atrium mean regurgitation of the respective atrioventricular valve. Tall V waves in the right atrium are seen also in atrial septal defect. The estimation of atrioventricular regurgitation may be difficult if the mean pressure in the atrium is high (because of congestive

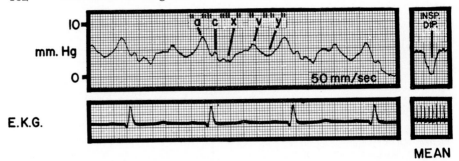

Figure 157. Normal right atrial pressure tracing. Note the A, C and V waves with the x and y depressions. Note also the dip in right atrial pressure on inspiration. The pressure here is mean pressure, electrically integrated. Compare this tracing with the jugular venous tracing in Figure 9.

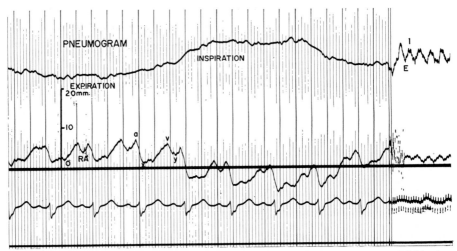

Figure 158. Changes in right atrial pressure tracing with respiration. Compare with inspiratory dip in Figure 157.

heart failure, atrial fibrillation or even stenosis of the atrioventricular valve).

A well marked y descent excludes atrioventricular stenosis. The ratio of the y descent to the height of the V wave is one of the ratios suggested for calculation of the degree of mitral incompetence.[544]

VENTRICULAR TRACINGS. Ventricular systole corresponds approximately to the Q-T interval of the electrocardiogram. Left ventricular systole begins with mitral closure and ends with aortic closure, whereas right ventricular systole is delineated by the corresponding events on the right side. Both ventricular tracings have an *isometric contraction phase* beginning with the atrioventricular valve closure and ending with semilunar valve opening. The first point is easy to identify by the beginning of ventricular upstroke, and the second by the onset of the rise of the central arterial (aorta or pulmonary artery) tracing, occasionally visualized on the ventricular tracing as an anacrotic notch. The *ejection* phase of ventricular systole begins with semilunar opening and ends with semilunar closure, identified by the dicrotic notch.

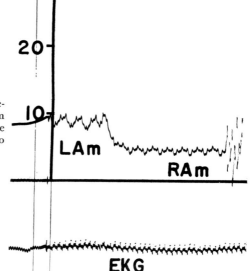

Figure 159. Withdrawal of catheter from left atrium to right atrium through the foramen ovale. Note the drop in mean pressure between the two atria. This is the normal situation.

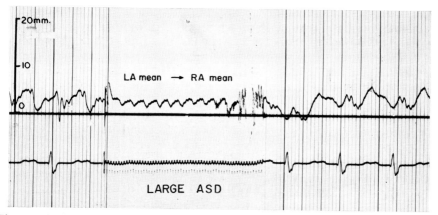

Figure 160. Equal left atrial and right atrial pressures in a patient with large atrial septal defect.

Ventricular diastole may be defined electrocardiographically as corresponding to the interval between the end of the T wave and the onset of the Q wave. Hemodynamically, it is the period between closure of the semilunar and closure of the atrioventricular valves. A drop in pressure to slightly below the diastolic level usually occurs after semilunar valve closure. After this dip some low frequency vibrations occur, followed by a steady diastolic low pressure level. Toward the end of diastole a small pressure rise may occur again, secondary to overdistention of blood from the atria (Fig. 161).

As indicated, under normal circumstances left ventricular systolic pressures are three to four times right ventricular pressures. The appropriate figures are indicated in Table 13 (p. 781). In patients having large ventricular septal defects, the pressures in the two ventricles are practically identical.

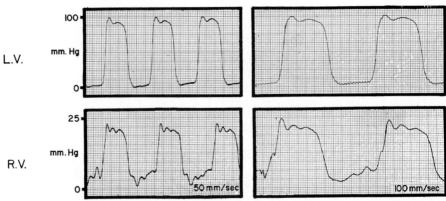

Figure 161. Normal right and left ventricular pressures. Note the identical contour, but that left ventricular systolic pressure is about four times the right ventricular systolic pressure. Diastolic pressure is down to zero in both instances. In the left side panels the pressure tracings are inscribed at 50 mm. per second, and in the right hand panel, at 100 mm. per second.

Extrasystoles change the normal systolic pressure, depending on diastolic filling time. If diastole is long, the pressure is high; if short, it is lower than normal. The height of the pressure corresponding to the extrasystolic and postextrasystolic beat depends not only on the amount of diastolic filling, but also on the time in the cardiac cycle when the irregular beat falls. Premature beats in patients having large ventricular septal defects do not result in significant differences between the pressures of the two ventricles.

An increase in right ventricular systolic pressure is observed in patients with pulmonic stenosis, ventricular septal defect and pulmonary vascular obstruction. An increase in left ventricular pressure occurs in aortic valve disease, coarctation of the aorta and systemic hypertension. Regurgitation of the atrioventricular valve is reflected in the ventricular tracing by some lowering of the systolic peak and an early, sharp diastolic dip.

An increase in diastolic pressure in either ventricle indicates congestive heart failure, semilunar regurgitation, or constrictive myocardial or pericardial disease.

ARTERIAL TRACINGS. The central arterial systolic pressure is identical with ventricular systolic pressure. When the pulmonic valve opens, the pulmonary arterial pressure climbs, steeply at first, then more gradually, and then goes into a steady decline as far as the dicrotic notch, indicating valve closure (Figs. 162, 163). No anacrotic notch can be seen in the pulmonary arterial pressure tracing, whereas on the aortic tracing a notch is commonly observed.

In pulmonic stenosis of appreciable degree, the pressure is low and resembles a mean pressure pulse without phasic variations. In pulmonary hypertension the systolic, diastolic and mean pressures may be elevated to varying degrees, according to the underlying physiology. The shape of the curve is usually grossly altered.

Pulmonary incompetence as part of the picture of pulmonary arterial hypertension, or as a manifestation of "idiopathic" pulmonary arterial dilatation, seldom causes appreciable changes in the pulmonary arterial tracing. The more significant the regurgitation, the less diastolic gradient there is between the pulmonary artery and the right ventricle.

High diastolic pressure in the systemic artery predisposes to more regurgitation and a truly rapid downstroke, with absence of the dicrotic notch. Significant aortic stenosis may result in slight lowering of the central aortic pressure, or narrowing of the pulse pressure, but more characteristically it results in slowing of the rate of upstroke. The anacrotic notch is clearly visible, and vibrations representing the murmur of aortic stenosis are superimposed on the tracing.

In both aortic and pulmonic stenosis the diagnostic clue is definitely

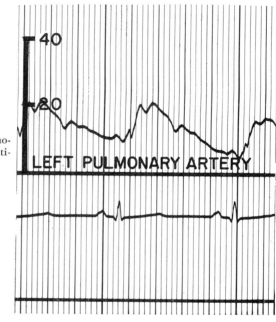

Figure 162. Normal pulmonary arterial pressure tracing critically damped.

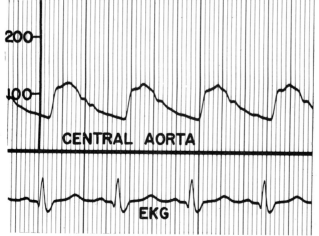

Figure 163. Normal central aortic pressure tracing. Note the dicrotic notch on the descending limb.

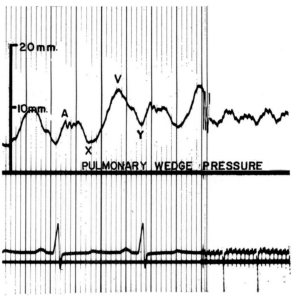

Figure 164. Normal pulmonary-capillary "wedge" tracing.

on the ventricular curve, not in the arterial tracing. The ventricular pressure is raised to maintain the necessary arterial pressure across a stenosed semilunar valve. In severe valvar (pulmonic or aortic) stenosis a so-called Bernouille effect can be noted in the central arterial tracing. This dip in pressure is caused by the negative suction of the jet of blood coming with high velocity through the narrow semilunar valve, past the tip of the catheter.

It should be re-emphasized that peripheral systemic arterial pressure is appreciably higher than central aortic pressure because of the reflected wave effect.

PULMONARY ARTERIAL WEDGE PRESSURE.   Dexter and his colleagues[192] made the observation that if the catheter is passed far out into the lung fields and "wedged" there, it reflects left atrial pressure. Although in most instances this is true in adults and normal animals, in many children and infants pulmonary wedge pressure is appreciably higher (5 to 10 mm. of mercury) than left atrial pressure. Still, with certain qualifications, pulmonary wedge "mean" and phasic pressures may be assumed to reflect left atrial pressure (Fig. 164).

PULMONARY VENOUS WEDGE PRESSURE.   Under certain circumstances, particularly in patients with maximal pulmonic stenosis or transposition of the great arteries, when the pulmonary artery cannot be entered, an approximate value of the pulmonary arterial pressure may be obtained by passing the catheter through the atrial septum into a pulmonary vein and "wedging" it as far as possible.

Resistance Calculations.   By relating the flow in a system to the pressure drop across it, a rough estimate of the resistance to flow may be obtained. Poiseuille's equation states that

$$(12) \quad R = \frac{\text{Pressure drop}}{\text{Flow}}$$

Within recent years it has been the custom in our laboratory to express the resistance in units and to relate it to the flow index rather than to the actual flow. By this method we believe that comparable values may be obtained from infants, children and adults.

Pulmonary vascular resistance:

$$(13) \quad R_p = \frac{PA_m - PC_m}{Q_p \text{ (index)}}$$

Systemic vascular resistance:

$$(14) \quad R_s = \frac{Ao_m - RA_m}{Q_s \text{ (index)}}$$

Normal values are between 1 and 3 units for the pulmonary vascular bed and between 10 and 20 units for the systemic circuit. If the resistance figure, calculated not on the basis of the cardiac index, but on the actual flow, is multiplied by eighty, the resistance is expressed in dynes, seconds and centimeters to the minus fifth power, the unit used in the previous edition of this volume.

It cannot be emphasized strongly enough that these calculated resistances are merely useful approximations of the cross-sectional area of the respective vascular beds. Berglund[75] and Rudolph[599] stressed the fact that in order to truly appreciate the significance of any given resistance figure, the actual flow and the actual pulmonary arterial and left atrial pressures must be taken into consideration.

Orifice Calculations. Valve sizes may be calculated with reasonable accuracy by taking into consideration the pressure gradient across the valve, the flow through it, and the time during which flow occurs. The basic formula was worked out by Gorlin[292] for the mitral valve, but it has been applied successfully to the pulmonic and aortic valves as well. More important than the actual accuracy of the prediction is the principle of introducing flow and time factors, in addition to pressure measurements, to the understanding of valvar stenosis. Thus the calculated size of the orifice becomes less of a contest between the cardiologist's slide rule and the surgeon's finger, arbitrated by the ruler of the pathologist, but rather one way of expressing physiologic information of comparative value. The formula for the mitral valve is as follows:

$$(15) \quad MVA = \frac{MVF}{31 \sqrt{Pc_m - LV_{dm}}}$$

MVA indicates mitral valve area in square centimeters. *MVF* indicates mitral valve flow, which equals cardiac output in cubic centimeters per minute over diastolic filling period in seconds per minute. Pc_m equals pulmonary capillary mean pressure or, preferably, left atrial mean pressure. Preferably, left ventricular diastolic mean pressure should be measured. If this is not possible, it may be assumed to be 5 mm. of mercury, i.e. left ventricular end-diastolic pressure. The diastolic filling period (*DFP*) in seconds may be measured directly from a left ventricular or systemic arterial pressure tracing. The diastolic filling period per beat should be multiplied by the beats per minute to calculate diastolic filling period per minute. Errors in calculation may occur because of an appreciable degree of mitral regurgitation and lack of a steady state. Normal area is about 5 square centimeters. Significant disease is present if the valve area is less than 1.5 square centimeters.

The aortic valve area may be calculated on the basis of the following formula:

$$(16) \quad AVA = \frac{AVF}{44.5 \sqrt{LV_{Sm} - A_{Sm}}}$$

$$AVF = \frac{\text{Cardiac output in cc./min.}}{\text{SEP (systolic ejection period) sec./min.}}$$

Normal values are between 3 and 4 square centimeters. Critical stenosis is less than 0.8 square centimeter. The formula for the pulmonic valve area is:

$$(17) \quad PVA = \frac{PVF}{44.5 \sqrt{RV_{Sm} - PA_{Sm}}}$$

Normal values are 2 to 4 square centimeters, and critical stenosis is less than 0.8 square centimeter.

ACQUIRED
HEART DISEASE

PART TWO

7

ACUTE RHEUMATIC
FEVER AND
RHEUMATIC
HEART DISEASE

ACUTE RHEUMATIC FEVER

Incidence and Etiology

Rheumatic fever is one of the two most important causes of heart disease in children. It is difficult to determine its incidence accurately, since there is no unanimity as to diagnostic criteria. Furthermore, the disease is not a reportable one in the United States. In countries where rheumatic fever is reportable, incidence varies between 11 and 30 per 10,000 persons each year. In our climate about 25 per cent of the adults with heart disease can clearly be classified as rheumatic.[728] In England, in 1927, it was estimated that 10 to 15 per cent of children less than 12 years old were affected by rheumatic fever or rheumatic heart disease.[746] School surveys in the United States within recent years place the incidence of rheumatic heart disease, in children 5 to 19 years of age, at between 2 and 6 per 1000, depending on geographic location.[338] More recent figures place the incidence in school children at between 1 and 4 per cent.[157] In Norway[569] the incidence of acute rheumatic fever has been reported to be approximately 3 cases per 10,000 persons. According to a recent report of the United States Public Health Service, the incidence of definite rheumatic heart disease among college students is approximately 7 per 1000 students. Finally, according to Metropolitan Life Insurance Company statistics, in 1944, rheumatic fever and rheumatic heart disease was the principal cause of death among persons 5 to 20 years of age.

Although proof pointing to the magnitude of the problem seems unequivocal, there is equally convincing evidence that rheumatic fever has been declining in incidence in the last fifty years. Glover[281] found that the crude death rate from rheumatic fever and rheumatic heart disease fell from 67 per million of population in 1901 to 22 per million in 1937 in England. In the urban population of Denmark the number of acute rheumatic fever cases declined from about 45 per 10,000 to approximately 5 per 10,000 between 1885 and 1945. It is interesting to note that the relatively low incidence in the rural population changed comparatively little during the same period. During a recent trip to Sweden I was amazed to find that, according to the pediatricians, acute rhematic fever among children is practically nonexistent there. A trip to Greece during the same period, the spring of 1961, indicated that in that country severe acute rheumatic fever is a common disease. One might possibly attribute these differences to the economic conditions in the two countries. There has been an equally steady decline in rheumatic mortality and morbidity in the United States during the past forty years, according to the Metropolitan Life Insurance Company.[338] The downward trend has increased significantly within the past twenty years. The same tendency may be discovered in statistics available from the United States armed forces; in World War II the incidence of rheumatic fever was only one tenth of that in World I. Whether this change has been brought about by the improved socioeconomic status of the population, by antibiotics or by unknown factors cannot be said with certainty.

The etiology of rheumatic fever is unknown, but certain factors play a decisive role in its causation. The association of rheumatic fever with group A hemolytic streptococci has clearly been established to the satisfaction of most observers in the field.[151, 551] Careful questioning can elicit a definite history of antecedent streptococcal infection in about 50 per cent of the cases of rheumatic fever occurring in adults. Epidemics of rheumatic fever usually follow epidemics of streptococcal infection in isolated communities and army camps. In rheumatic fever convalescent homes there has been no recurrence without the presence of hemolytic streptococcal infection.[405] Active rheumatic fever is almost invariably accompanied by unusually high antistreptolysin O titers.[672] Finally, the prevention of streptococcal infections by means of chemoprophylaxis practically eliminates rheumatic recurrences, whereas in carefully selected control groups the expected number of attacks have developed after streptococcal infection.[403, 487, 713]

The incidence of streptococcal infection obviously varies a great deal, depending on geography, age group, economic status, and so forth. Studies of Dingle and his co-workers in Cleveland[198] indicate that streptococci may be responsible for 1 to 3 per cent of all respiratory infections. According to one study,[671] the incidence in adults is approximately half that noted in adolescents living under the same circumstances. More recent figures from Chicago[642] indicate that although 47 per cent of more than 2500 children with nasopharyngitis had beta hemolytic streptococci in their throats, four fifths of which belonged to group A, in only half of them could the organism be typed serologically.

The incidence of rheumatic fever after known streptococcal infection has been estimated to be, on the average, 2 to 3 per cent. Apparently children are more susceptible than adolescents, and adolescents more than adults. The attack rate for rheumatic fever in children in the recent Chicago study was only 0.33 per cent, contrasting sharply with the 3 per cent figures relating to airmen at Warren Air Force Base, and corresponding closely to the clinical impression of pediatricians.

Although the streptococcus is clearly implicated in the etiology of rheumatic fever, it cannot be said to cause the disease as long as it can be recovered from throat cultures in only 50 to 60 per cent of rheumatic fever patients and practically never from the blood stream, the heart, the joints or the nodules of these patients. Furthermore, rheumatic fever cannot be produced by injection of hemolytic streptococci into animals. The present concept, then, accepted by most workers, is that rheumatic fever represents a particular host reaction to group A hemolytic strepto-cocci. Supporting this hypothesis is the work of Rich,[584] who found tissue reactions similar to Aschoff bodies in animals dying from anaphylactic shock.

The role of heredity in the etiology of rheumatic fever has been discussed repeatedly. May Wilson[734] and her group, studying several families with rheumatic fever on the lower East Side of New York City, came to the conclusion that the disease is inherited according to the mendelian recessive pattern. She stated unequivocally that if both parents are rheumatic, nearly every child is susceptible to rheumatic fever; if one parent is rheumatic and the other is a carrier (i.e. rheumatic fever is present in near relatives), each child has a 50 per cent chance of getting rheumatic fever. Though most observers cannot accept heredity as the sole etiologic agent, all agree that familial disposition unquestionably plays an important role in determining who will and who will not get rheumatic fever when attacked by group A hemolytic streptococci.

The geographic distribution of rheumatic fever suggests that climatic factors may have considerable influence on the development of the disease. According to a recent survey of school children, the lowest incidence may be found in areas as geographically distant as New York, Massachusetts, Virginia, Tennessee and Oklahoma. Relatively high rates are found in North Carolina, Kentucky, Nebraska and Washington. The Rocky Mountain states, Colorado, New Mexico, Wyoming, Montana, Utah, Idaho, Arizona, Nevada, South Dakota and Oregon, have the highest incidence, but this is almost matched by that of Pennsylvania and Indiana. This indicates that factors other than climate may have considerable influence on this geographic distribution. Recent figures from tropical climates, such as the Philippine Islands,[10] suggest that rheumatic heart disease may be almost as common in these geographic areas as it is in New England.

Age is a definite factor in the development of rheumatic fever. The disease seldom occurs in children less than two years of age, though within the last five years approximately six children in this age group have been treated for severe rheumatic carditis at The House of the Good Samaritan. Its incidence declines rapidly after puberty. The younger the patient, the more likely is the rheumatic fever to be severe. First attacks usually occur in children between six and eight years of age. Recurrences also follow an age patern; they are more likely to occur in the young, and are rare after the age of 25. Recurrences are much more likely within the first year after the initial attack; the longer the period following the original attack, the less likely is a recurrence.

Socio-economic influences on the development of the disease cannot be denied. Poor housing, crowding, dampness and poor diet—poverty, in short—predispose to rheumatic fever.

Seasonal incidence of rheumatic fever correlates well with that of hemolytic streptococcal infections. March to May is the high point of the year, whereas August and September seem to have the lowest incidence.

Pathology

The pathology of rheumatic fever will be discussed only briefly and only on the basis of data available in the literature. My personal experience with such pathologic material is not extensive or recent enough to be of significant value.

The earliest pathologico-anatomic changes in rheumatic fever are nonspecific, exudative ones. These are seldom observed today, since early deaths from fulminating forms of the disease are rare. Nevertheless reports of these cases point to edema, hemorrhage, tissue necrosis and round cell infiltration as the principal features. The changes occur throughout the body, but particularly in the heart, joints and lungs. The myocardium may be especially affected, and maximal cardiac dilatation without endocardial proliferation may occur.

In contrast to these early, nonspecific exudative changes are the chronic proliferative features of subacute and chronic rheumatic infection. Essentially, these changes consist in scar formation, the production of specific granulomas, and thrombosis. These lesions are found most characteristically in the heart, blood vessels, lungs, periarticular spaces, tendons and the central nervous system.

For obvious reasons, rheumatic changes in the heart have been described in the greatest detail. The endocardial changes consist principally in verrucose endocarditis, localized on the atrial surfaces of the mitral valve and the ventricular surfaces of the aortic valve. The tiny kernels, consisting of debris and fibrin, are found predominantly at the line of closure of the valve and on the chordae tendineae. The valves are swollen, edematous and distorted. The parietal endocardium is rarely involved. The myocardium is the site of perivascular round cell infiltration and specific Aschoff bodies; these are usually seen in the subendocardial myocardium, especially in the left atrium and the ventricles. The pericardium, if involved in the process, characteristically presents the picture of serofibrinous pericarditis, varying from the "bread-and-butter" type to the predominantly exudative form.

The development of these acute or subacute changes furnishes the anatomic basis of rheumatic heart disease. The verrucose lesions, at first easily removable from the valves, become more and more adherent. The valves themselves lose their elasticity or become scarified, and the leaflets adhere to each other. The papillary muscles and chordae tendineae thicken and become plastered with exudate. If there are recurrences in the rheumatic process, fresh vegetations and fresh exudates are produced irregularly on the already affected surfaces. As a result of the thickening and adhesion of the leaflets, stenosis of the mitral valve occurs within a matter of years (two to eight years, according to Cary Coombs[166]), though individual cases of mitral stenosis have been known to develop in less than one year's time. The shortening of the chordae and the papillary muscles prohibits the valves from closing completely; hence they become incompetent. This process, in contrast to the stenosis, may develop (at least in a functional sense) within a few weeks.

Aschoff bodies, the principal feature of myocardial involvement in the rheumatic state, have been thought to be short-lived. They seldom are seen within the first weeks of acute rheumatic fever and probably disappear within six months after their first appearance. During this short life span they undergo changes from "fibrinoid degeneration" to a granulomatous stage, and finally to scar formation. This concept that Aschoff bodies are short-lived and represent an acute rheumatic process has been challenged by the finding at biopsy of more or less typical Aschoff bodies in the atria of approximately 40 per cent of patients who were undergoing mitral valvotomy and in whom there was no evidence of rheumatic activity. If scar tissue develops around the conduction system, permanent conduction disturbance may result. If the myocardial involvement is severe and persistent, serious, and even fatal, cardiac dilatation may ensue without major valvular deformity.

Rheumatic pericarditis, although of severe prognostic importance in the acute stage, seldom leads to chronic pericardial disease. Constrictive pericarditis on a rheumatic basis seldom, if ever, occurs. If the heart can recover from the endocardial and principally the myocardial involvement, the pericardium usually heals without any significant residuum.

Other organs involved in the rheumatic process should be mentioned briefly. In the acute stage the lungs may be the site of pneumonitis of the hemorrhagic type. Rheumatic encephalitis with round cell infiltration around the basal ganglia has been described. The rheumatic joint is characterized by redness of the synovia, serous fluid accumulation in the joint spaces and fibrin deposits over the cartilage; Aschoff bodies may be found in the periarticular tissue and the synovia. Rheumatic subcutaneous nodules, attached to tendons or periosteum, may be found over joints, scalp and vertebrae. Histologically, they represent granulation tissue similar to Aschoff bodies. Nodules usually last several weeks or months.[486] They can be produced experimentally by injecting blood subcutaneously into rheumatic patients.

Clinical Picture

Since, as has been pointed out before, rheumatic fever is considered to be a specific host reaction to invasion by the group A hemolytic streptococci, it can easily be seen that the clinical picture, depending on the host, will be protean indeed. Depending on age, heredity, climate and economic factors, a number of rheumatic syndromes may present themselves.

Antecedent Infection. In about 50 per cent of children having rheumatic fever the parents describe a cold, a sore throat or even scarlet fever ten to fourteen days before the onset of illness. This was treated with an inadequate dose of an antimicrobial agent, only transiently, or not at all. The severity of this respiratory infection was average, and its duration usually no more than two to four days.

The Acute Attack. GENERAL SIGNS OF INFLAMMATION. These usually begin ten to fourteen days after the antecedent infection and consist of (1) fever. Characteristically, this is not high; it ranges between 101 and 103° F., and is of the relapsing type. High spiking temperatures, such as are seen commonly in rheumatoid arthritis, are rare. (2) Polymorphonuclear leukocytosis of moderate degree, (3) elevated erythrocyte sedimentation rate, positive C-reactive protein, and elevated antistreptolysin O titer, (4) mild (or occasionally severe) anemia secondary to depressed erythropoiesis, increased plasma volume, diminished red cell survival, and even severe nosebleeds, (5) lassitude, irritability and moderate weight loss.

SPECIFIC MANIFESTATIONS. These may best be discussed under the headings of individual syndromes, recognizing the fact that, commonly, not one but several of the syndromes, of varying intensity, make up the clinical profile.

Arthritis. Rheumatic fever involves several joints simultaneously or in succession. Monoarthritis almost never is a manifestation of rheumatic fever. The joints involved are usually the large ones: knees, ankles, wrists and elbows. Heat, redness, swelling, severe pain, and tenderness are the rule. If, as is the custom on many orthopedic services, the joint is tapped, clear, serous, sterile fluid of high protein and cell content is obtained. From this description of rheumatic arthritis it may be seen how sharply different it is from the vague muscle and tendon pains called "growing pains," the relation of which to rheumatic fever is questionable. Differentiation of the two conditions is possible by simply asking the mother what she is doing for the pains of the youngster. If she says that the child likes to have his limbs rubbed or massaged, one can be almost certain that one is not dealing with rheumatic arthritis. This condition, in its true form, makes the joints so tender that even the weight of a blanket may be intolerable.

Carditis. Definite evidence of carditis almost requires the diagnosis of rheumatic fever in children. Although accurate figures on the occurrence of carditis in unselected cases of rheumatic fever are not available, the incidence is usually considered to be about 50 per cent, and it is found in every fatal case.

For the evaluation of carditis, a knowledge of the condition of the patient's heart before the onset of the present illness is of great importance. This is particularly pertinent in trying to determine whether or not the presence of a murmur indicates acute carditis. If the murmur was clearly not present before the attack of rheumatic fever, the likelihood that it signifies carditis is strong. Apical systolic murmurs can be considered significant only if they last at least through the first half of systole and if the intensity is at least grade 3. Apical diastolic murmurs, always significant, are commonly found in acute carditis at a time when no organic mitral stenosis is present.[65] The origin of this murmur is not clear, but it is thought to be due to relative mitral stenosis caused by dilatation of the left ventricle. Aortic diastolic murmurs are also noted early in the history of carditis; in contrast to the diastolic murmurs in the mitral area, these are more likely to become permanent. All these murmurs may develop into permanent auscultatory features or may be entirely transient, and the heart, after recovering from acute carditis, may sound entirely normal.

The heart sounds in acute carditis often lose their luster and become distant, dull and muffled. Taran[680] emphasized the development of embryo-cardia, an equalization of the duration of systole and diastole, resulting in a tic-tac-like rhythm. Diastolic gallop is commonly present.

Cardiomegaly of appreciable degree can usually be demonstrated on physical examination. Serial radiograms give objective evidence, and are useful as guides to prognosis. At fluoroscopy the heart beat is usually feeble. Enlargement of the left atrium, demonstrated in the right anterior oblique view, is emphasized by Wilson[734] as a prime criterion of carditis.

Pericarditis can usually be detected by the presence of a friction rub. Sometimes, with the development of a large effusion, the friction rub disappears; at this stage, however, the massive cardiomegaly, the feeble heart sounds, poor cardiac pulsation, and evidences of tamponade usually reveal the diagnosis. On the other hand, rheumatic pericarditis is practically never seen without a significant murmur. Although pericarditis is of serious prognostic significance, it usually does not require paracentesis except occasionally for diagnostic purposes.

Evidences of congestive failure, i.e. distended neck veins, puffy face, hepatomegaly, pulmonary rales, low urinary output and even pitting edema, can all be regarded as evidences of carditis. Almost axiomatically, any child with rheumatic heart disease who is in failure must have active carditis. This is in contrast to older people, in whom congestive failure may be the outcome of the mechanical stress placed on the heart by rheumatic valvular involvement. *Right-sided failure, particularly involving facial edema, probably secondary to left-sided failure, is characteristic of congestive failure in rheumatic children.* Pure left-sided failure, on the other hand, is relatively rare. The accumulation of fluid in some of these youngsters may be so great that they have been known to be admitted to hospital wards as "nephrotics" (Fig. 165).

In discussing the characteristic features of active carditis, in addition to the specific signs of congestive failure—endocardial, myocardial or pericardial involvement—the less specific but nevertheless characteristic general signs and symptoms must also be mentioned. These children are anxious, frightened and perspiring; they show slight peripheral cyanosis, which improves in oxygen. The pulse is usually rapid and thready, although bradycardia has been found in 50 per cent of a series of adults with rheumatic fever.[339] Dyspnea, orthopnea with flaring of the alae nasi, is prominent.

The electrocardiogram is a sensitive index of active carditis.[548] (This statement has been challenged by Feinstein and his associates,[241] principally on semantic grounds.) The changes may be transient, however, and, unless frequent, even daily, electrocardiograms are taken, may be missed completely. Prolongation of the P-R interval (first-degree block) and the presence of the so-called Wenckebach phenomenon (second-degree block) (Fig. 166) are the most commonly mentioned abnormalities,

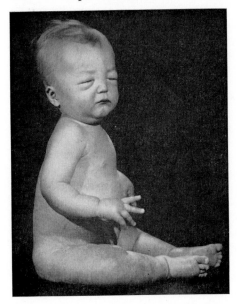

Figure 165. Photograph of little girl with congestive failure due to rheumatic carditis. Note the similarity to the features of patients with nephrosis.

T-wave changes and QRS abnormalities may be noted also. But *the presence of a prolonged P-R interval, per se, does not mean active rheumatic fever or carditis.* [579] Many cases of impaired atrioventricular conduction reflect only past rheumatic activity; in others it may be congenital in origin. In this respect a transient prolongation of the atrioventricular conduction time is more suggestive of an active process than is a permanent one. We have even seen second-degree block persist through the years without any evidence of active rheumatic fever. Taran[173, 249, 681, 746, 748] emphasized the importance of measuring the corrected Q-T interval in cases of suspected rheumatic fever; he regarded a QT_c of 0.42 second or more as definite evidence of active carditis. He also stated that, with obvious carditis, a QT_c of less than 0.42 second probably indicates pericardial involvement. Others have failed to find a high degree of correlation between active carditis and QT_c. [173, 249] Nodal rhythm, S-T and T wave changes, atrial fibrillation and bundle branch block are less common evidences of active carditis. Sinus tachycardia is the rule, as mentioned, with occasional instances of normal rate or even sinus bradycardia.

Chorea. In terms of immediate prognosis, chorea is the most benign of the rheumatic syndromes; whereas all patients who die with acute rheumatic fever have carditis, practically none has chorea. There has also been noted an antagonism between the presence of chorea and the other acute rheumatic syndromes; the simultaneous occurrence of polyarthritis and chorea is practically unknown. In spite of this, there can be little doubt that chorea is one of the rheumatic manifestations, since, according to various authors, from 50 to 75 per cent of patients with chorea exhibit other rheumatic manifestations at some time before or after its appearance. According to the well controlled series of Ash,[21] about a third of these patients had definite rheumatic heart disease ten years after the onset of the chorea. It should be mentioned, however, that these patients were not on chemoprophylaxis.

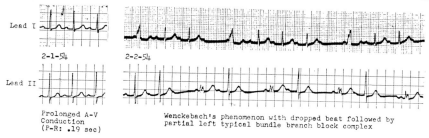

Lead I
2-1-54 2-2-54
Lead II
Prolonged A-V
Conduction
(P-R: .19 sec)
Wenckebach's phenomenon with dropped beat followed by
partial left typical bundle branch block complex

Figure 166. Electrocardiographic changes in acute rheumatic fever. Note in the tracing of February 1 the prolongation of the P-R interval, in the tracing of February 2 the Wenckebach phenomenon with left bundle branch block or aberrant interventricular conduction.

St. Vitus's dance is different from the other rheumatic syndromes, not only because it is a solitary event within the rheumatic cycle, but also because of the absence of general signs of inflammation (fever, leukocytosis) and of acute phase reactants (sedimentation rate, C-reactive protein).

The occurrence of an antecedent infection is more than usually difficult to determine because of the vague onset of the disease. Emotional disturbances are usually the first manifestations. The child, most often a girl between the ages of eight and twelve years, becomes difficult to live with. She tends to be extremely moody and irritable. At school she cannot concentrate; at home she refuses to do her chores. She fights incessantly with her siblings. Parents and teachers alike resent her attitude, and pressures are put on. This only aggravates the situation; the changes in mood become truly explosive.

A few weeks after the gradual onset of emotional instability, involuntary movements are first noted. They are quick and brusque, and involve all parts of the body. Voluntary movements become difficult to execute and bring on choreiform twitchings. The handwriting deteriorates and becomes almost illegible. Glasses and china are easily broken when the child helps with the dishes. She cannot unbutton her clothes or lace her shoes.

Signs of ataxia appear. The speech becomes slurred and gait hesitating; her movements lose all their grace and become jerky and angular. When sticking out her tongue at the time of the physical examination, she jerks it back suddenly and snaps her jaws. The tongue itself may show twitchings and fibrillary motion.

Evidences of weakness occur. Her grasp is hesitating and unsustained. She cannot play her favorite games, and tires easily.

All these signs of weakness and locomotor ataxia may be limited to one side of the body only (hemichorea).

Skin manifestations. The rashes seen in patients with rheumatic fever may include nonspecific lesions, such as urticaria, petechiae and erythema nodosum. On the other hand, erythema marginatum is, for all practical purposes, a specific and main manifestation of severe rheumatic fever. It consists of a circinate macular and erythematous rash appearing on the trunk or extremities, but not on the face, usually symmetrically distributed and of varying duration. The typical pattern consists of a wavy, thin red line surrounding an area of intact skin about 1 to 2 cm. in size (Fig. 4, p. 15). No itching or discomfort is associated with it.

Rheumatic nodules are definitely a major and specific manifestation of rheumatic fever. Similar to erythema marginatum, they occur almost exclusively in the severest types of rheumatic fever with carditis. They are never transient; if untreated, their duration is from several weeks to months. They occur symmetrically, singly or in clusters, loosely attached to joint capsules, tendon sheaths or the periosteum. They are freely movable under the skin. Most commonly they are seen over the joints, scalp and vertebrae. Initially, they may best be discovered by looking for them in an indirect light; later they can be felt without any difficulty. They are not painful or tender; their size varies from that of a small pea to a small almond (Fig. 3, p. 14).

Epistaxis. Severe nosebleeds commonly occur in acute rheumatic fever, although within the past decade their incidence at The House of the Good Samaritan in Boston has definitely been decreasing. Repeated nosebleeds in a child with rheumatic heart disease, but without any of the principal manifestations of the disease, are not especially rare.

Abdominal pain. Often the presenting symptom of a patient with acute rheumatic fever is abdominal pain. If this is accompanied by general signs of inflammation, a rigid abdomen and right lower quadrant localization, differential diagnosis from acute appendicitis may be difficult indeed. If an exploratory laparotomy is done, the peritoneum will be found to be moderately injected, with swollen mesenteric glands and a slight increase in the peritoneal fluid. Acute appendicitis is the admitting diagnosis in a number of patients with acute rheumatic fever referred to our hospital.

Pneumonia. Rheumatic pneumonia is rare and indicates severe rheumatic fever. Furthermore, it may be impossible to tell in any given case how many of the signs and symptoms of pneumonitis are caused by left-sided congestive failure, pulmonary hemorrhage, secondary infection or true rheumatic granulation tissue.

Differential Diagnosis

Jones, in a historic paper in 1944,[368] suggested definite diagnostic criteria for rheumatic fever. Although later he stated that publication of a set of definite criteria might introduce an element of unnecessary rigidity into the diagnosis of rheumatic fever, still for didactic purposes this represents an extremely useful classification. He divided the clinical syndromes into two groups, major and minor manifestations. The major manifestations were carditis, chorea, subcutaneous nodules and previous attacks of rheumatic fever. The minor manifestations were fever, adominal pain, precordial pain, rashes, epistaxis, pulmonary changes, anemia and high sedimentation rate; later an elevated antistreptolysin O titer was added to the list. Jones felt that the diagnosis of rheumatic fever could be made with certainty if any two major, or one major and two minor, manifestations of rheumatic fever were present. The least specific of these combinations is the presence of arthralgia with fever and elevated sedimentation rate.

More recently a committee of the American Heart Association modified these criteria in the following manner:[158] major criteria: (1) carditis, (2) polyarthritis, (3) chorea, (4) subcutaneous nodules, (5) erythema marginatum; minor criteria: (1) fever, (2) arthralgia, (3) prolonged P-R interval in the electrocardiogram, (4) increased erythrocyte sedimentation rate, presence of C-reactive protein or leukocytosis, (5) evidence of preceding beta hemolytic streptococcal infection, (6) previous history of rheumatic fever or the presence of inactive rheumatic heart disease.

Although in many instances the diagnosis of rheumatic fever can be made at the time of the first visit, in a number of cases observation extending to weeks or months is necessary before a definite opinion can be expressed. On the other hand, since the advent of hormone therapy, a number of investigators, especially Massell[484] and his associates at The House of the Good Samaritan, have stressed the necessity of early diagnosis. They believe that steroids in adequate doses, administered early in the disease—before the advent of carditis—may prevent the development of valvular deformities. Since, among the five major manifestations, arthralgia is the only one that is likely to precede carditis by an appreciable interval (chorea is usually not followed by carditis within the same cycle, and rheumatic nodules without carditis are extremely rare), a great deal of emphasis is placed on the early identification of arthritis as rheumatic. Thus the presence of polyarthritis, with signs of inflammation and an elevated antistreptolysin titer, should be regarded as prima facie evidence of rheumatic fever. It is difficult to argue against the validity of this concept in terms of diagnosis. Nevertheless, the therapeutic implications to be drawn from it represent, in my mind, a much more controversial point.

Probably all children in whom the diagnosis of rheumatic fever has been made on the basis of the criteria mentioned will have the disease. The only exceptions are patients having other collagen diseases, which are really cousins of rheumatic fever. Rheumatoid arthritis, or Still's disease, should be mentioned in detail. Children with rheumatoid arthritis may have either no fever at all or a spiking, septic type of temperature. Even if the fever is high, the patients are usually not sick in proportion to their febrile response. The joints involved are more commonly the smaller ones (metacarpal or metatarsal) or the unusual ones (sternoclavicular or mandibular). The inflammatory process is not as painful as that which we are accustomed to see in rheumatic fever; the joints are tender, but not excruciatingly so, and are only moderately red. The involvement is more chronic, the fluid accumulation lasting for weeks and months in the same joint. The affected fingers assume a spindly appearance (Fig. 167). Cardiac involvement is rare; if it occurs, it is more likely to attack the pericardium and the myocardium, leaving the endocardium intact. Aortic regurgitation is certainly seen, on a rheumatoid basis, in adults with spondylitis. It is my impression that murmurs of mitral regurgitation also occur in patients, even children, having what seems like a pure form of rheumatoid arthritis. To ignore these murmurs or to assume that they are due to separate and distinct rheumatic fever seems equally unrealistic. I would not be surprised if some time in the future mitral regurgitation may be considered a cardiac manifestation of rheumatoid arthritis, much as aortic regurgitation is now. Nevertheless, *murmurs or cardiac involvement of any kind is a rare manifestation of rheumatoid arthritis.* Far from the 50 per cent incidence of carditis in rheumatic fever, cardiac involvement in rheumatoid arthritis is probably less than 10 per cent. Pulmonary arterial hypertension caused by pulmonary vascular disease has been seen in patients with rheumatoid arthritis. Splenomegaly is fairly common. Fleeting rashes of the erythema multiforme type are seen momentarily; erythema marginatum is rare. Laboratory tests reveal mild anemia, marked leukocytosis and elevated sedimentation rate. The antistreptolysin titer may or may not be elevated.

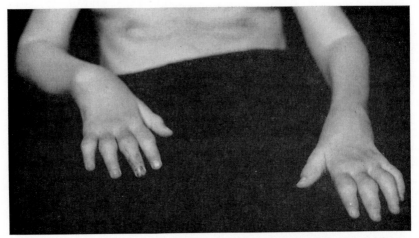

Figure 167. Typical joint involvement of patient with rheumatoid arthritis.

As can be seen from this brief description, the border between rheumatoid arthritis and rheumatic fever is not sharp. It is my personal belief that they may represent different host reactions to the same insult; everyone who has dealt with this problem to any extent has had the experience of seeing a patient with a clear-cut diagnosis of one of these conditions turn into an equally characteristic picture of the other. Nevertheless, from the practical, and principally prognostic, viewpoint the two entities should be kept separate. It may be said that rheumatoid arthritis is chronic joint disease without verrucose endocarditis.

Disseminated lupus erythematosus and periarteritis nodosa should also be mentioned as members of the collagen disease group in which widespread visceral and vascular lesions dominate, arthritis and carditis playing only minor roles.

A list of the referring diagnoses of patients who later turned out to have definite rheumatic fever may give some idea of the other problems in differential diagnosis. No detailed description of the distinguishing points will be given. Simply thinking about the entities will serve the purpose: appendicitis, poliomyelitis, toxic synovitis, osteomyelitis, nephritis, leukemia, tuberculosis and septicemia.

Course and Prognosis

Untreated rheumatic fever is a cyclic disease. Both the general signs of inflammation and the specific syndromes may wax and wane through weeks, months and perhaps years. Individual cycles are usually 6 to 12 weeks apart. Between these, although the disease seems quiescent, the sedimentation rate stays high, no significant weight gain occurs, and anemia persists. The patient does not seem to be quite himself, and the sleeping pulse rate may be high. It takes several months before one can be entirely certain that the disease has subsided. There is no single criterion to indicate when the acute attack has ended. Most centers taking care of large numbers of rheumatic patients require that a number of criteria be satisfied before they announce the process as being arrested. The principal requirements are as follows: (1) no evidence of major manifestations of rheumatic fever, (2) no signs of inflammation, (3) satisfactory weight gain, (4) normal erythrocyte count and hemoglobin, and (5) general sense of well-being, good disposition and good appetite. In an occasional child the sedimentation rate remains elevated, months beyond the subsidence of other criteria of activity, and may have to be disregarded.

The clinical course, as described, was considered to be the classic one in a child with rheumatic fever until approximately 1950. Within the past decade the profile of the disease changed. The change may have been a spontaneous one in the natural history of rheumatic fever, or it may have been brought about by advances in the fields of medicine and social welfare in the Western World. Whatever its cause, the change is striking. No longer are children staying in convalescent homes for months and years, their fever waxing and waning. The effective eradication of the streptococcus from the nasopharynx, the prevention of reinfection with the organism, and the potent antirheumatic and anticongestive drugs enable most children to return to their comfortable homes within a matter of a few weeks or months. The changing relation between the number of admissions to The House of the Good Samaritan and the average length of stay during the past 20 years graphically illustrates this change (Fig. 168).

With the termination of the acute attack, whatever end-point one may use, the question of recurrences and ultimate prognosis should be considered. The figures published by Bland and Jones on 1000 patients from The House of the Good Samaritan reflect the history of this disease as seen in Boston between 1920 and 1950.[63, 369]

The number of recurrences in their study depended a great deal on the time which had elapsed after the first attack. During the first 5 years there was a 20 per cent probability for recurrence; during the second 5 years the figure dropped to 10 per cent; during the third 5 years to 5 per

H.G.S. 1939-58

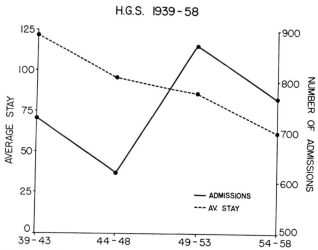

Figure 168. Total (first attack and recurrences) five-year admissions and average length of stay of patients with rheumatic fever at The House of the Good Samaritan in Boston. Changes between 1939 and 1958. Note the steady decline in the average stay from 125 days to approximately 70 days, with the fluctuation of total admissions between 700 and 775 per 5-year period.

cent; and finally between 15 and 20 years after the original attack, only 1.4 per cent had recurrences.

The long-term prognosis in the 1000 cases reviewed by Bland and Jones is summarized in Table 16 (p. 782). At the end of the first attack of rheumatic fever 65 per cent of 1000 patients had definite rheumatic heart disease. Of these children with definite heart disease, a third died within the first ten years and another sixth during the next ten years. To put it in another way, half of those who emerged from their first attack of rheumatic fever with heart disease were dead twenty years later. Most of these deaths occurred within five years after the initial attack.

In contrast to the poor prognosis of the group who acquire heart disease at the time of their first attack stands the favorable outlook of the 35 per cent who escape manifest cardiac damage initially. Of this group of 347 patients, none died as a consequence of rheumatic fever or rheumatic heart disease in the next 20 years.

Reviewing these mortality statistics according to specific rheumatic syndromes, it becomes obvious that gross cardiomegaly and congestive failure have the worst prognostic implications; 70 to 80 per cent of the patients with these conditions died within the first 10 years. In contrast, only 12 per cent of the children whose initial syndrome was chorea died within the same period.

The cause of death was acute rheumatic fever and congestive failure in 80 per cent, and subacute bacterial endocarditis in 10 per cent of the cases.

Of the total 1000 patients, about 650 were still alive 20 years after the initial attack, and three fourths of these were able to lead a relatively normal existence.

Somewhat less than half of the survivors (316 patients) had no residual heart disease at all. Two thirds of these were patients who escaped from their first attack without heart disease; however, a third of them (108 patients) were thought at the end of their first attack to have definite evidence of rheumatic heart disease, on the basis of apical, systolic or mid-diastolic murmurs, and even an occasional instance of faint aortic regurgitation.

Of the 650 patients in Bland and Jones's series who survived 20 years, 383 had definite rheumatic heart disease. The majority of these had acquired heart disease during their initial attack. But about 150 of them, mostly patients with chorea, had not had heart disease initially; in these mitral stenosis developed insidiously, without overt evidence of recurrence through the years.

Similar results were published by Ash and also by Wilson. Ash's[21] study of 537 children, followed up for 10 years, revealed an over-all mortality rate of 24.4 per cent. Among those with heart disease it was 42 per cent. She also found that about 10 per cent of the survivors of acute carditis, 50 per cent of the survivors of polyarthritis, and 66 per cent of the survivors of chorea had no residual heart disease 10 years after the initial attack. In this group more children died within the first year of the disease than in any subsequent year.

Wilson and Lim[735] reviewed data on more than 1000 children followed up during a 40-year period. Of those who reached the age of 20, 82 per cent would reach the age of 45, as compared with 95 per cent of the general population.

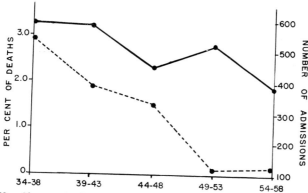

Figure 169. Changes in 5-year admissions of patients with rheumatic fever and percentage of death from first attack at The House of the Good Samaritan between 1934 and 1958. Note that the number of admissions for first attacks changed from about 550 to 390 per 5 years in the 25-year period, whereas the percentage of deaths dropped from about 3 per cent in the first 5-year period to practically zero in the last 10 years. In this figure the number of 5-year admissions is based only on first attacks; in Figure 168 all admissions are counted.

It seems, then, that in these studies, which preceded the antibiotic era, the over-all mortality was 25 to 35 per cent. It is also clear that most of the deaths occurred within the first five years, most likely within the first year of the disease.

There has not been enough time to collect a large amount of long-term follow-up data since the introduction of modern methods of treatment and prophylaxis. Nevertheless it is clear that children with first attacks of rheumatic fever seldom die in the hospital today. Figure 169 shows that at The House of the Good Samaritan of the Children's Hospital Medical Center, the 5-yearly death rate from a first attack of rheumatic fever is down from 3 per cent to practically zero, whereas the yearly admissions have not changed proportionately. Furthermore, as Massell and his co-workers[488] pointed out, 35 per cent of the patients discharged with a definite diagnosis of heart disease from The House of the Good Samaritan had no evidence of cardiac involvement 5 years later. This contrasts with about 10 per cent after the 20-year follow-up study of Bland and Jones,[63] from the same institution, in the preantibiotic era.

The larger the heart at the time of discharge, the louder the murmur, and the more extensive the valvular damage, the more likely is it that evidences of heart disease will persist. Feinstein and his associates[241] reported similar observations on several hundred children followed up from two to nine years. Among the patients with definite heart disease, 32 per cent had no evidence of cardiac involvement at the end of the study; of those with probable heart disease, 75 per cent seemed to have normal cardiac findings.

Treatment

Until the last ten years no specific treatment for acute rheumatic fever was available. There is still no unanimity about the effectiveness of various drugs on acute rheumatic fever, but an increasing number of clinicians believe that the course of the disease may be significantly influenced by a number of therapeutic agents. The use of hormones, salicylates, anticongestive measures and other therapeutic approaches will be discussed.

Hormones. The demonstration by Hench and his associates,[336] in 1949, of the beneficial effects of ACTH and cortisone therapy on patients with arthritis and other hypersensitivity states raised the hope that a cure for rheumatic fever might be at hand.

In order to make a scientific evaluation of the effects of the hormones on acute rheumatic fever, a combined study group was organized in the United States, Canada and Great Britain. This group included most of the large centers for study of rheumatic diseases in the respective countries and employed the talents of first-rate investigators and statisticians. A rigid schedule for case selection, dosage, and length of treatment was set up. Within a relatively short time 500 cases were collected; a third of these patients were treated with aspirin, another third with ACTH and a final third with cortisone. The three groups were selected in such a fashion that statistically significant comparisons could be made.

A detailed report of this study has been published,[581] indicating that there was no statistically significant difference in the results of the three plans of treatment. Aspirin seemed even slightly more beneficial than the hormones, and the pendulum swung away from hormone treatment. A five-year report from the same group confirmed the initial findings.[582]

While all this was going on, members of the study group made their own observations without the aid of IBM machines. Other investigators throughout the United States, Canada and England drew their own conclusions without statisticians, as physicians have done since time immemorial. The almost unanimous conclusion was that, from the clinical viewpoint, the hormones were immensely useful indeed. Though nobody could say with certainty that residual heart disease was less likely to develop in the hormone-treated patients, almost everybody felt that the sickest patients, the ones with pancarditis and congestive failure, were much more likely to recover with the use of the new agents than they would have been under the old treatment plan. There also seemed to be unquestionable and startling effects on fever, sedimentation rate, polyarthritis, pericarditis, subcutaneous nodules and electrocardiographic changes. No clearly significant effects on chorea or erythema marginatum were noted. The survey of the independent observations to date on the treatment of acute rheumatic fever with hormones has been admirably summarized by Massell.[484]

The opinion of most observers today is that hormones are a useful tool in the treatment of acute rheumatic fever. Obviously, they are not the whole answer to the problem, but the clinical impression prevails that the sickest children are much more likely to recover with hormones than they did before the advent of the steroid era.

As a matter of fact, I have the distinct impression that few children critically ill with acute rheumatic fever (pancarditis, congestive heart failure) are treated by responsible physicians without steroids. An excellent example of this is described in the publication of Kuttner and her associates[156] in the New England Journal of Medicine. A careful study was made in large centers on the Eastern seaboard, testing the efficacy of hormones versus salicylates in the treatment of acute rheumatic fever, using case selection by strict statistical methods. They concluded that there was no statistically significant difference in terms of residual heart disease between the various treatment schedules utilized. On the other hand, there were only six patients among the total who would be classified as being critically ill. Three of these were assigned to the steroid group and were so treated, and recovered. For three others, the statisticians assigned aspirin. One of these never received salicylates, in spite of the statisticians, because he was "too sick." He was given steroids and indeed recovered. A second one received aspirin for four days, at which time steroids were started because he was " too sick." He recovered as well. The third patient in the group received salicylates for nine days; then because of lack of clinical improvement he was switched to steroids, but died on the next day. I believe, then, that children with severe pancarditis have a much better chance to survive if treated with steroids than if treated with any other method presently available.

Whether a child who has acute carditis, but no pericarditis or congestive failure, is less likely to end up without residual heart disease if treated with steroids, rather than aspirin, is a much more difficult question to answer. Numerous investigators have looked at this question in numerous ways. I believe that at present there is no *conclusive* evidence that steroids prevent residual valvular damage. There is this to be said, though— the hormones accomplish their job of suppressing inflammatory signs more quickly, more certainly, than aspirin does. Hospitalization is shortened.[356] Furthermore, I know of no instance myself in which, if steroids had failed to control acute infection, aspirin would have been able to accomplish it. I do have personal experience with a number of cases in which the reverse was true. On the other hand, steroids may cause occasional serious complications (psychosis, peptic ulcer, hemorrhage with chickenpox). On the whole, I am in favor of steroid treatment in cases of acute rheumatic fever with carditis, with or without congestive failure and pancarditis. But, whereas in the pancarditis group I would consider it mandatory, in the others it should be left to the preference of the individual physician.

For a third group of patients, those with acute rheumatic fever without clinical evidence of carditis, I do not feel justified at this time in recommending hormone treatment. According to Bland and Jones,[63, 369] two thirds of their patients without initial carditis did not exhibit heart disease twenty years later. The patients in Bland and Jones's group, by virtue of the fact that they were referred to The House of the Good Samaritan, must have represented a collection of more seriously ill children than the ones the pediatrician is likely to see in his private practice today. If heart disease did not develop in two thirds of these patients, who were perhaps relatively sicker than the average, and who did not later benefit from chemoprophylaxis, one is scarcely justified at this point in recommending hormone treatment for the average patient with acute rheumatic fever who does not have cardiac involvement. Considerable evidence seems to have accumulated within recent years, indicating that if a patient has no evidence of heart disease when first seen within the framework of rheumatic fever, the chances are rather slim that it will develop during that attack at all. If 2 weeks after the onset he still shows no evidence of heart disease, there is a better than 90 per cent chance that no carditis will develop.[488] Feinstein's data indicate that if the patient escapes rheumatic heart disease during the first attack, it is unlikely to develop subsequently if adequate chemoprophylaxis is given. For all these statistical reasons and because of the well documented rare toxic effect of the hormones, it seems unwise at present to use these agents in the treatment of patients who have rheumatic fever without carditis. Recent observations indicate that intractable chorea, without carditis, may serve as an indication for hormone treatment.

In patients with chronic recurrent rheumatic fever the hormones, like anything else available at this time, are probably of no use. Hormone treatment should start early; there is considerable evidence that treatment instituted shortly after the initial attack has a much better chance to succeed than treatment administered later. Dosages should be high. A tentative schedule for cortisone and Meticorten, used presently at The House of the Good Samaritan, is included in Table 14 (p. 781). Wilson and his associates[736] recommended, instead of the long-term schedule outlined, a short course lasting on the average seven days. Among the forty-seven children these authors described, five required a second course of seven days. Large doses of steroids were recommended (hydrocortisone 300 mg., prednisone 100 to 150 mg.), the actual amount being determined by daily eosinophile counts. At the end of the seven- to eight-day period the drug was abruptly discontinued.

Dorfman and his co-workers[201] suggested hormone dosages equivalent to 2 mg. of hydrocortisone per kilogram of body weight for 9 weeks, with gradual tapering after that.

My own inclination is to take a middle ground between the very long and the very short courses. I would recommend that large doses of cortisone (200 to 300 mg.) or Meticorten (50 to 100 mg.) be used for 4 to 6 weeks, depending on the individual response. Then I would taper the drug in two weeks' time. I believe that in this way adequate hormone effect on the inflammatory process may be achieved without a disturbing maximal side effect.

A useful adjunct in the hormone treatment of acute rheumatic fever is careful control of the fluid intake to no more than 1000 ml. per day. The diet should contain no more than 50 to 100 mg. of sodium chloride daily. Potassium chloride in doses of 1.5 to 2 gm. should be added to the diet. Vigorous anticongestive measures, especially mercurials and digitalis, should be used if congestive failure is present. Antibiotics, probably penicillin or one of the broad-spectrum drugs, should be administered to guard against intercurrent infection and to eradicate any streptococci present in the nasopharynx.

There are definite drawbacks and dangers to hormone treatment. Cushing's syndrome (Fig. 170), with considerable weight gain, will develop in all patients treated according to the long schedule proposed. This will retrogress in almost all cases, but it is an unpleasant sight while it lasts. Unsightly striae accompany the weight gain. Bleeding peptic ulcers may develop. In some patients significant arterial hypertension develops to the extent that treatment cannot be completed. Glycosuria may appear; psychoses, although not common in children, do occur. The fluid retention inherent in steroid treatment may be disastrous to patients with congestive failure unless the beneficial effects of the hormones on the myocardium compensate for this.

One of the most serious complications of steroid therapy is its effect on infections. Haggerty and Eley[319] reported fatalities due to chickenpox

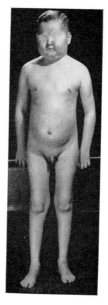

Figure 170.   Patient with fully developed
Cushing's syndrome.

in children receiving hormone treatment. Flare-up of latent tuberculosis has been reported in adults. I have seen bacterial endocarditis misdiagnosed as rheumatic fever and treated with steroids, resulting in the death of a patient with congenital heart disease.

One further drawback to hormone treatment is the development of the so-called rebound phenomenon. This consists in the appearance of a flurry of signs and symptoms of activity when hormones are discontinued. There is no good explanation for this phenomenon, but it seems somewhat more prevalent if short courses are given. It is possible that the "rebound" is nothing but the emergence of rheumatic activity, after cessation of the suppressive agent, and will last the length of the original cycle. This is a good argument against very short courses of treatment.

Salicylates.   For many years salicylates have been administered to achieve symptomatic relief in acute rheumatic fever. About 15 years ago Coburn[152] attempted to prove that intravenous administration of salicylates in doses raising the salicylate level to at least 30 mg. per 100 ml. of blood influences the course of the disease itself. This thought, although alien to the thinking of English and American physicians, has been widely accepted in Europe for a considerable time. Nevertheless an increasing number of physicians in this country are of the opinion that salicylates indeed have an "antirheumatic" effect over and beyond the obvious symptomatic relief they afford. Interestingly enough, this "renaissance" of aspirin resulted from the findings of the "combined study," designed primarily to investigate the efficacy of hormones, in which salicylates were used only as controls.[581] There is still no conclusive proof of the therapeutic effect of salicylates in rheumatic fever. The consensus today is that, when salicylates are administered, they too, much like the hormones, should be given in large enough doses for a long enough time.

The dosage used today at The House of the Good Samaritan is 1 grain (0.06 gm.) per pound of body weight per day in 4 to 6 divided doses.

The total dose should not exceed 10 gm. per day. This dosage should be continued for at least four weeks, when gradual "tapering off" may be introduced. Salicylate treatment should be continued, however, for at least six weeks, or until all signs of activity have disappeared. When salicylates are administered in large doses, vitamin C and vitamin K should be given simultaneously to prevent hemorrhage. If evidences of salicylate intoxication appear, the dose may have to be diminished or the drug entirely discontinued. Among the salicylate preparations, aspirin seems to be as effective as any. The enteric-coated tablets of sodium salicylate are palatable, but their satisfactory absorption cannot always be assumed.

Salicylates are the drugs of choice today for patients having acute rheumatic fever without carditis, except in cases of chorea, in which, even symptomatically, they are not effective. Whether salicylates should be used in addition to hormones in patients with severe carditis is debatable. It is important to note that when a patient with active rheumatic fever is switched from aspirin to hormone therapy, the aspirin should not be suddenly discontinued, but rather, gradually tapered with the onset of steroid administration.

Anticongestive Measures. The general principles of management of congestive failure will be discussed in a separate chapter (see p. 309). *Rheumatic fever patients in congestive failure should receive anticongestive drugs, in addition to steroids, in essentially the same fashion as do other patients with congestive failure.*

A great deal of controversy surrounds the use of digitalis in rheumatic carditis. Much of the argument centers around the point that a certain number of patients with acute rheumatic carditis die when digitalis is administered to them.[620, 621] Often it is forgotten that some of these patients are extremely sick and might die irrespective of the treatment. I believe that cautious, electrocardiographically controlled administration of digitalis is an extremely useful tool in the treatment of congestive failure associated with rheumatic carditis. Of course it must be remembered that these children may be extremely sensitive to the glycoside, and doses smaller than those usually given will be optimal in their treatment. It also should be pointed out that potassium depletion may develop in patients treated with corticoids, especially if mercury is administered simultaneously and potassium intake is low; it is well known that digitoxicity is more prone to develop in patients with low serum and intracellular potassium levels.[449] Consequently, if digitalis is given to a patient treated with steroids, an adequate potassium intake must be assured.

Eradication of the Streptococcus. The streptococcus carrier state can easily be treated with penicillin. Oral administration of one million units of penicillin per day in 4 divided doses for 10 days, or the single intramuscular injection of 600,000 to 1.2 million units of benzathine penicillin, accomplishes the purpose in practically all instances. After the eradication of the streptococcus, penicillin prophylaxis should be started immediately. Sulfonamides are apparently relatively ineffective in the treatment of streptococcal infections, although they may be used effectively for prophylactic purposes.

Bed Rest. One of the criticisms raised against the opinions expressed in the first edition of this volume was that the bed rest recommended for the treatment of acute rheumatic fever was too long and too strict. Reviewing the available evidence, it seems that the criticism was justified.

There seems to be no disagreement that during a florid, acute attack, with painful joints, congestive failure and pericarditis, strict bed rest is necessary. Under present day management this period does not usually last more than two weeks. As the acute danger and discomfort pass, bathroom privileges may be allowed.

At the end of a month, if the signs of cardiac embarrassment have disappeared and evidences of inflammation have been supressed, further increase in activities may be allowed. The speed with which a child should be allowed out of bed may be judged by observing his rebelliousness against bed rest. Usually, if these children are sick, they do not particularly want to get up. As they feel better, it is increasingly harder to keep them in bed. We usually start ambulation by allowing them one hour a day in a chair. Additional hours may be added to this, weekly, depending on the clinical progress. Often it becomes evident that "rest" is indeed much better accomplished by letting a child play quietly in a chair rather than jump up and down in bed.

Diet. The use of salt restriction in the diet of patients with congestive failure and those under hormone treatment has already been mentioned. During the feverish stage children do not want to eat, and they are better off with a liquid carbohydrate diet. When the fever has subsided, especially if they are under steroid treatment, the appetite will improve. They should be given a diet high in protein, carbohydrates and vitamin C. The appetites of some of the hormone-treated patients are astounding.

Prophylaxis

The use of chemotherapeutic agents for the prevention of rheumatic fever is predicated on the acceptance of two premises: one is the etiologic role of group A beta hemolytic streptococci; the other is the significance of the number of recurrences in the prognosis of rheumatic fever. If, as most people are willing to accept today, recurrent rheumatic fever damages the heart, and if recurrences are dependent on the presence of hemolytic streptococci, then it seems logical to try to prevent streptococcal infections, thus avoiding rheumatic recurrences and precluding further cardiac damage.

Massell and his group,[485] in a carefully controlled study at The House of the Good Samaritan, followed up a large number of children who received various penicillin preparations for long periods. Statistically, followup covered more than 12,000 patient weeks for rheumatic fever subjects, whereas the controls amounted to more than 16,000 patient weeks. Intramuscular benzathine penicillin, oral penicillin V and oral buffered penicillin G were used. All three preparations were effective to a high degree in preventing infection with group A hemolytic streptococcus. Nevertheless, the monthly intramuscular injection of benzathine penicillin seemed most effective in reducing clinical as well as subclinical streptococcal infections (91 per cent and 86 per cent reduction, respectively). Failure to prevent streptococcal infections by means of oral prophylaxis can always be blamed on the patient. "He probably did not take his medicine." This convenient explanation is not available if monthly intramuscular injections are given. In these cases, as in many others of oral prophylaxis, one must assume that the penicillin level achieved by the particular regimen was not adequate in the given patient. An increase in the dose of penicillin usually, but not invariably, accomplishes the desired result. There are a few patients, however, whose throat cultures remain positive even in the face of the most vigorous treatment with penicillin. These are rare instances of penicillin resistance. I am aware of only one such case in the patient population of The House of the Good Samaritan. It may be said, then, that with penicillin prophylaxis most patients may be kept free from group A hemolytic streptococcal infection, a small minority will need higher than average doses, and in still others a different antimicrobial agent may have to be used. Sulfadiazine, being a bacteriostatic rather than a bactericidal agent, may not be used for treatment of streptococcal infection, but is effective in prophylaxis, though less so than penicillin.

A second point to be discussed is the effectiveness of penicillin in eliminating rheumatic recurrence. The evidence is unequivocal. Bywaters and Thomas[122] indicated that sulfonamide prophylaxis reduced the mean incidence of recurrences from 5 or 6 per cent per year to 1.2 per cent. Penicillin reduced recurrences by 90 to 95 per cent.[489, 713]

Considerable controversy surrounds two points about the practical application of these principles. One concerns the duration of chemoprophylaxis, and the other the use of prophylactic measures in patients with throat infections who have not previously had rheumatic fever.

If the figures of Bland and Jones[63, 369] on the relation of rheumatic recurrences to the time elapsed since the original infection are valid, there seems to be no good reason to administer chemoprophylaxis longer than ten years after the first attack. Nevertheless, even if no more than 8 per cent of the patients have recurrences after 10 years, is it not worth preventing those? All that one may say is that every physician must make an individual decision in regard to each patient. There is a psychological point in the life of many patients at which getting rid of "pills" may be worth risking something in terms of rheumatic fever. Others do not mind taking medication ad infinitum. Fortunately for the pediatrician, this decision must be made by the internist in most instances. As far as pediatricians are concerned, anybody who has had acute rheumatic fever should be protected against streptococcal infection throughout childhood, probably for at least ten years.

Stollerman and his associates[671] pointed out that not only the time lapse from the last attack, but also the age of the patient, is important in this regard. They found that adolescents and adults are indeed less susceptible to streptococcal infections than children. Furthermore, even if older patients do become infected with the organism, recurrences are much less likely to occur in them.

The second controversial point concerns the treatment of sore throats in patients who have not had a previous attack of rheumatic fever. Every pediatrician sees, or talks on the telephone to the parents of, hundreds of children with sore throats, with or without fever. I do not believe that for practical purposes it would be feasible to treat all these for ten days with penicillin. The patient's patience, the druggist's bill and the psychological havoc are all limiting factors. A little common sense is extremely useful in this situation. Factors favoring the use of chemotherapy with ordinary sore throats are (1) family history of rheumatic fever, (2) evidence that the throat infection is streptococcal in origin (positive throat culture, presence of exudate, fever, leukocytosis, cervical lymphadenitis), and (3) crowded living conditions, i.e. boarding schools, army camps, and so forth. If none of these situations exists, I do not recommend that sore throats should be treated with antibacterial agents.

One further point should be disposed of briefly. It has been stated, and I could scarcely disagree more strongly, that all febrile illnesses at their onset should be treated with penicillin as a sort of diagnostic procedure. If the fever subsides within twenty-four hours, it was probably due to the hemolytic streptococcus; thus, according to this line of reasoning, the penicillin should be continued for ten days. If the fever does not disappear, I presume one ought to call a physician to find out what is the matter with the patient.

Any pediatrician knows that fevers of unknown origin, and of no particular consequence, make up a large part of his daily practice; he also knows that bed rest, fluids and mild antipyretics will keep the situation in hand in most instances. Although it has to be granted that an occasional case of rheumatic fever may result from this symptomatic regimen, it still seems to me the sensible course to follow because of the relative rarity of the disease, and the untold psychological, economic and even physical damage that would inevitably follow the continuous use of penicillin.

The drug of choice in chemoprophylaxis, at present, is penicillin. If a suspicion of acute streptococcal infection exists, the treatment schedule previously outlined for "eradication" of the carrier state should be used (see p. 190). This schedule should be followed by the prophylactic schedule of penicillin or sulfonamides. The recommended dose is either 1.2 million units of benzathine penicillin once a month, or 500,000 units daily of oral penicillin V or buffered penicillin G. Sulfadiazine or Gantrisin may also be used for prophylaxis, but not for treatment (0.5 to 1.0 Gm. per day).

Through the judicious use of penicillin, by one route or another, streptococcal infections may be eliminated.[98] It is worth mentioning that the earlier in the course of streptococcal infection this is accomplished, the less likely is it that rheumatic fever will occur. Still, if penicillin treatment is instituted as late as nine days after the onset of sore throat, the incidence of rheumatic fever will be significantly lower than in a control group.[503, 569] Continuous prophylaxis with penicillin or sulfonamides prevents streptococcal throat infections and thus significantly reduces the danger of recurrence of rheumatic fever.[403, 405, 487, 691, 713]

RHEUMATIC VALVULAR DISEASE

It may be possible for the internist to separate a chapter on rheumatic fever into two divisions, one dealing with the acute attack and the other with the mechanical consequences of rheumatic fever, i.e., rheumatic valvular disease. Histologic studies showing Aschoff bodies in the left atrial appendage in patients undergoing mitral commissurotomy,[693] however, strongly suggest that low-grade active disease may be present even in adults without clinical evidences of rheumatic activity.

In pediatrics it has long been known that every child having symptomatic rheumatic valvular disease should be strongly suspected of having some degree of activity. This is obviously not the case in all instances, but the burden of proof is on the physician who says that the rheumatic process is totally inactive in a child who is symptomatic with rheumatic heart disease. Consequently it seems wiser to discuss the entire rheumatic heart disease problem under one heading. In the following pages individual valvular lesions will be discussed as if they represented the only pathologic condition present, although the presence of acute rheumatic fever cannot, in most instances, be excluded with certainty.

DISEASES OF THE MITRAL VALVE

Evidences of mitral heart disease are obtained through auscultation in most instances. It is usually assumed that significant murmurs heard maximally at the apex of the heart are referable to the mitral valve; the assumption is also made that if no murmurs are heard at the apex, the mitral valve is intact. Although, as will be seen later, exceptions to these rules exist, still, by and large, they do hold true. The mitral valve alone, or in combination with aortic valvular disease, is involved in about 90 per cent of the patients with rheumatic heart disease.

According to the studies of Bland and Jones,[63, 369] it may be said that evidence of mitral heart disease appearing during an attack of acute rheumatic fever means permanent involvement of this valve in about 85 per cent of the cases. As stated earlier, however, more recent studies, obtained since the advent of antibiotics, give a more optimistic outlook for these patients. Massell's[488] and Feinstein's[241] data suggest that only 60 to 70 per cent of these children suffer permanent damage to the mitral valve.

Mitral Stenosis

Mitral stenosis is the most common single valvular lesion developing as a consequence of rheumatic endocarditis. Women are more commonly affected than men. The disease is rare in children. At least two, but probably more, years are needed for its development. A considerable number of patients with no evidence of valvular involvement in the acute attack will have mitral stenosis ten to twenty years later. The stenosis may vary from only slight narrowing of the orifice (mitral valve area of 2.0 to 2.5 sq. cm.) to a calcified buttonhole stenosis (mitral valve area of 0.5 to 1.0 sq. cm.). In children, calcification is extremely rare, although severe stenosis may occur.

Physiology

The principal hemodynamic difficulty in mitral stenosis is the imposition of a barrier between the left atrium and the left ventricle in diastole. The basic hemodynamic principles have been well worked out by Dexter, Gorlin and their associates.[293, 295, 296] These physiologic studies demonstrate that in order to overcome the obstruction at the site of the mitral valve, the pressure in the left atrium is raised and a gradient between left atrial mean and left ventricular end diastolic pressure is established. This elevated left atrial pressure is reflected in the "pulmonary capillary" pressure obtained at cardiac catheterization.

In the case of mild mitral stenosis (with an orifice of 2 to 2.5 sq. cm.) the left atrial (or "pulmonary capillary") pressure needs to be raised only to a level of 10 to 12 mm. of mercury to supply a normal cardiac output at a normal rate. This type of lesion allows for normal activity and is recognized only by careful examination.

Moderate stenosis (1.5 to 2.0 sq. cm.) still allows adequate function, since a normal resting output still may be accomplished at the price of an "acceptable" left atrial mean pressure of 10 to 20 mm. of mercury. Serious difficulties may arise, however, if such patients try to increase their cardiac output by violent exercise at the same time that the rapid heart rate diminishes the diastolic filling period. This results in an increase in left atrial and pulmonary capillary pressures to levels at which pulmonary edema may occur (Fig. 171).

Further constriction of the mitral orifice to an area of 0.5 to 1.0 sq. cm. (probably by scar formation rather than by smoldering activity) results in critical stenosis, so that the patient vacillates between the Scylla and Charybdis of unbearably high left atrial and pulmonary capillary pressures (30 to 40 mm. of mercury, which is well above the pulmonary edema level) and a cardiac output so low that it allows for virtually no effort. The high "pulmonary capillary" pressure may evoke reflex pulmonary arterial constriction, which, in effect, "protects" the patient from pulmonary edema, but at the same time causes pulmonary arterial and right ventricular hypertension and a restricted cardiac output.[748]

At right heart catheterization patients with mild degrees of mitral stenosis show little that is abnormal. With increasing severity of the disease the following changes may be noted: "pulmonary capillary" pressure increases, and pulmonary arterial hypertension occurs on exercise, later even at rest; cardiac output diminishes as the systemic arteriovenous difference increases; later the cardiac output becomes fixed; and, finally, right ventricular end diastolic pressure increases and right-sided congestive failure is present.

Clinical Picture

The first heart sound at the apex is accentuated, presumably because the cusps are held wide apart to the very end of diastole by the high left atrial pressure. As the ventricle starts its isometric contraction, the cusps are slammed like a wide-open door by a high wind. The first sound is also delayed, since the ventricular pressure has to rise to a higher than average level before it can close the valve. The interval between the Q wave in the electrocardiogram and the appearance of S_1 in the phonocardiogram has been used as a measure of the severity of mitral stenosis (see p. 111). The longer the Q-S_1 interval, the more severe the stenosis.[723]

The second sound at the pulmonary area is loud only if pulmonary arterial hypertension is present. It is usually only narrowly split. An opening snap (Fig. 123, p. 119), corresponding to the opening of the mitral valve, is almost invariably present at the lower left sternal border. This high-frequency vibration may have to be differentiated from the pulmonary com-

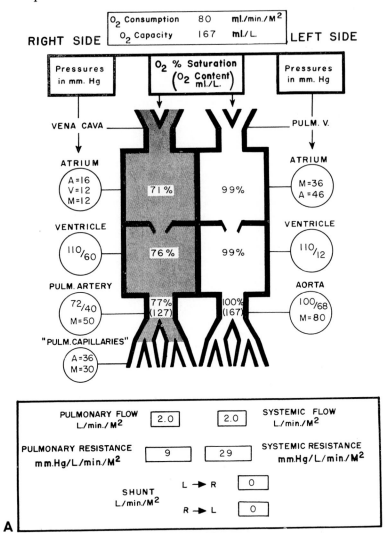

Figure 171.

ponent of the second or a third sound (see p. 118). The closer the opening snap is to aortic valve closure, the more severe is the mitral stenosis.

A low-frequency, rumbling, mid-diastolic murmur is audible at the apex; with the progression of the disease this murmur extends further and further into diastole, finally occupying presystole (Fig. 113, p. 113), where it assumes a crescendic configuration. This crescendic, apical presystolic murmur, often accompanied by a thrill, is the pathognomonic auscultatory finding in rheumatic mitral stenosis. Occasionally, rarely in children, a short, high-frequency, early diastolic blow can be heard over the pulmonary area (Graham Steell murmur). This is due to pulmonary regurgitation secondary to pulmonary arterial hypertension, although recent evidence points to the possibility that many of the so-called Graham Steell murmurs[605] may indeed represent mild aortic regurgitation.

Obviously, not all these phenomena are present in all cases. At the onset of mitral stenosis only a loud first sound at the apex may be audible

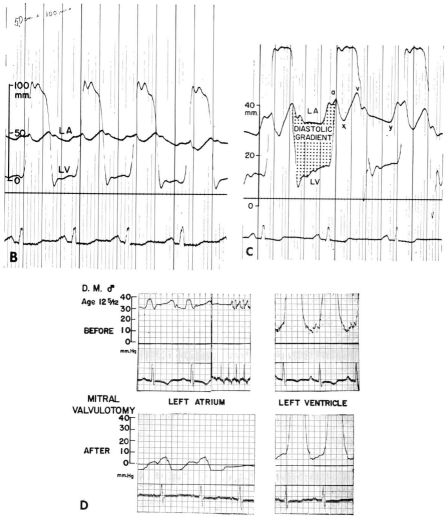

Figure 171. Left atrial and left ventricular pressure tracings in patient with mitral stenosis. *A*, Cardiac catheterization findings in patient with critical mitral stenosis. *B*, Low-sensitivity tracing indicates the constant pressure gradient between left atrium and left ventricle in diastole. *C*, High-sensitivity tracing indicates the magnitude of the gradient in the stippled area and also indicates that the gradient is maximal in presystole, corresponding to the A wave of the left atrial pressure tracing. Note also the gentle slope of the y depression, also characteristic of mitral valve obstruction. *D*, indicates operative relief of mitral stenosis. Note the large pressure gradient between left atrial and left ventricular diastole in the two upper panels and the absence of a significant gradient after mitral valvulotomy in the two lower panels.

at rest. This should arouse suspicion if the patient has a history suggestive of rheumatic fever. Having the patient exercise, turning him in the left lateral position, and listening with an open bell stethoscope may bring out the diastolic-presystolic murmur. Later, with the development of atrial fibrillation, the presystolic crescendic murmur always disappears, thus furnishing conclusive proof that, when present, it is due to the forceful atrial contraction squeezing blood through a tight mitral opening. The nightmare of all clinicians is the patient with maximal mitral stenosis and an output so low that no murmur may be heard at all.

The rest of the physical examination is less specific. Patients have high color; characteristically a malar flush with suggestion of peripheral cyanosis is described. Probably this is due to the low cardiac output and the high oxygen extraction in the capillaries. Left chest deformity usually is not severe. The cardiac impulse is of right ventricular nature. The pulse is usually small and shows a narrow pulse pressure.

The electrocardiogram in pure mitral stenosis of some severity shows right axis deviation, vertical heart and right ventricular hypertrophy. In adults more than forty years old or in children with active carditis, atrial fibrillation frequently occurs. If P waves are present, they are commonly abnormal. Their abnormalities consist in an increase in height and width in the standard limb leads, occurrence of diphasic, even inverted, P waves in lead V_1, and flat-topped or notched P waves in leads I and II.

The radiologic appearance of mitral stenosis is characterized by mild or moderate cardiomegaly with left atrial prominence (Fig. 172) and right ventricular enlargement. The pulmonary arterial segment becomes prominent as pulmonary arterial hypertension appears. Characteristically, the lungs show evidence of passive congestion, haziness, and engorged lymphatics (Kerley lines). Distended pulmonary veins may be seen entering the heart, and the congestion is greater in the lower than in the upper half of the lungs. Radioactive studies in these patients indicate that the upper pulmonary veins have a higher flow than do the lower ones.

Most of the so-called complications of mitral stenosis are seldom if ever seen in children. Hence they will be mentioned only briefly. (1) Atrial fibrillation, presumably the effect of overdistention of the left atrium, occurs frequently in patients more than forty years of age. If it is observed in children or adolescents, it almost invariably means active carditis. (2) Hemoptysis is the result of infarction, pulmonary edema, or rupture of a distended vessel into the bronchial tree. Occasionally hemoptysis occurs in very sick patients with acute carditis and "rheumatic pneumonia." (3) Bacterial endocarditis always should be thought of in conjunction with

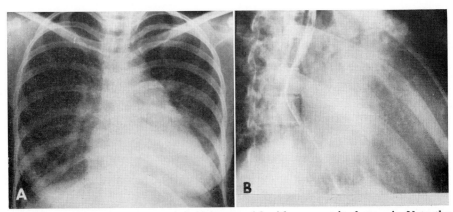

Figure 172. Roentgenograms of adolescent girl with severe mitral stenosis. Note the cardiac enlargement, the prominent main pulmonary artery segment in the posteroanterior view (A) and the large left atrium, pushing back the barium-filled esophagus, in the right anterior oblique view (B).

rheumatic heart disease, but actually its occurrence is rare in pure mitral stenosis, especially in children.

Differential Diagnosis

Mitral stenosis is usually easy to recognize in children; a recent history of rheumatic fever can be obtained more frequently than in adults, and a good mid-diastolic-presystolic murmur is present almost without exception.

For practical purposes, the only problem in differential diagnosis is presented by other conditions which give rise to apical diastolic murmurs. Among these should be mentioned acute rheumatic carditis without organic stenosis, the Austin Flint murmur of aortic regurgitation, and congenital heart disease with left-to-right shunt, especially atrial septal defect. If one remembers that it takes a considerable amount of time for organic mitral stenosis to develop, then the apical diastolic murmur appearing within the framework of acute carditis can be recognized as probably representing a "functional" murmur. The Austin Flint apical presystolic murmur, associated with aortic regurgitation, is almost impossible to differentiate from the murmur of true mitral stenosis, except by thinking about it in patients with free aortic incompetence. The apical diastolic murmur of the left-to-right shunt group may also be hard to differentiate from that of mitral stenosis. The presence of real presystolic accentuation, a diastolic thrill, an opening snap and a loud first sound favor the diagnosis of mitral stenosis, whereas a low-frequency murmur, without thrill and without opening snap, occupying early or mid-diastole in a patient with pulmonary vascular engorgement favors the diagnosis of congenital heart disease with a left-to-right shunt. In the latter group, if incomplete right bundle branch block is present in the electrocardiogram, atrial septal defect is the likely diagnosis.

One further point to be mentioned in the differential diagnosis is the separation of congenital mitral stenosis from mitral stenosis of rheumatic origin. This can be done only on the basis of age. If mitral stenosis occurs in an infant or very young child, one must assume that it is of congenital origin.

Course and Prognosis

Children with mitral stenosis, unless they have acute carditis, are usually asymptomatic. In rare instances they may show some fatigue and exertional dyspnea. According to Gorlin and his associates,[295] the clinical picture of advanced mitral stenosis, as seen principally in adults, is the result of an interplay between the narrowing of the valve, the pulmonary vascular obstruction consecutive to it, and the state of the myocardium. Patients in group I, those with the mildest stenosis, have a mitral valve area of more than 1.5 sq. cm. and normal pulmonary vascular resistance, and show only slight, if any, dyspnea on exertion. The cardiac output of these patients is within normal limits at rest and exercise. Patients in group II are characterized by a valve area of 1.0 to 1.5 sq. cm. and relatively normal vascular resistance. These patients have respiratory symptoms, some dyspnea on exertion, paroxysmal nocturnal dyspnea, and hemoptysis. The cardiac output is normal at rest, but does not rise sufficiently on exercise. Patients in group III have severe mitral stenosis (valve area of 0.5 to 1.0 sq. cm.) with moderately increased pulmonary vascular resistance and an impaired myocardium. Although these patients show considerable dyspnea on exertion or strenuous exercise, their main trouble is weakness, tiredness and easy fatigability. The cardiac output is low normal at rest and practically fixed on exercise. Finally, group IV is made up of patients with extreme mitral stenosis (valve area less than 0.5 sq. cm.), considerable increase in pulmonary vascular resistance, poor myocardium and fixed low cardiac output. These patients have dyspnea at rest, gross cardiomegaly and right ventricular failure.

The outlook for patients with asymptomatic mitral stenosis depends on the presence or absence of recurrences, diet, crowding, and climatic and genetic factors. On the whole, the prognosis of patients with mitral stenosis is perhaps less favorable than that of those having mitral or aortic regurgitation; the average age at death, in a series in which chemoprophylaxis had not been used, was between thirty-five and forty-five years.[36] Wood[748] placed the average age at death at approximately forty years. Bland and Jones's figures suggested that many patients die in acute carditis. Most of the deaths in their series occurred within five or ten years after the initial attack; most of those who survived the first ten years were still alive twenty years after their first attack.

Some patients with mitral stenosis survive in good health to the fourth and fifth decades, and even longer. Obviously, these figures vary tremendously, according to the patients analyzed. Statistical support may be found for any type of therapeutic program the physician or surgeon may be inclined to endorse. Suffice it to say that, as far as the pediatrician is concerned, most children with mitral stenosis are asymptomatic unless they have acute rheumatic fever. If they recover from the acute attack, if recurrences are prevented and they maintain a sensible outlook on life, they can look forward to many years of normal, active existence.

Treatment

The treatment of mitral stenosis has three principal parts. The most important of these is the prevention of recurrences by means of chemoprophylaxis.

The second therapeutic measure is the surgical correction of the stenosis by mitral valvuloplasty.[32, 325] Although until the last two years the approach to the mitral valve was almost exclusively through the left atrium, dissatisfaction with the results[372, 432] led many surgeons here and abroad to transventricular mitral valvotomy.[441] The results seem encouraging. Probably surgical correction is not necessary in most children; it should be advocated only if one can be certain that the symptoms are due to organic mitral obstruction rather than to myocardial factors. One must also be sure that severe organic mitral stenosis, and not combined valvular lesions, with or without active rheumatic carditis, is the principal cause of the patient's difficulties. A few successful cases of mitral surgery in youngsters between twelve and fourteen years of age have been reported in the literature.[458] We have had half a dozen patients less than fifteen years of age who underwent mitral valve surgery. The indications for surgery are (1) definite and progressive dyspnea on exertion, (2) attacks of pulmonary edema, and (3) paroxysmal dyspnea with hemoptysis.

The patients who benefit most from the various surgical procedures are those in whom the predominant difficulty is a mechanical block at the mitral valve.[245] These patients may be recognized physiologically by the presence of a low, fixed cardiac output and pulmonary hypertension with a significant rise on exercise. Conversely, patients with equally severe symptoms and clinical signs of mitral stenosis in whom the main difficulty is the inefficiency of the myocardium fail to respond well to mitral valvotomy; these patients also have a low and fixed cardiac output, but do not have significant pulmonary hypertension at rest or on exercise.

The technical aspects of mitral commissurotomy or valvuloplasty have been described adequately in many publications.[32, 325] The over-all mortality figures vary according to the condition of the patient, the accuracy of the diagnosis and the skill of the surgeon. On the whole, a mortality figure of about 1 to 5 per cent may be quoted for patients without congestive failure, whereas the others entail a 20 to 25 per cent mortality risk. The cause of death is mostly embolic, and not congestive failure. Among the postoperative complications should be mentioned, in addition to embolism, the so-called postcommissurotomy syndrome.[653] This peculiar cyclic disease, occurring in 15 to 20 per cent of patients after mitral commissurotomy, consists of fever, chest pain, pneumonitis and cardiomegaly. It had been thought to be due to reactivation of rheumatic fever, but recent evidence points more toward a nonspecific reaction secondary to opening of the pericardium, and possibly based on auto-antibody formation (postpericardiotomy syndrome).[227]

The patient who survives the immediate postoperative period and is kept on a strict medical regimen for a few months, including prophylactic chemotherapy and the judicious use of anticongestive measures, usually improves. More than 60 per cent of the survivors report considerable symptomatic relief, not always documentable by physiologic observations; the explanation of the discrepancy between symptoms and physiologic data belongs in the realm of psychosomatic medicine rather than in pediatric cardiology. In 5-year follow-up studies,[326] late deaths occurred in less than 5 per cent of the cases; reoperation was necessary in only a few patients.

The final considerations in the treatment of mitral stenosis in children are the assurance of good dental hygiene, adequate diet and a sensible attitude toward the disease.

Mitral Regurgitation

If the presence of a "significant" apical systolic murmur may be taken as definite evidence of mitral regurgitation, then it must be present in almost all cases of acute rheumatic carditis. As a matter of fact, without the presence of an apical systolic murmur the diagnosis of rheumatic carditis rests on tenuous grounds, according to Bland and Jones's study.[63] On the other hand, maximal mitral regurgitation may be present without a significant apical systolic murmur.

In the past about two thirds of the patients who, in their acute attack, had auscultatory evidence of mitral regurgitation, had definite mitral incompetence twenty years later. Recent observations on patients who have received chemoprophylaxis justify a more optimistic attitude about the long-term outlook. That mitral regurgitation as an isolated rheumatic valve lesion exists is suggested by the auscultatory findings in chronic rheumatic heart disease and is supported by the observations of surgeons whose palpating fingers, in left atrial exploration, occasionally encounter a regurgitant jet without evidence of mitral stenosis. In contrast to these clinical and surgical experiences are the observations of pathologists who maintain that pure mitral regurgitation is almost never found at post-mortem examination. Probably this means only that mitral regurgitation, per se, is not a fatal disease. In contrast to pure mitral stenosis, mitral regurgitation affects men more frequently than women.

Incompetence of the mitral valve, anatomically speaking, results from the rigidity and shortening of the valve cusps. In addition, the chordae tendineae, contracted through scar formation, also may impede complete closure of the mitral valve during ventricular systole.

Physiology

The principal difficulty in mitral regurgitation is that the left ventricle and the left atrium have to handle an increased volume of blood. This is necessary since a considerable portion, sometimes as much as 50 per cent, of the left ventricular stroke output is dissipated into the left atrium, and thus the left ventricular diastolic filling has to be increased to a point at which, in spite of the loss into the left atrium, the aortic flow still is in the required range. At right heart catheterization, usually, but not invariably, the "pulmonary capillary" pressure tracing shows unusually tall V waves; at left heart catheterization a large V wave is encountered in the left atrium (Fig. 173). The relation of the height of the V wave to the rate of descent of the y trough has been used as an index of the degree of mitral regurgitaton. Other methods suggested for quantitative estimation of mitral regurgitation include dye dilution curves and cine-angiograms. These approaches are satisfactory in a *qualitative* sense, but neither of them can be used for exact *quantitation* at present. The left atrial mean pressure, in spite of tall V waves, is usually not very high because of the deep and rapid y descent. Pulmonary vascular obstruction, if present at all, is less severe than in mitral stenosis. An increase in right atrial and right ventricular pressure is found only if the left ventricle fails. The cardiac output is moderately decreased.

Clinical Picture

The signs of mitral regurgitation are much less clear-cut than those of mitral stenosis. As has been mentioned, the principal auscultatory finding is the presence of an apical systolic murmur which probably means mitral insufficiency if (1) the murmur is grade 3 or louder, (2) it is heard best at the apex and is transmitted along the posterior axillary line to the left base, (3) it starts immediately with the first sound and lasts at least through the first half of systole, and (4) it does not change with position and respiration.

Other features of the physical examination are left chest deformity,

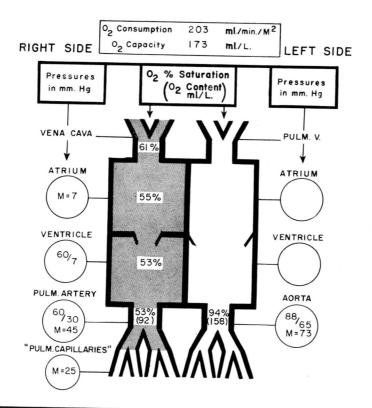

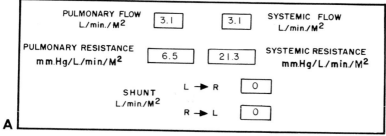

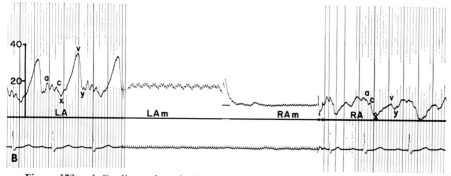

Figure 173. *A*, Cardiac catheterization findings on patient with severe mitral regurgitation. *B*, Pressure tracings of patient with mitral regurgitation. Note the difference between left atrial and right atrial phasic tracings, with the tall V wave and precipitous y descent in the left atrium.

203

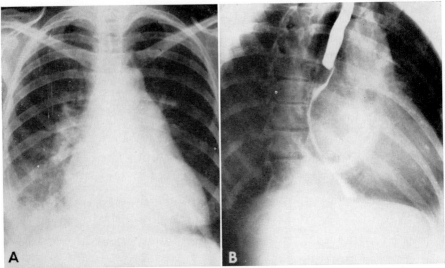

Figure 174. Roentgenogram of patient with mitral regurgitation. Note the large left ventricle in the posteroanterior view (*A*) and the large left atrium in the right anterior oblique view (*B*). Note also in *A* the haziness of the lower lung field as compared with the upper lung field.

a rocking, hyperdynamic left ventricular impulse, a moderately accentuated pulmonary second sound, a normal first sound, a loud third sound, and normal blood pressure and slightly widened pulse pressure. Hoarseness, due to pressure on the recurrent laryngeal nerve by the large left atrium, has been noted.

The electrocardiogram shows left ventricular dominance, or left ventricular hypertrophy, occasionally with "P mitrale."

Under the fluoroscope the heart seems overactive, particularly in the region of the enlarged left ventricle. Left atrial and left ventricular enlargement of significant degree is usually found in the more advanced cases (Fig. 174); as a matter of fact, the largest left atria in rheumatic heart disease are seen with mitral regurgitation. Systolic expansion of the left atrium is commonly noted. The pulmonary vasculature is within normal limits unless the left ventricle fails. The inaccuracy of all these clinical signs in indicating the presence of mitral regurgitation has been amply documented by surgeons who found significant mitral regurgitation on left atrial exploration in patients in whom none was preoperatively suspected, and vice versa.

Differential Diagnosis

All the conditions accompanied by an apical systolic murmur should be considered in the differential diagnosis of mitral regurgitation. First to be considered in this regard are patients with "insignificant" apical systolic murmurs. These murmurs are faint and short, and do not transmit, but may change with position or respiration. Using essentially the same criteria, though different nomenclature, Boone and Levine[74] studied two groups of patients, one with "organic" murmurs, the other with "functional" murmurs. Ten years later the group with the "organic" murmurs contained ten times as many patients with multivalvular involvement or significant cardiomegaly as did the group with "functional" murmurs. Kuttner and Markowitz,[404] in a similar study, found that after 8 years 48 per cent of the patients in the "organic" group showed significant heart disease, as compared to 13 per cent in the "functional" group. Although the nature of the murmur is important in the differential diagnosis, obviously the clinician ought to use all other tools, including a good history, physical examination, x-rays and the electrocardiogram, to determine the significance of an apical systolic murmur.

"Significant" apical systolic murmurs may be heard in patients with rheumatic heart disease other than mitral regurgitation. It has been reported[499] that frequently adults with aortic stenosis may show only an apical systolic murmur; in children this is rare because rheumatic aortic stenosis is rare. But it is true that certain cases of nonrheumatic aortic stenosis manifest themselves solely by an apical systolic murmur. Tricuspid regurgitation may give rise to a systolic murmur at the apex. This is also rare in children and practically never occurs as the principal valvular lesion. It may cause confusion, however, in that the murmur of tricuspid regurgitation accompanying definite mitral stenosis may be interpreted as indicating mitral regurgitation. The correct diagnosis may be suggested by the following points: (1) the jugular venous pulse indicates tricuspid regurgitation, (2) there is a right ventricular type of impulse, and (3) the murmur is maximal toward the lower left sternal border and may increase on inspiration.[617]

Patients with "pure" mitral stenosis may also have significant apical systolic murmurs, a fact which brings up the difficult question of differentiating by clinical means a predominantly stenotic type of lesion from a dominantly regurgitant one. The importance of this from the surgical viewpoint can scarcely be overemphasized. Fortunately for the pediatrician, surgically significant mitral stenosis rarely occurs in children. Nevertheless in an occasional adolescent the problem may arise. It may be said unequivocally that there is no single criterion which distinguishes, without fail, a predominantly stenotic mitral valve from one in which regurgitation dominates. A sustained left ventricular type of cardiac impulse, an intense systolic murmur transmitting well to the mid or posterior axilla and even to the back, the presence of systolic expansion of the left atrium, and an electrocardiogram indicating left ventricular hypertrophy would give the clinical impression of predominant regurgitation. Physiologic studies aimed at quantitative estimation of the relative degrees of mitral stenosis and mitral regurgitation, through left and right heart catheterization, are all more or less satisfactory in the clinically obvious cases.[406, 657] All may be misleading in borderline situations.[707] Neoclassicists in cardiology find the simple statement that "a loud systolic murmur transmitted to the posterior axilla and accompanied by a rocking left ventricular impulse indicates significant mitral regurgitation" is as good a criterion as any of the rather more complex physiologic observations.

Congenital heart disease, especially endocardial cushion defect, corrected transposition of the great arteries, and Marfan's syndrome may show convincing evidences of congenital mitral regurgitation. A loud, apical systolic murmur may be heard in many patients with left-to-right shunts and coarctation of the aorta. In these instances this may indeed represent functional or even anatomic mitral regurgitation. Finally, almost any other type of heart disease, acquired or congenital, may be accompanied by an apical systolic murmur of "significant" nature. All the ingenuity the pediatrician is able to muster may be necessary for accurate interpretation of a grade 3 apical systolic murmur.

Course and Prognosis

Most patients who have pure mitral regurgitation are relatively asymptomatic for a long time and have a good long-term prognosis. The symptoms—if no active carditis exists—consist mainly of fatigue and palpitation. Pulmonary edema or hemoptysis is seldom seen in patients with pure mitral regurgitation. Congestive failure is rare; life expectancy is satisfactory. Massell and his associates[363] reported a sizeable group of patients with benign mitral regurgitation of long standing. In contrast to the relatively rare occurrence of subacute bacterial endocarditis in pure mitral stenosis, its presence in patients with mitral regurgitation is relatively common.

About a third of the patients starting out with pure mitral regurgitation eventually have combined stenosis and insufficiency; in these, symptoms develop and the prognosis becomes grave.

Treatment

Medical treatment is essentially the same as that outlined in the section on mitral stenosis, and consists of adequate chemoprophylaxis for an adequate period. Within the past few years surgeons have made considerable progress in the treatment of the disease.[222] No uniform surgical procedure has been adopted as yet, nor can meaningful figures be quoted in terms of results or risks. In our hospital only the most serious cases have been considered for surgery, and the results may be called fair.

DISEASES OF THE AORTIC VALVE

Aortic valvular disease is diagnosed on the basis of murmurs heard in the aortic area, i.e. at the second right and fourth left interspaces. There is some pathologic evidence that in adults[499] aortic valve involvement may occur without any murmur at all. I have never seen this in an older child, but I do know that it occurs in infants with maximal congenital aortic stenosis.

Rheumatic aortic disease alone or in combination with mitral valvular disease is common. Fifty-eight per cent of the patients[63, 369] in whom rheumatic heart disease develops show evidences of aortic involvement. In contrast to diseases of the mitral valve, disappearance of aortic murmurs is rare.

Aortic Regurgitation

Aortic regurgitation is the dominant consequence of involvement of the aortic valve in rheumatic endocarditis. Men are more commonly affected than women. All degrees of the disease are known, from the faint early diastolic "whiff" without any peripheral signs, to the free aortic regurgitation represented by a loud murmur and a diastolic pressure near zero.

Anatomically, the valve ring is dilated, the semilunar cusps are shortened and deformed by scarring, and thus the valve edges fail to close the aortic orifice during ventricular diastole.

Physiology

The overload of aortic regurgitation is carried almost exclusively by the left ventricle. The increased volume work of this chamber is the consequence of the increased stroke output, which is caused by the fact that a certain proportion of the blood expelled into the aorta leaks back into the left ventricle. It seems clear, then, that the left ventricular stroke output must be large enough to ensure adequate aortic flow even with appreciable loss back into the ventricle. The degree of regurgitation depends on the size of the regurgitant opening and on the difference between aortic and left ventricular diastolic pressures. In severe cases of aortic regurgitation an increase in "pulmonary-capillary" mean pressure may be encountered at right heart catheterization. Paralleling this is an increase in left atrial and left ventricular end-diastolic pressures in aortic regurgitation, leading to congestive heart failure. Dye dilution curves, with injection into the pulmonary artery or left atrium and sampling from the systemic artery, have been used with more or less success for quantitative determination of aortic regurgitation.[409] Another approach, advocated by Braunwald and Morrow,[83] consists in the retrograde injection of indicator dye into the descending aorta and noting the appearance of the dye by cine-angiography in the left ventricle.

Significant peripheral vasodilatation is a regular concomitant of severe aortic regurgitation.[729] Thus the drain on the aortic pressure head is from two directions: part of the blood regurgitates back into the ventricle, and part dissipates rapidly into the dilated peripheral vascular bed. As a result of both these factors, aortic diastolic pressure is low; this interferes with adequate coronary filling.

A low aortic diastolic pressure not only impedes coronary circulation, but also interferes with the satisfactory nutrition of the tissues, since it lowers the mean arterial pressure at the periphery. In order to counteract the unfavorable effects of the low diastolic pressure on the mean arterial pressure, the systolic pressure is appreciably raised. This, then, results in a relatively satisfactory mean pressure with a wide pulse pressure. The increased systolic pressure adds a significant amount of pressure load to the already increased volume load of the left ventricle.

The high systolic and low diastolic pressure in the arterial system is reflected in the characteristic radial arterial tracing obtainable in patients with aortic regurgitation (Fig. 175).

The powerful musculature of the left ventricle is able to cope with the considerable flow and pressure work involved in aortic regurgitation for an appreciable length of time. Difficulties arise when the left ventricle fails or when angina develops as a result of poor diastolic filling of the coronary arteries. Both these consequences occur in adult life and should

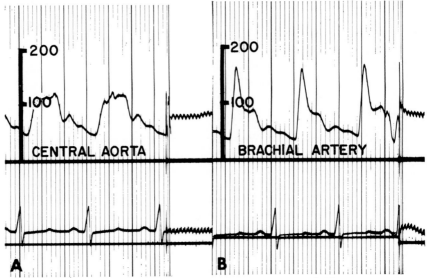

Figure 175. Pressure tracings of aortic regurgitation.

affect the thinking of the pediatrician only in terms of long-range prognosis rather than as events likely to occur within the first two decades of life.

Clinical Picture

The diagnostic sign of aortic regurgitation is the early insufficiency blow, which is best registered at the third to fourth left or the second right interspace. This consists in high-frequency vibrations immediately following the second sound in a decrescendo fashion, perhaps preceded for a short period by a slight crescendic phase. The stethoscope with the diaphragm type of chest-piece brings out the murmur best, particularly with the patient in a sitting position, slightly bent forward. Even though sometimes it may be almost impossible to time the murmur accurately, it still should be recognized as a high-frequency, metallic-sounding, almost "echo-like" murmur.

The rest of the physical examination is somewhat more characteristic in these patients than in those with mitral disease. Increased pulsations of the carotid arteries can be clearly seen and easily palpated; the powerful and sudden thrust of the left ventricle may rock the head, the chest, and even the bed of the patient with regurgitation. Considerable left chest prominence may be present. The cardiac impulse is forceful and of the left ventricular type. Occasionally there is a diastolic thrill, palpable at the third to fourth left interspace. On auscultation, in addition to the typical murmur described, a systolic murmur of varying intensity and sometimes of stenotic nature may be heard at the aortic area; these two murmurs assume a to-and-fro nature (Fig. 176) with a gap between the systolic murmur and the second sound. The aortic closure is usually accentuated, and unless congestive failure is present, it is louder than the pulmonary closure. An apical presystolic murmur (Austin Flint), practically indistinguishable from the murmur of true mitral stenosis, is often ob-

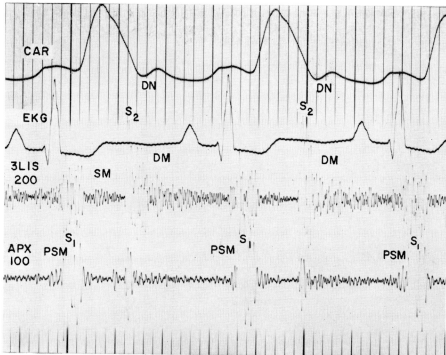

Figure 176. Pressure tracing of patient with severe aortic regurgitation. Note the low dicrotic notch on the carotid artery tracing *(top)*. On the sound tracing at the third left interspace, note the long decrescendo diastolic murmur ending with presystolic accentuation. Note also the relatively insignificant systolic murmur at the third left interspace.

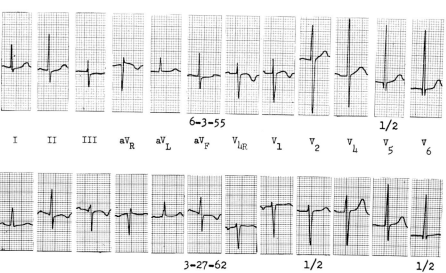

Figure 177. Progressive changes in the electrocardiogram of patient with aortic regurgitation. Note the change in the T waves in the seven-year period, particularly in leads I, II, aV$_F$ and V$_6$. This tracing indicates how patients with this lesion, a prototype of so-called diastolic overloading, may have cardiograms that could be classified as showing so-called systolic overloading.

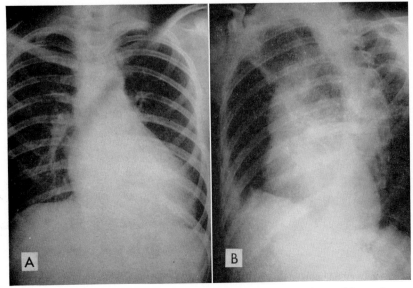

Figure 178. Posteroanterior and oblique roentgenograms of patient with aortic regurgitation.

served, but is not accompanied by a thrill. The pulses are full, and the pulse pressure is wide with high systolic and low diastolic readings.

The electrocardiogram may be entirely normal. In severe cases of long duration left ventricular hypertrophy may be present (Fig. 177). Typically, deep q waves and late R waves are present in the left ventricular leads. The T waves in V_5 and V_6 may be pointed, tall and symmetrical at first; later, depression of the S-T segment and inversion of the T wave ensue. P mitrale may be present in advanced cases.

Radiologically, cardiomegaly, principally left ventricular in type, can be seen (Fig. 178). If the left atrium is enlarged, left ventricular failure or associated mitral valve disease must be suspected. The aorta and the left ventricle show powerful pulsations under the fluoroscope; the pulmonary artery segment is relatively quiet. The ascending aorta and the aortic knob are prominent and have a collapsing type of beat.

Differential Diagnosis

The differential diagnosis of aortic regurgitation encompasses two main entities. One is the group of conditions with dissipation of the aortic pressure head (*aortic runoffs*). In this category should be mentioned thyrotoxicosis, severe anemia, peripheral arteriovenous aneurysm, patent ductus arteriosus, aortopulmonary fenestration, ruptured sinus of Valsalva, coronary arteriovenous fistula and ventricular septal defect with aortic regurgitation. The first three conditions have to be borne in mind if the problem of differential diagnosis arises; all three of them, by virtue of their extracardiac findings, can be recognized once they are brought to mind. The five latter conditions may be much harder to differentiate from rheumatic aortic regurgitation, though several points may be helpful. For one thing, three of these congenital heart diseases (patent ductus arteriosus, fenestration, and ventricular septal defect with aortic regurgitation) involve a left-to-right shunt; hence, radiologically, they are characterized by pulmonary vascular engorgement with a hilar dance and an overactive main pulmonary artery. Second, especially patent ductus arteriosus and aortopulmonary fenestration are accompanied by continuous systolic and diastolic murmurs, where the second sound is enveloped into the murmur. Of course a history of a murmur from the time of birth and the absence of a clear-cut rheumatic episode also help to identify the left-to-right shunt group. Yet in spite of all this, cardiac catheterization must sometimes be performed in order to establish the diagnosis.

The other group of patients to be considered in the differential diagnosis are those with *pulmonary regurgitation* (mitral stenosis, pulmonary arterial hypertension and idiopathic pulmonary regurgitation), in whom diastolic murmurs of a quality similar to that of aortic regurgitation may be noted. The murmur is usually less loud, however, and usually of lower frequency; it is maximal at the second to third left interspace and is not accompanied by an increase in pulse pressure.

Course and Prognosis

Much like mitral regurgitation, and in contrast to mitral stenosis, aortic regurgitation may occur early within the framework of acute rheumatic fever. Once an aortic diastolic murmur appears, the chances of its disappearance are slim (less than 5 per cent), although there are some suggestions in the most recent literature that treatment with corticoids may change the outlook.[484]

Children with free aortic regurgitation, but without active carditis, are usually asymptomatic. The powerful left ventricle is able to maintain compensation throughout childhood and most of adolescence unless rheumatic myocardial disease interferes with its efficiency. Severe aortic regurgitation in adults leads eventually to exertional dyspnea, anginal pain, pitting edema and intractable congestive failure. Like those with aortic stenosis, these patients "break late," but when they do, their downhill course is precipitous.

The severity of the lesion can probably best be judged clinically on the basis of the length of the diastolic murmur and the pulse pressure, the electrocardiogram and the roentgenograms and only to a lesser degree on the basis of the intensity of the murmur. The poor prognosis, to be measured in terms of years, must be contrasted with the good outlook and life expectancy for children with only a slight or moderate degree of aortic regurgitation. The average life expectancy of patients with aortic insufficiency is quoted as twenty to thirty years after discovery of the murmur.[746]

Treatment

There is no universally accepted surgical treatment for this disease. Hufnagel valves,[346] inserted in the descending aorta to abolish the effects of peripheral vasodilatation, have been recommended for adults. After initial enthusiasm, the use of these valves has been discontinued in most centers. More recently reconstruction, under direct vision, by means of the pump oxygenator has been undertaken with varying results. The use of plastic prostheses is currently being tried out in the experimental laboratory and even on patients. Hufnagel[347, 348] reported excellent short-term results in more than 100 patients in whom one or more of the deformed cusps were replaced by plastic prostheses. Similar results have been reported by Kay[373] from Cleveland and Muller[514] from Charlottesville. I have no doubt whatsoever that in the near future good surgical repair for aortic regurgitation will be available.

Chemoprophylaxis and regulation of living conditions are just as important as they are in diseases of the mitral valve. Furthermore, knowing that the left ventricle is capable of maximal effort for a long time without failure, but that when it fails, the end is rather near, I usually recommend that youngsters with aortic regurgitation abstain from competitive sports. Sometimes this is hard to enforce, since many of them are athletically inclined young males.

Aortic Stenosis

Rheumatic aortic stenosis, as an uncomplicated lesion, is practically unknown in children. There were only 2 patients in the group of 1000 studied by Bland and Jones[63, 369] in whom pure aortic stenosis developed within 20 years; both patients were more than 25 years old.

If signs and symptoms of pure aortic stenosis are found in a child, it must be assumed, for practical purposes, that it is congenital in origin. The problem of aortic stenosis will be discussed in detail in the section on Congenital Heart Disease.

DISEASES OF THE TRICUSPID VALVE

Rheumatic diseases of the tricuspid valve are rare and of no practical significance in pediatrics; they almost never occur as an isolated lesion and seldom as a dominant one.

Physiologically, the mechanisms elaborated on in connection with mitral stenosis and mitral regurgitation operate here, except that the burden falls exclusively on the right side of the heart. Right atrial pressure and jugular venous pressure tracings show prominent V waves in tricuspid regurgitation and tall A waves in tricuspid stenosis. In addition, characteristically, in cases of tricuspid stenosis, there is a gradient, on cardiac catheterization, between right atrial mean and right ventricular end-diastolic pressures.

Clinically, the systolic murmur of tricuspid regurgitation and the diastolic murmur of tricuspid stenosis are both heard best at the lower right sternal border. It is hard, almost impossible, to differentiate them from mitral murmurs transmitted from the apex. An increase in intensity on inspiration suggests that the murmur is of tricuspid origin. But absence of this sign does not exclude tricuspid disease. Careful observation of the jugular venous pulse and the pulsations of the liver aids a great deal in the differential diagnosis. Presystolic pulsations of the neck veins and the liver are characteristic of tricuspid stenosis, whereas vigorous systolic pulsations, and V waves of the jugular venous pulse and the liver are typical of tricuspid regurgitation. Roentgenologically, the huge right atrium is noted. Electrocardiographically, P pulmonale is in evidence.

COMBINED VALVULAR DISEASES

Involvement of more than one valve is the rule rather than the exception in rheumatic heart disease. According to White,[728] mitral diseases dominate in about three fourths of the cases, and aortic valve abnormality in about one fourth. Stenosis and regurgitation of the same valve usually occur together. Clinically, mitral regurgitation without stenosis is more common than mitral stenosis without regurgitation. If, especially in relatively acute cases, one cannot be sure which mitral lesion is predominant, the term "mitral involvement" is useful.

Aortic regurgitation without stenosis is common, whereas aortic stenosis of rheumatic nature without coexisting aortic regurgitation is practically unknown in children.

8

BACTERIAL ENDOCARDITIS

In contrast to the usually sterile inflammatory lesions of rheumatic endo-carditis, the vegetations of bacterial endocarditis contain microorganisms identifiable morphologically as well as culturally. The causative organism may be cultured in vivo from the blood stream in about 75 per cent of the patients with bacterial endocarditis; blood cultures from patients with rheumatic endocarditis, on the other hand, are sterile.

Bacterial endocarditis is commonly divided into two groups, subacute and acute, depending on the duration of the disease.[422, 728] At present this distinction seems almost meaningless, since many cases of so-called subacute bacterial endocarditis are recognized within a week after onset, and bacteriologic cure is accomplished within a month. Distinction on the basis of causative organisms is equally difficult, since a variety of pathogens may serve as etiologic agents, and in 10 to 20 per cent of the cases no organism may be isolated at all. Consequently I prefer to discuss the cases with pre-existing heart disease as one group and those without heart disease as another group.

BACTERIAL ENDOCARDITIS IN CHILDREN WITH HEART DISEASE
(SUBACUTE BACTERIAL ENDOCARDITIS, SBE)

In this section I shall discuss bacterial endocarditis occurring in children with rheumatic or congenital heart disease, with principal localization of the infection in the heart or the great vessels.

Incidence and Etiology

Subacute bacterial endocarditis, much like rheumatic fever, has been on the decline within the past decade; this trend is most likely explained by the widespread use of antibiotics for the treatment of respiratory infection and by dental prophylaxis in patients with heart disease. Littman and Schaaf[440] found that whereas, during the 3-year period from 1944 through 1946, 1.12 per thousand of the patients admitted to the Massachusetts General Hospital had subacute bacterial endocarditis, from 1947 through 1949 only 0.59 per thousand had this disease. On the other hand, within the first half of 1961, ten patients with bacterial endocarditis were treated at The Children's Hospital Medical Center, representing about 3 times the usual annual rate. Whether this indicates a real increase in the incidence of bacterial endocarditis cannot be stated with certainty, but informal conversations with other pediatric cardiologists indicate that this may be more than a chance occurrence.

Subacute bacterial endocarditis is primarily a disease of young adults. Men are more commonly affected than women. In White's[385] series of 250 patients only 2 per cent were children less than 10 years old, and only 17 per cent were in their second decade. At the Babies Hospital in New York the youngest patient with bacterial endocarditis was three months old, but eight out of fifty-eight were less than three years of age. Compared with the general incidence of subacute bacterial endocarditis in a general hospital, its frequency at The Children's Hospital in Boston is approximately 0.5 per thousand patients, an incidence similar to that reported by Blumenthal and his associates.[71]

The alpha streptococcus (viridans), the gamma streptococcus (enterococcus) and the staphylococcus are responsible for close to 95 per cent of all cases of bacterial endocarditis in adults.[259] More than two thirds of these are caused by *Streptococcus viridans*. In Blumenthal's series, four out of five were caused by the streptococcus, and one out of five by *Staphylococcus aureus*.

Our experience at The Children's Hospital in the past fifteen years supports the same figure. Other organisms, rarely implicated, are *Escherichia coli, Bacillus pyocyaneus*, pneumococcus, beta hemolytic streptococcus, and Pseudomonas. *Staphylococcus albus* infection has been reported after open-heart surgery; presumably the presence of silk, as a foreign body, predisposes to this type of infection in the heart or great vessels.

In adults rheumatic heart disease accounts for about 80 per cent of the cases; congenital heart disease is implicated in less than 10 per cent. On the other hand, on the basis of our experience and that of Blumenthal's,[71] about one third of the children with this disease have rheumatic valvular lesions; the other two thirds have congenital heart disease.

In our series of twenty-four cases three patients had ventricular septal defect, and three had coarctation of the aorta. Single cases of patent ductus arteriosus, pulmonic stenosis, endocardial cushion defect and aortic stenosis were encountered among the patients who did not have cyanosis. Five of the six patients with cyanotic disease had Fallot's tetralogy. One of the latter also had had a "shunt" operation performed some years previously. Since our original series was reported, we have seen a number of patients with tetralogy of Fallot who had had shunt procedures and in whom bacterial endocarditis did develop. Within the past year or two this has seemed common enough to give the impression that perhaps endocarditis is more likely to occur in patients who have had a shunt operation for tetralogy of Fallot than in those in whom no shunt procedure has been performed. This is simply an impression, however, and has no statistical confirmation. Seven of our eight patients who had rheumatic heart disease had mitral valve involvement.

According to White,[728] subacute bacterial endocarditis eventually occurs in about 5 per cent of all patients with rheumatic heart disease. Apparently, pure mitral stenosis is rarely the site of subacute bacterial endocarditis, but the disease commonly accompanies mitral or aortic regurgitation. Another interesting point in this regard is Levine's contention[421] that the disease is less likely to develop in patients with the severest type of rheumatic lesions (atrial fibrillation or congestive failure) than in patients with sinus rhythm who are relatively well compensated. Obviously, the valvular deformity itself, rather than the presence or absence of rheumatic activity, is the predisposing factor.

Among congenital heart deformities, bicuspid aortic valve, patent ductus arteriosus, coarctation of the aorta, ventricular septal defect and sometimes pulmonary or aortic stenosis are the most common lesions affected by alpha hemolytic streptococci. The fact that bacterial endocarditis may develop as a complication of open-heart surgery has plagued surgeons and cardiologists within the past four or five years. Every child who has persistent fever beyond the first week or so after open-heart surgery should be looked at with suspicion in this regard.[445] The incidence of infection, according to Gelfman and Levine,[272] is 6.5 per cent of all persons having congenital heart disease and 16.5 per cent of those who lived to be 2 years of age or more. Taussig[684] stated that the incidence of subacute bacterial endocarditis in tetralogy of Fallot, with or without an associated Blalock procedure, is about 8 per cent. The significance of these figures in the light of the extensive use of chemotherapy and chemoprophylaxis is not known. It is of considerable interest that atrial septal defect seldom is affected by this disease,[303] and also that small ventricular defects are more likely to be accompanied by endocarditis than larger ones. The assumption frequently made in the past that cyanotic congenital heart disease does not predispose to subacute bacterial endocarditis is no longer tenable. Of 24 patients with this condition seen at The Children's Hospital within an eighteen-year period, six had cyanotic disease.

Pathology

The characteristic lesions of subacute bacterial endocarditis are friable vegetations made up principally of bacteria and thrombi. Typically, there is little granulation tissue in the acute stage, and the vegetations are easily removable. It is thought that the infecting organisms settle on the damaged valves or the parietal endocardium from the blood stream at the time of a transient bacteremia. They are then embedded in a meshwork of thrombus formation from which the blood stream constantly snips off minute, infected emboli. The vegetations usually settle on the valve leaflets; the mitral valve is affected most commonly, and the aortic valve next. In patent ductus arteriosus the pulmonary orifice is the site of the vegetation; in ventricular septal defect the right ventricular side of the septum is usually involved; in coarctation of the aorta the infection is usually situated at the site of the aortic block. The vegetations may spread from the valve leaflets to the chordae tendineae; in fact, the valves themselves may become perforated. The parietal endocardium in the right ventricle, opposite a ventricular septal defect, may sometimes be the site of an infected thrombus.

Embolic phenomena may be observed in almost every organ. The kidneys may show embolic focal nephritis and even acute glomerulonephritis. The lungs may be the site of infarcts. The brain may be affected to varying degrees; in some cases only small areas of softening are found; in others gross hemorrhage and even diffuse meningoencephalitis are present. Vessels themselves may be destroyed by the infected emboli; the bacteria may invade the vessel wall, causing rupture or aneurysmal dilatation (mycotic aneurysm).

Splenomegaly is an almost indispensable feature of subacute bacterial endocarditis; the enlargement consists principally in lymphatic hyperplasia with enlargement of the malpighian bodies, and occasionally infarcts.

Clinical Picture

We saw 24 children with subacute bacterial endocarditis at The Children's Medical Center in Boston between 1944 and 1956;[177] the profile as described in the following paragraphs is based on observations made on these patients.

All our patients were children with known heart disease. Their ages ranged from eight months to sixteen years. Until the onset of subacute bacterial endocarditis they had all lived relatively normal and happy lives. The majority were going to school. Gradually the onset of fatigue, fever, night sweats and chills was noted. The fever followed a mild respiratory infection in most instances. In two cases a history of dental extraction was obtained. The following possible etiologic factors could be implicated in single instances: tonsillectomy, severe pyoderma, tonsillitis and pneumonia. Not included in the group under discussion was one adolescent seen recently in whom the onset of fatal endocarditis occurred about six weeks after diagnostic left heart catheterization for severe aortic stenosis. No other possible instance of endocarditis was observed in connection with more than 3000 cardiac catheterizations performed in our institution. In two patients the onset was sudden; one of these had a convulsion as the initial complaint, and the other was under observation in the hospital for cyanotic congenital heart disease when a sudden rise in temperature occurred.

The pertinent findings revealed by physical and laboratory examinations are summarized in Figure 179. It may be seen that there is no single criterion on which the diagnosis of subacute bacterial endocarditis can be based; a palpable spleen, anemia, fever and weight loss in a patient with known heart disease should make the pediatrician consider this disease seriously.

Most of the time the splenomegaly is considerable; some of the largest and hardest spleens in children are encountered in patients with subacute bacterial endocarditis. Pain in the splenic region may indicate an infarct.

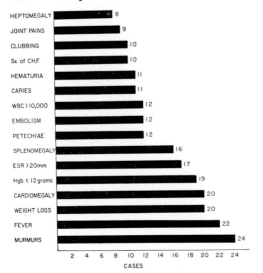

Figure 179. Clinical and laboratory findings in patients with bacterial endocarditis.[177]

The temperature most commonly is between 101 and 103° F., with considerable daily fluctuation. Severe dental caries is common.

The presence of petechiae clinches the diagnosis, although their absence does not preclude subacute bacterial endocarditis. Sometimes the petechiae are elusive and look like small freckles. It is worth while to mark the suspicious spots with a skin pencil and to follow them day by day to see whether they disappear or whether new ones occur. It is important to note that the petechiae of subacute bacterial endocarditis are widely scattered, not clustered around an area such as the neck or the antecubital fossa. Localized petechial spots suggest increased capillary permeability rather than embolic phenomena. Petechiae sometimes persist after bacteriologic cure of subacute bacterial endocarditis, and may last for several months without ill effect.

In twelve patients embolism occurred, frequently to the lungs or brain. At necropsy an embolus was found in the coronary artery of one patient and in the renal artery of another.

Clubbing is significant as a diagnostic aid only if the patient does not have cyanotic congenital heart disease; in this situation, however, it is practically pathognomonic if liver disease and lung abscess can also be excluded.

Congestive failure, especially right-sided, may be the first manifestation of subacute bacterial endocarditis in a patient with known heart disease. On the other hand, congestive failure may begin after bacteriologic cure of the endocarditis. In the latter instance it is usually blamed on the myocardial damage or more likely on the valve deformity subsequent to the localization of the infection on the valve cusps. Transient hemiplegia, with or without convulsions, in a patient with known heart disease should raise the suspicion of subacute bacterial endocarditis with consecutive emboli or small petechial hemorrhages.

The red and raised nonhemorrhagic Osler nodes and the tender fingers and toes often described in adults are seldom seen in children.

Anemia was present frequently in our patients; most had hemoglobin levels below 12 gm. and some below 8 gm. Whether the anemia is the result of interference with iron metabolism, such as is assumed to be the case in many infections, or whether a specific hemolytic or "toxic" effect is involved is not definitely known. A blood smear obtained from the ear lobes frequently shows a large number of histiocytes or macrophages.

Four of our patients did not have positive blood cultures, and in at least half of our patients the blood cultures were reported as positive only several days after the onset of treatment. Elevated sedimentation rate is a nonspecific manifestation of subacute or chronic infection, but it may be present even in the face of severe congestive heart failure. The high leukocyte count in twelve of the twenty-four cases was caused principally by an increase in polymorphonuclear leukocytes, but in three cases monocytes dominated the picture. Macroscopic hematuria was not present in any instance; microscopic hematuria was found in eleven. The electrocardiographic and x-ray changes were dependent on the underlying heart disease.

Differential Diagnosis

In trying to establish the diagnosis of subacute bacterial endocarditis, rheumatic fever should first be excluded. Among the major manifestations of rheumatic fever, only carditis may be present in subacute bacterial endocarditis. On the other hand, a number of the minor manifestations (fever, abdominal pain, precordial pain, rashes, epistaxis and similar laboratory findings) may frequently be found in both diseases.

A positive blood culture makes mandatory the diagnosis of subacute bacterial endocarditis; the presence of chorea, polyarthritis or subcutaneous nodules favors a diagnosis of rheumatic fever. Another clinical point may be helpful; namely, pericarditis almost never occurs in patients with subacute bacterial endocarditis, whereas it is commonly associated with the severe carditis of rheumatic fever. High antistreptolysin titers are rarely present in subacute bacterial endocarditis; on the other hand, severe anemia is a fairly common finding. The principal points in the differential diagnosis between subacute bacterial endocarditis and rheumatic fever are summarized in Table 16 (p. 782). As mentioned earlier, an elevated sedimentation rate in the face of congestive heart failure favors bacterial endocarditis.

Almost all the systemic and localized infections occurring in patients with heart disease should also be considered in the differential diagnosis, especially the enteric diseases, pyelonephritis, pneumonias.

Course and Prognosis

Before the introduction of sulfonamides, subacute bacterial endocarditis was practically always fatal. Lichtman, in 1943,[429] placed the spontaneous recovery rate at about 1 per cent. He also found a 5 per cent recovery rate when sulfonamides were used in the treatment. Today, because of penicillin and other potent antibiotics, the recovery rate is not less than 65 per cent. In our series of 24 children with this disease, all but 4 (17 per cent) survived. Blumenthal's figures are identical to ours.[71]

Apparently the success of treatment depends a great deal on how early the disease is recognized. According to Friedberg,[257] if intensive therapy is started within a month after the onset of illness, the recovery rate is 90 per cent or better, whereas, if the condition goes unrecognized for 3 months or more, as many as 50 per cent of the patients die.

Another factor to be taken into consideration is the age of the patient; older people are less likely to recover than younger ones. The isolation of a microorganism from the blood stream enhances the success of treatment considerably. Whether the poor prognosis for patients with negative blood cultures is due to the delay in treatment caused by a search for the etiologic agent, or whether the same set of circumstances that prohibits the bacteria from getting into the circulation prevents antibiotics from penetrating the vegetation, is not known. It is a fact, however, that patients with negative blood cultures have a poorer prognosis. Obviously, the more sensitive the isolated organism is to the commonly used antibiotics, the more successful the treatment will be.

In our experience the presence of congestive heart failure, embolic phenomena, or both, indicates a poor prognosis. In a recent study of adults with bacterial endocarditis, Bland[502] found rupture of a mycotic aneurysm or embolus to cerebral or coronary vessels to be the most common immediate cause of death. A clinical picture of congestive heart failure was the dominant feature in those who failed to survive. Postmortem findings suggested that severe endocardial destruction, superimposed on an already damaged heart, was the anatomic basis of congestive heart failure.

Treatment

In view of these factors there has been a tendency within the past five years to start treatment of patients suspected of having subacute bacterial endocarditis before the causative organisms have been identified. This policy is predicated not only on the advantages of early therapy, but also on the unlikelihood of obtaining a positive blood culture after the first few hospital days. Finland[250] stated that "from the bacteriologic point of view, however, a delay of more than forty-eight hours, or at most five days, is logistically unsound, and does not seem justified, provided the treatment is begun only after adequate samples of blood for culture have been obtained during this waiting period for later examination." The chance of obtaining a positive blood culture later in the disease, if it was impossible during the first five days, is practically nil. As a matter of fact, most of the positive cultures are obtained within the first forty-eight hours.

Our policy within the past few years, then, has been one of suspecting subacute bacterial endocarditis in all children with known heart disease who have fever of unknown origin of at least one week's duration. If, in addition to fever, one or more of the following criteria are present, the diagnosis of subacute bacterial endocarditis is made clinically: (1) splenomegaly, (2) embolic phenomena, and (3) clubbing in a patient without arterial unsaturation. Several blood cultures (at least six) are obtained within the first forty-eight hours, especially during chills or sudden elevation of temperature. At the end of a two- to five-day waiting period, during which all pertinent differential diagnostic possibilities are explored, penicillin treatment is begun, even if the cultures are not yet positive.

The drug of choice depends on the availability and the sensitivity of the organism. Since the alpha streptococcus is the commonest etiologic agent, penicillin alone or in combination with streptomycin is the most commonly used therapeutic agent. The dosage of penicillin should be between 5 and 10 million units per day, given preferably in a continuous intravenous drip or by the intramuscular route in six divided doses. The intravenous route, using a Number 24 short needle or threading a plastic catheter into the vein, is less likely to cause discomfort than the intramuscular route. As a rule, if a small dose of heparin is added, the continuous drip may be left in the same vein for two to four days at a time. If the sensitivity tests *in vitro* indicate that the addition of streptomycin is desirable, or if treatment is started before the organism is identified, 1 to 1.5 Gm. per day of streptomycin is added to the penicillin. On the basis of our own experience and of the theoretic considerations outlined by Finland,[250] we believe that aqueous solutions of sodium or potassium salt of penicillin should be used rather than the longer-acting repository form, at least for the first four weeks. Probenecid, a renal excretory inhibitor of penicillin, may be utilized to elevate the level of penicillin in the blood; 1 or 2 Gm. per day in 4 divided doses can be given by mouth. The use of this agent in children is limited.

Instead of penicillin and streptomycin, other drugs such as bacitracin, the tetracyclines, chloramphenicol, erythromycin or polymyxin may be used in cases in which the organism seems sensitive only to one of these agents. However, approximately *90 per cent of the cases of subacute bacterial endocarditis are caused by alpha or gamma streptococci, organisms extremely sensitive to adequate doses of penicillin.* Whatever drug is used, it should be continued for at least six weeks, except for streptomycin, which should be discontinued after one to two weeks. Recent reports suggest the combined use of penicillin and streptomycin for two weeks only; however, I consider the evidence in favor of such a short cure insufficient. It may be permissible, though, if the patient's condition progresses satisfactorily, to substitute one daily injection of a repository penicillin in comparable doses for the last two weeks of treatment. If *Staphylococcus aureus* is identified as the causative organism, high doses of staphcillin are recommended for treatment. This is also the drug of choice in patients with a positive blood culture in whom bacterial endocarditis has developed after open-heart surgery.

One of the most disturbing features in the treatment of subacute bacterial endocarditis is the persistence of a low-grade fever without positive blood cultures or any other signs of activity. In our experience this is commonly due to the local irritant effect of a large number of penicillin shots given intramuscularly to a child with a greatly wasted musculature, or to phlebitis due to the local effects of prolonged intravenous treatment. I feel that only with the utmost nursing skill, the use of the sharpest needles and a carefully mapped-out rotation of the injection sites can this be avoided. Even with the best of nursing care, local irritant action may be unavoidable. Sometimes only the complete cessation of treatment will effectively abolish the elevation in temperature (Fig. 180). To discontinue penicillin treatment in the face of persistent elevation of temperature is one of the hardest decisions to make; no definite guidance in this regard can be given. I can only draw the reader's attention to this phenomenon, and urge him to consider the possibility that the fever may be due to the inflamed injection sites.

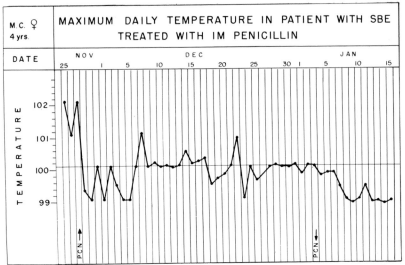

Figure 180. Temperature course of patient with subacute bacterial endocarditis treated with penicillin. Note the initial high fever before penicillin is started and the prompt drop occurring on institution of treatment. Then, less than 10 days later, another elevation of temperature that does not completely subside until penicillin is discontinued on January 3.

Another disturbing feature in the treatment of subacute bacterial endocarditis may be persistent showers of petechiae, or even pulmonary embolism, in a patient who otherwise is doing well. This phenomenon, by itself, ought not to be considered an absolute indication of persistence of infection; sterile embolic or petechial hemorrhages may occur several weeks or even months after the bacteriologic cure of subacute bacterial endocarditis.

Prophylaxis

The decline in the incidence of subacute bacterial endocarditis has been attributed largely to the widespread use of antibacterial agents for even minor manifestations of infection, and before and after even minor surgical procedures. This hypothesis, probably correct, although conclusive proof is still missing, has been accepted to the extent that prophylactic use of penicillin or some other antibacterial agent before and after dental extractions and during febrile illnesses is a required routine for all patients with organic heart disease. The danger of bacteremia developing after dental extractions has been demonstrated by Palmer and Kempf,[547] who found transiently positive blood cultures in fourteen of eighty-two patients after dental extraction.

It is recommended that 600,000 units of aqueous penicillin and 600,-000 units of procaine penicillin be administered 30 minutes before dental extraction or other oral surgery (tonsillectomy and adenoidectomy). An alternate method is to administer one million units of penicillin by mouth the day before, the day of and the day after oral surgery. Febrile illnesses of any sort in patients having congenital or rheumatic heart disease should be treated by some antibacterial agent for at least one week.

Although liberal chemoprophylaxis and chemotherapy are probably

extremely useful in preventing the development of subacute bacterial endocarditis, it must be pointed out that they are not uniformly successful and
may not be without danger. One must bear in mind the development of
resistant strains, the occurrence of sensitivities and a change in the bacterial
flora. Since well documented instances of penicillin-resistant alpha streptococci have been presented, I do not recommend continuous penicillin
prophylaxis for the prevention of bacterial endocarditis in patients with
congenital heart disease.

Complications

Since the introduction of effective agents against organisms causing
subacute bacterial endocarditis, it has become obvious that some patients
may not recover in spite of a bacteriologic cure. In a considerable proportion of these, death is caused by congestive failure; at postmortem examination no organisms can be cultured, but evidences of severe myocardial
damage are found. According to our experience, this does not seem to
be a serious risk in children; all the patients in whom we were able to
sterilize the blood stream recovered satisfactorily.

In one of our patients, however—a boy with true truncus arteriosus
who recovered from subacute bacterial endocarditis—polyarthritis, pericarditis and a typical picture of acute rheumatic carditis developed within two
months after his blood cultures had become sterile. He responded well
to treatment with ACTH. Whether this was a complication of subacute
bacterial endocarditis or whether it was true rheumatic carditis cannot be
stated with certainty. It is simply mentioned as an interesting and therapeutically approachable condition developing in the wake of bacteriologically cured subacute bacterial endocarditis.

In 1959 Bland[502] reviewed the long-term outlook of patients with
bacteriologically cured bacterial endocarditis. In 8.5 per cent of the patients
in his series, endocarditis recurred. Almost 15 per cent of his patients died
later, a few with recurrent endocarditis, but most because of severe structural disease involving principally the valves, and to a lesser extent the
myocardium. In other words, although an immediate cure may be accomplished in about 65 per cent of the patients, a sizable percentage of the
adults who are "cured" may have severe, even fatal, complications later.

ACUTE BACTERIAL ENDOCARDITIS WITHOUT PRE-EXISTING HEART DISEASE

Incidence and Etiology

Septicemia with invasion of the endocardium is called acute bacterial
endocarditis. It is a rare condition today; only about half a dozen such
instances have been seen at The Children's Hospital Medical Center
within the past fifteen years.

Acute bacterial endocarditis, in contrast to subacute bacterial endocarditis, should terminate favorably or unfavorably within two months.
Also, whereas the cardiovascular phenomena dominate the picture in
"subacute" bacterial endocarditis, in acute bacterial endocarditis these are

overshadowed by the general picture of sepsis. No single organism is implicated in the majority of cases, unlike "subacute" bacterial endocarditis, in which the alpha or gamma streptococcus is responsible. *Staphylococcus aureus,* beta hemolytic streptococci, pneumococci and *Escherichia coli* are the microorganisms most frequently encountered in this condition in children. Nevertheless, any other organism causing generalized blood stream infection may attack the endocardium.

Pathology

In acute bacterial endocarditis the picture is dominated by thrombotic masses (vegetations) consisting of fibrin and bacteria, which invade the valvular or parietal endocardium. Pre-existing heart disease is not a prerequisite, as it is in patients with "subacute" bacterial endocarditis. Further pathologic differences between the two conditions are the much more severe destruction, ulceration, perforation (endocarditis ulcerosa) and the purulent or serosanguineous pericarditis commonly present with acute bacterial endocarditis.

Any and all organs may be invaded in the septic process. Splenomegaly is the rule. Pneumonitis with abscess formation is common. The kidneys are involved in a high percentage of cases; they may show multiple abscesses, parenchymal or perinephric, and even evidences of glomerulonephritis or infarct. Meningitis and meningoencephalitis may be present as well.

Clinical Picture

Within the framework of generalized sepsis there may be only a few signs pointing to the involvement of the cardiovascular system. The most clear diagnostic finding is the appearance of a loud heart murmur in a patient with septicemia. Other less pathognomonic findings are progressive cardiac enlargement, congestive failure and the presence of embolic phenomena. Janeway spots—painless, hemorrhagic lesions on the palms or soles—are also characteristic of acute bacterial endocarditis.

Diagnosis

The diagnosis is almost solely of academic importance. It should be possible to make the diagnosis of a blood stream infection with ease; if the signs mentioned previously are present, a localization of the septic process in the endocardium must be suspected. It is interesting to note that among the forty-five patients in Bland's series who died with acute bacterial endocarditis,[502] in only two instances was an accurate diagnosis made before death.

Treatment

Whether or not there is cardiac involvement, the treatment of septicemia should be the same; it consists in adequate antibacterial treatment with penicillin, streptomycin or any other agent that proves to be effective, according to sensitivity tests. The dosage schedule outlined for penicillin and streptomycin in subacute bacterial endocarditis should be adequate in instances of acute bacterial endocarditis.

There are no mortality figures based on large series available in the pediatric literature. In 1947 Wilhelm and his associates[730] analyzed 40 cases of acute bacterial endocarditis in adults; a mortality rate of 60 to 80 per cent was noted, depending on the causative organisms. A recent report by Shubin and his associates[639] quoted a 74 per cent mortality rate. In Bland's series only 15 per cent survived. Our small experience with the disease suggests that at least a 50 per cent mortality rate must be expected at the present time.

9

ARRHYTHMIAS

The normal rhythm of the heart is dependent on sinoatrial impulses, discharged at regular intervals and spreading through the conduction system at conventional speeds. The impulse travels rapidly from the sinus node, through the atria, and arrives at the atrioventricular node. The passage through the atrioventricular nodal tissue is slow—about one fifth of the speed in the atria. From the atrioventricular node the impulse spreads at an increased speed down the bundles of His, stimulating the left side of the muscular septum first; then it is conducted through the Purkinje fibers and through the ventricular wall proper from endocardial to epicardial direction (Figs. 37, 38, p. 48).

In the healthy child this mechanism results in a regular rhythm at a rate of 80 to 180 beats per minute. The actual rate in the normal person depends a great deal on his age and his state of mind. On the whole, the younger the child, the more rapid is the pulse. Rates as high as 180 per minute are occasionally encountered at birth, though a significant drop usually occurs in 1 or 2 hours' time. During the first week of life the average rate is less than 140 beats per minute, and during the first year less than 120. By the time a child is 6 years of age the sleeping pulse rate is usually less than 100 beats per minute, and at puberty, as a rule, less than 80. Obviously, all these are average values subject to a great deal of fluctuation through crying, excitement, fear, and so forth. Consequently, *pulse rates,* to mean anything at all, *must be taken during sleep,* especially in children.

Changes in this regular rhythm at average rate are called arrhythmias. The arrhythmias will be discussed according to the following classification: (*a*) arrhythmias with sinus pacemaker, (*b*) arrhythmias with ectopic pacemakers, and (*c*) arrhythmias caused by conduction defects.

ARRHYTHMIAS WITH SINUS PACEMAKER

SINUS TACHYCARDIA

Sinus tachycardia is the rule rather than the exception in children being examined by a physician; most youngsters exhibit higher than normal pulse rates because of anxiety when they enter a physician's office. Exercise, fever, anemia or shock may also cause an increased pulse rate. Usually, but not invariably, rheumatic carditis is accompanied by a persistently elevated heart rate, even in sleep, which is out of proportion to the accompanying temperature. Congenital heart disease without cardiac insufficiency or cyanosis does not usually give rise to tachycardia. Thyrotoxicosis, a common cause of sinus tachycardia in adults, is rare in children; occasionally it may be encountered in girls at the age of puberty. Congestive heart failure (probably by means of the Bainbridge reflex and anoxia) is, of course, associated with tachycardia.

Clinically, sinus tachycardia is suspected if the heart rate is between 140 and 200 beats per minute and does not have a clocklike regularity and consistency. If one spends a few minutes listening to the heart or counting the radial pulse, minor changes of 10 to 15 beats per minute will frequently be observed. This is in contrast to the patient with paroxysmal atrial tachycardia whose heart rate is rigidly fixed and is almost always more than 180 beats per minute. Reflex vagal stimulation (eyeball pressure, carotid sinus stimulation or Valsalva maneuver) often causes slight but definite alterations in the heart rate of patients with sinus tachycardia.

Electrocardiographically, sinus tachycardia can easily be recognized by the well formed P waves with a normal P axis, a P-R interval of 0.1 to 0.2 second and a normal-appearing QRS complex (Fig. 75, p. 79).

In most instances sinus tachycardia does not require any specific treatment—only search for, and elimination of, the cause (shock or anemia). Digitalis has no influence on sinus tachycardia without underlying heart disease. Phenobarbital sometimes slows the pulse of a hyperexcitable youngster. Tranquilizers, particularly Reserpin, may be effective in slowing the heart rate in sinus tachycardia.

SINUS BRADYCARDIA

Sinus bradycardia in adults is commonly defined as a heart rate of less than 60 beats per minute. It is obvious from the previous discussion of the normal heart rate of healthy children that no such clear-cut definition is possible in the field of pediatrics. By and large, rates of less than 100 in infants and 80 in children should be considered bradycardic.

Sinus bradycardia is rare in healthy children, but is seen occasionally in athletes and in patients with rheumatic fever, increased intracranial pressure, increased systemic blood pressure, typhoid fever or hypothyroidism. The appearance of atropine-resistant sinus bradycardia during cardiac surgery is an ominous sign which may indicate profound anoxia, leading gradually to cardiac standstill and death. Electrolyte disturbances, especially potassium intoxication, may also be accompanied by profound bradycardia.

The clinical differentiation of sinus bradycardia from a slow pulse rate resulting from nodal rhythm is impossible. On the other hand, in second- or third-degree heart block, a fairly common cause of bradycardia, careful observation of the jugular venous pulse reveals atrial pulsations (A waves) during ventricular diastole. On scrupulous auscultation the intensity of the first heart sound at the apex shows definite changes in patients with atrioventricular dissociation or heart block (see p. 113).

The effect of exercise or a dose of amyl nitrate is revealing in this regard. The rate in patients with complete heart block changes little, if at all. In patients with sinoatrial block the rate may double. In patients with nodal rhythm, sinus bradycardia or second-degree heart block the rate increases appreciably, but without a clear mathematical ratio.

In most instances the electrocardiogram is essential in making a definite diagnosis of sinus bradycardia. The tracing is characterized by a normal P wave, a P-R interval of less than 0.20 second and a normal QRS complex (Fig. 76, p. 79).

Sinus bradycardia in children does not require symptomatic treatment; careful search for the underlying cause should be made, however.

SINUS ARRHYTHMIA

Sinus arrhythmia is a phasic change in the rate of discharge of sinus impulses, resulting in a rhythmic speeding and slowing of the heart rate. The change in rate may be coordinated with respiration (slowing on inspiration) or may be independent of it. The presence of sinus arrhythmia is predicated on increased vagal tone and therefore is almost never present in young infants, but is pronounced in adolescents. Slow rates predispose to sinus arrhythmia, and fast rates abolish it. By and large, sinus arrhythmia is a sign of good cardiac reserve, although it has been noted with congenital as well as rheumatic heart disease.

The diagnosis is easily made without the use of the electrocardiograph. The pathognomonic feature is a phasic variation of the heart rate, which may or may not be synchronous with respiration. It can readily be abolished by the tachycardia caused by exercise.

Electrocardiographically, the QRS complexes and the P-R intervals are regular and unchanging, whereas the P-P and R-R intervals are different at various portions of the tracing (Fig. 77, p. 79).

The degree of sinus arrhythmia has been expressed by means of a so-called frequency index.[618] The mean values ranged around 20 with heart rates of 90 to 96 in a study of normal children at The House of the Good Samaritan.[370]

No treatment is indicated.

ARRHYTHMIAS WITH ECTOPIC PACEMAKERS

All parts of the conduction system, from the sinus node to the Purkinje fibers, have basic impulse-forming properties. Under ordinary circumstances the sinus node, because it discharges impulses most rapidly, is the pacemaker of the heart. All other potential pacemakers have an inherently slower discharge rate; hence they do not usually have an opportunity to take over the lead.

Under certain circumstances, however, such as decreased irritability of the sinus node (sinus bradycardia or sinus arrhythmia), blockage of sinus impulses (sinoatrial block) or acquired hyperirritability of one of the lower centers, the sinus node may lose control of the rhythm of the heart. Under these conditions one of the ectopic pacemakers in the atria, in the atrioventricular node or in the ventricle proper may become the governing body of the heart temporarily or permanently. If the reign of the ectopic pacemaker lasts for one or two beats only, ectopic or premature beats occur. If the sinus node relinquishes its control for several cycles in succession, ectopic tachycardia results.

ECTOPIC BEATS

Ectopic beats appear to be less common in children than in adults, but no recent figures on their incidence are available. Lyon and Rauh[462] found ectopic beats in 0.06 per cent of a large series of healthy newborns and in 2.2 per cent of healthy school children. Landtman[407] in his detailed book on arrhythmias of children found ectopic beats in 1.53 per cent of his cases. Supraventricular premature beats are more common in children than ventricular ectopic beats.

Physiologically, the premature beat is a less than completely effective

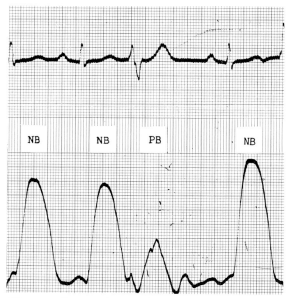

Figure 181. Electrocardiogram (top) and right ventricular pressure tracing obtained at cardiac catheterization (bottom). The first electrocardiographic beat is followed by a normal beat in the right ventricle. The second QRS complex is equally followed by a normal ventricular complex. The third QRS complex is a premature one and is followed by a low pressure tracing within the ventricle. After this a compensatory pause follows, and the beat following the compensatory pause shows considerably higher pressure in the right ventricle than the normal beat and the premature beat.

contraction because of the shorter than normal diastolic filling of the ventricle. In contrast, the succeeding normal beat, if separated from the ectopic one by a compensatory pause, is a stronger than average contraction because of the extra-long diastolic filling time (Fig. 181) and the super-normal phase of excitation.

Etiology

The majority of patients with ectopic beats have normal hearts. However, rheumatic fever, endocardial fibroelastosis, myocarditis and drugs (digitalis, quinidine, cyclopropane, chloroform and epinephrine) may all contribute to their occurrence. Fortunately for the pediatrician, coronary disease, pregnancy, alcohol and tobacco—all common causes of premature beats in adults—do not have to be considered in the etiology of this arrhythmia in the majority of children.

Clinical Picture and Differential Diagnosis

Premature beats usually cause no symptoms, although older children may find them annoying if they occur several times per minute. It may be of interest to mention that the extra-strong postextrasystolic beat is often noted by the patient as a "thump," whereas the premature beat itself may pass by unobserved. Supraventricular, i.e. atrial or nodal, premature beats should be suspected from the clinical examination if less than a complete compensatory pause is present. In contrast, ventricular premature beats are followed by a complete compensatory pause. One further point in differential diagnosis is that, whereas the first sound of the supraventricular premature beat is always accentuated, the first sound of the ventricular premature beat varies from normal to loud to diminished,[170] depending on the time interval between the QRS complex and the preceding P wave. If the atrial contraction occurs only a short time (less than 0.12 second) before the QRS, the first sound will be loud. If the P-R interval is long, the first sound will be dull.

Electrocardiographically, the ectopic beat is always premature and may or may not be bizarre in contour. If the QRS configuration is like that of the normal beat, the premature beat is supraventricular. Within this group a P-R interval of 0.10 second or more indicates an atrial origin, whereas a shorter P-R interval, with a P axis of —60 to —90 degrees, points to nodal origin.

If the QRS complex is bizarre and is different from the normal complex, one may be dealing with a ventricular premature beat. In this case no premature or abnormal P wave precedes the premature complex. If a bizarre P wave does precede a bizarre QRS complex, one probably is dealing with a supraventricular premature beat and aberrant intraventricular conduction.

Ectopic beats originating from a normal heart are usually easy to distinguish from those occurring in a diseased heart. To begin with, premature beats are seldom, if ever, the sole manifestation of heart disease in children; if carefully searched for, other evidences of cardiac abnormality (murmur, cardiomegaly, electrocardiographic evidence of hypertrophy, or elevated sedimentation rate) are demonstrable if there is underlying heart disease. Exercise abolishes premature beats originating from a normal heart, whereas they are commonly exaggerated on exercise if heart disease is present. The presence of heart disease should be suspected if the premature beats show varying configuration (suggesting multifocal origin) in the electrocardiogram. On the whole, ventricular premature beats are relatively more common in children with heart disease than in those whose cardiovascular system is intact.

Excess digitalis administration usually causes supraventricular premature beats in children, although the occurrence of ventricular premature beats, particularly in bigeminal rhythms, is practically diagnostic of digitoxicity. Quinidine intoxication is more likely to cause ventricular than supraventricular premature beats.

A series of ectopic beats (usually though not invariably supraventricular in origin) may be encountered in newborn babies. Keen obstetricians have discovered the presence of this arrhythmia when listening to the fetal heart. The ectopic beats may be so numerous that the rhythm is totally irregular, but the over-all rate is seldom more than 140 to 160 beats per minute. The prognosis of this "arrhythmia of the newborn" is usually good, and the arrhythmia, if not accompanied by other evidences of heart disease, usually disappears without treatment within the first ten days of life. It should be electrocardiographically differentiated, however, from congenital atrial flutter, a rare and serious abnormality usually associated with endocardial fibroelastosis.

The diagnosis of premature beats should usually be based on the electrocardiogram. Sinus arrhythmia, sinoatrial block and occasionally even atrial flutter or fibrillation may have to be considered in the differential diagnosis. Although exercise tests, inspection of the jugular venous pulse and careful observation of the heart sounds may aid in determining the nature of the arrhythmia by clinical means, in most instances the little effort and expense spent on the electrocardiogram, in return for an accurate, authoritative explanation of the child's condition, are fully appreciated by the parents.

Treatment

Premature beats, in themselves, unless they occur frequently, require no treatment, but the question of underlying heart disease should be given careful therapeutic consideration in every instance. Ventricular premature beats are always more worrisome than supraventricular ones because of their possible extension into ventricular tachycardia.

Whereas ectopic beats originating from a clinically normal heart are not worrisome at all, their occurrence in children with known heart disease should cause some concern. I have seen patients with congenital heart disease (aortic stenosis, endocardial cushion defect) in whom the appearance of numerous ventricular premature beats was the sole indication of the severity of the disease. Furthermore, one of our patients, an adolescent boy with rheumatic aortic regurgitation, who had no evidence of active rheumatic fever, but who had frequent ventricular premature beats, died suddenly at home. The assumption was made that ventricular fibrillation developed.

If the ectopic beats are clearly the result of psychological factors in an unstable adolescent, reassurance and the judicious use of phenobarbital or

Reserpin may abolish them. If treatment by these simple methods is not successful and the arrhythmia is of concern to the patient, then specific cardiac drugs may be administered, depending on the site of the pacemaker. Supraventricular premature beats should be treated with digitalis, ventricular premature beats with quinidine or Pronestyl. Potassium chloride, administered orally, may be effective for both supraventricular and ventricular premature beats. The dosages are outlined in Table 17 (pp. 783–786). Before either digitalis or quinidine is administered, the physician must be certain that these drugs do not, in fact, cause the arrhythmia. If any doubt exists, it is a good policy to discontinue all medication for a period of days or weeks.

ECTOPIC TACHYCARDIA

A series of premature beats at rapid rates is called ectopic tachycardia. The duration of the ectopic rhythm may be from a few seconds to several years.

Simple Paroxysmal Tachycardia

Usurpation of the normal sinus rhythm by an ectopic focus results in simple paroxysmal tachycardia; characteristically, the paroxysm begins and ends suddenly, much as one would abruptly shift the gear of an automobile from a lower to a higher speed. Paroxysmal tachycardia is not a common condition in children. At The Children's Hospital Medical Center in Boston the yearly admission rate of new patients with paroxysmal tachycardia is about two. The average pediatrician may see one such case every five years or so. Nevertheless it may be worth while to spend considerable time in discussing this arrhythmia, since it is one of the real, treatable cardiac emergencies in children.

For obvious reasons there are not many physiologic studies of people with paroxysmal tachycardia. A brave soul would he be who would attempt cardiac catheterization under these conditions. A few studies are available, however, indicating considerable increase in the arteriovenous oxygen difference and some decrease in the arterial saturation during a paroxysm.[195] Animal experiments point to a decrease in the coronary blood flow and the mean arterial pressure during the attack. These changes are more pronounced with higher rates. Ventricular tachycardia results in a greater change in the coronary circulation than supraventricular tachycardia at a comparable rate.[719]

Clinical Picture

Paroxysmal rapid heart action may be supraventricular or ventricular in origin, and a clinical differentiation of the two types is often possible. The rate of supraventricular tachycardia is perfectly steady from one minute to the next, whereas ventricular tachycardia may show small variations in rate. Reflex vagal stimulation (eyeball pressure, carotid sinus stimulation, Valsalva maneuver) may influence supraventricular tachycardia, whereas it has no demonstrable effect on ventricular tachycardia. At auscultation the intensity of the first heart sound is increased but unchanging in supraventricular tachycardia, whereas recurrent changes in intensity are often noted in ventricular tachycardia.

A clinical differentiation between the two principal types of supraventricular tachycardia, i.e. atrial flutter and atrial tachycardia, is difficult. Reflex vagal stimulation, if effective at all, converts atrial tachycardia into normal rate and rhythm, whereas its effect on atrial flutter is only one of altering the atrioventricular conduction, resulting in an arithmetical division of the rate, such as halving. Exercise, by the same token, does not change the rate of paroxysmal atrial tachycardia at all, whereas in paroxysmal flutter it may cause the rate to increase in a mathematical ratio by one third or one half, through changes in atrioventricular conduction.

The following clinical profile of simple paroxysmal tachycardia is based on our observations of forty-one cases seen at The Children's Hospital Medical Center during a twenty-year period.

The etiology of paroxysmal tachycardia often is not known. Slightly more than 10 per cent of our patients showed electrocardiographic evidences of the Wolff-Parkinson-White syndrome; another 20 per cent had congenital heart disease. About 20 per cent of the patients had infections, injuries or heart tumors, or were under the influence of drugs, at the time tachycardia occurred. Whether or not any of these findings had anything to do with the occurrence of paroxysmal tachycardia would be hard to prove, but in 50 per cent of the patients not even such circumstantial evidence was available to explain the occurrence of paroxysmal rapid heart action.

Analysis of the age at onset in our forty-one patients resulted in the interesting observation that the disease was more likely to start within the first four months of life than throughout the rest of childhood (Fig. 182). Also, in most cases occurring in young infants no etiologic factors could be detected. Conversely, in older infants and children factors were frequently present that might explain the occurrence of the tachycardia. Finally, when the etiologic factors were correlated with the sex incidence, it was learned that most patients with "idiopathic" paroxysmal tachycardia were males (Fig. 183). Thus, on the basis of age, sex and the presence or absence of possible etiologic factors, paroxysmal tachycardia in children divides itself into two groups, one consisting of males less than four months of age without concomitant disease and the other of older infants and children of either sex who may or may not have demonstrable etiology for tachycardia.

Seven of our forty-one patients were not sick, and their paroxysmal tachycardia was discovered during a routine physical examination. The majority of the infants, however, were very ill indeed, the picture resembling that of severe pneumonia or septicemia. These babies were irritable and restless, with ashen-gray or cyanotic color and cold, clammy skin. Respirations were rapid and labored, and often a hacking cough was present. Cardiac enlargement was manifest, and the heart rate was rapid, even uncountable, with a thready pulse. Rales were heard over the chest, and the liver was enlarged. Peripheral edema and puffiness of the face were noted in some.

Fever was noted occasionally. In a few instances it could be explained on the basis of infection alone; in others it was assumed to be due to congestive failure.

A systolic murmur was present during the attack in almost half of the patients, but in only a quarter of this group—all with murmurs of at least

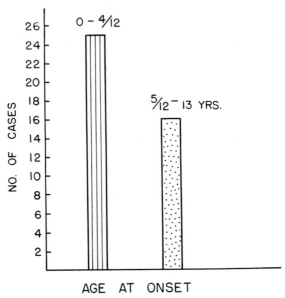

Figure 182.   Age at onset in forty-one patients with paroxysmal tachycardia.[527]

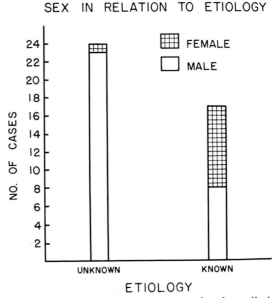

Figure 183.   Sex in relation to etiology of paroxysmal tachycardia in children.[527]

grade 3 intensity—did the murmur persist after cessation of the attack. No diastolic murmurs were observed.

Results of laboratory examinations were usually not of much assistance. Leukocytosis, if present, could be explained by infection or congestion.

The radiologic findings were those of congestive failure with "non-specific" cardiac enlargement of varying degree and pulmonary congestion. Isolated left atrial prominence was occasionally demonstrable. The cardiac beat under the fluoroscope was rapid and feeble.

Congestive failure developed in slightly more than 50 per cent of our patients with paroxysmal tachycardia; most of the signs and symptons described are manifestations of combined left and right ventricular failure. Analysis of our cases revealed that 3 factors seemed to influence the development of heart failure: (1) the rate—failure did not develop in any patient with paroxysmal tachycardia in whom the rate was less than 180 beats per minute; (2) the duration of the tachycardia (Fig. 184)—the longer the paroxysm lasted, the more likely was it to lead into congestive failure; (3) the age of the patient—the younger the child, the more likely was congestive failure to develop, perhaps because the manifestation of cardiac failure was the first symptom noted by the mother of a baby too young to complain.

The electrocardiograph is the only consistently reliable tool for the accurate analysis of these arrhythmias. About 95 per cent of our cases fell into the category of supraventricular tachycardia, i.e. paroxysmal atrial tachycardia (Fig. 82, p. 82) or paroxysmal flutter. Only 5 per cent of the patients showed characteristics of ventricular tachycardia (Fig. 88, p. 87).

The heart rate during the attack varied between 160 and 330 beats per minute. Patients with rates of 300 or more almost always exhibited flutter (f) waves in leads II and III. P waves were rarely identifiable; they were either absent or superimposed on the preceding T wave. If P waves were present, the P-R intervals varied from 0.08 to 0.13 second. In practically all instances of supraventricular tachycardia the QRS complexes were normal in configuration and similar to the ventricular complexes between attacks. Occasionally, however, because of the presence of intraventricular conduction block, abnormal QRS complexes, resembling those of ventricular tachycardia, may be present in patients who have, in fact, paroxysmal atrial tachycardia. In these cases exact determination of the P-QRS relation or observation of the effect of vagal stimulation helps to identify the type of tachycardia accurately. The QRS complexes in ventricular tachycardia are, by definition, bizarre and wide and unlike the complexes seen between attacks. The T waves, as mentioned, usually blend with the preceding atrial waves; hence it is difficult to describe their characteristics.

After cessation of the paroxysm the majority of the children in our series showed normal electrocardiograms for their age. In some, evidences of left and right atrial hypertrophy persisted for a few days. In others, electrocar-

DURATION OF TACHYCARDIA AND DEVELOPMENT
OF *CONGESTIVE FAILURE

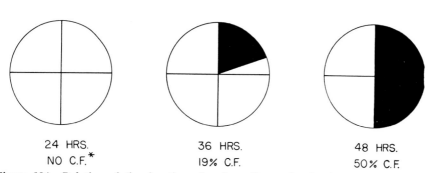

24 HRS.
NO C.F.*

36 HRS.
19% C.F.

48 HRS.
50% C.F.

Figure 184. Relation of the duration of tachycardia to the development of congestive failure.[527]

diograms characteristic of the Wolff-Parkinson-White syndrome were found. In a few, short P-R intervals without corresponding widening of the QRS complex were observed.[448] Diphasic or inverted T waves in leads I and II, with depressed S-T segments, were noted in some cases immediately after cessation of severe tachycardia of long duration; these changes, much like the P wave abnormalities, lasted for a few days only. We believe that the P wave changes are due to increased atrial pressure caused by congestive failure; the T wave abnormalities may be an expression of myocardial ischemia.

Treatment

Simple paroxysmal tachycardia can be successfully treated in almost every instance. Before treatment is begun it is extremely important to ascertain whether the tachycardia is supraventricular or ventricular in origin, since the therapeutic approaches to the two groups are entirely different.

The treatment of supraventricular tachycardia should begin with reflex vagal stimulation. First, carotid sinus pressure should be tried, by palpating the carotid artery as high up the neck as possible and pressing it against the vertebral column; first the right side, then the left, should be pressed, never both sides at the same time. The pressure or massage should be sustained for about thirty to sixty seconds, with the stethoscope on the chest, and released immediately when the rhythm changes. If this maneuver is not effective, eyeball pressure should be attempted. The pressure should be applied on the closed lids just below the supraorbital ridge, one side at a time for about thirty seconds. In older children, if neither of these procedures is effective, an effort may be made to stimulate the vagus nerve by asking the patient to perform a Valsalva maneuver or making him vomit by the administration of 1 or 2 teaspoonfuls of syrup of ipecac.

In our experience reflex vagal stimulation by the methods described is usually successful for paroxysms of short duration, without congestive failure. Only rarely, however, were we able to abolish the paroxysm in critically ill, small babies by these methods.

Drug therapy is the next step in the treatment of paroxysmal supraventricular tachycardia. In our opinion digitalis is the drug of choice. We have used digitoxin, Digoxin and Cedilanid equally successfully, but in recent years Digoxin has been the drug of choice. All three of these digitalizing drugs may be given parenterally; digitoxin and Digoxin may be administered orally as well. For the appropriate digitalizing dose, see Table 17 (pp. 783–786). In most instances the calculated dosage can be given throughout an eighteen-hour period in three divided doses. The oral or intramuscular route is recommended for the average patient, but in an emergency the intravenous route may be used safely. If the calculated digitalizing dose does not convert the rhythm to normal, more digitalis should be given cautiously; about one sixth of the calculated amount may be administered every four hours until either the desired effect is achieved or evidences of toxicity appear. Incidentally, carotid sinus stimulation may be worth attempting after full digitalization; it may be effective under these circumstances even if it had no effect before digitalization.

Digitalis, if given in appropriate doses, has been successful in the treatment of all but one of our patients with paroxysmal supraventricular tachycardia during the past twenty years. Only one person did not respond to

digitalis, but she responded easily to Prostigmin administered subcutaneously after full digitalization.

Our experience in the treatment of paroxysmal atrial tachycardia with
other drugs is limited. Quinidine and procaine amide are recommended by
some authors, but in our experience their principal use is in the treatment
of paroxysmal ventricular tachycardia. Mecholyl has also been recommended for the treatment of this condition; our experience with this drug
is limited, but rather unfavorable.

Continuous electrocardiographic tracings obtained during postoperative development of paroxysmal atrial tachycardia have revealed the
electrocardiographic patterns of conversion in a few instances. They are
frightening electrocardiograms, indeed, consisting of prolonged asystoles,
appearance of atrial flutter with block, later supraventricular or ventricular premature beats, and finally appearance of normal sinus rhythm.
Hellerstein and his associates[335] observed these and other changes during
conversion by means of carotid sinus pressure.

Ventricular tachycardia, in contrast to supraventricular tachycardia,
does not respond to reflex vagal stimulation. Treatment with digitalis is
contraindicated in most instances, though it has been successful on occasion
when all other measures failed. Quinidine and Pronestyl, administered
orally or parenterally, are the drugs of choice in this arrhythmia.

In our experience, after a test dose of 25 to 50 mg., 100 mg. of quinidine
every 2 hours should be given for 8 doses. If this does not work, the next
day 200 mg. should be given every 2 hours, again for 8 doses. The dose should
be gradually increased in this way until either the tachycardia is abolished or
toxic effects are noted. Among the clinical signs of toxicity, nausea, tinnitus
and vomiting should be mentioned. The toxic effects are manifested on the
electrocardiogram by widening of the QRS complex by more than 50 per
cent of its original duration.

Obviously, if the patient is critically ill, this leisurely schedule of oral
administration of the drug cannot be adhered to. In these instances quinidine should be given in progressively larger doses at hourly intervals,
starting with 100 mg., and continuing up to 200, 300, 400 or even 500 mg.,
until either therapeusis or toxicity is achieved. In an emergency the drug
may even be given intramuscularly.

If quinidine is not effective in controlling ventricular tachycardia, procaine amide, given orally or intramuscularly, should be tried. The oral dose
is 7 mg. per pound of body weight, to be given every 2 to 4 hours. Intramuscular administration, for the sicker patient, should start with 50 to 100
mg. and should increase by increments of 50 mg. every 2 hours until the
arrhythmia is controlled or toxicity supervenes. The principal toxic effects
of procaine amide are hypotension or the development of multifocal ventricular premature beats. In an emergency Pronestyl may be given intravenously under continuous electrocardiographic control. At first 100 mg. should
be administered during a period of 5 minutes; this should be followed by
the same dose every 5 minutes until either the arrhythmia is controlled or
toxicity occurs (Fig. 185). This is a dangerous procedure and may produce
ventricular fibrillation, but if it is used cautiously, it may serve as a lifesaving measure. Seldom should more than 1.0 Gm. be administered during
one hour, even for adolescent patients.

Within the past year electric, external countershock has been used in

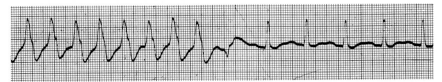

Figure 185. Successful use of Pronestyl in reverting ventricular tachycardia to normal sinus rhythm (lead II). Conversion occurred after the administration of 3 gm. of Pronestyl given over a period of one hour. Note (1) sudden reversion occurring within 2 beats; (2) ventricular tachycardia at rate of approximately 140 before reversion; (3) reversion to normal sinus rhythm with first-degree heart block (P-R interval, 0.28 second).

the treatment of resistant tachycardias in adults.[766] I have had no experience with this method except as it is used in the operating room, internally, for patients recovering from open-heart surgery. In the ensuing years it may well find wide application.

Ventricular tachycardia caused by digitoxicity should be treated by withdrawal of the glycoside and administration of potassium chloride or Pronestyl.

Through the judicious and intelligent use of these rather simple tools, most paroxysmal tachycardias in children may be reverted to normal rhythm without difficulty. This, of course, is different from experience with adults. The difference may be due to the structurally intact heart underlying most cases of paroxysmal rapid heart action in children. One cannot emphasize often enough that if these children are treated rationally, they should recover without difficulty, and that there is no reason for drastic and hurried "catastrophe reactions" when such a problem arises. Of forty-one patients with simple paroxysmal tachycardia treated at our hospital, all but three recovered. (One patient who died was treated with Mecholyl and one with an unusually high dose of digitalis, accompanied by bilateral carotid sinus pressure. The third patient died from a cerebrovascular accident presumably caused by arterial embolism. This complication, with recovery, has since been seen in one other child; hence it may not be as infrequent an event as was thought previously.)

In addition to the efforts aimed at conversion of the ectopic rhythm to normal sinus rhythm, the treatment of paroxysmal tachycardia should also consist in the administration of oxygen, antibiotics and perhaps morphine for restlessness.

The change in a desperately sick baby after the cessation of the tachycardia is truly remarkable. Within a few hours the color returns, the restlessness and cough disappear, and the sensorium clears. Within twenty-four to forty-eight hours the baby loses its edema, occasionally with a weight loss amounting to as much as 10 per cent of the total body weight. In a matter of days the liver returns to normal size, and the transient, post-tachycardic P wave and T wave changes disappear. Usually, x-ray examination shows clearing of the pulmonary congestion within a few days, but the heart may not return to normal size for seven to ten days.

Prophylaxis

The drug used to convert the rhythm to normal should be administered for at least a month for prophylactic purposes, after which it may be abruptly

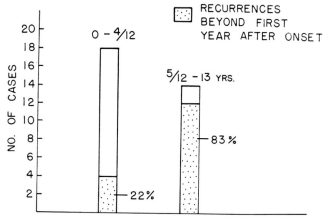

Figure 186. Recurrences of tachycardia in relation to age at onset in 32 cases of paroxysmal tachycardia followed for more than one year.[527]

discontinued. If recurrences are noted, it should be resumed for at least another six months. At this point sudden cessation should again be attempted.

Digitalis, in maintenance doses, is usually effective in preventing the recurrence of supraventricular tachycardia. Patients with the Wolff-Parkinson-White syndrome should probably receive quinidine for prophylaxis in doses of 200 to 400 mg. 4 times a day. On occasion, heroic doses (400 to 800 mg. 5 times a day) of quinidine and digitalis are needed to prevent frequent recurrences. Ventricular tachycardia may be successfully warded off by treatment with either quinidine or Pronestyl. The finding of a high uptake of I^{131} by the erythrocytes in euthyroid adults with normal protein-bound iodine levels has led some investigators to treat refractory cases of paroxysmal atrial tachycardia with radioactive iodine.[168] Of twenty-five patients so treated, twenty obtained good results. So far I have not tried this approach in children with recurrent paroxysmal atrial tachycardia, but it may well be an avenue worth exploring if conventional methods for prevention do not suffice.

Recurrences

Figure 186 demonstrates the importance of age at onset of the disease in determining the frequency of recurrences. In the idiopathic simple paroxysmal tachycardia of young infants, recurrences are rare beyond one year after the first attack, although during this period many episodes may occur. In contrast, older infants and children may continue to have attacks several years after the initial one.

Chronic Ectopic Atrial Tachycardia

Classic attacks of "simple paroxysmal tachycardia" in children are characterized by sudden onset and termination, fixed rates of more than 180 beats per minute lasting from hours to days, and a response to adequate treatment in terms of return to normal sinus rhythm. We have seen ten cases of supraventricular tachycardia at The Children's Hospital Medical Center in Boston which in one respect or another did not correspond to the typical picture described. For one thing, these patients had tachycardia lasting several months or even years. The second unorthodox feature was the change in rate without a change in pacemaker; in a baby a waking rate of 200 beats per minute would slow down to 130 during sleep, without change in the electrocardiogram (Fig. 187). Finally, some of these children responded initially to treatment with digitalis by maintaining their rapid ectopic atrial rhythm, but developing 1:2 or 2:3 atrioventricular block and thus slowing the ventricular rate.

Some of these cases correspond to what Parkinson and Papp[549] called repetitive tachycardia (Fig. 83, p. 83), a transition between extrasystoles and paroxysmal tachycardia. In effect these are repetitive premature beats, continuing throughout a period of several months or years, either occurring in short bursts or lasting several minutes, but always interspersed by periods of normal sinus rhythm (Fig. 188).[330] According to these authors, in a long tracing an occasional premature beat may be seen, alternating with short runs of tachycardia, then again a few premature beats. The ultimate prognosis in all Parkinson and Papp's cases was good, although in one instance the attacks lasted as long as ten years. They recommended quinidine as the treatment of choice.

One of our cases occurred in a newborn infant, but the others occurred in older infants or children.[501] Digitalis was effective only in slowing the ectopic pacemaker and decreasing the frequency of the bursts. Quinidine abolished the ectopic focus in some instances, but not with any regularity (Fig. 189).

Our other patients never had normal sinus rhythm while under our

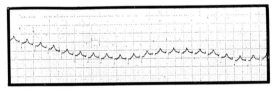

10 A.M.   Lead II
Awake
Atrial rate 170
1:1 AV response

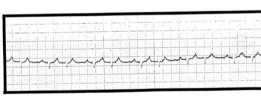

3 P.M.   Lead II
Awake
Atrial rate 155
2:1 and 1:1 AV response

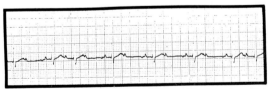

10 P.M.   Lead II
Asleep
Atrial rate 120
2:1 and 1:1 AV response

Figure 187.   Tracing of patient with chronic atrial tachycardia exemplifying the change in rate depending on the state of consciousness. The slowing during sleep is determined mostly by the slowing of the atrial pacemaker, and to a minor extent by the ventricular response to the atrial impulse.

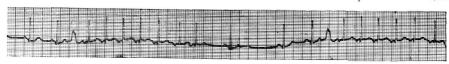

II 4/21/58

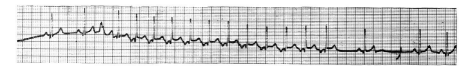

II 5/8/61

Figure 188. Persistence of chronic supraventricular tachycardia. Two tracings, taken at three-year intervals, repeat essentially the same patterns.

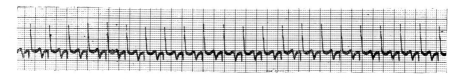

NO RX HR 165/M SUSTAINED TACHYCARDIA

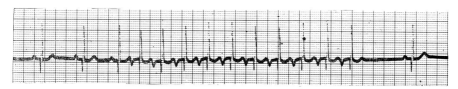

AFTER DIGITALIZATION HR 140/M "REPETITIVE" TACHYCARDIA

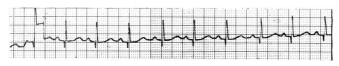

DIGITALIS AND QUINIDINE NORMAL SINUS RHYTHM

Figure 189. The influence of drugs on the pattern of chronic ectopic tachycardia. The top tracing shows a "sustained pattern." With digitalis, the sustained pattern is converted into a "repetitive" configuration, and administration of digitalis and quinidine, in combination, was accompanied by conversion to normal sinus rhythm.

care. This type of patient was referred to by Schacknow[634] as having "persistent supraventricular tachycardia." I prefer the term "sustained ectopic tachycardia." The P waves are always abnormal, even at slow rates. In one case digitalis was able to reduce the ventricular rate by producing a second-degree atrioventricular block (Fig 189) while a fast atrial rate persisted; Serpasil in combination with digitalis slowed the pacemaker and maintained a 3:1 atrioventricular block, resulting in the satisfactory ventricular rate of 80 to 100 beats per minute. In another patient (Fig. 190) digitalis

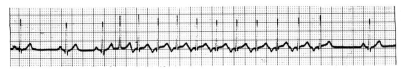

11/24/58 NO RX

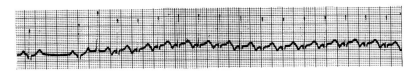

12/22/58 TWO WEEKS 0.3 mg RESERPINE PO qd

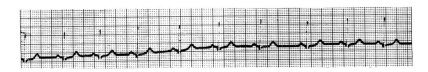

1/18/59 SIX WEEKS RESERPINE; FOUR WEEKS DIGOXIN

Figure 190. Chronic supraventricular tachycardia treated with reserpine and digitalis. The upper tracing shows a clear-cut repetitive pattern, essentially uninfluenced by reserpine. Later, conversion occurred with the administration of a combination of the two drugs, as shown in the lower tracing.

alone eventually slowed, but did not change, the atrial pacemaker. Quinidine, Pronestyl, potassium and Prostigmin were not effective in these patients. The rhythm in these children today, one at least ten years[8] and the other at least five years after they were first seen, is still under the control of an ectopic pacemaker (Fig. 191).

Both types of atrial arrhythmia, the one with repetitive appearance of the ectopic focus and the other with sustained ectopic pacemaker, may be seen in children. Their prognosis from the cardiac viewpoint, at least throughout childhood, is good. Nevertheless, one of our patients (and another one described in the literature by Schacknow) suffered a cerebral vascular accident, presumably due to cerebral embolism. Furthermore, congestive heart failure developed in two of our patients. Thus it may be worth while to try to treat these patients. Although control of the ectopic pacemaker may not be accomplished, still, slowing it and increasing the atrioventricular block may result in an over-all slowing of the ventricular rate, which may well prevent the development of congestive heart failure.

Paroxysmal Atrial Tachycardia with Block

A transitional stage between flutter and paroxysmal atrial tachycardia is an irregularity called paroxysmal atrial tachycardia with block. Electrocardiographically, the arrhythmia consists in regular-looking P waves at a rate of 150 to 250 and normal QRS complexes at a rate of 100 to 150, separated from the P waves by varying, but always prolonged, P-R intervals.[447, 449] In

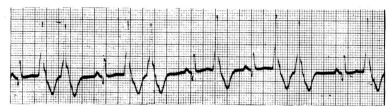

III 4/29/49 ADM.

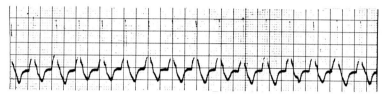

III 12/17/51 NO RX

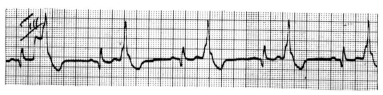

III 2/16/60 DIGOXIN

Figure 191.   Chronic repetitive tachycardia in a patient followed up over a twelve-year period. Note the maintenance of essentially similar ectopic complexes throughout this time. There is definite diminution, however, in the number of the ectopic beats.

contrast to atrial flutter, an isoelectric base line is seen between P waves. The P-R interval is variable. First- or second-degree atrioventricular block is always present (Fig. 85, p. 85). This arrhythmia is commonly present in patients with digitoxicity, although we have seen it in children with primary myocardial disease who had never received digitalis and in whom the arrhythmia was abolished by administration of the glycoside.

Because the ventricular rate is only moderately rapid, the arrhythmia itself probably never leads to congestive failure. But, reflecting the status of the myocardium or the presence of severe digitoxicity, paroxysmal tachycardia with block has serious prognostic implications. According to this line of thought, the management of this arrhythmia should be directed principally toward establishing whether digitalis may have played a role in its causation. If this is the case, withdrawal of the glycoside and administration of potassium chloride are indicated. It is recommended that adults receive 5 Gm. (67 mEq.) of potassium chloride, by mouth, as the first dose. In children, smaller doses are indicated, proportionate to weight, of course. Half the initial dose may be repeated twice at four-hour intervals. In critically ill patients, particularly if they are vomiting, potassium chloride should be given intravenously under continuous electrocardiographic control. The drip should be promptly discontinued if evidences of potassium intoxication (see p. 89) appear. The intravenous solution should contain 1.0 Gm.

of potassium chloride in 250 ml. of a 5 per cent solution of dextrose and water. The entire amount may be infused into a 100-pound child in one hour; proportionately less should be given to smaller children. The necessity of electrocardiographic monitoring can scarcely be overemphasized.

It is also important to stress that in a patient with an arrhythmia induced by digitalis, not only should the administration of the glycoside be discontinued, but diuretics should also be withheld temporarily. If cessation of anticongestive drugs and administration of potassium chloride do not control the arrhythmia, procaine amide should be administered by mouth or intravenously in adequate doses (see p. 237). If digitalis cannot be implicated in the etiology of paroxysmal atrial tachycardia with block, and if it cannot be controlled by administration of Pronestyl, cautious digitalization may be attempted.

Atrial Flutter

One of the supraventricular arrhythmias most commonly associated with severe heart disease is atrial flutter. The atria here are in continuous regular activity at a rate of 200 to 350 beats per minute. The condition is rare in adults (one in eighty patients with heart disease)[473] and is even rarer in infants and children.

In its most benign form atrial flutter may occur in a previously normal heart and manifest itself as paroxysmal supraventricular tachycardia with a 1:1 response and a ventricular rate of 300 beats per minute or more. In this form it is no different from other types of simple paroxysmal tachycardia.

In contrast, atrial flutter accompanying rheumatic heart disease is of serious prognostic importance, since in a child it indicates, almost without exception, the presence of active carditis. The association of flutter with congenital heart disease is of equally ominous significance; only the severest lesions, usually accompanied by congestive failure and gross atrial enlargement (large atrial septal defect, total pulmonary venous anomaly, Ebstein's disease and, particularly, corrected transposition of the great arteries) manifest this arrhythmia. Occasionally we have seen atrial flutter appearing transiently as a postoperative complication of closure of atrial septal defects. Finally, we have encountered this arrhythmia in conjunction with endocardial fibroelastosis; in one fatal instance this was the first manifestation of heart disease in a newborn infant, and in another fatal case it was associated with digitalis intoxication.

The electrocardiographic features of atrial flutter have been discussed and illustrated previously (see p. 84 and Fig. 50, p. 60).

Two prevailing theories on the nature of impulse formation in flutter will be mentioned. The older and, in the eyes of many, the best explanation for the rapid atrial activity is the one proposed by Lewis.[426] Elaborating on theories of others, he proposed that no single focus is responsible for the presence of flutter, but that the atria are in one continuous "circus movement"—a wave of impulse incessantly going around the two atria. Prinzmetal,[567] using cinematographic techniques, seriously challenged the validity of Lewis's views and proposed his "unifocal" theory, according to which the impulses in atrial flutter, much as in paroxysmal tachycardia, originate in one ectopic focus somewhere in the atria. According to this theory of the atrial arrhythmias, paroxysmal tachycardia and flutter are not qualitatively, but only quantitatively, different from each other.

The proponents of this unifocal theory seem to increase in number with the years. The only pertinent observation I can make on this subject, also favoring Prinzmetal's theory, is to point out the surprising ease with which paroxysmal tachycardia, flutter and fibrillation may convert into each other within a matter of a few minutes or hours.

Clinical Picture

The suspicion of atrial flutter should be raised in any patient who has a regular pulse rate of 180 beats per minute or more. If, by carotid sinus stimulation, the rate can be decreased to one half or one third, or if, by exercise, the rate can be increased in the same proportion, the clinical diagnosis of flutter can be made with assurance. Absence of these vagally induced changes does not, however, exclude the diagnosis of atrial flutter.

The clinical profile is not significantly different from that discussed in the section on Simple Paroxysmal Tachycardia, except that, because of the relatively frequent association of this condition with structural heart disease, the symptoms may occur earlier and in more severe form.

The effect of flutter on the circulation depends largely on the ventricular rate. If only one third or one fourth of the impulses are carried to the ventricles, the arrhythmia is tolerated relatively well, although the patient feels better when it is converted to normal sinus rhythm. If the ventricles respond in a 1:1 or 1:2 fashion, congestive failure ensues.

Treatment

The drug of choice in the treatment of flutter is digitalis. One effect of the glycoside is to increase the atrioventricular conduction time and, by so doing, to increase the ratio between atrial and ventricular beats; by virtue of this ventricular slowing alone, the patient's symptons may improve a great deal, and congestive failure may disappear. Perhaps even more important, digitalis may convert atrial flutter either directly into normal sinus rhythm or, more commonly, first into fibrillation and then to normal sinus rhythm. Digitalis in the dosages indicated (Table 17, p. 783) should be used.

If flutter does not change into normal sinus rhythm after administration of an adequate amount of digitalis, sudden cessation of the drug for two or three days may result in the desired effect. If flutter or fibrillation still persists, administration of digitalis in doses resulting in 1:3 or 1:4 block should be resumed, and quinidine should be added to the regimen, according to the schedule outlined on page 237. Quinidane should not be used in the treatment of flutter (or fibrillation) without previous digitalization, since it may result transiently in a higher ventricular rate. External electric countershock may be used in desperate, refractory situations.

Results of treatment vary with the underlying heart condition. Almost all cases of flutter originating from a normal heart and manifesting themselves as paroxysmal atrial tachycardias can be successfully treated with digitalis. Conversion in the patient with severe rheumatic or congenital heart disease cannot be expected in more than 50 per cent of the cases. If atrial flutter persists in the face of rigorous attempts at conversion, one ought to aim at maintaining a 1:3 or 1:4 atrioventricular block with digitalis.

Embolic complications in conversion of ectopic tachycardia are rare in children, although they have occurred at least twice in the last twenty years at The Children's Hospital Medical Center.

Atrial Fibrillation

The severest type of supraventricular arrhythmia is atrial fibrillation. The atria are in continuous, irregular motion at a rate of 400 to 700 beats per minute. The ventricular response, depending on the atrioventricular conduction, is always only a fraction of the atrial rate, but is equally and totally irregular.

Although "idiopathic atrial fibrillation," i.e. fibrillation originating from an anatomically "normal" heart, does, reportedly, exist in adults, fibrillation in children always means structural heart disease, usually severe active rheumatic carditis. Severe congenital heart disease, specifically atrial septal defect, ventricular septal defect, Ebstein's anomaly of the tricuspid valve or corrected transposition of the great arteries, may also be associated occasionally with this irregularity. On the whole, it is not a common arrhythmia. It occurs in less than 5 per cent of children with rheumatic heart disease[276] and considerably less frequently in patients with congenital heart disease.

The electrocardiogram in fibrillation has been discussed and illustrated previously (p. 85 and Fig. 51, p. 60). The controversy mentioned in the section on flutter between the supporters of Lewis and those of Prinzmetal exists in regard to fibrillation as well. Lewis explained atrial fibrillation on the basis of a hypothetic "circus movement"; according to Prinzmetal, fibrillation is the result of a combination of a rapidly discharging ectopic atrial focus and a complete breakdown of the normal spread of impulse through the atria, resulting in completely chaotic activity.

Clinical Picture

The diagnosis of fibrillation is predicated on the finding of an "irregular irregularity" of the heart. On listening, there is no pattern whatsoever to the rhythm of the heart sounds; the total rate is usually between 100 and 150 beats per minute. The sounds are not only totally irregular, but also vary considerably in intensity. Sounds following a relatively long pause are loud, whereas the rapid succession of beats is characterized by dull heart sounds. Exercise may increase the total rate and exaggerate the arrhythmia. The murmur accompanying the underlying heart disease undergoes profound changes with the onset of fibrillation. To mention only the most significant features, the presystolic crescendo murmur of mitral stenosis always disappears, and the systolic murmur, although persisting, changes from cycle to cycle, depending on the ventricular rate. Comparing the apical heart rate with the radial pulse rate, one becomes aware of a definite "pulse deficit" in most cases; the less effectual ventricular contractions are not transmitted as pulse waves to the periphery. The effectiveness of the heart action can be measured by determining the size of the pulse deficit; the smaller the deficit, the more effective the heart action may be considered.

The consequences of fibrillation are inseparable from those inherent in the structural heart disease always accompanying this condition. Congestive failure is the obvious consequence of rapid ventricular rates, especially if the heart muscle is already diseased. But reversal to normal sinus rhythm is accompanied by a sense of well-being even without significant change in the ventricular rate. Carefully controlled catheterization studies in adults with atrial fibrillation indicate that a change from fibrillation to sinus mechanism results in increased cardiac output even if the ventricular rate stays essentially the same.[324] Embolic phenomena are common in adults; in children they are rare.

Treatment

The purpose of treatment of atrial fibrillation is twofold. In the first place, the ventricular rate should be slowed; this may be accomplished with digitalis. Second, fibrillation should be converted, if possible, to normal sinus rhythm; digitalis may accomplish this occasionally, but quinidine is much more effective.

Digitalization is indicated in all patients with fibrillation unless the ventricular rate is less than 70 beats per minute. If, at these slow rates, congestive failure is present, diuretics should be used in preference to glycosides. If, during the course of digitalization, the ventricular rate drops to less than 70 at rest and does not exceed 110 on moderate exercise, the drug should be discontinued. The dosage of digitalis is the same as that indicated in Table 17 (p. 783).

Once congestive failure has improved and the ventricular rate has slowed, the decision must be made whether or not to attempt conversion to normal sinus rhythm. Considerations favoring conversion are numerous: (1) Patients with continued fibrillation usually have limited life expectancy. (2) Studies of cardiac output, venous pressure, and so forth, amply demonstrate the relative ineffectiveness of the circulation during fibrillation. (3) The longer the arrhythmia persists, the greater are the hazards of embolic phenomena. Arguments against conversion are as follows: (1) Increased numbers of embolic incidents appear at the time of conversion. (2) Deleterious effects may follow quinidine toxicity. Taking all these factors into consideration, I believe that at least one vigorous attempt at conversion should be made in every patient who has fibrillation. I also believe that quinidine should be given only to patients with slow ventricular rates, preferably those under the effect of digitalis. In adults, quinidine is effective in achieving restoration of normal sinus rhythm in about 50 per cent of the cases.

According to these principles, then, the treatment of fibrillation should consist in (1) digitalization to slow the ventricular rate to 100 beats per minute or less and treatment of congestive failure with diuretics, if necessary; (2) quinidinization, according to the schedule outlined on page 237, and maintenance dose of digitalis during this period to keep the ventricular rate between 70 and 100; (3) maintenance doses of quinidine for at least 3 months after conversion; and (4) electric countershock in severely ill patients, if the foregoing fail.

Ventricular Flutter and Fibrillation

Clinical Picture

In essence, this arrhythmia consists in rapid and almost totally ineffective contractions of the ventricles. No clear distinction between flutter and fibrillation can be made; if the rate is only moderately rapid, if some semblance of regularity can be obtained, and if the QRS complex in the electrocardiogram vaguely resembles a normal complex, it is called ventricular flutter. If, on the other hand, the tracing is totally chaotic and no effective circulation can be maintained spontaneously, ventricular fibrillation is present. Ample experience with this type of arrhythmia in children has been obtained in recent years during cardiac surgery and, occasionally, during cardiac catheterization. Before this era, only older people with coronary disease, Adams-Stokes attacks, digitalis intoxication or terminal phases of any heart disease were known to have this arrhythmia. Since no satisfactory cardiac output is maintained during ventricular fibrillation, survival is possible for only a few minutes. Most observers feel that full recovery, in terms of an intact central nervous system, is not possible if ventricular fibrillation exists for three minutes or more without cardiac massage. Recovery, in a cardiac sense, has been reported after considerably longer periods of ventricular fibrillation.

Ventricular fibrillation cannot be diagnosed clinically, but it may be suspected if a child, during anesthesia, operation or cardiac catheterization, suddenly loses completely his blood pressure, his peripheral pulses, and heart sounds. About 10 per cent of the patients with cardiac arrest have ventricular fibrillation.

If one is fortunate enough to have an electrocardiogram connected to the patient, one may follow these stages in ominious succession: (1) occasional ventricular premature beats, some with long Q-T intervals; (2) development of a series of ventricular premature beats into ventricular tachycardia; (3) appearance of ventricular flutter—the QRS complexes of ventricular tachycardia widen until they appear as a continuous regular sine wave at a rate of about 200 beats per minute without a clear-cut distinction of QRS complexes and T waves; and (4), finally, these complexes become irregular in size, shape and rhythm. This is called ventricular fibrillation.

Treatment and Prevention

Prompt and well organized treatment of this condition is of utmost importance; the patient's survival depends on action within sixty seconds. The plan of treatment for cardiac arrest will be discussed later (see p. 255).

Almost more important than the treatment of ventricular flutter and fibrillation is their prevention. Since the occurrence of this often fatal arrhythmia in children is almost always dependent either on an operation, cardiac or otherwise, or on cardiac catheterization, and not primarily on myocardial disease, certain preventive measures are possible: (1) Choose the proper anesthetic and method of induction. (2) Avoid anoxia by the administration of an extra amount of oxygen at critical periods, as when dye is injected during angiography or when ventricular premature beats appear during operation. (3) Prophylactic injection of procaine into the pericardial sac and into the myocardium if this is going to be incised. Pronestyl should be administered intravenously if ventricular premature beats appear in any appreciable number. (4) The electrocardiogram should be used continuously during operation to indicate the danger signals.

ARRHYTHMIAS CAUSED BY CONDUCTION DEFECTS

SINOATRIAL BLOCK

The absence of a P wave caused by failure of the impulse to reach the atrium from the sinus node is called sinoatrial block. Since the only indicator of the activity of the sinus node is the contraction of the atrium and the electrical phenomena connected with it, it is obviously impossible to distinguish between failure to form impulses within the node and failure of a sinus impulse to reach the atrium. By convention, then, disappearance of the P waves in the electrocardiogram through one or several cycles is called sinoatrial block.

The mildest degree consists in an occasional dropping out of a P wave (Fig. 80, p. 81). In other instances the halving of the rate may persist for several minutes, giving rise to bradycardia and even to Adams-Stokes syndrome. Persistent sinoatrial block is almost unknown in children; however, occasional dropped beats occur relatively frequently in patients having rheumatic carditis, primary myocardial disease or digitalis intoxication, and also in persons without heart disease, especially in the newborn.

No symptoms result from this arrhythmia in children. I have never seen Adams-Stokes attacks resulting from it, although obviously they do occur in adults.

The diagnosis usually rests on the electrocardiogram, although bradycardia responding to atropine administration or exercise by a doubling of the rate should suggest it, even without an electrocardiogram.

Sinoatrial block does not require treatment unless the underlying heart disease needs attention.

ATRIOVENTRICULAR BLOCK

Atrioventricular block is an interference with the normal conduction of the impulses from the atria to the ventricles through the atrioventricular node. There are several degrees of block.

First-Degree Block

First-degree atrioventricular block is defined electrocardiographically as a P-R interval longer than that expected from the patient's age and heart rate. It cannot be emphasized strongly enough that a prolonged P-R interval does not necessarily indicate heart disease; as a matter of fact, in at least one study[579] 90 per cent of the patients with first-degree block had no other evidences of heart disease. Among the etiologic factors should be mentioned rheumatic carditis, congenital heart disease (atrial septal defect, Ebstein's anomaly corrected transposition), primary myocardial disease, diphtheria, digitalis and, much less commonly, quinidine intoxication. Long P-R intervals of rheumatic carditis may be reverted to normal by the administration of atropine,[442] perhaps indicating the vagal rather than myocardial origin of this phenomenon. First-degree heart block, per se, does not cause symptoms or require treatment.

Second-Degree Block

In second-degree atrioventicular block an occasional P wave is not conducted to the ventricles at all. This may happen haphazardly, or it may occur once every three, four or five beats. It may also be noted as a so-called Wenckebach phenomenon, within a series of progressively prolonged P-R intervals, culminating in the complete blocking of one atrial impulse (Fig. 53, p. 62).

Second-degree block is not common in patients without heart disease, but I can remember at least four children who had this condition for years and in whom no other evidence of heart disease existed (Fig. 192). The etiologic factors responsible for first degree block are the most significant factors causing second-degree block as well. No treatment is necessary, except as indicated by the underlying heart disease. Recently I saw an adolescent boy with second-degree heart block and symptoms strongly suggestive of Adams-Stokes disease. The therapeutic dilemma posed by this problem can hardly be overstated.

Third-Degree Block

In third-degree atrioventricular block (complete heart block) the atria and the ventricles beat independently. Their rates are different, and, in contrast

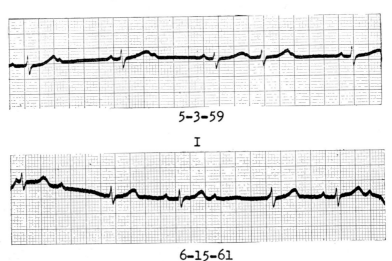

Figure 192.   Chronic Wenckebach phenomenon in a little girl with no heart disease. The tracings were taken two years apart.

to atrioventricular dissociation, the ventricular rate is always the slower of the two.

Physiology

The ventricular rate in children with complete heart block is considerably faster than in adults with acquired heart block. The pulse rate is usually fixed between 40 and 80 beats per minute; it is less than 40 in only about 10 per cent of the cases. A change of more than 20 beats per minute, after exercise, is noted only rarely, although an increase of 10 to 20 beats per minute occurs frequently. Because of the increased stroke volume and the secondary peripheral vasodilatation, wide pulse pressure will be noted. Of twenty-seven patients with complete heart block studied at The Children's Hospital Medical Center none had a pulse pressure of less than 33 mm. of mercury, while the average was 56.

We have studied twelve patients with complete heart block by means of right heart catheterization.[554] In three of these an atrial left-to-right shunt was demonstrated, and in one a patent ductus arteriosus was found. There was no significant increase in oxygen saturation in the right heart chambers of any of the remaining eight patients, in spite of the clinical suggestion of a left-to-right shunt. Pressure measurements on these eight children showed normal right atrial, slightly increased right ventricular systolic, and normal diastolic pressures. Tall A waves, cannon waves, could be seen in the right atrium if atrial systole occurred at a time when the atrioventricular valves were closed (Fig. 10). The cardiac index was within normal range in all but one patient. Obviously, since the heart rate was considerably slower than average, this implied that the stroke volume was considerably increased (63 to 119 ml. per square meter per stroke), and the circulation seemed effectively compensated. It is interesting to contrast these physiologic observations in children with data obtained in four elderly subjects who had complete heart block.[662] In the older people, although there was no clinical evidence of heart failure, the hemodynamic data were consistent with moderately severe congestive heart failure (low output, wide atrioventricular difference, increased systemic and pulmonary resistance, and right ventricular hypertension).

Etiology

Complete heart block in children is usually congenital in origin. Rheumatic heart disease seldom, if ever, causes third-degree block in this age group. Of our twenty-seven patients, two had definite cyanotic congenital heart disease (one with diminished and the other with increased pulmonary vasculature). Two patients were thought, on clinical grounds, not to have associated heart disease (no murmurs, no symptoms, normal roentgenograms and electrocardiograms). In the remaining twenty-three patients various associated congenital cardiac anomalies were suspected (ventricular septal defect, atrial septal defect, aortic stenosis and pulmonary stenosis), but in eight of these, right heart catheterization failed to reveal any left-to-right shunt. In four a left-to-right shunt was demonstrated.

It has been assumed[102] that congenital heart block is commonly associated with ventricular septal defect. Much of the evidence on which this assumption is based is purely clinical: namely, the presence of a harsh systolic murmur at the lower sternal border. From the embryologic viewpoint it seems rather unlikely that an isolated small ventricular septal defect, usually located high and anterior in the membranous septum, would interfere with the development of the bundle of His, which runs posteriorly and is well developed before the formation of the septa.[755] In fact, a few cases of congenital heart block with ventricular septal defect, confirmed at postmortem examination, have been described, but certainly far fewer than would be suspected on clinical grounds; when it does occur, it is likely to be associated with corrected transposition.

One further etiologic factor to be mentioned is endocardial fibroelastosis, which has been found at postmortem examination in patients with congenital heart block and may well explain the clinical and physiologic findings in some of these patients.

Briefly, then, on the basis of our own experience and a review of the literature, I do not believe that simple ventricular septal defect is likely to be associated with complete heart block. Third-degree heart block may well be associated with a variety of cyanotic or acyanotic congenital heart diseases, or even endocardial fibroelastosis. In our experience atrial defect of the ostium primum variety and corrected transposition are probably the two most common lesions associated with complete heart block. We have observed at least two families in which congenital heart block occurred in several members. This has been described in the literature as well.[712] One family is of particular interest in that some of the members have second- and others third-degree block (Fig. 193).

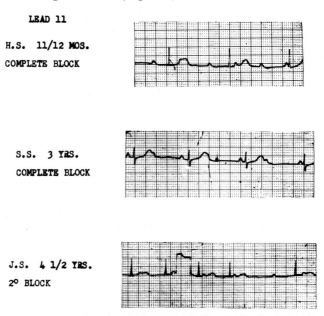

Figure 193. Familial occurrence of atrioventricular conduction disturbance. The two upper tracings indicate that two members of the family had complete block. The lower tracing, from the third member, indicates second-degree atrioventricular block.

A sizable number of children with congenital complete heart block have no other demonstrable heart disease, although auscultation may suggest a left-to-right shunt. Of course, the commonest cause of heart block today is intracardiac surgery. This will be discussed separately.

Clinical Picture

In the majority of instances the condition is discovered during a routine physical examination, although, on close questioning, a history of fatigue may be obtained in about half of the children. In two out of twenty-seven children seen at The Children's Hospital Medical Center, heart block was suspected by the obstetrician before delivery. In a few instances the irregularity of the heart beat or the appearance of "spells" is noted by the parent. Some of these patients are underdeveloped and have a history of occasional cyanosis. We had not seen true Adams-Stokes attacks in any of these youngsters until recently. This past year we lost one teen-age boy in a classic Adams-Stokes attack; we have two other children under observation who have suggestive symptoms. Two patients had evidences of congestive failure.

A grade 3 or 4 harsh, ejection type of systolic murmur was heard at the left sternal border in all but two of the children in our series (Fig. 194). Low-frequency early or mid-diastolic murmurs were also noted in the majority. Three patients showed no murmurs at all and had normal roentgenograms and electrocardiograms.

The changing intensity of the first heart sound, depending on the proximity of the QRS to the preceding P wave, has been noted repeatedly and is characteristic of complete atrioventricular block. An atrial or fourth heart sound often can be detected by the stethoscope and demonstrated by phonocardiograms. A third sound can commonly be heard.

Roentgenologic evidence of cardiac enlargement was found in more than half of our patients. In most instances the enlargement involved the left ventricle. Additional right ventricular and left atrial enlargement could be seen in some patients. Pulmonary vascular engorgement with or without hilar dance was observed only in patients with demonstrable left-to-right shunts.

The electrocardiogram, of course, shows complete heart block. In our series the atrial rate varied from 75 to 150 beats per minute, and the ventricular rate from 42 to 85. The majority of these patients had normal mean electrical axes, a few had right, others left axis deviation. P pulmonale was

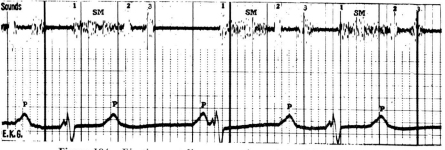

Figure 194.   Ejection systolic murmur in patient with heart block.

observed in about a third of the patients. As a rule, the voltages indicated left ventricular hypertrophy. An rsR′ pattern was seen in patients with coexisting atrial septal defects. The QRS duration was normal. Atropine, ephedrine and Isuprel increased the ventricular rate by 10 to 30 beats per minute.

Course and Prognosis

On the whole, the course of this group of patients is rather satisfactory. Only three of our twenty-seven patients died—one with tetralogy of Fallot, one with familial congenital heart block and an atrial septal defect, and one additional adolescent with a probable Adams-Stokes attack. The others lead normal, active lives with few, if any, limitations. Campbell and Thorne[134] followed up seven patients for twenty-five years and observed no significant changes in cardiac status. Obviously, the presence and the nature of the associated cardiac anomaly determine to a great extent the ultimate fate of these children. Congestive failure is more likely to be caused by the coexisting heart disease than by the heart block itself. Adams-Stokes attacks are common in adults.

One of our two patients with cyanotic congenital heart disease has now reverted to sinus rhythm. This phenomenon in patients with congenital heart disease and complete heart block has also been mentioned by Campbell and Thorne.[134]

Treatment

Since most of our patients with complete heart block are relatively symptom-free, we have not believed we were justified in attempting to increase the ventricular rate. In adults, in whom Adams-Stokes attacks are common, the continuous oral administration of ephedrine may be necessary. Digitalization and other anticongestive measures may be indicated if cardiac failure occurs. On the whole, however, because of the effects of digitalis on atrioventricular conduction, digitalization should be undertaken only if it is absolutely necessary. Within recent years the administration of chlorothiazide has been used in some patients who have a slow ventricular rate and complete atrioventricular block. This helps partly by reducing edema and partly by causing potassium diuresis, resulting in a low total body potassium level. This, in turn, increases cardiac irritability and causes a higher ventricular rate with essentially the same atrial pacemaker.

The occurrence of Adams-Stokes attacks in a few of our patients has made me assume a somewhat less philosophic attitude toward them than I had before. If there are any symptoms suggesting Adams-Stokes disease, and if the pulse rate drops to less than 40 any time of the day or night, I now prescribe Isuprel or ephedrine, with or without chlorothiazide. So far we have never felt called upon to insert an artificial pacemaker into the heart of a child with congenital atrioventricular block. This, of course, is done extensively for adults and patients with postoperative block. I would not be surprised if, in the future, with technical improvement in the pacemakers, such a step may be considered justifiable even for children with congenital block.

CARDIAC ARREST

Complete cessation of the circulation can be regarded as the most serious arrhythmia imaginable; hence it may be discussed in this chapter on the disturbances of rhythm.

Close to 90 per cent of cardiac arrests are based on complete mechanical and electrical asystole; in the other 10 per cent ventricular fibrillation is the underlying mechanism.[667] Differentiation between the two is impossible without an electrocardiogram. At the operating table the heart may seem to be entirely motionless on direct inspection, but the electrocardiogram may still show fibrillary activity.

Cardiac arrest has occurred much more frequently in children since the introduction of cardiac surgery. Johnson and Kirby,[366] discussing principally adults, placed the incidence at about one in 5000 operations. Before the era of thoracic surgery the etiologic factors of significance were anoxia and vasovagal reflex, i.e. sudden cardiac standstill during paracentesis or introduction of an intratracheal tube.

The physiologic effects of cardiac arrest concern primarily the brain. Lack of an adequate supply of oxygen to the central nervous system for three minutes or more usually results in irreversible damage (blindness, convulsions, severe mental deficiency), even if the circulation is later restored.

The clinical recognition of cardiac arrest during operation rests on the absence of blood pressure and pulse and on the cessation of bleeding. Dilatation of pupils, respiratory arrest and generalized cyanosis are late signs. Zoll and his associates[765] recommended the use of a cardiac monitor for instantaneous recognition of asystole during operation.

The most important point in the management of cardiac arrest is its prevention. Adequate preventive measures have been outlined in the section on Ventricular Fibrillation (see p. 248).

If cardiac arrest does occur, however, early recognition and prompt treatment, within three minutes, according to a well rehearsed plan are of the utmost importance.

The first step in the treatment of cardiac arrest is the establishment of an adequate airway, through an intratracheal tube. Pure oxygen (10 to 15 mm. of mercury pressure) can be administered through this, within less than one minute. If this is not accomplished within the allotted time, mouth-to-mouth breathing may be substituted.

While the airway is being introduced, external stimulation of the heart may be undertaken. If the chest is closed, this may be accomplished (1) by pounding the left precordium, (2) by using the external compression method developed by the group at Johns Hopkins Hospital,[317, 401] (3) by using a cardiac pacemaker,[371] and (4) by thoracotomy and cardiac massage.

The external compression method developed at Johns Hopkins consists of firm, rhythmic pressure applied to the sternum, compressing the heart between the sternum and the vertebral column. In this way adequate blood flow and pressure may be maintained for several minutes or even an hour. This allows time for an electrocardiograph to be connected to the patient to determine whether there is ventricular fibrillation or cardiac standstill. Once this is determined, a pacemaker and defibrillator are connected to the patient while external massage is going on. If the basis of the cardiac arrest is standstill, the patient may be driven for at least 60 minutes by an external pacemaker delivering 1.5 to 2 amperes. If ventricular fibrillation is revealed by the electrocardiograph, electric countershock should be applied. If cardiac action is not re-established by these means, thoracotomy and cardiac massage may or may not be resorted to, according to the underlying heart disease.

By the prompt use of these resuscitative methods a certain number of patients may be restored to life. Kirby and Johnson[366] were able to resuscitate ten of nineteen adults, most of whom did not have cardiac disease. In larger series only 25 to 35 per cent recovery is reported. Obviously, a patient without heart disease responds better and more promptly than one in whom there is a cardiac defect. Equally clearly, the sooner the resuscitative measures are started, the better the results will be.

10

MYOCARDIAL DISEASES

Diseases affecting principally the myocardium will be discussed in this chapter. Myocardial disease thus is contrasted with rheumatic fever and bacterial endocarditis (in which endocardial involvement is almost a sine qua non), with pericarditis, the arrhythmias (which are purely functional derangements) and with congenital heart disease (typical examples of structural defect).

PRIMARY MYOCARDIAL DISEASE

As a purely clinical entity, primary myocardial disease is characterized by changes in the myocardium not associated with any other known disease. These patients have (1) cardiac enlargement without significant murmurs and (2) electrocardiographic abnormalities, principally changes in the S-T segments and T waves.

None of them have (1) evidences of left-to-right or right-to-left shunts, (2) pericarditis, (3) paroxysmal atrial tachycardia, (4) arterial hypertension, (5) renal disease, (6) neuromuscular diseases (Friedreich's ataxia or muscular dystrophy) or (7) infections (streptococcal infections, diphtheria, acute exanthemas, and so forth) preceding or associated with the disease. Most of these conditions can easily be excluded from the differential diagnosis, but occasionally the presence of fever, pulmonary rales and harsh breath sounds makes the differential diagnosis between congestive failure consecutive to myocardial disease and myocardial disease secondary to pneumonitis an exceedingly difficult one. Knowing the rarity of heart failure in even the severest attacks of pneumonia, I believe that in most of these cases the myocardial involvement probably precedes the infection. This contention finds a practical demonstration in the beneficial effect of anticongestive measures on the pulmonary changes of these patients.

Some years ago, in order to learn the etiology of primary myocardial disease, Rosenbaum, Neuhauser and I collected forty-five cases with clinical syndromes of the disease from the files of The Children's Hospital Medical Center.[592] Twenty-six of these children died and were examined post mortem. The five pathologic entities producing this clinical syndrome and their frequencies are listed in Table 18 (p. 787). It may be seen from this table that most of the patients had endocardial fibroelastosis or myocarditis (Fiedler's).[248]

Nineteen of the forty-five patients were living and well at the time of completion of the study. What the anatomic diagnosis is in these patients can only be surmised. However, they are likely to fall into the category of either myocarditis or endocardial fibroelastosis because of their survival, and even improvement, through months and years. As will be pointed out later, an accurate differential diagnosis in vivo between these two conditions is extremely difficult.

In the following pages the five etiologic entities encountered at postmortem examination will be described first, and then a discussion of our nineteen living patients will be presented.

GLYCOGEN STORAGE DISEASE OF THE HEART

Biochemical Classifications

Cori and her associates[169] first devised a biochemical classification for the various types of glycogen storage diseases. They all have in common an increase in glycogen content of the various organs, demonstrable histologically as well as chemically.

Cori's type I is the classic form of von Gierke's disease, the hepatorenal type; the glycogen accumulation is probably due to a deficiency in glucose-6-phosphatase, and heart disease is not a feature of the condition.

Cori's type II is generalized glycogen disease in which the striated, as well as the cardiac, muscle has a high glycogen content. This is known as Pompe's disease[564] and is commonly referred to as cardiac glycogenosis, although, in addition to the muscles, the liver has a high glycogen content as well. Interestingly enough, no enzyme deficiency can be detected in these patients, and the glycogen seems structurally normal. Furthermore, glycolysis takes place in vitro at a normal rate.

Cori's type III is referred to as limit dextrinosis; here a deficiency of the so-called debrancher enzyme may be demonstrated. As a rule, these patients do not have heart disease.

Finally, Cori's type IV includes patients with cirrhosis of the liver in whom large amounts of a structurally abnormal glycogen are found in the hepatic cells (Table 19, p. 787).

Pathology of Generalized or Cardiac Glycogen Storage Disease (Cori II)

In cardiac glycogen disease the heart is greatly enlarged. Microscopically, the individual muscle cells are filled with large vacuoles, easily stained by Best's carmine. The ventricles are thick and heavy, and endocardial fibroelastosis may be seen inside the left ventricle.[737] Chemical analysis of fresh specimens shows 5 to 10 per cent of the wet weight to be glycogen.

Striated muscle, liver and other organs show a similar microscopic picture and increase in glycogen content. Muscle biopsies show glycogen contents varying from 1.5 to 9 per cent (normal wet weight 0.1 to 1 per cent) and liver biopsies, 10 to 17 per cent (normal wet weight 2 to 6 per cent).

Clinical Picture

Cardiac glycogen disease is a rare condition. Only four such patients have been given this diagnosis at The Children's Hospital Medical Center during the past twelve years. Keith[380] accepted twenty-four cases from the literature as bona fide. Rossi[594] recognized forty well documented cases.

Clinically, a baby with this condition usually looks pale and sick and has a large tongue and flabby musculature. The last such patient I saw was brought to the hospital with severe, generalized muscular weakness (Fig. 195). This, in conjunction with the large tongue, results in real feeding difficulties. The heart is big, but evidences of congestive heart failure are missing, and the liver is not particularly enlarged. This fact clearly differentiates Pompe's disease from von Gierke's, the latter being characterized by maximal hepatomegaly with only slight, if any, cardiac enlargement. It also tends to distinguish glycogen storage disease of the heart from the other forms of primary myocardial disease, in which a

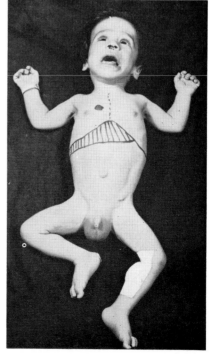

Figure 195. Photograph of patient with glycogen storage disease of the heart. Note the large liver outlined over the abdomen, the frog-like position, indicating general hypotonia, and the large tongue.

large heart is almost always accompanied by hepatomegaly as an expression of congestive heart failure.

In addition to a large tongue, weakness and a large heart, anorexia, coughing, vomiting, poor weight gain, and abscesses may dominate the clinical picture. No murmurs are heard, as a rule. In two patients I have observed, atelectasis, secondary to compression of the lung by the tremendous heart, dominated the clinical profile.

The disease is commonly a familial one and may be sex-linked.

Results of laboratory examinations aimed at determining the adequacy of glycogen metabolism (fasting blood sugar, glucose tolerance,

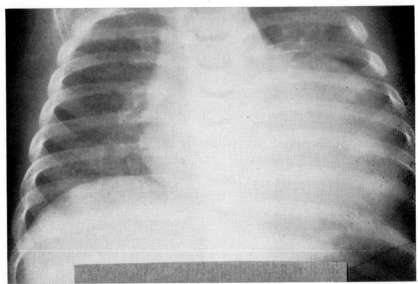

Figure 196. Roentgenogram of patient with glycogen storage disease of the heart. Note the tremendous cardiac enlargement and the passive congestion in the lung field.

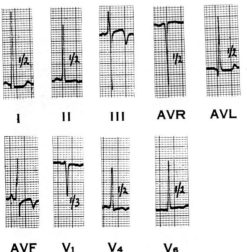

I   II   III   AVR   AVL

AVF   V₁   V₄   V₆

Figure 197. Electrocardiogram of the same patient with glycogen storage disease of the heart whose photograph and roentgenogram were shown in Figures 195 and 196. Note the high left ventricular voltages and the changes in the T wave.

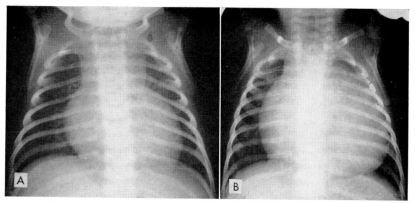

Figure **198.** Posteroanterior roentgenogram of a baby with glycogen storage disease of the heart. (*A*) At birth. (*B*) At three weeks of age.

epinephrine tolerance and urinary acetone determination) are usually within normal limits. The radiologic picture is characterized by diffuse cardiac enlargement, normal pulmonary vasculature and a poor beat at fluoroscopy (Fig. 196). Electrocardiographically, evidences of left ventricular hypertrophy with changes in the S-T segments and T waves are noted (Fig. 197).

The diagnosis is established at biopsy by the demonstration of an abnormally high glycogen content in muscle or liver, or both. In this type of glycogen disease the concentration of glycogen in the erythrocytes is normal, in contrast to the concentration in types III and IV.[641]

A personal observation about the time of development of the changes is of particular interest. At The Children's Hospital Medical Center we had cared for two siblings with glycogen storage disease. The family notified us immediately after delivery about the arrival of a third child. Physical and radiologic examinations and electrocardiographic studies showed the newborn to be perfectly normal in all respects. Cardiomegaly and electrocardiographic changes first appeared when the child was three weeks old, and death in ventricular fibrillation ensued at four weeks (Fig. 198).

According to the literature, symptoms never occur at birth, but are always present by the sixth month of life, and sudden death with or without congestive failure almost always occurs before the child has reached one year of age. Therapy is usually of no avail, but digitalization may be tried. Anabolic hormones have been suggested also for the treatment of this condition.

ABERRANT ORIGIN OF THE CORONARY ARTERY

This is another rare anomaly; fewer than seventy-five cases have been reported. Because of a developmental anomaly in the embryologic division of the common arterial trunk, the left coronary artery originates from the pulmonary artery rather than from the aorta. In other and even rarer cases the right, or even both, coronary arteries may originate from the pulmonary trunk. The former is of minor significance, but the latter is incompatible with life for more than a few weeks.

The physiologic handicap resulting from an aberrant left coronary artery has been radically reappraised within the last few years. Edwards and his associates[213] furnished pathologic proof, and Sabiston and his co-workers[608] clinical evidence, that the flow of blood in the left coronary artery, in at least some instances, is *toward* the pulmonary artery. In other words, this represents, in effect, a coronary arteriovenous fistula; aortic blood is ejected into the right coronary artery; this drains through anastomoses into the left coronary artery and finally into the pulmonary artery. Thus a constant pressure and oxygen gradient exists between aorta, right coronary artery, left coronary artery and pulmonary artery. If correct, this hypothesis has important therapeutic implications.

Pathologically, the left ventricle of a patient with an aberrant coronary artery seems thin and fibrosed. At the operating table one is impressed by the pallor of the apex and the left ventricular portion of the anterior surface. One may also see that the pulsations in this region are feeble, even paradoxical. Microscopically, fibrous displacement of the myocardial fibers and fibroelastosis dominate the picture.

The clinical picture was first described by Bland, White and Garland.[64] Symptoms usually occur between the second and sixth months of life, and death ensues before one year of age. The characteristic symptoms are episodes of colicky pain, pallor, cyanosis, tachycardia, tachypnea and perspiration. These are likely to occur at feeding time and last for a few minutes; they resemble anginal attacks of adults. Between these spells the infant is usually well, although the heart is large. There are no murmurs. The heart rate and respiratory rate are rapid. Often there is a considerable amount of wheezing. An enlarged liver, indicating right-sided congestive failure, is rarely, and only terminally, noted.

Radiologically, generalized cardiac enlargement, characteristic of the entire myocardial disease group, may be seen (Fig. 199). The only distinguishing feature on the radiogram may be the occurrence of a localized aneurysmal bulging in the area of the left ventricle.

The electrocardiograms are characterized by deep inversion of the T waves in the standard limb leads and left precordial leads. These patterns, much like the x-ray picture, are no more characteristic of this condition than of the other members of the primary myocardial disease group. If, however, in addition to the T wave changes, deep Q waves occur in lead I and aV_L, and QS or QR complexes in V_{2-4} or the left chest leads, indicating necrosis, or a "hole," in the myocardium, then the diagnosis of anomalous origin of the left coronary artery seems justifiable on the basis of the electrocardiographic picture alone (Fig. 200). One of my patients with anomalous left coronary artery had electrocardiographic evidences of complete left bundle branch block (Fig. 201).

Physiologic studies may confirm the clinical diagnosis. (1) Failure to demonstrate a left coronary artery, with good visualization of the right coronary artery, on retrograde aortography suggests this anomaly. (The contrast material should be injected immediately above the aortic valve.) (2) If there is retrograde visualization of the left coronary artery when contrast material is injected into the pulmonary artery, the diagnosis of an aberrant coronary artery may be considered established. (3) An increase in oxygen content at the pulmonary arterial level in a patient who has primary myocardial disease, but no evidence of a patent ductus arteriosus,

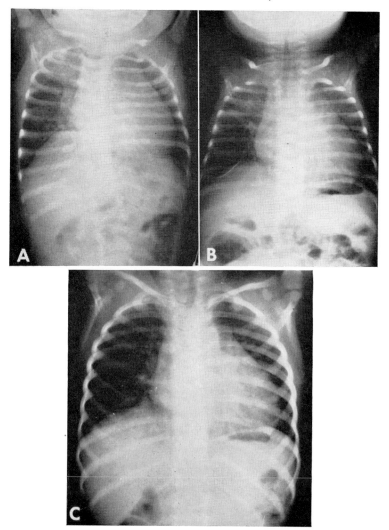

Figure 199. Serial roentgenograms in patient operated on for anomalous left coronary artery arising from the pulmonary artery. Operation was performed after *A* and before *B*. *C* was obtained two years after operation.

again suggests this anomaly. None of these methods is infallible, and it is better to make the diagnosis on the basis of the characteristic clinical and electrocardiographic picture. It is important that the diagnosis be made early, since the probability of successful surgical treatment is strongly dependent on the extent of myocardial damage.

Within recent years surgical correction of the anomaly has been attempted.[266] Transplantation of the coronary artery has been uniformly unsuccessful. The Johns Hopkins Hospital group,[608] following the new physiologic concept of the disease, successfully ligated the left coronary artery at its entrance into the pulmonary artery. It was hoped that this would ensure a better coronary supply to the entire heart by forcing blood

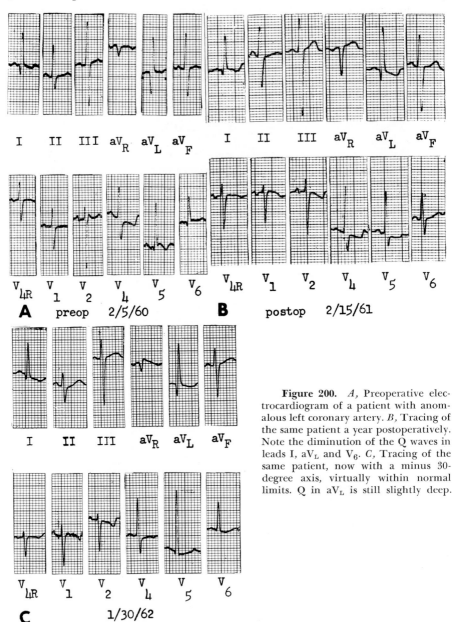

I   II   III   aV_R   aV_L   aV_F   I   II   III   aV_R   aV_L   aV_F

V_4R   V_1   V_2   V_4   V_5   V_6   V_4R   V_1   V_2   V_4   V_5   V_6

A   preop   2/5/60   **B**   postop   2/15/61

I   II   III   aV_R   aV_L   aV_F

Figure 200. *A*, Preoperative electrocardiogram of a patient with anomalous left coronary artery. *B*, Tracing of the same patient a year postoperatively. Note the diminution of the Q waves in leads I, aV_L and V_6. *C*, Tracing of the same patient, now with a minus 30-degree axis, virtually within normal limits. Q in aV_L is still slightly deep.

V_4R   V_1   V_2   V_4   V_5   V_6

C   1/30/62

into the collaterals. This type of operation is indicated, obviously, only in cases in which a drainage of coronary artery blood *into* the pulmonary artery may be assumed. One of our patients survived ligation of the left coronary artery at its entrance into the pulmonary artery. This baby had the characteristic anginal attacks and the typical electrocardiogram (Fig. 200) and roentgenograms (Fig. 199) of the disease. It is now over two years since this operation, and the child is asymptomatic and his x-ray studies and cardiograms are improving, although they are not yet normal. Inter-

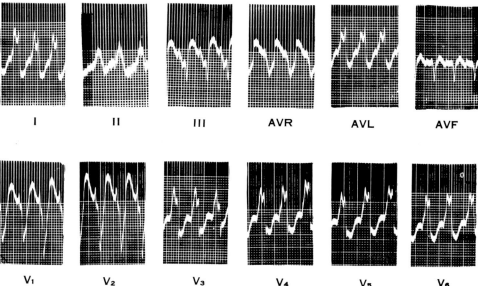

I **II** **III** **AVR** **AVL** **AVF**

V₁ **V₂** **V₃** **V₄** **V₅** **V₆**

Figure 201. Electrocardiogram from patient with anomalous left coronary artery who died at two and one half years of age. Note the left bundle branch block pattern.

estingly enough, he underwent successful repair of an inguinal hernia about six months after his cardiac surgery.

MEDIAL NECROSIS OF THE CORONARY ARTERIES

This is the rarest of the five conditions being discussed; less than thirty such cases have been reported. Pathologically, a generalized vascular disease with medial necrosis, intimal proliferation and eventually arterial occlusion is the underlying abnormality. In addition to the coronary arteries, the pulmonary and the renal vessels are also likely to be involved.

As may be expected, this is an extremely severe condition, usually leading to death at less than three months of age. The symptoms are anorexia, vomiting, respiratory infection, pallor, cyanosis and, terminally, congestive failure. The roentgenograms and electrocardiograms are much the same as have been described in the previous two conditions, but the deep Q waves characteristic of anomalous coronary arteries are usually absent.

The patients in this group are distinguished from those having other types of primary myocardial disease by the presence of associated congenital anomalies and by the involvement of the renal arteries.

ACUTE MYOCARDITIS

The patients to be discussed here represent all who have principally an inflammatory disease of the myocardium.[610, 688] Patients who have myocardial complications of diphtheria and other well known infectious diseases will be discussed separately. In the previous edition of this volume the word "idiopathic" preceded myocarditis in the heading. With the identification of a number of agents, viral or otherwise, in the etiology of myocarditis, the word "idiopathic" may safely be omitted. Keith and his associates used the term "isolated myocarditis" for these cases. This is not tenable, either, since in many cases the myocarditis is part of a generalized systemic disease.[673] It may be fair to make the further prediction that in the unlikely event of a third edition of this book, myocarditis will be discussed only under specific etiologic entities. This would represent considerable progress from the publication of Fiedler's original paper on the subject in 1900.[248]

Etiology

In spite of the number of etiologic agents identified as causative organisms of the disease, *in most instances the etiology is not known.* That an infectious agent may indeed be responsible has been most dramatically demonstrated by the occurrence of the epidemic form of the disease in Munich in 1952[670] and in Johannesburg in 1956.[362] Among the agents already identified as causing myocarditis, the following should be mentioned: Coxsackie B,[387] trichinosis,[247] psittacosis,[361] toxoplasmosis,[321] vaccinia,[461] infectious mononucleosis[718] and probably influenza. In the tropics, Chagas's disease should be considered in the differential diagnosis.

In addition to infective agents, allergic mechanisms have also been invoked to explain the occurrence of myocarditis.

The pathologic picture, depending on whether one is dealing with an acute or subacute phase of the disease, may show interstitial edema, diffuse perivascular round cell infiltration or even fibroplastic, granulomatous changes. Macroscopically, in rare instances, the heart may look normal. Ordinarily it is dilated, overweight, flabby and pale.

The clinical picture is usually characterized by the sudden onset of left- and right-sided congestive failure. In the fulminating cases a child, usually six months old or older, who was perfectly well a few hours before, becomes desperately ill, with dyspnea, pallor, cyanosis and a hacking cough. In less acute situations the onset may be more gradual; first, the patient has a "cold" which lasts longer than usual, shortness of breath is marked, lassitude appears gradually, and puffiness of the face is noted. The temperature is moderately elevated. Pulmonary rales appear, and the liver is enlarged. Definite cardiac enlargement is present, and the heart sounds are muffled. Gallop rhythm without a murmur is noted. Characteristically, the symptoms and signs are not episodic; the child is continually and severely ill.

Roentgenograms shows features common to the entire primary myocardial disease group (Fig. 202). The electrocardiographic changes are also characteristic of the entire group; low voltages and conduction disturbances (atrioventricular and intraventricular) may be present more commonly in this condition than in the others (Fig. 203). Conversely, severe left ventricular hypertrophy is rare. In the differential diagnosis, pneumonitis, septicemia and paroxysmal tachycardia should be considered.

Although this is the clinical picture of myocarditis in infants and children in general, a fairly specific pattern of Coxsackie B myocarditis in the newborn was described recently by Kibrick and his associates.[387] Most

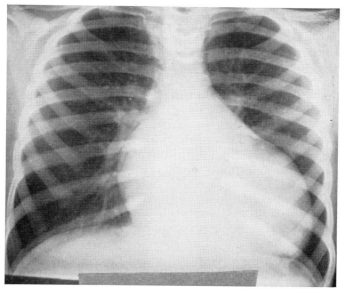

Figure 202. Roentgenogram of patient with acute myocarditis proved at postmortem examination.

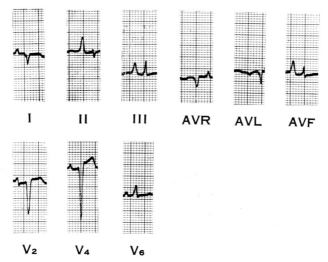

Figure 203. Electrocardiogram of patient with acute myocarditis proved at postmortem examination. Note the tall P waves in leads II and III and aV_F, and the low voltages and flat T waves throughout.

of these infants became sick within the first two weeks of life, none beyond the third week. A maternal respiratory infection was commonly noted a few days before delivery. Feeding difficulties, fever, lethargy, cyanosis, shock and respiratory distress were the most common presenting symptoms. Convulsions or other signs of disease of the central nervous system occurred in a third of the patients. Evidences of heart disease, cardiomegaly, tachycardia or electrocardiographic changes were described in only half of the patients reported, but it is not clear how thorough a search was made for these signs. Three fourths of the twenty-five infants described by these authors died within a week of admission, irrespective of treatment. The others recovered in two to three weeks. This, then, is the typical picture of the disease in the newborn. Although an occasional instance of myocarditis of less fulminating nature due to Coxsackie B virus has been described in older children,[469] on the whole, for certain immunologic reasons, it is rare. Pericarditis due to this agent is, of course, relatively more common (see p. 301).

In all cases of suspected myocarditis an attempt should be made to determine the etiologic agent. Blood culture, nose and throat cultures and skin tests, in conjunction with careful histories, should disclose the common bacterial and virus infections (diphtheria, measles, mumps, chickenpox, vaccinia, poliomyelitis, toxoplasmosis). Nose and throat washings and fecal specimens should be submitted for viral studies, and two specimens of serum should be collected, six weeks apart, for the identification of neutralizing antibodies. Stool specimens should be searched for parasites. Blood smears and agglutination tests should be made for infectious mononucleosis.

In some cases of myocarditis, irrespective of etiology, treatment may be extremely effective. Although conclusive proof is missing, I believe that many, if not most, of our successfully treated cases of primary myocardial disease may fall into this category. Oxygen and antibiotic therapy should be given routinely. The principal drug to be used, however, is digitalis administered in average, or slightly lower than average, doses and maintained for several months or even years (Table 17, p. 783). The response is just short of miraculous in many instances. Careful electrocardiographic control is necessary because some of these children are susceptible to digitoxicity. Within a few hours or days the pulse rate and respiratory rate slow, the color improves, and good diuresis occurs. Roentgenologic examination shows that pulmonary congestion has disappeared, though the heart is still large. Usually, within a few weeks, months, or at the latest in a year or

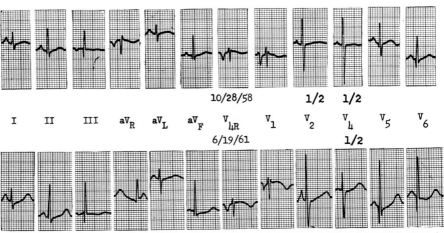

Figure 204. Two electrocardiograms, almost three years apart, in patient with chronic myocardial disease. Note the persistence of the mean electrical axis at approximately plus 60 degrees, the improvement in the T waves in the limb leads, the persistence of atrial hypertrophy from V_{4R} to V_2, and the deepening Q waves in V_5 and V_6.

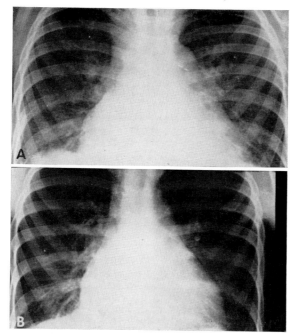

Figure 205.   Roentgenograms of patient with chronic myocardial disease. Note the persistence of cardiac enlargement through a period of almost three years.

two, the heart size and the electrocardiogram return to normal. In exceptional instances, however, after good initial response to anticongestive measures, the heart stays enlarged and episodes of congestive heart failure recur weeks and even months later (Figs. 204, 205). The prognosis in these cases is almost uniformly poor; almost invariably, death from heart failure or arrythmia occurs within a few months or years. At postmortem examination diffuse myocardial fibrosis is present. In still other patients, although symptomatic recovery is complete, the electrocardiogram never returns to normal, even though the heart seems to be normal by physical and roentgenologic examination. It is problematical what the ultimate fate of these patients will be.

Within recent years steroids have been used in some patients with the presumptive diagnosis of "idiopathic" myocarditis. At present I see no reason to abandon the therapeutic regimen consisting of digitalis with supportive treatment. As more is learned about hormone therapy, it may well be used with increasing frequency.

ENDOCARDIAL FIBROELASTOSIS

This is one of the commonest types of primary myocardial disease. Dennis and his associates[191] in 1953 collected 149 cases from the literature. Many cases have been reported since. Keith[380] estimated that it occurs in 1 per cent of all patients with congenital heart disease.

Pathologically, the condition is characterized by a milky appearance of the parietal endocardium, involving principally the left atrium and the

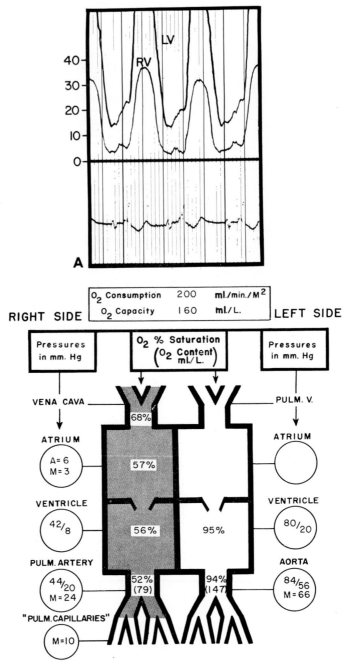

Figure 206.

left ventricle. Frequently there is associated involvement of the mitral or aortic valve, or both. Involvement of the right heart chambers is rare. The heart is considerably overweight.

Histologically, the endocardium is two to three times thicker than normal, with endocardial and subendocardial fibroelastic proliferation, a picture similar to that seen in "collagen disease." The myocardial fibers are often hypertrophied, but signs of inflammation are strikingly absent. Electronmicroscopy reveals that the surface layers of the endocardium are composed principally of fibrin-like fibers.[669]

In 1956 Anderson and Kelly[17] reviewed the pathologic picture of endocardial fibroelastosis with or without associated congenital heart disease. They concluded that in patients who have endocardial fibroelastosis secondary to structural deformities of the heart, endocardial thickening is progressive with age, and its location is constant and characteristic for the individual malformation. They attributed its occurrence to a combination of increased intracardiac pressure (jet effect), vibration and anoxia. Edwards emphasized the stretch effect of various structural abnormalities of the heart, causing secondary fibroelastosis. The majority of patients with congenital heart disease showed some degree of endocardial fibroelastosis,[70, 240, 306, 405] but the lesions most commonly associated with diffuse endocardial fibroelastosis are the hypoplastic heart syndrome,[536] coarctation of the aorta, and pulmonic stenosis or atresia.

In contrast to the patients with congenital heart disease are the infants with primary endocardial fibroelastosis in whom diffuse endocardial thickening, principally of the left ventricle and the left atrium, is the only important cardiac lesion. These are the patients to be considered in the primary myocardial disease group, excluding not only those with other congenital malformations of the heart, but also those with myocarditis, glycogen storage disease, and so forth. Anderson and Kelly stated that primary endocardial fibroelastosis represents a congenital, sometimes familial, metabolic defect, leading to myocardial weakness, dilatation and endocardial fibroelastosis. According to Anderson's study of primary endocardial fibroelastosis, the oldest age at death reported in the literature was four and a half years. Others[26, 703] described the disease in adolescents and adults.[695] Whether this represents the same primary disease entity as the one found in infants, or whether it should be regarded as secondary to nutritional disorders, infections or other processes, cannot be stated.

One interesting pathologic complication of endocardial fibroelastosis described by Thomas and his co-workers[694] should be mentioned briefly. These authors described two infants with primary endocardial fibroelastosis, mural thrombi and coronary emboli leading to infarction and calcification.

Detailed physiologic studies are few. Using catheterization of the right side of the heart, we studied three patients who had a clinical diagnosis of fibroelastosis. All had mild elevation of "pulmonary capillary" and pulmonary arterial pressures. Similar observations have been made by others.[4]

Figure 206. *A,* Right ventricular and left ventricular pressure tracings, at high sensitivity, emphasizing the diastolic pressure in a child with endocardial fibroelastosis which was proved at postmortem examination. Note the high end-diastolic pressure in the left ventricle, about 20 mm. of mercury. The right ventricular pressure is within normal range, both at systolic and diastolic levels. Electrocardiogram is used as a reference tracing. *B,* Catheterization data in patient with endocardial fibroelastosis.

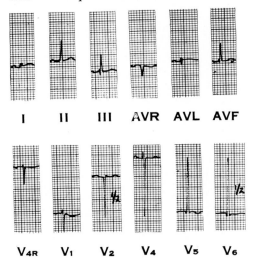

I   II   III   AVR   AVL   AVF

V4R   V1   V2   V4   V5   V6

Figure 207. Electrocardiogram of patient with endocardial fibroelastosis. This is the tracing reputed to be typical of this condition, with high left ventricular voltages reflected as S waves in V_2 and V_4, and R waves in V_5 and V_6. In addition, note the S-T and T wave changes over the left precordium.

In one instance a pathologically proved case of endocardial fibroelastosis was studied by combined left and right heart catheterization. The data are shown in Figure 206. If the observations made on patients with myocardial fibrosis and constrictive pericarditis by Burwell and his associates[119] can be considered to apply to this group, it may be assumed that the pathologic process results in an elevation of the diastolic pressure and impairment of systolic ejection of the left ventricle, with a narrowing pulse pressure. It results in "constrictive endocarditis," similar physiologically to constrictive pericarditis. The poor diastolic emptying of the left ventricle in a case of endocardial fibroelastosis has been demonstrated angiocardiographically by Gasul and his associates.[270] Linde and his co-workers[498] showed prolonged retention of contrast medium in the left ventricle and little change in volume between systole and diastole.

Often the clinical picture of endocardial fibroelastosis cannot be distinguished from that of other members of the primary myocardial disease group; the similarity to primary myocarditis is particularly striking. Approximately 50 per cent of these patients have symptoms within the first 6 months of life, and, according to Blumberg and Lyon,[70] in 95 per cent of the cases symptoms become manifest within the first year. But *in some cases of pathologically confirmed subendocardial sclerosis the patients were completely asymptomatic until they were five to six years of age.* Left- and right-sided congestive failure dominates the picture. The children may be cyanotic, but the cyanosis may improve considerably when 100 per cent oxygen is administered. Pulmonary rales, and dullness, with a hacking cough, suggest the presence of pneumonitis or pulmonary edema. Peripheral edema is rare, but hepatomegaly and distended neck veins are common. On auscultation the heart sounds are clear, gallop rhythm is not too common, and murmurs are faint or do not exist. The infants are usually underdeveloped and undernourished.

Electrocardiographically, evidences of left ventricular hypertrophy with T wave changes can be seen (Fig. 207). Right atrial hypertrophy may be present (Fig. 208). Low voltage (Fig. 209) and conduction disturbances are rare. Occasionally complete heart block occurs. I cannot subscribe to

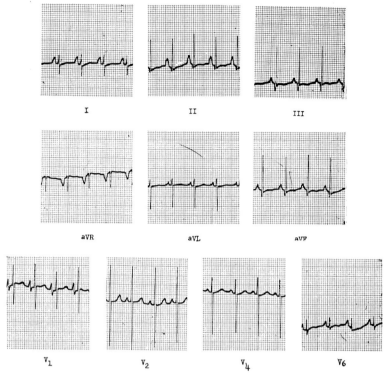

Figure 208. Electrocardiogram in patient with endocardial fibroelastosis. Note the atrial hypertrophy as revealed in leads II, aV$_R$ and V$_1$.

the thesis that electrocardiographic evidence of left ventricular hypertrophy with strain distinguishes endocardial fibroelastosis from other forms of primary myocardial disease, particularly myocarditis. I am sure that this pattern is more frequent in patients with endocardial fibroelastosis and am also convinced that low voltage and conduction disturbances are more common in myocarditis, but I have seen enough overlapping between the groups not to take this as a pathognomonic sign.

Radiologically, there is an enlarged heart, with involvement of all chambers, and a poor beat under the fluoroscopic screen. There are usually evidences of pulmonary congestion or infection (Fig. 210).

Treatment should consist of anticongestive measures, principally the administration of digitalis and mercurials with oxygen and antibiotics. The similarity of the histologic findings to those in collagen disease has suggested the use of steroids in this condition; however, I am not acquainted with any sizable series of patients treated with hormones.

Results of treatment are extremely hard to judge. Some patients with a clinical picture practically identical to the one described respond well to digitalization; others with the same clinical profile die in spite of vigorous treatment. So far there are no reliable criteria to indicate which patients will or will not respond to present-day therapeutic regimens. It seems that the younger the infant and the more severe the respiratory symptoms, the worse the prognosis is likely to be. Also, if, after an initially favorable response to treatment, the symptoms recur, the ultimate prognosis seems

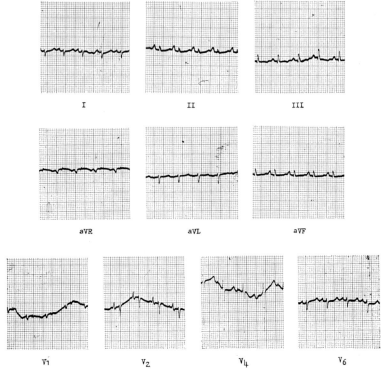

I   II   III

aVR   aVL   aVF

V₁   V₂   V₄   V₆

Figure 209. Low-voltage tracing in a patient with endocardial fibroelastosis proved at postmortem examination. Note the similarity of this tracing to that in Figure 203.

worse. Patients who eventually get better usually respond promptly and have no recurrences.

PATIENTS WITH PRIMARY MYOCARDIAL DISEASE WHO RECOVER

As indicated at the beginning of this section on primary myocardial disease, nineteen of the forty-five patients with primary myocardial disease seen at The Children's Hospital were living and well at the completion of that particular study.[592] Since no anatomic basis for a definite diagnosis in these patients exists, they cannot be discussed under any of the previous subheadings. At the same time, on the basis of the clinical definition of the syndrome, they do belong in this general category. They all had cardiac enlargement, without significant murmurs, and changes in the S-T segments and T waves in the electrocardiogram.

If one were to speculate about the anatomic diagnosis in these patients, one would feel compelled to exclude glycogen storage disease, anomalous coronary arteries and medial necrosis of the coronary arteries by virtue of the fact that these children recovered. There is practically no instance in the literature of a patient surviving beyond the first year of life who was proved to have had any one of these three entities. Therefore these living patients must belong to the myocarditis or endocardial fibroelastosis group,

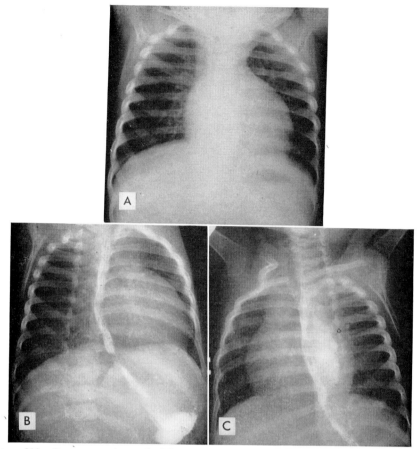

Figure 210.   Posteroanterior and oblique roentgenograms in a patient with endocardial fibroelastosis.

unless they represent another entity outside the scope of the etiologies suggested by our pathologic material.

Patients with "reversible" primary myocardial disease are encountered at our hospital about as frequently as those with paroxysmal atrial tachycardia—i.e. two or three times a year. The age at which symptoms begin varies from birth to seven years. Almost half of the patients were one year old, or older, when they first became sick. This is the most suggestive evidence that many of these youngsters belong in the myocarditis group.

The clinical picture in the typical case is characterized by the sudden appearance of symptoms of congestive failure—dyspnea, cyanosis, anorexia and vomiting. The picture may resemble that of pneumonia, especially if cough and fever are also present. In rare cases the onset is insidious, congestive failure being preceded for several months by anorexia, failure to gain weight, irritability and profuse perspiration.

On examination, many of these children are well developed and well nourished; some are actually chubby; this, again, suggests that the etiology is less likely to be a congenital anomaly than an acquired inflammatory disease. Generally, these patients look very ill; their color is pale, with cyanosis, their respirations are rapid and labored, and peripheral edema may be present. Rales are commonly heard, and there is almost always significant hepatomegaly. The heart sounds are distant and "mushy," with a gallop rhythm. There are no significant murmurs; deformity of the left side of the chest may be present, but is not too common. The temperature may be slightly elevated, but a fever higher than 102° F. is rare. The roentgenograms and electrocardiograms cannot be distinguished from those in the rest of the primary myocardial disease group.

Response to treatment is dramatic. Thirteen of our nineteen children received digitalis, and one received cortisone. In addition, Mercuhydrin was administered to the children with peripheral edema. All received general supportive measures, such as oxygen and antibiotics. Within twenty-four hours considerable clinical improvement occurred, and in one week these youngsters were practically asymptomatic. The electrocardiograms returned nearly to normal within six to twelve months (Figs. 211, 212); the hearts were considerably reduced in size within six months, but did not return to normal for one or two years. Digitalis therapy was routinely maintained for six months, after which an attempt usually was made to discontinue the drug suddenly. If the child started having symptoms again, the administration of the glycoside was resumed and continued for another year at least.

It should be mentioned here that not only are these patients benefited greatly by digitalization, but they also show toxic effects readily. Electro-cardiographic evidences of digitoxicity are often seen with average or lower than average doses of the glycoside; this is most emphatically not an absolute indication for discontinuance of the drug if good therapeutic effects are accomplished. Rather, an attempt should be made to diminish the dose to a point at which maximal therapeutic effects are achieved with minimal effects of toxicity.

Although the short-term prognosis for a child who shows dramatic initial improvement to anticongestive measures is good, obviously the long-term outlook cannot be predicted. Considerable encouragement may be gained from the fact that many of these children who have been followed

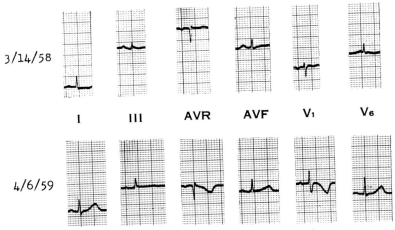

3/14/58

I   III   AVR   AVF   V₁   V₆

4/6/59

Figure 211. Electrocardiogram of patient with spontaneously improving myocardial disease. Note the improvement in P waves in leads I, aV_F and V_6.

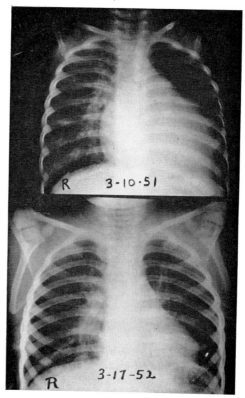

Figure 212. Upper, the heart in a patient at the height of his primary myocardial disease. Lower, one year later after complete disappearance of signs and symptoms of heart disease.

up for five years or more are now asymptomatic and have normal hearts as judged by physical examination, roentgenograms and electrocardiograms. These children are being encouraged to lead normal lives, although I am inclined to discourage participation in competitive athletics in high school or college.

A personal and wholly unsubstantiated view in regard to the etiology of the disease in these children is that myocarditis rather than endocardial fibroelastosis is the usual pathologic change. I can scarcely believe that the thick layer of constrictive subendocardial elastic tissue can disappear as a result of anticongestive measures any more than constrictive pericarditis is "cured" by such means. The age and good nutritional state in these patients also suggest myocarditis rather than primary endocardial fibroelastosis. On the other hand, Keith and Manning[379] stated that most of these patients have endocardial fibroelastosis. The diagnosis in their surviving patients is based on the electrocardiogram.

MYOCARDIAL DISEASE ASSOCIATED WITH DIPHTHERIA

The heart is affected in approximately 10 to 20 per cent of all patients who have diphtheria. Because of the rarity of the disease in the northeastern part of the United States today, my personal experience with diphtheritic myocarditis in the past fifteen years is nil. I have, however, seen a number of bizarre electrocardiograms obtained from children with diphtheria in Greece, where the disease is still rampant.[7] In some states in the southernmost part of the United States, an appreciable amount of diphtheritic myocarditis still occurs.

According to the reports in the literature, about 50 per cent of those who succumb to diphtheria have associated myocardial involvement.[726] Diphtheria bacilli are not found in the heart, and apparently the cardiac effects of the disease are caused by exotoxins liberated by the bacilli. The typical pathologic picture is one of fatty and hyaline degeneration, with only a small degree of cellular infiltration.

Circulatory derangements associated with diphtheria may present themselves in the form of early peripheral collapse or late myocardial injury.

Circulatory collapse is probably caused by the effects of the toxin on the peripheral vasculature and is characterized by evidences of shock. The patient's blood pressure drops precipitously, the pulse rate rises, and the skin looks gray and feels cold and clammy. This state of shock usually occurs toward the end of the first week of the disease; the earlier it occurs, the more severe is the prognosis. There are usually no electrocardiographic changes. Treatment consists in serum therapy of the underlying disease and shock treatment of the vasomotor collapse by administration of plasma, Neo-Synephrine or Levophed.

Diphtheritic involvement of the myocardium occurs most commonly toward the end of the second or the beginning of the third week, usually when convalescence is well under way. One of the few personal recollections I have of this condition is that of a boy, six to seven years old, who was convalescing from diphtheria and playing happily in his crib at the hospital, when he suddenly became pale, cried out, and died. He may have had an Adams-Stokes attack, or he may have succumbed to ventricular fibrillation. Fortunately, things are not always this sudden or catastrophic. Electrocardiographic changes—specifically, depression of the S-T segment, T wave inversions, atrioventricular block; bundle branch block, ventricular tachycardia and fibrillation—all may be seen at the onset of the myocardial involvement. The conduction disturbances are rare, but relatively specific to diphtheria, and they signify a more ominous prognosis. Changes in the S-T segments and T waves, on the other hand, may be seen in practically any kind of myocarditis with a less severe general outlook.

At physical examination the heart may show either severe tachycardia or bradycardia. There are no murmurs. The heart sounds are distant, and gallop rhythm may be present. In rare instances right-sided congestive failure occurs terminally.

The prognosis of diphtheritic myocarditis is grave; the mortality rate is placed at about 50 per cent by most authors.[560] If the patient survives, recovery is usually complete. Levine[121] believes that many of the cases of complete heart block first manifesting themselves when the patient is beyond the age of fifty are late sequelae of diphtheritic myocarditis. White[696] denies this contention.

Treatment is apparently not satisfactory. Serum, if not administered before, can be given at this stage, but the dangers of serum reaction must be considered carefully; indeed, this may prove to be catastrophic in a patient with a weakened and irritable myocardium. Digitalis is not recommended except in the rare instances of frank congestive failure, when cautious administration of a rapidly excreted preparation may be advisable if one is fully cognizant of the dangers involved in its use.

MYOCARDIAL DISEASE ASSOCIATED WITH FRIEDREICH'S ATAXIA

Although the chance of a pediatrician, in his general practice, ever encountering a case of Friedreich's ataxia is remote, those of us working in a children's hospital with an active neurologic service see it fairly frequently. The late Bronson Crothers, formerly head of the Neurological Service of The Children's Hospital in Boston, first drew my attention to this entity.

Friedreich's ataxia is a hereditary, familial disorder characterized by cerebellar and posterior column ataxia, weakness, areflexia and terminal dementia. Characteristic skeletal deformities include scoliosis and high-arched feet. The disease begins during childhood, and death usually occurs at puberty or in the early twenties. The age at onset as well as the age at death may be characteristic for one family.

Friedreich's original series, in 1863, included 6 patients, 5 of whom had clinical evidences of heart disease. Since then a number of authors have drawn attention to this association.[236, 522, 606] Apparently, electro-cardiographic abnormalities—particularly left ventricular S-T and T wave changes (Fig. 213)—are the most common evidences of cardiac involvement, occurring in at least one third of all cases of Friedreich's ataxia. Recently I saw a patient with Friedreich's ataxia in whom the electrocardiographic abnormality was limited to evidences of right ventricular hypertrophy (Fig. 214). This observation, coupled with a loud pulmonic closure and no murmur, suggested the presence of pulmonary hypertension. No cathe-

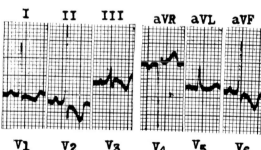

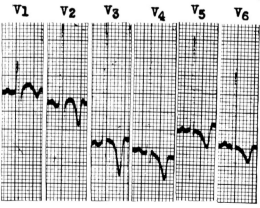

Figure 213. Electrocardiogram of patient with Friedreich's ataxia. Note the maximal T wave inversions in all the chest leads, bipolar limb leads and aV$_F$.

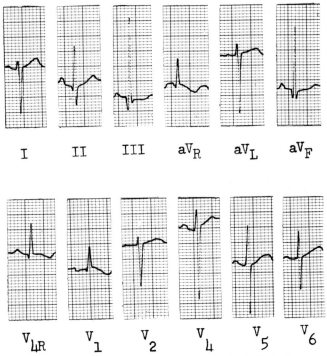

I   II   III   aV_R   aV_L   aV_F

V_{4R}   V_1   V_2   V_4   V_5   V_6

Figure 214. Electrocardiogram of a patient with classic clinical picture of Friedreich's ataxia. Note the mean electrical axis of plus 135 degrees and the right ventricular hypertrophy in the chest leads. This patient had no murmurs, but the pulmonic closure was accentuated. She has not been catheterized.

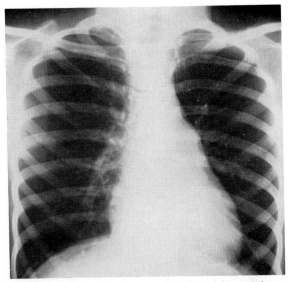

Figure 215. Roentgenogram of patient with Friedreich's ataxia and the previously described cardiogram (Fig. 214) with right ventricular hypertrophy. Note the prominent main pulmonary artery segment.

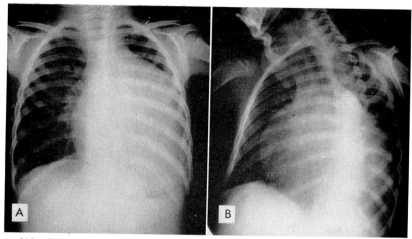

Figure 216. Posteroanterior and left anterior oblique roentgenograms in patient with Friedreich's ataxia and pericardial effusion.

terization studies were available to enable further elaboration on the diagnosis. Figure 215 shows a roentgenogram of this patient. Arrhythmias —parasystole and atrial fibrillation—have been described. Pericardial effusion has been seen (Fig. 216), and anginal pain occurs. Congestive failure is rare.

The few pathologic studies available indicate the prevalence of coronary arterial changes and evidences of myocardial fibrosis.

No treatment is available for either the cardiac or the neurologic aspects of this disease. The electrocardiogram may be a useful diagnostic tool, however. Whether these patients die because of the cardiac involvement or not is difficult to tell. The terminal stages of the disease are characterized by a virtual disintegration of the organism. The few postmortem observations described in the literature do suggest, however, that myocardial fibrosis, with or without coronary disease, may at least be a significant contributing factor in the death of these patients.[522, 606]

MYOCARDIAL DISEASE ASSOCIATED WITH PROGRESSIVE MUSCULAR DYSTROPHY

Another heredofamilial disease causing wasting, and even paralysis, of the skeletal muscles is progressive muscular dystrophy. This is a rare disease, and cardiac complications have been reported with various frequencies by various authors. I am aware of four such patients within the past ten years at The Children's Hospital Medical Center (Figs. 217, 218). One was a six-year old boy with progressive muscular dystrophy who was known to have had the disease from the time he was two years old; he died in congestive failure. Postmortem examination revealed cardiac enlargement with endocardial thickening of the left ventricle and the left atrium. Microscopic study showed fatty degeneration, scarring and lymphocytic infiltration. Two other patients were siblings; both died in their teens in severe left- and right-sided heart failure approximately one year after the onset of their cardiac symptoms. Cardiac catheterization data are available for one of these (Fig. 219). It is interesting that the involvement of the striated muscle in the disease was not severe enough to make the diagnosis certain without postmortem examination in one instance and muscle biopsy in the other. At first both patients were suspected of having unrecognized paralytic poliomyelitis. A fourth patient had muscular dystrophy which manifested itself only in scoliosis. Thus, at first, heart failure was thought to be secondary to pulmonary heart disease, whereas at postmortem examination, heart failure was proved to be secondary to muscular dystro-

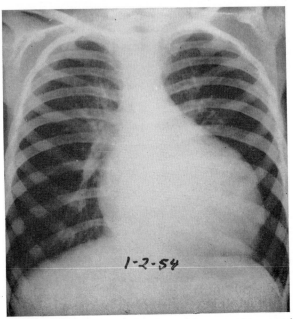

Figure 217. Posteroanterior radiogram of patient with progressive muscular dystrophy.

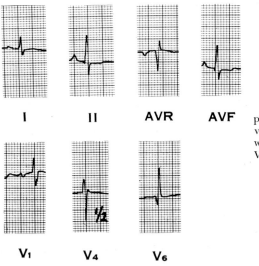

I   II   AVR   AVF

V₁   V₄   V₆

Figure 218. Electrocardiogram of patient with muscular dystrophy involving the heart. Note the flat T waves throughout, the deep S wave in V_4, and the wide Q wave in V_6.

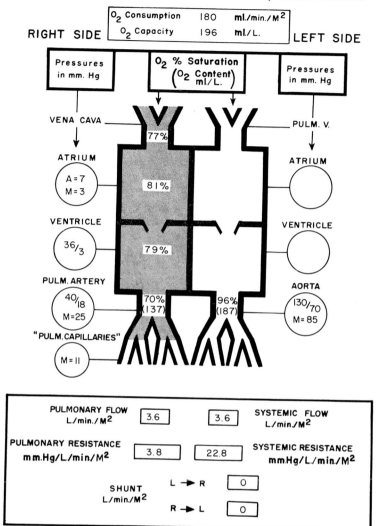

Figure 219. Catheterization findings in a patient with muscular dystrophy involving the heart.

phy, partly on account of the involvement of the heart muscle in the dystrophic process and partly because of the respiratory difficulties caused by the poor respiratory muscles and scoliosis.

Two interesting papers were published in 1952 on this subject.[597, 721] The consensus seemed to be that about 50 per cent of the cases examined post mortem show some degree of involvement of the myocardium similar to that seen in the striated muscle. Among the clinical manifestations of dystrophic heart disease, congestive failure, as well as tachycardia, arrhythmias, T wave changes and abnormal Q waves, should be mentioned. A temporary remission of the congestive failure can be achieved in these patients with anticongestive measures. Crandell, in 1956,[174] studied 16 patients with progressive muscular dystrophy and found only one with specific right ventricular myocardial disease. On the other hand, Manning and his associates,[477] in 1958, found abnormal electrocardiograms in 70 to

75 per cent of their 28 patients with dystrophy. Finally, in 1959, Kilburn and his co-workers[388] studied 17 patients with progressive muscular dystrophy and found that pulmonary function was impaired in all, probably secondary to muscle weakness. These authors concluded that circulatory impairment was probably secondary to the hypoventilation syndrome and to myocardial involvement in the dystrophic process. Our last-mentioned patient bears out this hypothesis. Recent evidence indicates that fetal myoglobin may be present in the skeletal as well as the cardiac muscle of these patients.*

MYOCARDIAL DISEASE ASSOCIATED WITH INFECTIONS

There are two interesting and diametrically opposing trends in pediatrics today in relation to the significance of cardiovascular involvement in acute infections.

In the older textbooks "toxic myocarditis" was blamed for the death of babies with bronchiolitis, bronchopneumonia and acute infectious diseases, including the exanthemas. There was talk about "scarlet fever heart," and prophylactic digitalization was widely recommended. Within the past twenty-five years most pediatricians have become rather skeptical about the validity of these observations on "toxic myocarditis." It may well be that the antibiotics are successfully combating infections to the point at which myocardial involvement no longer occurs. It is also possible that the widespread use of accurate diagnostic tools has made us interpret our observations more correctly. Whatever the reason, most pediatricians today are able to treat infectious diseases successfully without the use of digitalis or diuretics, and, by and large, people have stopped worrying about "toxic myocarditis." It has also been learned that if the circulatory system is involved in acute infections, the result is usually peripheral vascular collapse, a condition requiring shock treatment rather than anticongestive measures. A recent report of cardiac catheterization performed during attacks of severe bronchitis and pneumonia attests to the absence of demonstrable evidences of cardiac impairment.[761]

The opposing trend was started by the pathologists, especially Saphir and his associates,[290] who found myocardial changes at postmortem examination in a large number of persons who had died from infectious disease. They and others brought forward histologic proof of myocardial involvement in tuberculosis, hepatitis, poliomyelitis, encephalitis, pneumonia, tularemia, meningococcemia, infectious mononucleosis, rickettsial diseases, influenza, mumps, yellow fever and everything else one can think of. These pathologic studies were followed by widespread electrocardiographic studies in patients with infectious diseases. They showed transient T wave changes and some intraventricular conduction disturbances in a large percentage of children who had poliomyelitis, measles, hepatitis and infectious mononucleosis.

Although the presence of histologic or electrocardiographic changes in infectious disease can scarcely be doubted, their interpretation requires

* C. M. Whorton, P. C. Hudgins, J. J., Connors and A. S. Nadas: The Myoglobin Molecule and Its Structural Alterations in Diseased States of Skeletal and Cardiac Muscle. Presented before the Section on Pathology, Southern Medical Association, Miami Beach, Nov., 1962.

considerable caution. Remember that most of these patients have a high fever, their nutrition may be poor, and the peripheral circulation is certainly affected. In poliomyelitis, anoxia and difficulties in the autonomic nervous system play a significant role. Finally, with all this laboratory evidence, the clinical proof of insufficiency of the circulation, in terms of either congestive failure or significant arrhythmia, is lacking in most instances.

For practical purposes, it is well to treat acute infections in the young without too much concern for the myocardium unless definite evidences of significant arrhythmia, definite cardiac enlargement or congestive failure appear. On the basis of the evidence available in the literature, it is doubtful whether the state of the myocardium influences the prognosis of infectious diseases today in most instances. One exception to this statement, of course, is bacterial endocarditis, and possibly also infectious mononucleosis. The latter, a protean disease, may produce serious cardiac damage similar to that caused by rheumatic carditis.[495]

MYOCARDIAL DISEASE ASSOCIATED WITH ACUTE GLOMERULONEPHRITIS

Cardiac involvement in acute glomerulonephritis has been of considerable interest during the past two decades. Pediatricians who see children with acute glomerulonephritis are well aware of the possibility of the sudden catastrophic onset of pulmonary edema which terminates fatally within a few hours.

It is clear that although the majority of patients with acute nephritis have arterial hypertension, this alone cannot be blamed for cardiac failure, since the relation between the two is not close. Elevated venous pressure and increased blood volume have been found in a number of instances, and these indubitably contribute significantly to the circulatory embarrassment. Gore and Saphir[291] described significant myocardial changes at postmortem examination in 10 per cent of their series of patients who died after acute or subacute glomerulonephritis.

How often cardiac failure actually occurs in glomerulonephritis is a matter of considerable controversy. Ash and her associates[22] described evidences of congestive failure in twenty-two of fifty patients they studied. On the other hand, Keith reported that only 4 per cent of his patients had definite evidences of congestive heart failure; others place the incidence as high as 25 per cent. I think that much of the discrepancy between the reports of various authors may be due to varying definitions of congestive heart failure.

Peters[559] stated that congestive failure is common and that the edema of acute nephritis is due principally to this mechanism. I believe that nephritic edema is probably due to two factors: the increased venous pressure secondary to cardiac insufficiency and hypervolemia and the low plasma proteins inherent in renal disease.

Electrocardiographic changes (Fig. 220), especially depression of the S-T segment and inversion of the T wave, are seen in almost 75 per cent of the patients who have acute glomerulonephritis.[22] Prolonged Q-Tc is seen occasionally.

Radiologic evidences of cardiac failure are cardiomegaly and pulmonary congestion, which rapidly clears as the patient improves (Fig. 221).

The treatment of cardiac failure in acute glomerulonephritis should be aimed at reducing the load on the heart and improving myocardial efficiency. The former can be achieved by eliminating the hypertension with magnesium sulfate or hydralazine (0.1 to 0.15 mg. per kilogram of body weight) and reserpine (0.15 mg. per kilogram of body weight) administered intramuscularly, and by trying to reduce the circulating blood volume with a low salt diet. Venesection and application of a tourniquet to the extremities may even be necessary if pulmonary edema develops. Digitalis in a rapidly excreted form may be used to improve the myocardial effectiveness, but mercurial diuretics should be avoided for obvious reasons.

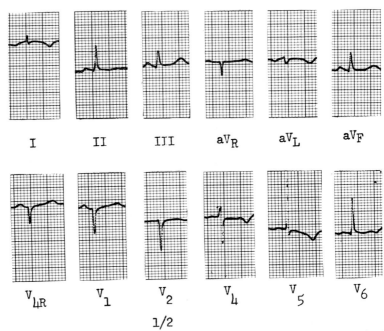

Figure 220. Electrocardiogram of patient with acute glomerulonephritis. Note the inverted T waves in lead I and the left chest leads. The voltages are low throughout.

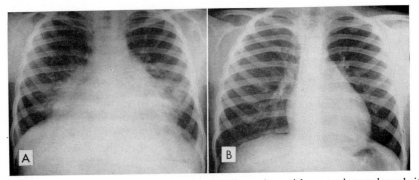

Figure 221. Posteroanterior roentgenograms of a patient with acute glomerulonephritis. The two films were taken three weeks apart, and the second one shows diminution of the heart size and of the pulmonary congestion.

The prognosis of acute glomerulonephritis is good in 95 per cent of the cases. The circulation is restored to normal after the disease has subsided.

FAMILIAL CARDIOMYOPATHY

The familial incidence of certain congenital cardiac deformities is well known. A familial disposition to rheumatic fever has been stressed by

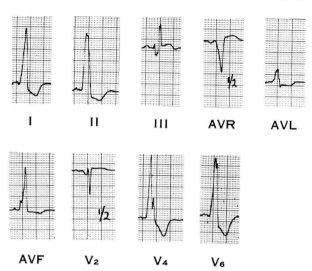

Figure 222. Electrocardiogram of patient with familial myocardial disease, with the Wolff-Parkinson-White syndrome.

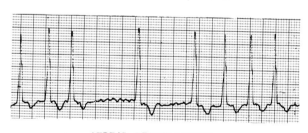

ATRIAL FIBRILLATION

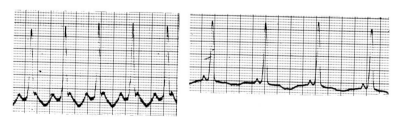

P.A.T. WITH BLOCK   REGULAR SINUS RHYTHM

Figure 223. Variety of arrhythmias ranging from atrial fibrillation, through paroxysmal atrial tachycardia with block, to regular sinus rhythm in a patient with familial myocardial disease and the Wolff-Parkinson-White syndrome.

Wilson and her co-workers.[734] Friedreich's ataxia, muscular dystrophy, glycogen storage disease, and even endocardial fibroelastosis, all have familial occurrences.

Excluding these well defined entities, there are still a number of families in which several members have evidences of myocardial disease. Evans[234] reported one family with three members, and another with two members, having myocardial disease. Campbell and Turner-Warwick[135] described two families, one with two, the other with three members affected. Familial cardiomegaly associated with the Wolff-Parkinson-White syndrome has been described by Schiebler and his associates.[615] Reviewing the electrocardiograms of Evans and Campbell's cases, Schiebler interpreted two of these as also having had the Wolff-Parkinson-White syndrome. Familial occurrence of obstructive cardiomyopathy resulting in critical aortic stenosis has been described by Hollman,[341] Goodwin[289] and Brent.[87]

Among our own material, most of these varieties of familial myopathy have been encountered. Some, with Friedreich's ataxia, glycogen disease, progressive muscular dystrophy and endocardial fibroelastosis, have already been discussed. Those with obstructive myopathy will be classified under

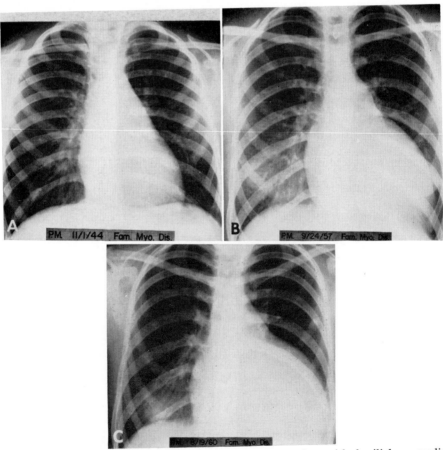

Figure 224. Progressive cardiac enlargement in a patient with familial myocardial disease and the Wolff-Parkinson-White syndrome throughout a 16-year period, from 1944 to 1957, to 1960.

aortic stenosis (see p. 565). At least three families still remain who at present may not be classified among any of the other entities. Two adolescents in one family have the Wolff-Parkinson-White syndrome (Fig. 222), attacks of paroxysmal atrial tachycardia (Fig. 223), cardiomegaly (Fig. 224) and angina. One of these siblings died, and at autopsy, as in patients with muscular dystrophy, fetal myoglobin was found in the heart muscle. (See reference in muscular dystrophy.) The mother of these two children has idiopathic atrial fibrillation. In the second family two children were also affected. One died at the age of twelve years; the second is alive, but symptomatic, at eleven. Both were mentally retarded and short in stature, and had webbing of the neck, but endocrine studies failed to show evidences of Turner's syndrome. The electrocardiograms did not indicate the Wolff-Parkinson-White syndrome, but showed right ventricular hypertrophy, combined atrial hypertrophy and changes in the S-T segment and the T waves (Fig. 225). Roentgenologic examination disclosed a very large heart and evidences of left- and right-sided congestive failure. Postmortem examination on the patient who died revealed diffuse nonspecific fibrosis.

We have physiologic data on three such patients. The cardiac outputs varied from 2 to 4 liters per square meter. Right atrial, right ventricular and pulmonary arterial systolic pressures varied from normal to moderately elevated levels. They all showed more or less elevation of diastolic pressure in the right ventricle and pulmonary artery. The left atrial and left and

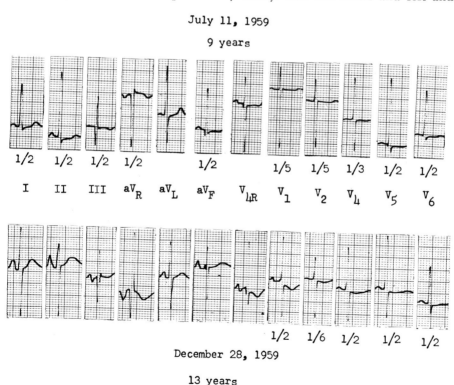

July 11, 1959

9 years

| 1/2 | 1/2 | 1/2 | 1/2 | | 1/2 | | 1/5 | 1/5 | 1/3 | 1/2 | 1/2 |
| I | II | III | aV$_R$ | aV$_L$ | aV$_F$ | V$_{4R}$ | V$_1$ | V$_2$ | V$_4$ | V$_5$ | V$_6$ |

| 1/2 | 1/6 | 1/2 | 1/2 | 1/2 |

December 28, 1959

13 years

Figure 225. Two electrocardiograms from two siblings who had familial myocardial disease, but not the Wolff-Parkinson-White syndrome. Both tracings were taken in 1959, when one of the children was 9 and the other 13 years old.

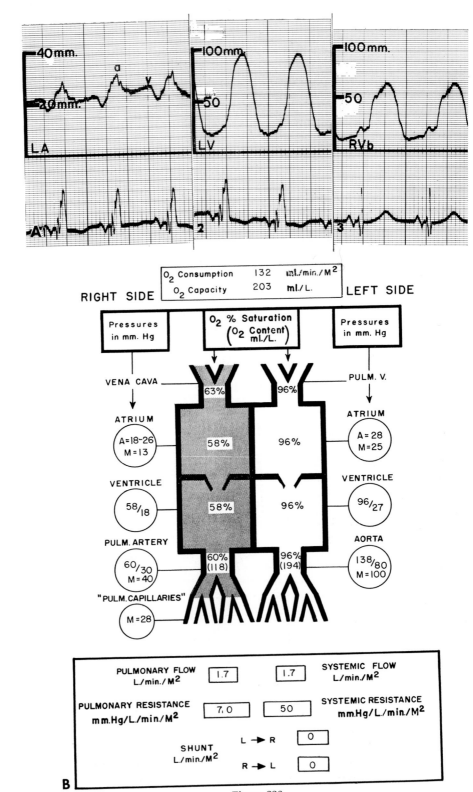

Figure 226.

right ventricular end-diastolic pressures were elevated in those in whom adequate studies were made (Fig. 226). As far as the physiologic data are concerned, the differences between these patients and patients with classic constrictive pericarditis were mostly quantitative, though the appreciable gradient between the right atrial and left atrial or pulmonary capillary pressure described by Wood[751] was noted in three of the four patients for whom adequate information was available.

In spite of the search for "specific" genetic chromosomal or metabolic abnormalities in these patients, no definite etiologic processes could be found. Undoubtedly, as more accurate tools for the investigation of these defects become available, a better etiologic classification will be made. For the time being they should be considered examples of familial cardiomyopathy.

As indicated, the clinical picture is variable. Arrythmias, congestive heart failure and syncope are the most common presenting symptoms. On physical examination cardiomegaly without murmur is noted. The roentgenologic features are similar to those seen in other primary myocardial diseases. With or without the Wolff-Parkinson-White syndrome, the electrocardiograms are characterized by arrythmias, changes in the S-T segment and T waves, and hypertrophy of one or both ventricles.

Treatment with anticongestive and antiarrhythmic measures may bring temporary relief. Steroids have been tried without spectacular success. The prognosis is poor. Most of our patients died in their teens. Reports indicate that survival to adulthood is possible, and Campbell[135] emphasized the "extreme variability of survival times, irrespective of the initial cardiographic and radiologic findings."

CHRONIC CARDIOMYOPATHY

In contrast to the instances of acute myocardial disease discussed under the heading of Primary Myocardial Disease, there are a number of children who have a chronic form of cardiomyopathy. These are patients whose clinical profile is not too different from that seen in adults with constrictive pericarditis. There is a history of repeated episodes of chronic left- and right-sided failure. The heart sounds may be muffled and gallop rhythm may be pronounced, particularly during the exacerbation of congestive heart failure. The second sound is usually narrowly split, and the pulmonic component is accentuated if pulmonary hypertension, secondary to left-sided failure, is present. Usually murmurs are not present, but in certain instances apical systolic and even mid-diastolic murmurs or stenotic murmurs at the second right interspace are clearly evident. In the latter situation the differential diagnosis from rheumatic mitral and congenital aortic lesions may be extremely difficult (see Muscular Aortic Stenosis).

Figure 226. *A,* Catheterization findings in sibling with familial cardiopathy without the Wolff-Parkinson-White syndrome. Pressure tracings from the left atrium, left ventricle and right ventricle. Note the high mean pressure in the left atrium with tall A waves and shallow x and y depressions. Note the high end-diastolic pressure in the left ventricle, corresponding to the left atrial pressure. There is moderate elevation of right ventricular pressure with a transmitted A wave and a high anacrotic shoulder. *B,* Cardiac catheterization findings in patient with familial cardiomyopathy.

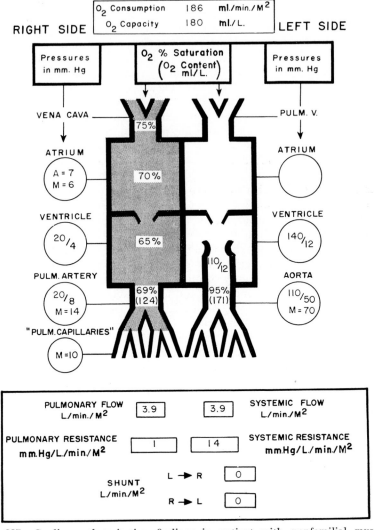

Figure 227. Cardiac catheterization findings in patient with nonfamilial myocardial disease, with some left ventricular obstruction.

The electrocardiogram is characterized by left or combined ventricular hypertrophy, changes in the T waves and conduction disturbances. The x-ray film shows varying degrees of cardiomegaly involving principally, if not exclusively, the left ventricle and left atrium. On screening, the pulsations are diminished. Pulmonary venous congestion is evident in the lung fields. Cardiac catheterization studies show the changes described in the section on Familial Cardiomyopathy; they are similar to those encountered in constrictive pericarditis (see p. 306) (Fig. 227).

The similarities of chronic cardiomyopathy to constrictive pericarditis are so close that often the differential diagnosis can be made only after thoracotomy. Constrictive pericarditis, of course, is a rare condition in children; still, since this is a surgically correctible disease and since no cure for chronic cardiomyopathy is available at present, surgical exploration is recommended unless pericardial constriction can clearly be excluded on other grounds.

Other conditions, less difficult to distinguish in the differential diagnosis, are (1) coarctation of the aorta and congestive failure, clearly recognizable by blood pressure measurements, (2) congenital aortic stenosis (to be discussed later), and (3) left atrial disease (mitral stenosis, cor triatriatum, left atrial myxoma, and even a ball valve thrombus). These conditions may be excluded by careful left and right heart catheterization studies (particularly through a comparison of the left atrial A wave with left ventricular end-diastolic pressures) and by good cine-angiograms.

Once the diagnosis of chronic cardiomyopathy has been made, principally by exclusion, an etiologic classification may be attempted with the full knowledge that it can be achieved in only a minority of the cases at present. Burwell and Robin,[120] describing diffuse myocardial fibrosis in adults, stated that the most frequent cause is coronary artery disease. Clearly this is not true in the pediatric age group. Certain specific steps are recommended for those attempting to obtain an etiologic classification for these patients: (1) careful family history to exclude familial cardiopathy, (2) neurologic examination to identify Friedreich's ataxia and the muscular dystrophies, (3) muscle biopsy to exclude glycogen disease and the dystrophies, (4) chromosome counts to discover abnormal genetic patterns, (5) plasma fractionation and urinary amino acid excretion tests to uncover metabolic disease, (6) stool examination for parasites, and (7) the Congo red test for amyloid disease.

Most likely, after all these tests, no definite cause for chronic cardiomyopathy will be discovered. Nevertheless it may be worth while to list the entities we have encountered in the past twelve years giving rise to the clinical profile described in this chapter: (1) familial cardiopathy, (2) chronic myocarditis, (3) primary endocardial fibroelastosis, (4) glycogen disease, (5) pulmonary hemosiderosis,[167] (6) Friedreich's ataxia, and (7) muscular dystrophy.

Other conditions, not seen by us, but described in the literature, are: (1) toxoplasmosis, (2) trichinosis, (3) amyloid disease, (4) scleroderma, and (5) sarcoidosis.[565]

11

DISEASES OF THE PERICARDIUM

Classification

Pericardial disease is usually a manifestation of some systemic condition; except for rare traumatic pericarditis or the presence of an isolated pericardial cyst, it never occurs as an isolated disease.

For practical purposes, unless proved otherwise, pericardial involvement indicates rheumatic carditis in children. Other common causes of pericarditis are (1) pyogenic organisms, (2) rheumatoid arthritis, (3) acute viral pericarditis, (4) uremia, and (5) neoplastic disease. Less common etiologic factors to be considered are (6) tuberculosis, (7) disseminated lupus, (8) chronic constrictive pericarditis, (9) congenital hypoplastic anemia, (10) Mediterranean anemia, (11) Friedreich's ataxia, and (12) ulcerative colitis.

Pathology

Pathologically speaking, pericardial disease can be divided into acute and chronic forms. Acute pericarditis, according to the nature of the exudate, may be serous, fibrinous, serofibrinous, purulent, hemorrhagic or neoplastic. Chronic pericarditis always involves fibroplastic proliferation. The various clinical entities differ in the extent and nature of the involvement.

Physiology

The physiologic effects of pericarditis depend to a great extent on the competence of the underlying myocardium and the nature, volume and speed of accumulation of the exudate. If the myocardium is intact and the serous exudate accumulates slowly, several hundred cubic centimeters of intrapericardial fluid may be tolerated without obvious interference with the circulation. On the other hand, in rheumatic pancarditis the sudden accumulation of only 100 to 200 cc. of exudate may cause serious circulatory embarrassment.

Cardiac tamponade is a clinical syndrome caused by the accumulation of fluid within the pericardial sac. Obviously, the more rapidly this fluid accumulates, the larger the amount, and the more rigid the pericardium, the more serious the consequences will be. A number of direct effects of the compression of the heart and a number of compensatory mechanisms are involved in the causation of the clinical syndrome (Table 20, p. 787). Perhaps the first thing that happens is that the ventricles cannot fill adequately during diastole because of the external pressure of the fluid. To counteract this, the right and left atrial and systemic, as well as pulmonary, venous pressures increase. Since this compensatory mechanism is not completely successful, and the stroke volume is still relatively small, an attempt to maintain an adequate cardiac output is made by increasing the heart rate. Finally, to obviate the drop in systolic blood pressure caused by the inadequate cardiac output, the diastolic pressure is raised by peripheral vasoconstriction, thus achieving a satisfactory mean pressure at the expense of a narrow pulse pressure. It may be worth emphasizing that the signs most commonly identified with cardiac tamponade, such as increased venous pressure, increased pulse rate and narrow pulse pressure, all represent compensating mechanisms and, therefore, should not be "corrected" lest the cardiac output drop even further. For this reason the treatment of cardiac tamponade consists solely in evacuation of the fluid. Therapeutic maneuvers aimed at lowering the venous pressure (venesection), slowing the pulse rate (digitalis) or decreasing the peripheral resistance (external heat) not only are ineffective, but also occasionally may even prove harmful.

Clinical Picture

On the whole, acute, dry or fibrinous pericarditis of the "bread and butter" type may be uncomfortable and painful, indeed, but it seldom causes failure of the circulation. Conversely, accumulation of a serous exudate of 200 cc. or more, especially if it develops rapidly, obstructs the work of the heart noticeably and causes cardiac tamponade. Accumulation of purulent pericardial exudate may cause not only tamponade, but also empyema-like symptoms characteristic of a septic focus.

Pericardial pain, if present, may be of two kinds. One is the dull, aching, nauseous, poorly localized "visceral" variety, involving the precordium and probably resulting from the stretching of the pericardial sac. The other is a sharp, stabbing, referred type of pain, localized to the left chest, shoulder, neck and scapula; it is exaggerated by lying down and relieved by sitting up. This type of pain is probably the result of the involvement of the diaphragm and the pleura, since there are no sensory nerves in the pericardium proper.[138]

A patient with acute rheumatic fever who suddenly starts complaining of precordial or referred pain is almost certain to show evidences of pericarditis within a few hours or days. Shortness of breath, grunting respirations, bothersome dry cough, and orthopnea with a tendency to lean forward, are all characteristic symptoms of the patient with pericardial disease. The symptoms of pericardial tamponade are those of acute congestive failure in a patient with pericarditis. Large effusions may cause swallowing difficulties. The symptoms of septicemia are characteristic of purulent pericarditis.

On physical examination the most typical feature of pericardial involvement is the presence of a friction rub. The characteristics of this have been mentioned previously; *it is not restricted to any heart cycle or any point of auscultation, and it may be evanescent.* It should be pointed out that it may on occasion be difficult to differentiate a friction rub from a high-frequency early diastolic blow; the rub may be heard best with the patient sitting up or leaning forward and with the bell chest-piece pressed hard against the precordium. Geiger[271] recommended auscultation in the knee-chest position during held inspiration. Occasionally, clear-cut synchronism between respiration and the friction rub is noted, in which case probably a pleuropericardial friction rub is present. Although friction rub is best heard in patients with dry fibrinous pericarditis, its presence does not exclude the existence of a large pericardial effusion. If the pericarditis is of rheumatic origin, the heart sounds are rather muffled, and significant murmurs are always present.

An increase in cardiac dullness is usually demonstrable, and the rather overrated Ewart's sign (a triangular dullness below the angle of the left scapula) is continuously sought for by medical students, to the great delight of their instructors. A possibly more useful sign is the fact that, in spite of the large size of the heart, the cardiac impulse is quiet and hypodynamic.

Classically, cardiac tamponade manifests itself in distention of the veins in the neck, enlargement of the liver and peripheral edema. The systolic blood pressure is lower than normal, and the pulse pressure is narrow. One of the most useful signs of cardiac tamponade is the paradoxical pulse, consisting in a drop in systolic pressure of more than 10 mm. of mercury at the end of deep inspiration. Frequently this may be noted by simply feeling the radial pulse, but accurate evaluation is possible only with the sphygmomanometer. These patients generally appear anxious and distressed; they are cyanotic and dyspneic, and look terribly sick.

As Williams[732] aptly pointed out, none of the "classic" signs is indispensable in the diagnosis of cardiac tamponade. Occasionally the venous distention is so severe that the top of the jugular venous column may not be seen below the ear lobe even when the patient is sitting up. In still other patients, vigorously pulsating neck veins, with a sharp, quick y or x descent, or both, may be seen as an expression of the rapid filling (with a small amount of blood) of an indistensible right ventricle by the high right atrial pressure. The heart sounds may not be muffled, the friction rub may not be abolished, the cardiac impulse may not be damped, and the pulse pressure may not be narrowed. In other words, in patients with the clinical diagnosis of pericarditis, who are critically ill and show evidences of congestive heart failure, tamponade should be strongly suspected even if the evidence is not clear-cut. Probably less harm is done by an occasional, unnecessary pericardial paracentesis, or even quick exploration, than by omitting relief of critical fluid accumulation. Pericardial tamponade is a real cardiac emergency.

It should also be mentioned here that a paradoxical pulse is not pathognomonic of pericarditis. Patients with dyspnea and increased negative intrathoracic pressure (emphysema, asthma, post-thoracotomy states) may have an appreciable lowering of the systolic pressure on inspiration without accumulation of fluid in the pericardium. Similarly, patients with cardiomyopathies may have paradoxical pulses of 10 to 20 mm. of mercury, but seldom more.

Routine laboratory examination reveals a moderate degree of leukocytosis, varying degrees of anemia, and normal urine.

Pericarditis is recognizable by radiologic means only if a sizable effusion is present; dry pericarditis cannot be identified by roentgenogram. Pericardial effusion manifests itself radiographically by an enlarged cardiac silhouette of "water-bottle" shape (Fig. 13, p. 30), with blunting of the cardiophrenic angle and shortening and widening of the supracardiac shadow. The lung fields are unusually clear and lack all evidences of congestion. Characteristically, the cardiac enlargement appears within a few days and disappears after treatment, or even spontaneously, with equal rapidity. At cardiac fluoroscopy the pulsations are feeble and undulating. By changing the patient's position from vertical to horizontal (by means of a tilt table), the size and shape of the effusion may be changed as well; this test has been described in several textbooks, but has been of no particular assistance to us. By introducing a cardiac catheter or contrast material (angiography), or even carbon dioxide, into the right atrium and right ventricle, the presence of an extracardiac mass (fluid) can clearly be identified. This is the only way by which pericardial effusion can be differentiated with certainty from massive cardiac enlargement radiologically. With the introduction of the image intensifier into fluoroscopic technique, it is often possible to delineate the pulsatile myocardium within the pericardial sac filled with fluid. So far, our experience with this method has been limited, but it may well prove to be the simplest and best way of identifying pericardial effusion.

The electrocardiographic changes of pericarditis have already been mentioned in detail (p. 93). Briefly summarized, they are (1) low voltage, (2) elevations in the S-T segment without reciprocal relation between leads I and III, and (3) diffuse T wave inversion, which appears last after the onset of pericarditis and may persist for several months after all other evidences of pericardial involvement have disappeared.

Occasionally the only way to find out whether pericardial effusion is present is to explore the pericardial sac by either paracentesis or thoracotomy. At The Children's Hospital Medical Center the Surgical Service believes that quick thoracotomy with a small incision is, on the whole, a safer procedure than blind exploration of the pericardial sac with a big trocar. With an excellent team of surgeons, anesthetists and operating room personnel in continuous attendance, this arrangement has worked well through the years. At the same time, at another hospital without a large personnel trained in cardiovascular surgery, the exploration of the pericardium by needle may be an extremely useful and simple procedure. The site of pericardial exploration should be at a point 2 cm. inside the left border of the cardiac dullness at the fifth intercostal space, or occasionally, in cases of large and presumably purulent effusion, at the angle between the xiphoid and the lower left costal margin.

Strict surgical asepsis should be observed. The patient should receive morphine subcutaneously fifteen minutes before the start of the procedure. Local anesthesia with 2 per cent procaine is used. A 3-inch, short-bevel trocar (number 16 to 18) connected with a 20-cc. syringe is used for a diagnostic tap. If the approach is through the fifth intercostal space, the needle should be directed to the right and toward the spine, whereas in the xiphoid approach one should proceed upward and backward, to the left. The needle enters between the ribs, and it is usually possible to feel it suddenly penetrate the pericardial sac 2 to 4 cm. from the skin. Usually only 20 to 40 cc. of fluid are removed for diagnostic purposes. If tamponade is present, the removal of 150 cc. or more may be a lifesaving maneuver. In this case the use of a three-way stopcock may prevent air from penetrating the pericardial sac; this saves the trouble of detaching and attaching the needle continuously.

Differential Diagnosis

The differential diagnosis of pericardial disease is not a difficult one. In children the only great problem is in distinguishing acute pericardial effusion from a large heart associated with one of the acute myocardial diseases. Features common to both are (1) congestive failure, (2) large, feebly pulsating heart without murmur and with muffled heart sounds, and (3) changes in the S-T segments and T waves on the electrocardiogram. If pericardial friction rub is present, the diagnosis is clear. In the absence of such, pulsus paradoxus favors the diagnosis of pericardial effusion, though we have seen pulsus paradoxus of 10 to 20 mm. of mercury with myocardial disease. In the roentgenogram, in addition to the help given by the image intensifier, the nature of the pulmonary vasculature may be helpful. In the myopathies pulmonary venous congestion is the rule, whereas in patients with pericardial effusion the lung fields are relatively clear, particularly considering the extent of cardiomegaly. If in doubt, it is suggested that intensive decongestive measures be undertaken for one to two days, and a careful record be kept of blood pressure, heart size and the patient's general condition. If speedy improvement does not follow these steps, catheterization, and even exploration of the pericardial sac, is recommended.

The only other differential diagnostic problem to be considered is the distinction between constrictive pericarditis and chronic cardiomyopathy. These two conditions have in common (1) moderate cardiac enlargement without significant murmur, (2) chronic, severe, right-sided congestive failure, and (3) catheterization data revealing (a) low cardiac output, (b) similarity of right atrial mean, right ventricular end-diastolic and pulmonary diastolic pressures, (c) deep x or y troughs, or both, in the right

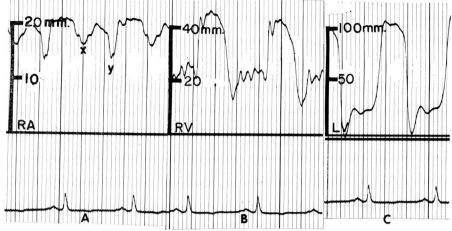

Figure 228.   Pressure tracings of patient with constrictive pericarditis. Note right atrial, right ventricular and left ventricular tracings. Note in the right atrium the high mean pressure with brisk x and y depressions. Note the high end-diastolic pressure in both the right and left ventricular pressure tracings, and the early diastolic dip in both ventricular tracings.

atrial tracings, (*d*) early diastolic dip, corresponding to the y trough of the atrial pressure pulse in the right ventricular tracing (Fig. 228) and (*e*) high pulmonary capillary and left atrial pressures.

Although, as mentioned before, often these two conditions may be distinguished definitively only by pericardial exploration, the young age of the patient, the absence of calcifications, the appreciable gradient between right atrial and left atrial or pulmonary capillary pressures and the relatively poor cardiac output all favor myopathy over constrictive pericarditis.

SPECIFIC PERICARDIAL DISEASE ENTITIES

RHEUMATIC PERICARDITIS

As mentioned before, rheumatic pericarditis is the commonest form of pericarditis in children; it is invariably accompanied by many of the manifestations of acute rheumatic fever. I have never seen a patient with rheumatic pericarditis who did not, at the same time, have a loud apical systolic murmur. Consequently, if a patient with pericarditis has no significant murmur, a diagnosis other than rheumatic fever must be considered. Rheumatic pericarditis is usually of the fibrinous or serofibrinous variety, and it is characterized more by pain and friction rub than by large fluid accumulation. As a rule, paracentesis is not advocated in patients with rheumatic pericarditis unless tamponade is imminent. The diagnosis is usually clear enough, and antirheumatic treatment is successful today in a high percentage of cases. The rare instance of cardiac tamponade, however, should be treated by paracentesis or thoracotomy. This represents a real cardiac emergency, and early decisive action may be lifesaving.

Since rheumatic pericarditis is always part of pancarditis, pulmonary congestion secondary to left-sided myocardial involvement is always present in addition to right-sided failure.

It has been mentioned that pericarditis is an ominous sign of acute rheumatic carditis. In my opinion, steroid treatment is mandatory. If properly treated, pericarditis will seldom last longer than one to two weeks.

PURULENT PERICARDITIS

Purulent pericarditis is usually associated with bacterial pneumonia, left-sided empyema, pyelonephritis, osteomyelitis or tonsillitis. It may be seen in infants as young as five weeks old. It is a rare but therapeutically important disease. These patients show the striking combination of pericardial tamponade with the septic picture of localized accumulation of pus. Chemotherapy has little, if any, effect on these youngsters. Emptying the pericardial sac, on the other hand, dramatically solves both problems. In this age of extensive chemotherapy, organisms are rarely cultured from the exudate, but the literature mentions pneumococci, streptococci, staphylococci, E. coli and H. influenzae[731] among the pathogenic organisms. Figure 229 shows the course of a patient with purulent pericarditis; Figure 230 shows the roentgenograms of this child before and after evacuation of the purulent exudate. Whether constrictive pericarditis will develop later in these patients, once they have been cured, cannot be stated with certainty. My personal feeling, based on limited experience, is that constrictive disease probably rarely follows in the wake of successfully treated purulent pericarditis.

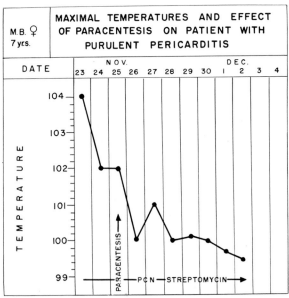

Figure 229.   Temperature chart and effect of paracentesis on patient with purulent pericarditis.

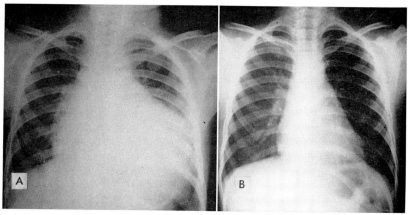

Figure 230.   Posteroanterior roentgenograms of a child with purulent pericarditis (*A*) before and (*B*) after thoracotomy.

IDIOPATHIC OR VIRAL PERICARDITIS (ACUTE BENIGN)

This is a relatively recently described disease.[43, 140] The initial case reports concerned young adults principally, but within the last few years children with this condition have also been described.[34, 76, 263, 469, 470]

The disease usually follows an upper respiratory tract infection. Occasionally it occurs in families or communities where there is an epidemic of pleurodynia, usually in August or September. The first symptom is fever, with pericardial pain and dyspnea. At physical examination these patients may appear very sick, sitting up in bed, short of breath, anxious-looking, leaning forward, perhaps even clutching a pillow against the chest. On auscultation a friction rub without murmur is heard, and the heart is enlarged. Electrocardiograms characteristic of pericarditis are obtained in almost every case. The sedimentation rate is increased, and leukocytosis is common, but cardiac tamponade is rare. The radiogram commonly shows pleural fluid accumulation.

Coxsackie B virus may be isolated from the stool specimens of these patients, and neutralizing antibodies may be found in paired serum specimens. During influenza epidemics, cases of pericarditis due to this agent have been described.[3] In all the reported cases due to Coxsackie virus, the outcome was favorable, though constrictive disease may develop.[34] Infections due to the influenza virus are much less "benign," and fatalities in adults have been reported. The illness lasts for several weeks. Chemotherapy, by and large, is not effective. Aspirin, oxygen and, occasionally, morphine give satisfactory symptomatic relief. The use of steroids has been advocated.[263]

Although the cessation of the individual attack within a matter of a few weeks can safely be predicted, the disease commonly recurs within a few weeks, months or even years. I have seen a boy who had three attacks of "idiopathic pericarditis" within two years. For recurrent attacks the prophylactic use of Achromycin and the therapeutic administration of steroids can be advocated, perhaps more on an emotional than an intellectual basis.

The differential diagnosis should be directed principally toward excluding rheumatic fever. Only secondarily should other causes of pericarditis be considered and identified by appropriate means.

PERICARDITIS ASSOCIATED WITH RHEUMATOID ARTHRITIS

Pericarditis associated with rheumatoid arthritis, or Still's disease, should be mentioned as one of the cardiac complications of this syndrome. Other circulatory disturbances associated with rheumatoid arthritis are (1) aortic regurgitation, (2) mitral regurgitation, (3) myocardial disease, and (4) pulmonary vascular obstruction.

The clinical findings are the same as those listed in the general description of pericarditis. Tamponade is rare; the incidental discovery of a pericardial friction rub is often the only sign of pericardial involvement in rheumatoid arthritis. The outcome depends on the prognosis of the associated disease. Steroid therapy may be indicated for the sickest of these children.

TUBERCULOUS PERICARDITIS

Tuberculous pericarditis is a disease of old people, but it has been noted in children occasionally.[561] We saw two adolescents with tuberculous pericarditis in our 10-year survey and an additional one in 1948.[521] The pericardial involvement is always the result of a direct spread of the infection from the adjoining lung field. It consists of serofibrinous or hemorrhagic exudate, followed by the development of granulation tissue and extensive scarring. A considerable body of opinion attributes the presence of constrictive pericarditis to long-standing tuberculous involvement.[19, 118] In the patient we saw in 1948, constrictive pericarditis developed before our eyes within a period of six months, while he was being treated for proved tuberculous pericarditis.

Until recently the prognosis was very poor. Tamponade occurs. With the newer chemotherapeutic advances in the treatment of tuberculosis the prognosis has improved a great deal. The pericardial involvement is only a small part of the generalized severe tuberculosis.

UREMIC PERICARDITIS

In the later stages of chronic glomerulonephritis uremic pericarditis occurs. It is a manifestation of the chemical irritation of the serous membranes by the high nonprotein nitrogen content of the plasma. Usually there are no symptoms. The diagnosis is based on the appearance of a friction rub in a patient dying with uremia.

NEOPLASMS

Neoplasms, such as lymphosarcoma, Hodgkin's disease or primary carcinoma of the lung, may invade the heart and give rise to a hemorrhagic exudate. This is usually a terminal event, and the involvement of the pericardium does not influence the clinical picture appreciably.

PERICARDITIS WITH BLOOD DYSCRASIAS

In children with chronic, long-standing anemias (Cooley's and hypoplastic anemias) pericardial effusion may develop in the course of the disease. The circulatory effects of a sudden accumulation of fluid in the pericardium on a myocardium weakened by anemia, and possibly hemochromatosis, may be disastrous. Sudden, life-threatening tamponade may be relieved only by pericardiocentesis. Whether the hemosiderin deposits, or the splenectomy performed because of the anemia, are responsible for the pericardial fluid accumulation is not known. The fluid is usually clear and straw-colored. Fluid accumulation may recur several times.

PERICARDIAL CYSTS

Pericardial cysts discovered on routine chest roentgenograms, and commonly giving no symptoms whatsoever, have been seen occasionally at The Children's Hospital. The tremendously enlarged heart, giving no symptoms and accompanied by no circulatory involvement and a normal electrocardiogram, presents a striking picture.

The radiologic and electrocardiographic findings in a boy with a pericardial cyst, which was successfully removed, are presented in Figures 231 and 232. Apparently most of these cysts are benign, and surgical removal is easy and is followed by complete recovery.

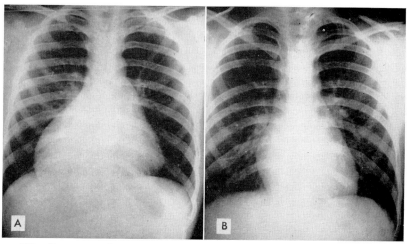

Figure 231.   Posteroanterior roentgenograms of a boy with a pericardial cyst (A) before and (B) after removal of the mucilaginous structure.

I   II   III

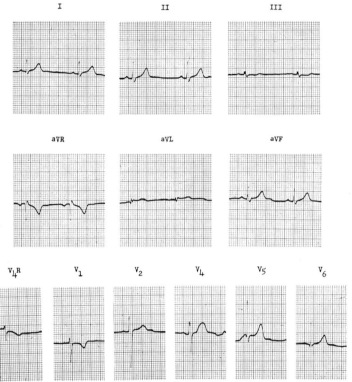

aVR   aVL   aVF

V_4R V_1 V_2 V_4 V_5 V_6

Figure 232. Electrocardiogram of a patient with pericardial cyst. Note the entirely normal tracing.

THE POSTPERICARDIOTOMY SYNDROME

In 1961 Engle and Ito,[227] in an article on this topic, estimated that this syndrome develops in 30 per cent of the survivors of open-heart surgery. Our experience, although not based on as thorough a follow-up as theirs, indicates that 10 to 15 per cent may be a more reasonable figure for our material.

Etiology

The first description of this entity attributed it to rheumatic recurrence.[654] Since no other evidence of active rheumatic fever is present in these patients, and since it occurs in patients undergoing cardiac surgery for congenital heart disease as well, the theory of rheumatic etiology has been discarded by most authors. The similarity of the clinical picture to that seen in acute viral pericarditis and the postmyocardial infarction syndrome suggests either a viral etiology or a nonspecific hypersensitivity reaction.

Clinical Picture

Fever occurring two to three weeks after cardiac surgery, chest pain, pleural and pericardial friction rub, cardiac enlargement due to effusion and electrocardiographic evidences of pericardial involvement dominate the picture. The sedimentation rate is elevated, and there is polymorphonuclear leukocytosis. The disease is self-limited within ten to twenty days. We have seen three recurrences within a year in one patient.

Treatment

Treatment is symptomatic and includes bed rest, aspirin, sedation and, rarely, pericardial tap. The use of steroids has been recommended, but we have not usually been forced to use them; however, short courses of steroid therapy may be given if the patient is very uncomfortable.

CHRONIC CONSTRICTIVE PERICARDITIS

Constrictive pericarditis must always be considered in the differential diagnosis of chronic congestive failure of unknown etiology. We have seen only a few cases of this disease at The Children's Hospital Medical Center in Boston, but we have had ample opportunity to see adults with this crippling condition in hospitals adjoining our institution. The youngest patient with constrictive pericarditis described by White was ten years old.[728] We have seen one two-year-old girl with constrictive pericarditis caused by tuberculosis. Keith[380] reported only one case of constrictive disease among 235 children with pericarditis. The Mayo Clinic group reported 8 patients less than 15 years old in a 25-year period.[637]

Tuberculosis is considered by most authors to be the most common etiologic agent. Occasionally, acute viral pericarditis may lead to constrictive disease.[34] Recently, *Histoplasma capsulatum* was implicated,[753] and purulent pericarditis and even, rarely, traumatic pericarditis are believed to lead to constriction.

The physiologic handicaps of constrictive pericarditis are the same as those discussed under pericardial tamponade (see p. 295). The catheterization findings have been discussed and contrasted to those found in the myopathies (see pp. 289–91) (Fig. 233). The edema and ascites are attributed by some to hypoproteinemia secondary to protein loss through the gastrointestinal tract.[186]

The clinical picture is characterized by the triad of a small heart, elevated venous pressure, and ascites. The ascites is out of all proportion to the edema elsewhere. The patients are not as sick as one would expect from the evidence of right-sided failure; they may be able to do a moderate amount of exercise, and orthopnea is rare.

The jugular venous pulse shows no giant waves; a dominant y trough or x depression can be seen clearly. A paradoxical pulse of more than 10 mm. can be observed easily. Blood pressure is low; pulse pressure, narrow. The cardiac impulse is quiet, but an early pericardial knock, synchronous with the opening snap or the third sound, may be palpable.

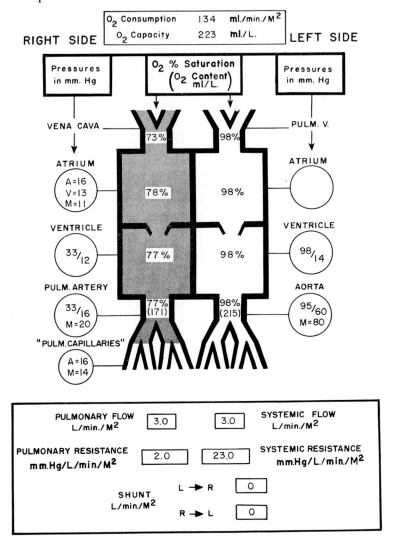

Figure 233. Cardiac catheterization data from patient with constrictive pericarditis.

Radiologic examination reveals a heart that is only moderately, if at all, enlarged (Fig. 234). Dalton and his associates[180] reported enlargement in 50 per cent of their 78 patients. Calcification in the pericardium is pathognomonic and occurs in as many as 55 per cent of the patients in some series.[556] At fluoroscopy the cardiac beat is diminished, sometimes more on the right than on the left side. The electrocardiogram shows low voltage T waves almost without fail, and a broad, notched P wave in about 75 per cent of the patients (Fig. 235).

Constrictive pericarditis, if it leads to the clinical syndrome here described, should be treated surgically. Radical pericardiectomy, as advocated by Holman and his associates,[343] is the preferred approach to the problem. This consists in decortication of the pericardium beyond the left, right and inferior cardiac borders, including liberation of the venae

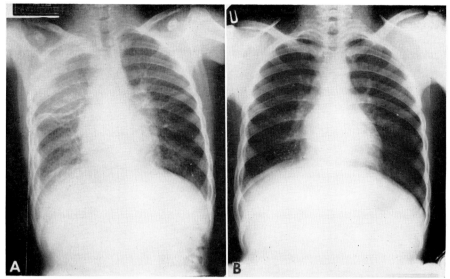

Figure 234. Roentgenograms, preoperative (*A*) and postoperative (*B*), of patient with constrictive pericarditis. Note the clearing of the lung fields and diminution of the cardiac silhouette after operation.

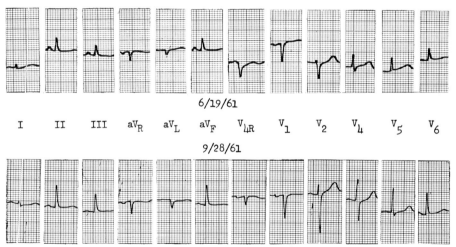

6/19/61

I   II   III aV_R aV_L aV_F V_{4R} V_1 V_2 V_4 V_5 V_6

9/28/61

Figure 235. Preoperative and postoperative electrocardiograms of patient with constrictive pericarditis. Note the low voltage T waves in the limb leads and the left chest leads preoperatively, with good upright T waves in the chest leads postoperatively. Note also the generalized increase in the QRS voltages after operation.

cavae. The results were good in fourteen of the twenty-six patients in Holman's latest series. Four of the twenty-six died. In Wood's[751] series of 30 patients who underwent surgery, 11 per cent died and 50 per cent showed excellent results. Dalton and his associates[180] reported follow-up studies on forty-five survivors of pericardiectomy from the Massachusetts General Hospital. All patients followed up for twenty years were still leading normal lives. Improvement can be measured largely in terms of a decrease in venous pressure and increase in cardiac output.

The postoperative course of these patients may be marred by the development of severe congestive failure which, however, responds well to conventional anticongestives. The muscular atrophy described by the Mayo Clinic group[197] in patients with constrictive pericarditis may well be the reason for postoperative congestive heart failure.

12

CONGESTIVE FAILURE

Definition and Physiology

Congestive failure, in the light of newer knowledge of circulatory physiology, is increasingly hard to define. Lewis[427] regarded cardiac failure as "inability of the heart to discharge its contents adequately." This was a perfectly good definition until it was recognized that in many instances of chronic congestive failure the ventricle does fulfill its obligation, but is able to do so only by invoking compensatory mechanisms, such as tachycardia, increased diastolic filling pressure or cardiac hypertrophy. Lewis's classic definition was further qualified when, on the basis of animal experimentation, it became clear that relatively minor impairments of cardiac function may be reflected solely in the increased renal tubular reabsorption of sodium, and only later in decreased glomerular filtration rate.[39, 41, 42]

Since, at present, no precise physiologic definition is available, it might be well to regard congestive failure simply as a clinical syndrome associated with heart disease in which the heart is either unable to supply the body with the cardiac output it demands or is unable to dispose adequately of the venous return, or, most likely, a combination of the two. Left-sided failure is characterized by weakness, fatigue, dyspnea on exertion, orthopnea, cardiac asthma, pulmonary edema, chronic hacking cough, pulmonary rales, accentuated pulmonary closure, gallop rhythm, hydrothorax and pulsus alternans.

In contrast, right-sided failure is identified by increasing systemic venous pressure, enlargement of the liver, dependent edema, right hydrothorax, hydropericardium, ascites and oliguria.

Cardiac enlargement is present in both left-sided and right-sided failure, with few exceptions, as are cold extremities; cyanosis may or may not be present in either.

The congestive failure syndrome is frequently encountered in pediatric hospitals; the age distribution is of some interest. In patients with congenital heart disease, failure is most likely to develop within the first six months of life. Keith stated that 90 per cent of the cases occur within the first year of life. If this period is survived without evidences of congestion, it is not likely to occur until at least two years of age or most likely considerably later. On the other hand, congestive failure associated with rheumatic heart disease usually does not occur before the age of four to five years, and it always indicates an active rheumatic process. Paroxysmal atrial tachycardia and primary myocardial disease—two relatively common causes of congestive failure in childhood—usually manifest themselves within the first year or two of life.

Among the congenital cardiac lesions most commonly causing congestive heart failure may be mentioned, in order of decreasing frequency, transposition of the great arteries, coarctation of the aorta, ventricular septal defect, hypoplastic left heart syndrome, total anomalous pulmonary venous drainage, endocardial cushion defect, endocardial fibroelastosis and patent ductus arteriosus.

The two most commonly quoted theories of congestive failure are the backward and forward failure concepts. According to the theory of backward failure,[328] the heart, consisting of two independent pumps (the left and the right ventricles), fails when one pump cannot forward the load offered to it by the other. For instance, a failing left ventricle, being unable to put out all the blood the right ventricle offers, acts as a dam behind which the blood rapidly accumulates, increasing the volume and later the pressure in the left atrium, pulmonary veins and even the pulmonary artery and the right ventricle. This theory would explain very well the clinical syndrome referred to as left-sided failure, consisting principally in pulmonary congestion and its consequences. The reason this explanation holds so well for left-sided failure is the rather limited capacity of the pulmonary vascular bed, where even a few hundred extra cubic centimeters of blood may cause considerable trouble.

If, on the other hand, one tries to explain the phenomena observed in right-sided failure, i.e., systemic congestion, on the basis of backward failure alone, one encounters a considerable amount of difficulty. The principal obstacle to this explanation for failure of the right ventricle is the fact that even if the entire contents of the pulmonary circuit—roughly one tenth of the circulating blood volume—were transferred to the systemic circuit, this, by itself, should not cause any trouble; the systemic reservoir is so large that simply shifting some (or even all) of the blood from the lungs should not cause an elevated systemic venous pressure any more than a good-sized blood transfusion would. Furthermore, ligation of the inferior vena cava, performed therapeutically as well as experimentally, does not produce evidences of systemic congestion with any regularity.[107] Finally, complete destruction of the right ventricle in animal experiments is tolerated relatively well, and certainly without evidences of failure.[666]

Proponents of the forward failure theory[493] maintain that the congestive failure syndrome is due to a low cardiac output, resulting in an inadequate supply of oxygen to the tissues, increased capillary permeability and renal failure. This, then, would give rise to increased blood volume, edema and other manifestations of congestive failure. The most obvious difficulty in accepting this theory is the observation that severe anoxic states, such as cyanotic congenital heart disease, may exist for many years without any evidence of congestion; furthermore, no really good evidence of increased capillary permeability in cardiac failure exists, nor is there a straight line correlation between the absolute level of cardiac output and the presence or absence of failure, nor between cardiac output and renal blood flow. As a matter of fact, as mentioned before, the increased sodium retention characteristic of early congestive heart failure depends on increased tubular reabsorption rather than on diminished renal blood flow.

Since neither of these two theories alone explains the phenomena described, perhaps a combination of several factors may result in a more acceptable hypothesis. Burch,[105] Altschule[14] and others[258] have proposed theories that fit in broadly with the concepts to be presented. The entire thought, however, is based on Starling's[665] fundamental work on the heart-lung preparation, expanded by the more recent work of McMichael,[472] Sarnoff[611] and Katz.[371]

Perhaps the outstanding feature of congestive failure is the failure of the cardiac output to meet all the demands placed on it by the metabolism of the body. At first this may manifest itself only if the demands are significantly increased, as with severe exercise. Later the demands may not be met even at rest, and finally the low cardiac output becomes incompatible with life itself.

When the cardiac output becomes relatively inadequate, the first mechanism that comes into play is a reflex increase of the heart rate. Thus, even with an unsatisfactory stroke volume, the cardiac output per minute may be adequate. This is an inefficient type of compensation, however, since the tachycardia, by and large, is achieved by shortening diastole, the resting period of the cycle, during which the coronary arteries fill.

A more efficient way the heart can try to increase its lagging stroke volume is by increasing the end-diastolic pressure in the ventricles; this is achieved by raising atrial and venous pressures. It has been pointed out before that this may be achieved easily in the pulmonary veins and the left atrium by merely shifting the blood volume. In order to increase the pressure in the systemic veins and the right atrium, however, the increase in systemic blood volume alone is not enough. One must assume the presence of a reflex increase in the tone of the veins as well. The increase in blood volume is the result of sodium and water retention, a renal component of cardiac failure. The regulation of water excretion is an amazingly complex mechanism. I only wish to mention here that water diuresis probably is under the control of, among other things, the pituitary antidiuretic hormone, which responds to the stimulation of osmoreceptors in the vascular tree and pressure receptors in the left atrium and pulmonary vein. Saluresis, on the other hand, may be influenced by aldosterone, a steroid under control of right atrial pressure and extracellular fluid volume, which also has been shown to improve the function of isolated heart preparations. It is possible that salt retention may be a price the body has to pay to have the beneficial effect of increased aldosterone excretion in the heart. It is also possible that instantaneous water diuresis, following left atrial distention, may be a defense mechanism against impending pulmonary edema. Finally, the sodium retention secondary to increased aldosterone excretion may result in water retention by stimulating the antidiuretic hormone secretion through the osmoreceptors. All this is only speculation, simply pointing to the factors that may be involved in regulating water balance.

It should be pointed out here that the cardiac output—or stroke volume—achieved by the ventricle at the price of the increase in ventricular diastolic and venous pressures is not commensurate with the output achieved by a corresponding increase in venous pressure in a normal heart. The failing heart is an inefficient motor needing the artificial stimulus of increased venous pressure to achieve average or normal cardiac output. The continuous increase in diastolic filling results first in dilatation of the ventricle, and later gives rise to hypertrophy. The hypertrophied heart is reputedly a more efficient organ than the dilated one, although good experimental evidence to this effect is missing.

Through these mechanisms of tachycardia, increased diastolic pressure and myocardial hypertrophy, the failing heart can maintain compensation; i.e., it is able to achieve a more or less satisfactory cardiac output for a while. As the condition progresses, however, cardiac efficiency becomes less and less adequate. The amount of work performed per cubic centimeter of oxygen consumed diminishes. Higher and higher venous pressure is needed to put out relatively small stroke volumes. Finally, a point is reached at which the stroke volume actually declines with further increase in venous pressure. The heart muscle has arrived at the declining part of Starling's curve; compensation cannot be further maintained, the cardiac output becomes inadequate for the maintenance of vital functions, and death ensues.

Starling's[665] law of the heart says that increasing the length of the myocardial fibers by means of increased diastolic volume and increased filling pressure results in an increased cardiac output *up to a point*. That point is reached when the fibers are "overstretched"; thereafter any further increase in pressure results in a drop in output.

Starling also found experimentally that a "tired heart" needed a higher filling pressure to accomplish the same cardiac output than a "fresh heart."

This same phenomenon is evident in the failing hearts of people; they need a higher filling pressure to accomplish an adequate cardiac output. But one cannot simply equate high atrial filling pressure and high ventricular end-diastolic pressure with congestive heart failure, since well compensated examples of aortic or pulmonic stenosis with thick ventricular walls need a higher filling pressure to accomplish their work. This means that normal musculature and hypertrophied musculature operate on different "Starling curves." Sarnoff and Berglund[611] demonstrated that there is really a family of Starling curves, one for the left ventricle, another for the right ventricle, one for a hypertrophied heart, one for a heart damaged with coronary disease, and, of course, one for a failing heart. The last will be a practically flat curve, one in which a basal output is performed only with a high filling pressure and in which any further increase of filling pressure and overdistention of the ventricle will result, actually, in a diminished output.

According to this concept, digitalis and catecholamines by improving cardiac function (tone, metabolism), in effect shift the ventricular function from a less efficient to a more efficient Starling curve. Venesection, tourniquets or diuretics, on the other hand, by reducing the blood volume and venous pressure of patients with congestive failure, shift the heart back to a more efficient portion of the same curve. Therefore with a low filling pressure a higher output will be accomplished. Physiologically, then, the failing heart may be characterized by a combination of the following features: (1) a dilated heart with high atrial and ventricular end-diastolic pressures at rest, in which further increase in filling pressure will not result in the expected increase in cardiac output, (2) a low cardiac output, particularly in relation to demands, and (3) a wide arteriovenous difference at rest. The last phenomenon may well be due to shifting cardiac output, by means of vasoconstriction, from low oxygen extraction areas (kidneys, skin and brain) to high extraction organs (active muscle, heart) so that the regional blood flows are uniformly low and extractions uniformly high. Finally, in severe congestive failure the cardiac output is almost completely fixed, and the increase in oxygen consumption is accomplished entirely by further widening of the arteriovenous difference. The limitations of this mechanism are obvious. It should be re-emphasized, however, that congestive heart failure is a clinical syndrome and that any one of the foregoing points may be absent in specific instances of congestive failure or may be present in patients who do not have heart failure. The presence of a high filling pressure in patients with fully compensated pulmonic stenosis has already been mentioned. An athlete with an optimal myocardium may have a high arteriovenous difference. Patients with thyrotoxic hearts have high outputs.

Within recent years some light has been shed on the metabolism of the failing heart. In a recent symposium Bing and his associates[183] maintained that in the usual forms of chronic congestive heart failure, myocardial oxygen consumption, as well as the utilization of other substrates, and energy production do not seem abnormal. By exclusion they believe that energy utilization is at fault. Olson and his associates[540] found differences in molecular weight and configuration between the myosin of normal and that of failing hearts. Bing indicated that the contractility of actomyosin bands of the failing heart is impaired.

Clinical Picture

How do the phenomena just discussed explain the clinical features of congestive failure?

Systemic venous hypertension is the cardinal sign of right-sided failure. Its significance and measurement have been described previously (p. 18). The contribution of the increased venomotor tone and the increased circulating blood volume to this phenomenon has already been discussed as well. *Hepatomegaly* is an expression of the increased venous pressure and may lead to cardiac cirrhosis, impaired liver function and jaundice. *Splenomegaly* is caused by the same mechanism, though with not nearly the same regularity as hepatomegaly. A *reversible nephrotic syndrome* with proteinuria, hypoproteinemia, massive edema, and so forth, has been described by Burack and his co-workers[103] as an expression of right-sided failure. *Edema* is probably a consequence of the increased venous pressure overpowering the normal or lowered oncotic pressure of the plasma proteins. Since the lymph flow is also hindered by the increased venous pressure, probably there is not only an increased production of interstitial fluid, but also a slower removal through the thoracic duct. Finally, the retention of salt and water by the kidneys in congestive heart failure has already been mentioned. Among the sites of edema in children with right-sided congestive failure, facial edema must be mentioned first. Ascites and anasarca are relatively late manifestations, and they usually occur after considerable enlargement of the liver has been noted. Hydrothorax and hydropericardium are rare.

Pulmonary venous hypertension explains many of the features of left-sided failure. *Dyspnea on exertion* is due principally to the decreased compliance of the lungs, secondary to pulmonary venous congestion. The lungs become stiff and hard to move, and rapid, shallow respirations are probably the most economical way of producing a satisfactory minute volume. Furthermore, the stretch receptors located in the left atrium and the pulmonary veins are also stimulated and induce dyspnea. The stimulation of chemoreceptors by anoxia and hypercapnia, secondary to the presence of transudate between alveoli and capillaries, probably plays only a minor role, except in instances of frank pulmonary edema. *Orthopnea* is probably the result of the maximal diastolic volume inherent in the supine position, plus an increase in circulating blood volume, secondary to reabsorption of fluid from the dependent parts, at night.

Cardiac asthma with pulmonary edema is an expression of maximal pulmonary venous congestion, the hydrostatic pressure in the lungs overpowering the oncotic pressure of the plasma. This results in alveolar fluid accumulation, rales, cyanosis, and often death. That the central nervous system also has a part in the production of pulmonary edema has been proved experimentally[546] and suggested therapeutically by the relief afforded by morphine. But under ordinary circumstances an increase in left ventricular volume or pressure load explains satisfactorily the occurrence of pulmonary edema.

A *chronic, hacking, irritable cough* is probably secondary to congestion of the bronchial mucosa. This may be secondary to the interference with the bronchial circulation caused by the increased pulmonary venous pressure.

A diminished cardiac output may be common in left- or right-sided failure. *Cold extremities,* resulting from the redistribution of blood in the venous reservoir, are an excellent clinical expression of this phenomenon. *Fatigue* and *weakness* are noted if the cardiac output is limited and cannot be increased on effort. *Oliguria* is secondary to poor renal blood flow, and a *cloudy sensorium* is present if cerebral blood flow is inadequate.

Cyanosis in congestive failure may be due either to decreased oxygen intake through congested lungs or to increased deoxygenation by the oxygen-hungry tissues during a prolonged circulation time in the dilated capillaries.

Pulsus alternans (see Fig. 6, p. 18) of the systemic arteries—an evidence of left ventricular failure—can best be detected when the patient's blood pressure is being taken. As the sphygmomanometer is slowly released, at one point every second arterial beat will come through the stethoscope. As the pressure in the manometer is dropped another 5 to 10 mm. the number of sounds heard per minute suddenly doubles and becomes equal to the apex beat. It is believed that the alternation is due to the weakness of the individual cardiac fibers, resulting in the alternately slower and weaker contractions.

Within recent years pulsus alternans of the pulmonary arterial system has been noted at cardiac catheterization in patients with right ventricular failure.[244]

X-ray evidence of cardiac enlargement is almost a sine qua non of the diagnosis of congestive failure. Usually the enlargement is generalized, involving all chambers. At fluoroscopy the cardiac beat is poor. The enlargement and the poor beat are thought to be due to the increased diastolic volume and the poor stroke output. In left-sided failure pulmonary congestion can be easily detected by roentgenogram.

Electrocardiographic evidences of congestive failure are furnished by the presence of P waves suggesting atrial hypertension.

The classic picture of congestive failure in children is one of right-sided or combined right- and left-sided failure; dramatic evidences of pure left-sided failure, such as pulsus alternans, orthopnea or paroxysmal nocturnal dyspnea, are rarely observed. Pulmonary rales, however, can be heard in at least half of the patients with frank right-sided failure, and gallop rhythm is commonly encountered.

Right-sided failure in its pure form may be seen in the following conditions: pulmonary vascular obstruction, pulmonary valvular obstruction, tricuspid valve disease, atrial septal defect, pulmonary venous anomaly and various types of cyanotic congenital heart disease (transposition, aortic atresia, and so forth).

Pure left-sided failure may be observed in severe systemic hypertension (renal disease), coarctation of the aorta, aortic stenosis, mitral valve obstruction and patent ductus arteriosus.

A combination of left-sided and right-sided failure, the systemic congestion dominating, is the commonest form of congestive failure in children. All the conditions which may cause pure left-sided failure may also cause combined failure. In addition, the hypoplastic left heart syndrome, ventricular septal defect, single ventricle and truncus arteriosus should be mentioned among the congenital conditions which may cause combined failure. For the most part, the diseases in this group, and all conditions causing congestive failure, are those which basically involve both ventricles, such as rheumatic fever, primary myocardial disease, paroxysmal atrial tachycardia and acute glomerulonephritis. Constrictive pericarditis, a rare condition in youngsters, also results in combined ventricular failure.

Treatment

Before the advent of cardiac surgery and the various therapeutic and prophylactic measures directed against rheumatic fever, treatment of congestive failure was about all one could offer for children with heart disease. Obviously the picture is different today; still, the successful management of congestive failure is one of the severest tests of the skill of the pediatrician.

Symptomatic Treatment. When the pediatrician sees a patient with congestive failure, his first task is to make the child more comfortable. Usually, sedation—morphine, phenobarbital or even chloral hydrate—is

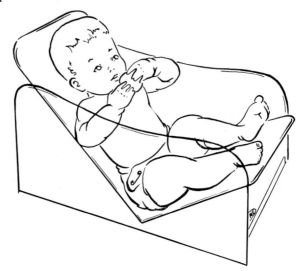

Figure 236. Cardiac chair. Children, particularly babies, with pulmonary congestion, seem more comfortable in the sitting position.[520]

indicated, since many of the older children are fretful, apprehensive and frightened, and the babies are irritable. Sedation need not be continued for a long time, but a little morphine sulfate for the first day or two gives much needed rest and invaluable support to the patient. It also lessens the impact of the various and inevitable therapeutic or diagnostic procedures to which the patient is subjected when his disease is first discovered.

Although the therapeutic value of oxygen in congestive failure has not been proved conclusively, the symptomatic relief afforded by it is unquestionable. Babies too small to worry about an oxygen tent, and children whose fears have been alleviated by sedation and appropriate explanation, will relax, breathe easier and act a great deal happier in a cool oxygen tent with about 50 per cent oxygen concentration. Nasal oxygen is bothersome and inefficient, and should be used only if a tent is not available. Since the prime purpose of oxygen administration is to make the child more comfortable, it does not make sense to insist on its administration for a child who is terrified of the tent. I feel strongly that, unless the child can be sedated or reassured to a sufficient degree, the use of a tent, by causing terror and apprehension, may actually be harmful. The use of a cardiac "chair" (Fig. 236) designed for babies may help them to breathe better in the sitting position.

Decreasing the Load of the Heart. If the assumption that congestive failure is connected somehow with inadequate cardiac output is correct, then it is desirable to decrease the demands made on the circulation.

One way to accomplish this is by keeping the patient in bed.[106] For adults and older children this is the procedure of choice in almost all instances; in small babies the problem does not arise. Toddlers and young children, however, may need special consideration. If one realizes that bed rest is desirable only as a means of achieving as much rest as possible, then it becomes obvious that if a child is upset and frustrated by being kept in bed, this therapeutic maneuver, much like the oxygen tent under certain circumstances, defeats its own purpose. In other words, rest should be interpreted as broadly as possible. Most children with failure actually welcome being put to bed. On the other hand, some overactive youngsters rest better by sitting in a high chair, being read to, looking at television or playing in a play pen. The physician's individual judgment about each patient should supersede here—as in most medical decisions—any preconceived ideas obtained from dogmatic textbooks.

If arterial hypertension of significant degree is present, as in renal disease, lowering of the blood pressure by hypotensive drugs is indicated.

Decreasing the load on the kidneys in congestive failure may be achieved by restricting the sodium intake to 500 mg. or less per day. This may be accomplished by not adding salt to the food, by using milk with a low sodium content and by avoiding heavily salted foods (bacon, and so forth). Water may be taken ad libitum as long as the salt intake is controlled.

Drugs. DIGITALIS. As a matter of principle, every child with obvious evidence of congestive failure should be digitalized. The only possible exceptions to this general rule may be patients whose cardiac failure is of a "high output" nature (anemia, thyrotoxicosis) or is caused by pericardial tamponade. Even in these situations digitalization probably does not do any great harm. The only true contraindication to the use of digitalis in congestive failure is the presence of digitoxicity.

The effect of digitalis on the heart has been discussed by internists, pharmacologists and physiologists for many years.[228, 446] The use of this glycoside in pediatrics has recently been summarized.[520] Digitalis causes an increase in myocardial responsiveness, an increase in contractile force, a slowing of the pulse rate, a decrease in venous pressure and shortening of the circulation time.

The digitalis preparation to be used depends a great deal on the experience of the individual physician. All digitalis preparations put out by reputable drug companies today can be used effectively and safely. The difficulty arises from the multiplicity of drugs with similar names (almost all using the prefix "dig" in some fashion) and radically different absorption and excretion patterns, as well as toxic effects. Every physician should become familiar with one rapidly acting parenteral preparation and one slowly or moderately rapidly acting drug that can be used orally as well as parenterally. The frequent and judicious use of only a few preparations enables the pediatrician to learn by personal experience the mode of action of the drug, its toxic manifestations and its therapeutic efficacy. It is hard to resist the lure of advertisements flooding the medical periodicals with a newer and better drug every month, each one supported by more and more learned quotations from the literature. In order to preserve one's own sanity, as well as to promote the patient's welfare, one should reject these wonderful new adventures in digitalization and persist with the few drugs one has learned to work with through the years. I usually use one of three drugs.

Digitoxin. Digitoxin is a relatively slowly acting glycoside which may be administered orally, intramuscularly or intravenously. Oral absorption is virtually complete; hence the great advantage that oral and parenteral dosages do not differ significantly. Oral preparations are available in liquid and tablet form.

The maximal effect of the drug occurs four hours after intravenous administration and six to eight hours after oral administration. Most of the glycoside is excreted within ten to fourteen days, but elimination may not be complete for three weeks. The slow excretion of digitoxin has the disadvantage that toxicity, once it occurs, persists for a relatively long time; the advantage is easy maintenance of digitalization.

A satisfactory dosage schedule (Table 17, pp. 783–786) may be obtained if the age and the weight of the patient are taken into consideration. Patients less than 2 years old need 0.02 to 0.03 mg. per pound of body weight, whereas children more than 2 years of age can be digitalized with 0.01 to 0.02 mg. per pound. This amount should be given in 3 divided doses within a 24- to 36-hour period. Digitalization can be maintained by one tenth of the total digitalizing dose.

Cedilanid. Cedilanid is a rapidly acting parenteral drug, primarily designed for intravenous administration, but it may also be given intramuscularly.

Appreciable effects of the drug may be demonstrated ten to fifteen minutes after intravenous administration, and maximal effects are achieved within one hour. Virtually complete elimination occurs in twenty-four to thirty-six hours. Such rapid action and excretion offer great advantages in the handling of emergencies, such as occur in the operating room, and they make this an ideal drug to use when one cannot be sure whether the patient has had too little or too much digitalis.

The total digitalizing dose is about the same, maybe 10 per cent more, than that outlined for digitoxin (Table 17). If the patient is to be maintained for several days or weeks with intravenous injections of Cedilanid, one quarter of the digitalizing dose should be given every six hours. It is a much better policy, however, to use Cedilanid only as the initial rapid digitalizing agent and then to maintain the level of digitalization with a slowly acting drug administered orally or intramuscularly. If this is to be done, the patient should be cautiously redigitalized with the slower-acting preparation, using the lower dosage scales, within twenty-four to thirty-six hours after the last dose of Cedilanid. Maintenance doses then can be calculated on the basis of the slower-acting glycoside alone.

Digoxin. Digoxin is a good all-round preparation. It may be used orally as well as parenterally, in emergencies as well as in chronic situations. Within recent years I have used this drug almost exclusively.

In terms of rapidity of absorption and excretion, it stands midway between digitoxin and Cedilanid. Full effects of Digoxin may be demonstrated four hours after its oral administration. A significant portion of the initial dose is excreted within twenty-four hours; most of it disappears within forty-eight to seventy-two hours. A debatable point has been the completeness of absorption from the gastrointestinal tract, which would obviously affect the relative size of oral and parenteral dosages. My impression is that parenteral dosages should be calculated at about 75 per cent of the oral dose.

The oral dose, administered in liquid or tablet form, is about 0.03 to 0.04 mg. per pound of body weight for children less than 2 years of age, and 0.02 to 0.03 mg. per pound for those more than 2 years old (Table 17). Daily maintenance doses can be calculated at 25 to 30 per cent of the digitalizing dose. The immaturity of the excretory systems of prematures may explain the increased sensitivity of these tiny patients to the glycosides; 0.02 to 0.03 mg. per pound may be adequate digitalizing dose for them.

Effectiveness. It cannot be emphasized strongly enough that the dosage schedules outlined for these three digitalis preparations can serve only as guide posts. *The digitalization of every patient should be an individual experiment.* For the first eighteen to twenty-four hours the lower of the two dosages suggested should be administered. If, at that time, the therapeutic goal has not been reached and there are no signs of toxicity, digitalis to the amount suggested by the higher of the two figures should be administered within the next twelve hours. If toxicity or therapeutic effects still are not noted, further increments should be given, cautiously checking one's position every twelve hours, until either the desired effect is obtained or evidences of overdosage are noted.

One of the best indices of therapeutic effectiveness is slowing of the pulse. A significant drop in heart rate with disappearance of gallop rhythm may often be evidence of good digitalis effect. Other, and equally significant, therapeutic aims are a decrease in the size of the liver, disappearance of pulmonary rales and edema, diminishing respiratory rate, and improvement of color, appetite and disposition. In older children weight loss is a significant index of successful digitalization. In small infants, however, because of the relatively small absolute amounts involved and the general inaccuracy of weighing methods, weight loss cannot be used as a sensitive measure of effectiveness of digitalization.

In contrast to the general accuracy of clinical observations, the electrocardiogram is of no use whatsoever in determining whether digitalization has been successful in the alleviation of congestive failure. There is almost nothing more exasperating to an electrocardiographer than to be asked by a colleague, "Has this patient been fully digitalized yet?" As pointed out in a previous chapter (p. 90), the electrocardiogram can show only whether there is some or too much digitalis in the myocardium; it is totally unable to gage whether there is enough present.

Ordinarily, evidences of digitoxicity may be readily obtained from the electrocardiogram. In addition to the cardiographic changes, digitalis toxicity may cause vomiting, headache and visual disturbances. Vomiting is the only common clinical manifestation of overdosage, however.

The response of infants and children in congestive failure to proper digitalization depends a great deal on their type of heart disease. On the whole, infants with cyanotic congenital heart disease respond poorly, whereas patients with paroxysmal atrial tachycardia, myocarditis, fibroelastosis, acute glomerulonephritis, coarctation of the aorta or patent ductus arteriosus respond relatively well. Patients with atrial septal defect, ventricular septal defect and pulmonary stenosis may derive some benefit from the drug, but no complete alleviation of the symptoms is usually noted. Whether children with active rheumatic carditis respond to digitalis or not has been a subject of heated debate for a long time. I believe that a patient with rheumatic heart disease and congestive failure should be treated with digitalis; although the results may not always be as striking as in other conditions, they may be rewarding indeed. It may be worth while to mention that patients with exclusively or predominantly left ventricular failure seem to have a better chance to respond favorably to digitalis than those in whom congestion is exclusively right-sided.

In our experience the patients who derive the most benefit from the glycosides are the ones who are most likely to show evidences of intoxication. It almost seems as though therapeusis and toxicity were related to each other. In effect, the children most commonly showing digitalis intoxication were the ones with definite myocardial involvement (primary myocardial disease or rheumatic heart disease). It is also interesting to note that these patients had received relatively small doses of digitalis when they showed evidences of toxicity. Most of the toxic effects were electrocardiographic and have been discussed before (p. 90). Vomiting occurred rarely and only in patients receiving large doses (more than 0.03 mg. of digitoxin per pound of body weight).

Treatment of digitalis intoxication. Treatment of digitalis intoxication consists in immediate withdrawal of the drug. If the atrial arrhythmia resulting from digitoxicity is severe enough to warrant treatment (paroxysmal atrial tachycardia with block), oral administration of potassium salts (potassium chloride) in doses of 1 to 2 Gm. per day is indicated. If the arrhythmia is of worrisome proportions, or if, accidentally, a large overdose was given, intravenous administration of a potassium solution (see p. 243) in appropriate fluid volumes is warranted, checking carefully the serum potassium level and being mindful of the renal function. Of course gastric lavage, if the overdose was administered orally, or incision and cooling of the injection site in case of intramuscular administration, is clearly indicated with accidental poisoning. In instances of severe ventricular arrhythmia, Pronestyl may be administered intravenously in addition to the potassium chloride, and external electric countershock may be considered an emergency measure. One cannot emphasize strongly enough that accidental ingestion of large amounts of digitalis is very serious business and ought to be treated with utmost caution. Even in the absence of any arrhythmia the following precautions are indicated: (1) continuous electrocardiographic monitoring, (2) start of an intravenous drip with dextrose and water, (3) emergency equipment (external defibrillator, Pronestyl, potassium chloride solution) at bedside, (4) physician in attendance.

Diuretics. Diuretics are indicated if digitalis, rest and sodium restriction do not quickly and effectively control congestive failure. In markedly edematous children, as well as in patients with pulmonary edema, it may even be desirable to start the administration of a diuretic simultaneously with the administration of digitalis. As a rule, however, it is wise to administer digitalis first in order to establish a reasonable glomerular filtration rate.

Until the past few years, in the modern physician's therapeutic armamentarium diuretics have been practically synonymous with mercurial diuretics. Although occasionally acidifying salts (ammonium chloride) and xanthine derivatives (Theocalcin, aminophylline) are used as diuretics by themselves, in most instances they are given only as adjuvants with mercurials.

The effect of mercury is directed principally toward the kidney; the site of action is most likely the distal end of the convoluted tubules. Here, by means of enzymatic inhibitory action, mercury slows down the reabsorption of electrolytes (chloride and sodium) and water. In addition, it inhibits tubular reabsorption of potassium, resulting in increased loss of potassium in the urine.

Since water diuresis is probably secondary to a negative electrolyte balance, and since tubular function is dependent directly on glomerular filtration and renal plasma flow, it is necessary that the glomeruli offer the tubules a sufficient amount of plasma of average electrolyte content to ensure a good mercurial diuresis. It follows, then, that if the plasma chloride level is low, administration of mercury may not result in satisfactory diuresis.[305] Correction of the plasma chloride level makes these patients "mercury-sensitive." People with poor cardiac output and poor renal plasma flow may become equally "resistant" to mercury, a condition sometimes easily corrected with digitalization. Finally, in some "mercury-resistant" patients good diuresis occurs if the administration of the diuretic is followed half an hour or an hour later by an intravenous dose of aminophylline, improving the glomerular filtration rate. The skillful use of ammonium chloride also may enhance the effectiveness of mercurial diuretics.

The two mercurial preparations which I use most frequently are Mercuhydrin for intramuscular, and Thiomerin for subcutaneous administration. For practical purposes, mercury should never be given intravenously. Sudden deaths have been reported after administration of the drug in this fashion.

The amount of mercury to be given (Table 17, p. 783–786) is the minimal dose achieving the desired effect; the dose of Mercuhydrin and Thiomerin is about the same. One should start with 0.1 ml. as a test dose, to be followed the next day by a dose of 0.25 ml. in infants and children less than 4 years old, and 0.5 ml. in older patients. If this dose results in effective diuresis, it should be repeated every 2 to 3 days; if it is not effective, the dose may be increased by 0.25 ml. increments until a maximum of 1 ml. is reached in the younger ones and 1.5 ml. in the older children.

Injections of mercury should be continued until the patient reaches his so-called dry weight, i.e. a weight without visible edema and without further weight loss after continued administration of the same doses of mercury.

The amount of mercury necessary to keep the patient at this dry weight varies considerably and can be determined only by accurate daily weighings. Some patients, once they have reached the dry weight level, may be kept there indefinitely with only digitalis and a low salt diet. Others may need mercury once a week, while still others may have to have it two or three times a week. Accurate charting of the patient's weight is the only way to assess critically the need for diuretics. Attempts to measure the urinary output and fluid intake, particularly in small children, are useless, inaccurate and time-consuming. Mercury injections, as a rule, should not be given at night; the ensuing diuresis interferes with the patient's sleep.

Mercury should almost never be given more often than every second day because of the possible cumulative effect on the renal parenchyma. Prolonged administration of mercury should be accompanied by frequent determinations of the plasma electrolyte levels. It is easy to see how prolonged electrolyte depletion of the organism by diuretics, accompanied by a limited salt and liberal water intake may lead to severe electrolyte disturbance, the so-called low salt syndrome. The relation of potassium depletion to digitoxicity has been alluded to previously.[446]

To counteract the electrolyte-depleting effect of the diuretics and to potentiate its effectiveness, intermittent administration of ammonium chloride for two-day periods, preceding the administration of mercury, has been recommended. The average dose for children is between 1 and 2 Gm. daily. To avoid digitoxicity, by maintaining a satisfactory plasma potassium level, continuous high potassium intake (either a quart of orange juice or 1 to 2 Gm. of potassium chloride daily) is recommended if mercury is to be used for a long time. As mentioned before, serum chemistry determinations every week, or every two weeks, are necessary with an aggressive plan of treatment of this sort.

Aminophylline, in doses of 0.1 to 0.2 Gm., may increase the effectiveness of mercurials, presumably by increasing the glomerular filtration rate and the renal plasma flow. In "resistant cases" I have been using aminophylline, given intravenously, diluted in 10 to 25 ml. of a 5 per cent solution of dextrose and water, injected slowly 1 to 2 hours after administration of mercury, with good effect for many years. There was one instance when sudden death occurred one to two hours after intravenous administration of aminophylline, but I am not at all sure that this was attributable to the drug. It should be mentioned, however, that many internists prefer to use aminophylline by rectum, considering the intravenous route too dangerous. At present, in regard to children, I cannot concur with this opinion.

Severe toxic effects of mercury are rare with intramuscular administration. Chills, fever, rashes and arrhythmias have been reported. These may be avoided by using the principle of the test dose before administration of therapeutic doses. I know of one patient who was recovering from bacterial endocarditis in whom fever developed a few hours after intramuscular administration of Mercuhydrin. Subsequent skin tests did not show any allergic reaction. Consequently a few days later mercury was again given intramuscularly. Again it was followed in a few hours by fever and, this time, death. Whether this patient, suffering from severe congenital heart disease and recovering from bacterial endocarditis, died as a result of mercury intoxication cannot be proved, but such a possibility exists. Several instances of sudden death minutes after intravenous administration of the drug have been reported.

Other side effects to be mentioned are (1) local irritation and (2) electrolyte disturbance. Under electrolyte disturbance should be considered (a) potassium loss, occurring particularly if ammonium chloride or Diamox is administered. In addition to weakness, lassitude and cramps, these patients may exhibit evidences of digitoxicity (arrhythmia). (b) Hypochloremic alkalosis due to excessive urinary chloride loss, (c) hyperchloremic acidosis due not to mercury itself, but to excessive administration of ammonium chloride, (d) low salt syndrome (to be discussed later).

Mercury should not be given to patients with obvious renal disease, either acute or chronic. It is a good rule of thumb never to use mercurials if there is a nonprotein nitrogen level of more than 50 mg. per 100 ml. of blood.

Within recent years another potent diuretic has been made available to the physician, the chlorothiazide (Diuril) group. Chlorothiazide, in vitro, is a carbonic anhydrase inhibitor, but at present this does not seem to be the mechanism of its diuretic action. It causes equal degrees of sodium and chloride loss with some potassium loss, probably through inhibition of tubular reabsorption. The drug is administered orally in approximate doses of 125 mg. twice daily in infants, and 250 mg. 2 to 3 times daily for children. If administered for long periods, provisions for increased potassium intake should be made. It has been our custom to use chlorothiazide in appropriate doses for five days a week. None is given through the weekend. This somewhat intermittent administration may minimize the potassium loss. There is no evidence that drug tolerance develops on daily administration.[253]

Up to the present time Diuril has not replaced mercury in our routine diuretic treatment. Thus far I have never seen a patient who would have been "resistant" to mercury and "susceptible" to Diuril, and the opposite is not too uncommon. Consequently we continue to use mercurials as the principal diuretic agent in the treatment of acute congestive heart failure. If the patient reaches his dry weight in this fashion and further long-term diuretic therapy is indicated, then we turn to the chlorothiazide group, which provides a safe, convenient, oral diuretic. But in the acute situation we continue to rely on mercurials, with or without potentiating agents. In support of this principle, Gold[282] found chlorothiazide to be only 40 per cent as effective as meralluride in comparable doses. A newer member of the chlorothiazide group, Saluron, was found by this New York group to be about 60 per cent as effective as mercurials. My experience with this latter drug has been slight, but I do not seem to find it too different from Diuril.

Treatment of the Underlying Disease. As mentioned previously, at least in terms of pediatric cardiology, the concept that congestive failure could be treated by attacking the underlying disease, rather than by alleviating symptoms, is only twenty years old.

The first things to be mentioned in this regard are the miracles of cardiac surgery! Mitral stenosis, aortic stenosis, constrictive pericarditis, congenital arteriovenous aneurysms, patent ductus arteriosus, pure pulmonary stenosis, atrial septal defect, ventricular septal defect and even coarctation of the aorta may all result in congestive failure in children, and all can be treated surgically. Of course surgery under these circumstances is fraught with more than the usual amount of danger; nevertheless the risk is obviously well worth taking. The dangers of surgery may be considerably lessened by intelligent anticongestive treatment preoperatively; in this regard, however, one should be careful to use a quickly eliminated digitalis preparation so that the cardiac hyperexcitability caused by digitalis will not predispose to arrhythmias at the time of operation. It may be best to stop digitalis therapy for twenty-four hours before operation. It is equally important to ensure, as far as possible, an optimal electrolyte profile in the preoperative and postoperative periods.

Another disease causing congestive failure in children for which etiologic treatment may be available is acute rheumatic fever. The pros and cons of steroid therapy have already been outlined, and the tentative indications and dosages have been proposed (p. 186). Occasionally, in a case reported in the literature, it is suggested that hormone therapy may have its place in the management of the primary myocardial disease entities as well.

Thyrotoxicosis seldom causes congestive failure in children. If it does, a course of thiouracil therapy, possibly followed by surgery, is the choice of etiologic treatment.

Congestive failure associated with anemia can, of course, be corrected by increasing the circulating hemoglobin level. I am certain that in a book written primarily for pediatricians the importance of slow and gradual transfusions for severely anemic patients does not need to be stressed. These patients have too little hemoglobin and too much blood volume; hence small amounts (50 to 100 cc. at a time) of packed cells should be given several times, twelve to twenty-four hours apart, rather than one large transfusion, which may be just too much for a heart already under maximal stress.

The Treatment of Acute Pulmonary Edema. This is an emergency of the first order. Action within minutes may be lifesaving. The measures to be undertaken are (1) administration of morphine, parenterally, (2) placing the patient in a sitting position, (3) administration of oxygen, possibly under positive pressure, (4) placing tourniquets on three extremities in a rotating fashion, (5) venesection, (6) administration of aminophylline, intravenously, and (7) administration of digitalis and mercurials, if they have not already been given.

The Low Salt Syndrome

Low plasma sodium concentrations are not too uncommon in patients with advanced congestive heart failure. The wide recognition of the effectiveness of a low sodium diet in the treatment of heart failure and the advent of potent diuretics both contribute to the more frequent occurrence of this phenomenon in the past ten years. The causes of the low salt syndrome have been summarized by Luckey and his associates[452] as follows: (1) cardiac insufficiency. This need not be elaborated on and may, perhaps, be amenable to correction (digitalis, and so forth). (2) Renal impairment, evidenced by rising nonprotein nitrogen levels and caused, possibly, by a sudden decrease in cardiac output. Correction of this factor must await improvement in cardiac function. (3) Sodium restriction in the diet. Slight liberalization of sodium intake may improve this situation if there is evidence that the total body sodium is diminished. This applies to patients with congestive heart failure who do not have edema. On the other hand, according to our experience and that of others, intravenous administration of a hypertonic saline solution should be condemned as a *dangerous procedure.* (4) Excessive water intake and decreased excretion of water by the kidneys. Correction of this also must await improvement of the circulation. Under these circumstances it is wise to restrict water intake to the insensible water loss. (5) Excessive antidiuretic hormone activity.

For the treatment of the low salt syndrome, Luckey and his co-workers recommended (a) reassessment of digitalis therapy, with possible increase in the administration of the glycoside, (b) correction of hypochloremia by the administration of large doses of ammonium chloride, (c) fluid restriction, and (d) mercurial diuretics. *These patients are desperately ill and, even under the most skillful management, more often than not they are not salvageable.*

13

MISCELLANEOUS DISEASES

HYPERTENSIVE HEART DISEASE

Etiology

Essential hypertension, the principal cause of persistently elevated blood pressure in adults, is rare in children. Renal disease, diseases of the central nervous system, coarctation of the aorta and endocrine disturbances are more common etiologic factors.[302, 464] The technique of obtaining accurate blood pressure readings and the normal values for various ages have already been discussed (see p. 15). Table 21, p. 788, lists the most important factors causing high blood pressure in children, with appropriate diagnostic tests for their identification.

Renal Disease. The most important cause of elevated blood pressure in children is renal disease. In addition to the laboratory tests enumerated in Table 21, a history of kidney disease is an important feature in the diagnosis, even when results of urinalysis and renal function tests are normal.

Diseases of the Central Nervous System. As outlined in Table 21, diseases of the central nervous system can usually be diagnosed by the clinical picture and results of laboratory tests, including studies on the cerebrospinal fluid, roentgenograms of the skull, and electroencephalograms. Pneumoencephalograms are rarely necessary. The syndrome of familial dysautonomia[587] can usually be recognized by the labile hypertension, absence of tearing, repeated febrile episodes, hypesthesia, motor disturbances and mental retardation.

Cardiovascular Diseases. The cardiovascular diseases listed in Table 21 have been amply discussed in appropriate chapters.

Diseases of the Endocrine System. The most frequent endocrine cause of hypertension today is prolonged administration of cortisone. Obviously, the clues to this diagnosis are a history of steroid administration and the appearance of Cushing's syndrome.

Pheochromocytoma is difficult to diagnose; it is also extremely rare in children, only 34 cases having been reported in the literature in patients less than 14 years of age by 1957.[160] At The Children's Hospital Medical Center only two authenticated cases have been found. The classic picture, caused by an increase in the amount of epinephrine and norepinephrine in the blood, consists in paroxysmal hypertension, intermittent sweating, dilated pupils, headaches, nausea, vomiting, tachycardia and pallor. In children the hypertension is more likely to be persistent. Occasionally an abdominal mass may be palpated, compression of which may induce the symptoms described. Among the specific tests mentioned in Table 21, an increase in urinary and blood catechol amines is the most reliable one. If the values for epinephrine and norepinephrine in the blood are normal and suspicion of the disease is strong, the determination should be repeated under the conditions of a cold pressor test. Possibly, under these "stress" situations abnormally high values may be obtained. Intravenous pyelography, which may reveal a mass in the region of the kidney, is perhaps the easiest and most helpful of the clinical laboratory tests, even though it does not demonstrate those pheochromocytomas lying outside the adrenal area (approximately 12 per cent). The Regitine and benzodioxane tests are useful if the patient has significant hypertension at the time of testing; an appreciable drop in systolic blood pressure may occur when one of these drugs is administered.[278, 286] The histamine test, causing an appreciable elevation of the blood pressure in patients with pheochromocytoma, should not be performed unless an intravenous dose of Regitine is held in readiness for an emergency. As a matter of fact, it may be worth while keeping a needle filled with Regitine in the vein as one does in the histamine test.

It may be interesting to mention that we have seen two patients who had von Recklinghausen's disease, with hypertension, in whom the diagnosis of pheochromocytoma was suspected, but never proved by the tests outlined. One of these has recently been successfully operated upon for unilateral renal artery constriction.

Poisonings. Poisonings that produce hypertension can usually be excluded on the basis of the history, the physical examination and the laboratory tests indicated in Table 21.

Essential Hypertension. Essential hypertension is principally a diagnosis of exclusion; if a child with significant hypertension does not have any of the conditions enumerated so far, one must assume that his hypertension is essential. No specific diagnostic test for essential hypertension exists.

As mentioned previously, this is a rare disease in children; we have seen nine patients with this disease less than fourteen years of age at The Children's Hospital Medical Center.[320] A critical evaluation of the English and American literature in 1956 revealed only another 10 well authenticated cases.

The ages of our patients ranged from seven months to thirteen years. Five of these children had severe hypertension (pressures consistently higher than 160/110) and secondary circulatory changes (cardiac enlarge ment, left ventricular hypertrophy and hypertensive retinopathy). The blood pressure of the other 4 patients was never found to be higher than 160/110. No secondary circulatory changes were present. All the members of the group with mild hypertension had a family history of essential hypertension, whereas only one in the group of five with higher elevation of the blood pressure had a family history of such. The disease in the former group may well be related to essential hypertension in adults, whereas the severe hypertension in the latter group may represent a completely different etiologic entity.

The prognosis of the mildly hypertensive group throughout childhood is good. On the other hand, two of our five patients with severe hypertension died.

Treatment

Obviously, the individual entities within the general hypertensive group should receive etiologic treatment if possible. In patients with unilateral renal disease removal of the affected kidney may give miraculous therapeutic results. Among patients with primary disease of the central nervous system the hypertension either may subside with the disappearance of the underlying inflammatory disease or may be cured by successful removal of a neoplasm. Surgical treatment of the congenital heart diseases causing hypertension can effect a cure relatively easily. Cessation of ACTH or cortisone therapy or removal of a pheochromocytoma may permanently lower the elevated blood pressures caused by these factors. Elimination of the poisons from the environment obviously will relieve hypertension caused by ingestion of mercury or lead.

The treatment of essential hypertension is as difficult a problem in children as it is in adults. Mild sedation, weight reduction and sustaining psychotherapy have been and still are the mainstays of treatment. Moderate physical activity is not only harmless, but even beneficial in many instances.

If these relatively simple measures do not control hypertension, drug therapy should be considered for its immediate therapeutic and future prophylactic effects. Table 21 (p. 788–789) lists the various drugs available, their dosages, toxic effects and indications for their use. At first, in our clinic, patients with mild hypertension are usually given Rauwolfia serpentina in doses indicated in Table 17 (pp. 783–786). Every 2 to 3 weeks the dose is increased by $\frac{1}{2}$ to 1 tablet a day until either the desired hypotensive effects are achieved or prohibitive side effects (drowsiness, nausea, diarrhea or nasal stuffiness) occur. If side effects appear, the dose is slightly reduced, and the patient is maintained on this dosage. If no significant reduction of blood pressure is achieved after several weeks, first chlorothiazide, and in a few weeks Apresoline (hydralazine) is added in appropriate doses.

If a combination of Rauwolfia, Diuril and Apresoline does not achieve the desired purpose, hexamethonium or other ganglionic blocking agents (Ismelin, Inversin) are added to the previous drugs. These drugs often significantly lower the blood pressure in patients in whom the others had had no effect. Patients taking hexamethonium must be warned about constipation and urinary retention. At the first sign of any of these the dosage should be reduced, and cathartics should be given. A certain degree of postural hypotension is probably an inevitable concomitant of the administration of ganglionic blocking agents. The dosage schedule should be adjusted so that this unpleasant "side effect" is minimized.

For patients with severe essential hypertension who are not benefited by any of these drugs, sympathectomy is recommended. Four of our five patients with severe hypertension had this formidable surgical procedure; in two cases the results were good, but in the other two there was no change in blood pressure. At present it is impossible to predict which patient will or will not respond to sympathectomy.

One further word about the treatment of patients with so-called hypertensive encephalopathy, such as is seen in acute and chronic glomerulonephritis, lead poisoning, chronic poliomyelitis or coarctation of the aorta. The therapy of these patients taxes the ingenuity of the pediatrician. Perhaps the most useful drug to start with is magnesium sulfate in controlled intravenous drip (Table 17), 0.1 ml. per pound of body weight of a 3 per cent solution, but no more than 75 to 100 mg. per hour. Other drugs recommended are Apresoline (hydralazine) and reserpine, intramuscularly, (see Nephritis, p. 286) and Arphonad. If these do not reduce the pressure, protoveratrine should be administered intravenously, with extreme caution, starting with 0.5 to 1 microgram per pound of body weight, and increasing the dose by minute amounts every 30 minutes. If the correct intravenous dose is determined, one can switch to intramuscular administration of protoveratrine or magnesium sulfate supplemented by and later substituted for the oral administration of Rauwolfia and chlorothiazide.

ANEMIC HEART DISEASE

Anemia may affect the circulatory system in two ways. Sudden loss of large quantities of blood (more than 20 per cent of the circulating blood volume) results in shock; this topic is probably not within the scope of a textbook on pediatric cardiology. On the other hand, a gradual loss of blood over a long period may cause circulatory alterations by increasing the load on the heart at the time when its efficiency is diminished because of poor coronary circulation.

Etiology

The most common causes of anemic heart disease in children today in the United States are sickle cell anemia, leukemia, hypoplastic anemia and Mediterranean anemia; anemia of parasitic infection and nutritional or infectious anemia are common in the tropics (kwashiorkor).

The degree of anemia required to cause demonstrable evidences of heart disease depends on the duration of the disease and the functional status of the heart. It stands to reason that a heart riddled with rheumatic infection will be less able to cope with the extra work imposed on it by the anemia than a healthy heart would be. It also seems logical that a moderate anemia of three weeks' duration will have fewer circulatory consequences than the same degree of anemia lasting for six months or more. With these qualifications, it may be stated that serious disturbances probably do not occur with hemoglobin levels higher than 7.0 gm. per 100 ml. of blood.[78]

Physiology

The physiologic consequences of anemia are based on the diminished oxygen capacity of the blood and the consecutive tissue anoxia. This lowered oxygen supply to the tissues by itself, and the compensatory mechanisms involved, may cause profound alterations in the circulation. The following observations have been made on adults with severe anemia by various authors: (1) shortened circulation time,[72] (2) increase in cardiac output,[78] and (3) increase in percentage of oxygen extracted from the arterial blood.[433]

Clinical Picture

The clinical picture of anemic heart disease is dominated by palpitation, dyspnea and fatigue. On physical examination one notes a murmur, moderate or severe cardiac enlargement and the distended neck veins. The cardiac impulse is left ventricular in nature and may be maximally hyperkinetic. It should be stated emphatically that there is practically no murmur that could *not* be caused by severe anemia; it is totally useless to attempt to determine whether a patient's murmur is "organic" or "functional," "significant" or "insignificant" in the face of severe anemia. Evidences of left-sided and right-sided cardiac enlargement, and even pitting edema, may be present. The electrocardiogram may show changes in the S-T segments and T waves over the left ventricle, as well as evidences of mild left ventricular hypertrophy. Blood pressure determinations characteristically show a wide pulse pressure with a significant decrease in the diastolic level and an elevation of the systolic level.

It should be mentioned here that, to the best of my knowledge, the changes in the heart in sickle cell anemia are limited to those just described, and no increased incidence of rheumatic heart disease exists.[640]

Excellent hemodynamic studies of adults with severe anemia exist.[78, 415, 636] I am not aware of cardiac catheterization studies on any large series of anemic children.

Treatment

The treatment of anemic heart disease consists in slow transfusion with packed cells. Extreme caution should be exercised not to correct the severe anemia of these patients too rapidly lest one provoke left ventricular failure and pulmonary edema. Small increments of cells administered frequently (probably no more than 5 to 10 ml. per pound at a time every 8 to 12 hours and possibly accompanied by removal of an equal amount of the patient's blood) will correct the anemia and abolish the picture of anemic heart disease.

CARDIAC TUMORS

Tumors of the heart should be mentioned briefly. This subject has been well reviewed by Engle and Glenn.[226]

Apparently metastatic tumors (bronchogenic carcinoma, malignant melanoma, and so forth) are more common than primary ones in adults.

Among the primary tumors, intracardiac myxomas arising in the atria are the most common; others worth mentioning are sarcomas, teratomas and rhabdomyomas.

The clinical picture in secondary tumors obviously will be dominated by the primary neoplasm. Primary tumors may cause symptoms by obstructing the mitral,[284] tricuspid or even the aortic orifice.[465] They also may cause conduction disturbances, congestive failure and progressive cardiac enlargement. Significantly enough, murmurs are not usually present. The electrocardiogram shows progressive evidence of myocardial damage, and angiocardiograms may show filling defects. Probably cardiac catheterization is not of much use in the diagnosis of cardiac tumors, except in the negative sense.

Various clinical syndromes may be caused by cardiac tumors. *Rhab-*

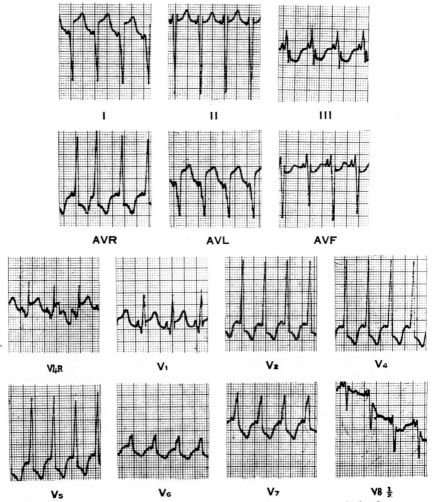

Figure 237. Electrocardiogram of patient with rhabdomyoma of the heart at ten days of age. Note the tachycardia, the mean electrical axis of minus 50 degrees, the right ventricular hypertrophy, the intraventricular conduction disturbance, and the T wave changes. Wolff-Parkinson-White syndrome?

domyomas may be suspected if there are neurologic findings suggesting tuberous sclerosis associated with cardiac enlargement, arrhythmias and severe conduction defects in the electrocardiogram (Fig. 237).

Atrial myxomas originate from the left atrium in about 75 per cent of the patients, and may simulate the clinical picture of mitral stenosis with posturally induced syncopal attacks, pulmonary edema and chronic left- and right-sided failure. Bizarre symptoms of the central nervous system have been described[344] and were thought to be due to tumor emboli. This diagnosis should always be considered in the unusual case of mitral stenosis or when it occurs in the very young. Cine-angiography may reveal the correct diagnosis, and successful surgery has been reported.[146, 164, 613, 702]

Asymmetrical hypertrophy of the heart in young adults, considered to be a hamartoma and affecting principally the intraventicular septum, has been described by Teare.[687] One of the eight patients described had two siblings with similar signs and symptoms. Syncopal attacks were common. Others had palpitation and evidences of congestive heart failure. I would suspect that these patients may be similar to those to be described later under Functional Subaortic Stenosis (see p. 565).

PULMONARY HEART DISEASE

Cor pulmonale is a syndrome encompassing the effects of primary lung disease on the circulation. Harvey and Ferrer[329] considered cor pulmonale to be present only if pulmonary disease was associated with cardiac enlargement or failure. It seems to me that the problem cannot be defined as simply as this.

To the pathologist cor pulmonale indicates right ventricular enlargement or hypertrophy associated with primary pulmonary disease. In a study published some years ago,[526] in patients with cystic fibrosis, we tried to assess heart weight in relation to age, body weight and kidney weight. In the same study we also compared right ventricular thickness with that of normal controls.

For the physiologist pulmonary arterial hypertension with pulmonary arterial mean pressure higher than 25 mm. of mercury, at rest or at exercise, is the sine qua non of cor pulmonale. This may or may not have pathologically or clinically appreciable effects. Similiarly, cor pulmonale may be defined as a decrease of the pO_2 to less than 60 mm. of mercury and an increase in pCO_2 to more than 50 mm. of mercury. The latter definition, in my mind, implicates only the respiratory pattern and does not really reflect the state of the pulmonary circulation.

Finally, the clinician may appreciate cor pulmonale if right ventricular enlargement is present on roentgenologic examination, if right ventricular hypertrophy manifests itself in the electrocardiogram, or if evidences of right-sided failure are on hand. A survey encompassing the pathologic, physiologic and clinical aspects of cor pulmonale in children is sorely needed.

Etiology

In adults emphysema is the most common cause of pulmonary heart disease; other causes to be mentioned are (1) kyphoscoliosis, (2) pulmonary embolism, (3) silicosis, (4) chronic bronchiectasis, (5) neuromuscular disease, (6) pulmonary fibrosis (Hamman-Rich syndrome), (7) pneumonectomy, and (8) extreme obesity.

No good survey of the causes of cor pulmonale in children exists. Obviously, idiopathic emphysema is extremely rare. The number of published cases of children with idiopathic kyphoscoliosis in whom there was time for clinical cor pulmonale to develop is only a handful. I am convinced that if detailed studies were available, cystic fibrosis would be recognized as the number one cause of cor pulmonale in children; we have seen a number of adolescents with cystic fibrosis dying in congestive heart failure.

The neuromuscular diseases (Friedreich's ataxia, muscular dystrophy) may affect the circulation partly through ventilating disorders caused by kyphoscoliosis or by muscular causes, and partly through direct involvement of the myocardium in the disease process. Occasionally a case of Hamman-Rich syndrome has been reported in children,[194] and extreme obesity, leading to the so-called Pickwickian syndrome through alveolar hypoventilation, has been described (Fig. 238).[142]

Physiology

Numerous, ingenious schemata indicating the mechanism of cor pulmonale exist in the literature. Suffice it to say that the principal mechanism creating cor pulmonale is *alveolar hypoventilation*. This results in anoxia and hypercapnia, which then leads to reflex pulmonary vasoconstriction,

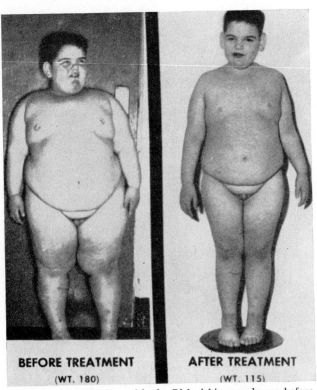

BEFORE TREATMENT   **AFTER TREATMENT**
(WT. 180)   (WT. 115)

Figure 238.   Picture of a fat boy with the Pickwickian syndrome before and after treatment.[142]

hypervolemia, high cardiac output, and polycythemia. Anatomic curtailment of the pulmonary vascular bed is rare, and probably is only a minor contributing factor, except in the rare case of embolism or fibrosis.

In early cases an elevated pulmonary arterial pressure is found at cardiac catheterization on strenuous exercise only. In more advanced cases, pulmonary arterial pressure is elevated at rest and increases steeply with effort; the pulmonary arterial resistance is elevated, *but pulmonary capillary or left atrial pressure is normal.* At this stage left atrial and systemic arterial oxygen saturation is low, but it may be raised to more than 100 per cent with inhalation of pure oxygen; cardiac output is high, the level of pO_2 is low, and that of pCO_2 is high. This may be referred to as compensated cor pulmonale. In still more advanced cases, patients have much arterial unsaturation, high pulmonary arterial pressure, and an increase in right ventricular end-diastolic and right atrial pressures. This may be referred to as decompensated cor pulmonale.

Clinical Picture

In patients with cystic fibrosis, the principal cause of pulmonary heart disease in children, the onset of cardiac symptoms cannot be sharply separated from the long-standing pulmonary disease. For many years these children have been short of breath and have had persistent coughs; infectious flare-ups have been common. As cor pulmonale appears, dyspnea becomes more severe, they become very tired, edema and anasarca develop, and cyanosis becomes more serious. Often an infectious episode, perhaps more severe than the average, heralds the onset of congestive failure.

On physical examination the expression is anxious, and there is severe shortness of breath and orthopnea. Severe cyanosis and clubbing are noted. The face is puffy, there is edema of the ankles, hepatomegaly is present, and often ascites. The neck veins are distended. There is choking of the disks. The extremities are warm except in the most severe cases of pulmonary vascular obstruction. The cardiac impulse is hyperkinetic, the chest is emphysematous, and many rales can be heard. Auscultation of the heart is almost impossible because of the emphysema and the rales, but tachycardia is obvious, gallop rhythm may be present, and pulmonic closure is loud.

Roentgenograms (Fig. 239) show the usual picture of cystic fibrosis in the lungs. Cardiomegaly involving the right atrium, right ventricle and pulmonary artery may be considerably masked by the low diaphragm and the overinflated lungs, and actually may not be obvious unless previous films are available for comparison. The rapid change in heart size is a characteristic feature.

The electrocardiogram is not nearly as sensitive an index of right ventricular hypertension and right ventricular hypertrophy in these cases as it is in congenital heart disease. The low diaphragm contributes to the swing of the mean frontal plane axis to the left; the increased anteroposterior diameter of the chest results in relatively low voltages in the chest leads (Fig. 240). Patients with severe cor pulmonale may have relatively normal tracings with low voltage, possibly because of the emphysema. Right axis deviation of $+90$ to $+115$ degrees may only be the expression of emphysema. Beyond this point it suggests right ventricular hypertrophy. The significance of an rsR' pattern is difficult to judge in these children. Definite

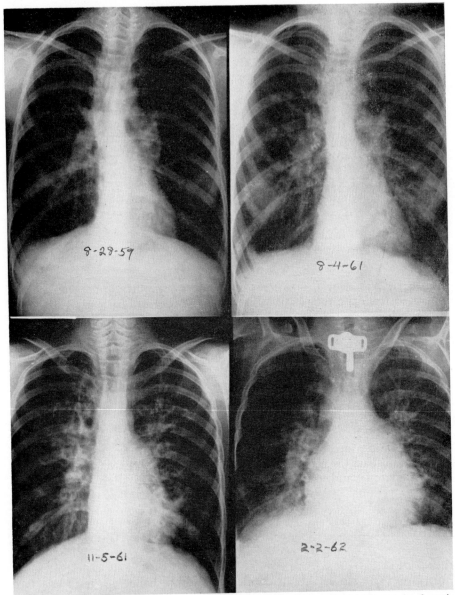

Figure 239. Serial posteroanterior films of the chest in a patient with maximal cystic fibrosis. Note the small heart through August, 1961, with dilatation beginning in November, 1961, and maximal cardiomegaly in February, 1962, just a few days before death.

evidence of right ventricular hypertrophy is rare. The T waves in the right chest leads may become more sharply inverted in acute anoxic states, but this again is hard to appreciate unless serial tracings are available. P pulmonale may be noted, and atrial arrhythmias are relatively common.

Differential Diagnosis

In patients with pancreatic fibrosis the onset of cor pulmonale may be extremely hard to detect. The distention of the neck veins may be due to

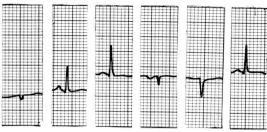

Figure 240. Electrocardiogram of an eighteen-year-old girl with maximal cystic fibrosis and presumable cor pulmonale, obtained just before death. Note the mean electrical axis of plus 105 degrees and the absence of any good evidence of right ventricular hypertrophy.

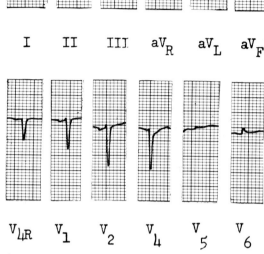

changes in intrapleural pressure, the hepatomegaly may be more apparent than real because of the low diaphragms, the cardiac enlargement may be masked by the emphysema, and the electrocardiogram is not very dependable in the diagnosis. Even in the presence of clear-cut fluid accumulation one may have to insist on unquestionable cardiac enlargement in the roentgenogram to prove the diagnosis. If the arterial oxygen saturation is less than 75 per cent and the carbon dioxide content is greater than 70 volumes per cent, the stress on the circulation is considerable. We have seen patients with a low level of pO_2 (less than 60 mm. of mercury) and a high level of pCO_2 (more than 50 mm. of mercury) who were grossly edematous, without an enlarged heart. Treatment of these patients with digitalis and mercurials may not result in any loss of fluid. Nevertheless vigorous correction of the profound respiratory acidosis results in diuresis and disappearance of edema. In other words, in the absence of cardiac enlargement, or pulmonary arterial hypertension at cardiac catheterization, even the presence of edema may not be taken as conclusive evidence that decompensated cor pulmonale is present. If, in spite of the emphysema, there has been significant cardiac enlargement, then probably one is dealing with decompensated cor pulmonale.

Treatment

Although one's first inclination when encountering a patient with decompensated cor pulmonale is to put him in an oxygen tent, a strong note of caution should be sounded. Many of these children have appreciable hypercapnia, blunting the efficacy of the respiratory center. Consequently their respiratory efforts are stimulated by anoxia alone; if, through the administration of oxygen, this anoxic stimulus disappears, respirations may become even less effective, there is further accumulation of carbon dioxide, and the patient may become unconscious and actually die. Consequently, *oxygen should be given only with simultaneous use of a respirator or with the administration of respiratory stimulants* (such as nickethamide).[383] Probably the onset of respiratory failure is also secondary to infection; consequently, vigorous antibiotic treatment is indicated. Bronchospasm is another contributory factor to respiratory difficulties; thus a bronchodilator, administered through aerosol, or aminophylline by rectum, is helpful. Bed rest is mandatory. Sedation should be given with great caution, if at all. Direct support of the circulatory system through low sodium diet, digitalis, diuretics and, if the hematocrit value is more than 65 per cent, through venesection is indicated. *In these patients the pulse rate should not be used as an index of full digitalization;* anoxia, per se, without evidence of failure, causes tachycardia, and if one persists in increasing the digitalis dosage until the heart rate slows, digitalis intoxication may occur. Over and above all this, correction of the respiratory failure by means of a respirator, preferably through a tracheotomy, is probably the most effective treatment of the situation.

Prognosis

As a rule, the outlook for children with decompensated cor pulmonale is very poor. Their life expectancy is surely no more than a few months or one to two years. As a matter of fact, most of those whom we have seen at The Children's Hospital Medical Center with cardiac enlargement, edema and high pCO_2 levels have not lived more than a few weeks in spite of vigorous respiratory and cardiac treatment. Patients with compensated cor pulmonale may survive for many years.

CONGENITAL
HEART DISEASE

PART THREE

14

GENERAL PRINCIPLES

Congenital heart disease is a structural abnormality of the heart, probably present from birth. There are two qualifying statements in this definition. The word "structural" excludes cardiac arrhythmias which, although they are often present at birth and may give rise to serious cardiac insufficiency, once they are abolished, may not recur, and the patient may be left with a normal circulation for the rest of his life. The statement that these malformations are "probably" present from birth seems at first glance unnecessarily vague. But since a considerable portion of congenital heart diseases, even in this age of excellent pediatric care, are not discovered until several weeks or even months after birth, there is some question as to when these malformation actually do take definite shape. Furthermore, as will be brought out later in the discussion of the individual malformations, a number of rather common lesions, such as patent ductus arteriosus, coarctation of the aorta or tetralogy of Fallot, although perhaps recognized as congenital heart disease from the beginning, do not assume their pathognomonic characteristics until many months or years later. Consequently the question arises whether some of these serious congenital malformations may not, in fact, develop through the first months or years of extrauterine life from a heart that is only slightly abnormal at birth. This point is brought up because I believe that the kind of thinking which assumes that the malformation is the same at birth, at ten years and at twenty years of age may actually hamper our understanding of the natural history of these anomalies.

For purposes of classification and simplification, the group of primary myocardial diseases, although probably present at birth and certainly representing structural abnormalities, has been discussed elsewhere.

The lesions to be discussed within the framework of congenital heart disease are (a) the abnormal communications betweens the systemic and pulmonary circuits, which include primarily the left-to-right shunt group, (b) the valvular and vascular lesions encompassing the right-to-left shunts together with the obstructive lesions, and (c) the transposition of great arteries, veins or individual cardiac chambers. These anatomic entities form the basis of our classification; the physiologic variants of each will be discussed separately.

Incidence

The importance of congenital heart disease in pediatric cardiology can scarcely be overemphasized. Until the last two decades it was believed that rheumatic heart disease was by far the most common form of cardiac disease in children. Within recent years, however, it has become obvious that rheumatic and congenital heart diseases occur with about equal frequency in this age group;[377, 574] as a matter of fact, in many cardiac centers congenital heart disease is the more common of the two. The shift of emphasis toward congenital heart disease in children is due to several factors. As has been mentioned before, rheumatic fever is on the downgrade. Also, the spectacular advances in the surgical treatment of congenital heart disease have prompted physicians and parents to seek help for infants with congenital cardiac malformations who, twenty years ago, would have died at home without any specific diagnosis.

No accurate large-scale figures are available for comparing the two conditions in the general population. But at least ten times as many new patients with congenital heart disease are admitted yearly to the Boston Children's Hospital Medical Center as are admitted with rheumatic heart disease. Figures from the Toronto Cardiac Registry[377] indicate that they find more than twice as many children with congenital heart disease as with rheumatic heart disease and that deaths from the former are about seven times as common as from the latter. The over-all incidence of congenital heart disease is placed at about 3 per 1000 at birth and one per 1000 at 10 years of age, according to British authors.[471] Richards and her associates,[585] studying 60,000 babies in New York, placed the over-all incidence at 0.83 per cent, including stillbirths. In 1960 Pleydell[562] reported on 62,224 births with 195 cases of congenital heart disease; this again is similar to MacMahon's[471] figures (3 out of 1000).

The frequency of the individual lesions is difficult to determine accurately. Different figures are obtainable, depending on whether one discusses living patients or results of postmortem examinations; in addition, each author's series varies in terms of age or type of disease. Abbott's[1] analysis of 1000 postmortem examinations, in respect to the more important congenital heart lesions, is presented in Table 22 (p. 790). In contrast to these data are the clinical results in Paul Wood's[748] series of 900 patients, excluding infants, studied by cardiac catheterization (Table 23, pp. 790–791). Table 24, compiled from the autopsy files of the Boston Lying-In Hospital,[538] shows the frequency of the lesions causing death in the early neonatal period. Keith's table (Table 25) gave the incidence in patients ranging in age from birth to fourteen years. Table 26 summarizes the cases of congenital heart disease at The Children's Hospital Medical Center, in which the diagnosis was proved either at cardiac catheterization, operation or postmortem examination. Obviously, most of our patients were children, and the interest of our medical and surgical staff is slanted toward the acyanotic group in general.

The rather wide discrepancies in patient selection between these various statistics is obvious at first glance. It seems to me simplest and most accurate to say that ventricular septal defect, alone or in combination with pulmonic stenosis, is the most common defect. Among the others each of the following make up 10 to 15 per cent of the total number of patients with congenital cardiac defects: atrial septal defect, patent ductus arteriosus, coarctation of the aorta, pulmonic stenosis, aortic stenosis and transposition of the great arteries. The other lesions are not common, and accurate statistical appraisal of their occurrence is not presently available.

Etiology

The etiology of congenital heart disease is unknown in most instances. Hereditary factors may play a role, since the incidence of congenital heart disease in siblings is significantly higher than in the general population. Polani and Campbell[563] in a study of 377 families of children with congenital heart disease found the incidence to be 2 per 100 families. In our experience the same lesions are likely to be repeated in siblings of the same sex; we have seen patent ductus arteriosus, atrial septal defect, pulmonary stenosis and tetralogy of Fallot, each in two siblings. We have also encountered patent ductus arteriosus in a mother and daughter, both successfully operated upon. Taussig[682] described a family in which the father and four children all had patent ductus arteriosus. Walker and Ellis,[711] reviewing the literature, found forty-eight families in which more than one sibling had congenital heart disease. In our series of approximately 2500 patients we have 15 families in which 2 siblings have congenital heart disease. The familial occurrence of cardiomyopathies has been discussed earlier (see p. 287).

Other congenital malformations associated with congenital heart disease will be mentioned only briefly. Mongolism is commonly associated with cardiac malformations. Berg and his associates[53] thoroughly reviewed this subject and came to the conclusion that an average of 19 per cent of patients with mongolism have some congenital cardiac deformity. They also pointed out, however, that in the literature, incidences varying between 70 and 7 per cent are quoted, depending on the age range of the patient and the criteria utilized for diagnosis. Rowe,[595] in a recent publication, placed the incidence at 40 per cent, including an anomalous right subclavian artery as a sole lesion. Berg stressed that a wide variety of cardiac deformities are associated with mongolism, but that endocardial cushion defects and atrial septal defects of the ostium secundum type are probably more common than any other. Interestingly enough, they noted that transposition of the great vessels, infantile coarctation of the aorta, and dextrocardia were not found in Mongols, and lesions found less frequently than in the controls included tetralogy of Fallot, "Eisenmenger's complex," persistent truncus arteriosus, coarctation of the aorta, aortic and pulmonic valve anomalies and fibroelastosis. Turner's syndrome often includes coarctation of the aorta or atrial septal defect and, in our experience, pulmonic stenosis with an intact ventricular septum, as well. Transposition of the abdominal viscera, with or without dextrocardia, is commonly accompanied by septal defects and transposition of the great vessels. Marfan's syndrome predisposes to aortic regurgitation, mitral regurgitation, atrial septal defect, dilatation of the pulmonary artery, and even endocardial fibroelastosis. The Ellis-van Creveld syndrome (ectodermal dysplasia, chondrodysplasia and polydactyly) is frequently associated with a single atrium. Deformities of the forearm are seen in patients with ventricular septal defect. Mental retardation and cleft palate, with harelip, seem to me to be more common in children with congenital heart disease, although no statistical confirmation of this clinical impression is available.

Environmental influences during pregnancy may be implicated. Mothers who contract German measles within the first three months of pregnancy are likely to give birth to children with multiple congenital anomalies, including congenital heart disease.[674] Among these patients patent ductus arteriosus is the most common lesion, but atrial septal defect, tetralogy of Fallot and pulmonary stenosis have also been encountered. Polani and Campbell[563] stated that mothers between the ages of forty and forty-four years are more likely to give birth to children with tetralogy of Fallot than are younger mothers. Animal experiments[650, 714] indicate that noxious influences, such as anoxia or vitamin deficiency, induce pregnant rats to give birth to litters with multiple congenital anomalies, including congenital heart disease. In Peru the incidence of cardiac anomalies, especially patent ductus arteriosus and atrial septal defect, seems higher in patients living at high altitudes and low oxygen pressures than in those born at sea level.[15] Certain congenital anomalies are more common in one sex than in the other; lesions involving the aorta (coarctation, aortic stenosis), and also transposition of the great vessels, seem more common in males, whereas atrial septal defect and patent ductus arteriosus are seen more commonly in females. Seasonal influences are significant only in that patients with patent ductus arteriosus are more likely to be born between October and January than at any other time of the year, according to Rutstein and his associates.[607] This is due to the prevalence of German measles in the late winter and early spring months.

How these and perhaps many other factors operate in the production of the individual case of congenital heart deformity is impossible to tell in most instances. Usually, even after taking the most careful family and prenatal history, the pediatrician cannot give a satisfactory answer as to why the child has congenital heart disease. Further pregnancies should be encouraged, however, especially if the parents are young. The chances that the next child will also have congenital heart disease are only about 2 per cent, as stated previously.

Embryology

The embryology of congenital heart disease will be touched on only briefly. At the second intrauterine week, when the embryo is only 1.5 mm. long, the heart begins to take shape. A functional circulatory system has been established by the fourth week; the ventricular septum is fully developed by the eighth week. Consequently any radical alteration of the architecture of the heart must occur between the second and eighth weeks of intrauterine life.

The primitive cardiac tube in the three-week embryo is a vertical structure attached dorsally by pericardial folds at its two ends. It consists of four chambers, from caudal to cranial direction: the sinus venosus, the atrial canal, the ventricular canal and the bulbus cordis. This originally straight cardiac tube undergoes changes consisting in torsions, kinkings, development of septums, and so forth, and at the same time it maintains the circulation of the embryo. By about six weeks all the prinicipal components of the human heart are clearly discernible.

The sinus venosus, into which the umbilical veins and the vitelline veins drain, is absorbed into the right atrium and eventually contributes to the formation of the sinus node. The anterior cardinal veins fuse into an inferior vena cava; the posterior cardinal veins contribute to the inferior cava and the coronary venous system.

The common atrial canal is divided into left and right atria by a septum primum growing down from the roof of the atrium at the end of the third or the beginning of the fourth week (5-mm. embryo). There are two openings in the septum primum—a foramen primum, which is in the lowest aspect of the septum, posteriorly, in the neighborhood of the atrioventricular valve, and a foramen secundum, which is high in the septum primum, approximately where the foramen ovale will be later. Under ordinary circumstances the growth of the septum primum and its attachment to the endocardial cushion of the atrioventricular valve completely abolishes the low foramen primum. The foramen secundum, on the other hand, is closed only partially by the growth of a newly formed septum secundum. This septum secundum develops about the fifth or sixth week and grows from the posterior wall of the atrium in a crescent shape, anteriorly, to the right of the septum primum. It partially covers the foramen secundum, leaving a slitlike opening, the foramen ovale. As long as the pressure in the right atrium is higher than that in the left atrium, this opening allows the flow of oxygenated placental blood from the inferior vena cava into the left atrium.

Thus the defects in the atrial septum developing between the fourth and sixth weeks may originate from the foramen primum or secundum. A foramen primum defect is low, principally posterior, and involves a defect of the atrioventricular valves as well. In contrast, the true atrial septal defect, which develops because the foramen secundum was not closed by the septum secundum, is usually high, dorsal, and accompanied by normal mitral and tricuspid valves. A patent foramen ovale develops if the septum primum fails to fuse with the posterior edge of the normally developed septum secundum.

The common ventricular canal is divided by an intraventricular septum (septum inferius) which starts at the same time as the septum primum of the atria and grows upward and backward toward the common atrioventricular orifice, which it divides into the mitral and tricuspid valves. This septum is muscular and is an outgrowth of the ventricular wall itself. It does not reach the floor of the bulbus cordis, and an opening in the ventricular septum is left in the center, high up, with a downward convex border. This opening is closed by a membranous structure growing down partly from the bulbus cordis and partly from the endocardial cushions on the side. The ventricular septum, as mentioned, is usually completely closed by the seventh or eighth intrauterine week.

In order for the ventricular septum to divide the common atrioventricular orifice evenly, this must shift toward the right; failure of this orifice to shift results in tricuspid atresia, and an excessive shift gives rise to mitral atresia. Failure of the bulbar ridges or the endocardial cushions to form the membranous part of the septum results in most common forms of ventricular septal defect. Defects of the muscular septum are usually ventral and high near the aortic orifice; only rarely do they occur in the neighborhood of the apex.

The bulbus cordis, the most cranial part of the primitive cardiac tube, participates in the formation of the aortic and pulmonary orifices, the membranous portion of the ventricular septum and the infundibulum of the right ventricle. The extracardiac continuation of the bulbus cordis is the truncus arteriosus.

The development of the bulbus cordis, at the five to seven week period, through a spiraling endocardial ridge, and its attachment to the divided ventricular cavity is difficult for medical students and cardiologists alike to understand. I never really understood it until a cartoon-like motion picture demonstrated it very simply. I shall not attempt to explain this development of the bulbar part of the heart, except to say that failure of the correct bulbar development may give rise to congenital aortic and pulmonary stenosis, transposition of the great vessels or ventricular septal defect with overriding aorta. If the septum in the truncus communis fails to develop entirely, persistent truncus arteriosus results. If there is a localized defect in the bulbar ridges, aortopulmonary fenestration results.

The blood vessels develop at approximately the same time as the heart. The principal structures are four large vessels, the two ventral and the two dorsal aortas. The two ventral aortas grow cephalad from the bulbus cordis, parallel with each other. In the cervical region they bend backward, forming the first branchial artery, and grow down both sides of the spine. This occurs at the second to third week of intrauterine life. Within the next two to three weeks five more connections between the ventral and dorsal aortas develop; thus six pairs of branchial arches are formed. All these branches never exist simultaneously, however; their appearance and disappearance are conditioned by the flow of blood, and by the time one pair develops another may disappear. The first four branchial arches are present at the end of four weeks; the next two develop at the end of six weeks. The fifth branchial arch disappears quickly in its entirety, without normally participating in the formation of any of the extrauterine vessels. Eventually the ventral aortas form the ascending portion of the aortic arch and the two external carotids. The internal carotids are made up of the third branchial arches and the dorsal aortas. The arch of the aorta is the fourth left branchial arch, and the descending aorta is the left dorsal aorta. The pulmonary arteries are derived from the ventral part of the sixth branchial arch, whereas the ductus arteriosus originates from the dorsal part. Variations in this normal development form the basis of the many anomalies of the aortic arch.

The Fetal Circulation and Its Adjustments after Birth. The intrauterine circulation in the human fetus differs from that of extrauterine life in a number of respects: (1) Oxygen is not obtained through the

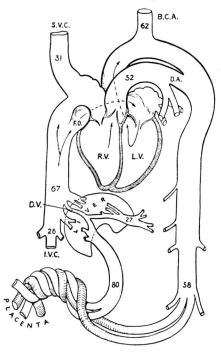

Figure 241. Diagram of the fetal circulation. Note the direct communication between inferior vena cava and foramen ovale and the passage of blood from there through to the left atrium. Figures indicate per cent of oxygen saturation. Note that the carotid arteries receive blood that is 62 per cent saturated, which is almost identical with the saturation of the blood entering the foramen ovale (67 per cent). Contrast this with the blood reaching the lower part of the body, which is only 58 per cent saturated, only slightly more than that found in the ductus arteriosus.[189]

pulmonary circulation, but from the placenta, through the umbilical vein and the ductus venosus. (2) Oxygenated blood does not enter the left side of the heart directly, but is emptied into the right atrium through the inferior vena cava. From here it is transferred to the left atrium by means of preferential streaming through the foramen ovale. As a matter of fact, Dawes[189] suggested that inferior vena cava blood is dumped directly into the left atrium through the foramen ovale (Fig. 241). (3) The ductus arteriosus is open and carries blood from the pulmonary artery into the aorta. This "right-to-left" shunt is dependent on the fact that the pulmonary resistance is higher than the systemic resistance in the fetus. (4) Because of these various shunts, pulmonary and systemic circuits do not receive equal amounts of blood. Toward the end of gestation the lungs receive 10 per cent, the fetal tissues minus the lungs 35 per cent, and the placenta 55 per cent of the total combined ventricular output.[190]

The studies of Barcroft[38] and Dawes[190] on newborn lambs and Lind and Wigelius's,[437] data on human fetuses suggest the following description of the fetal circulation. The superior vena cava carries blood, about 30 per cent saturated, from its usual drainage places into the right atrium. Here it is mixed to a certain extent with blood pouring in through the inferior vena cava, which is about 65 per cent saturated. This inferior vena cava blood represents a mixture of fresh placental blood through the ductus venosus (80 per cent saturated) and reduced systemic venous blood (25 per cent saturated).

The mixing in the right atrium, as indicated, is not complete. Most of the blood from the inferior vena cava enters the left atrium through the foramen ovale, and most of that from the superior vena cava enters the right ventricle through the tricuspid valve. The right ventricular

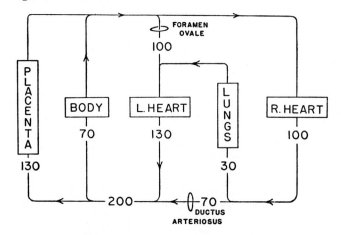

L. heart: left heart   R. heart: right heart

Figure 242. Schematic view of the fetal circulation. The figures indicate the volume of the blood flow through the heart and the great vessels. Note that only 30 per cent of the blood from the right side of the heart goes through the lungs. The rest passes through the ductus arteriosus. Of the 200 ml. entering the systemic circulation, 130 ml. go to the placenta and only 70 ml. to the rest of the body.[189]

output, representing a mixture of inferior and superior vena cava blood (50 per cent saturated) enters the pulmonary artery; slightly more than half of the pulmonary arterial blood enters the descending aorta through the patent ductus arteriosus, and the rest circulates through the lungs and enters the left atrium.

Left atrial blood, then, consists of a mixture of pulmonary arterial blood entering through pulmonary veins (one fifth) and inferior vena cava blood entering through the foramen ovale (four fifths). The oxygen saturation of the mixture in the left ventricle, supplying the head and the right arm, is about 60 per cent. In contrast, the left arm and the lower part of the body are supplied by a mixture of left ventricular and patent ductus arteriosus blood with an oxygen saturation of less than 60 per cent. As indicated, more than half of the combined ventricular output circulates through the placenta via the umbilical arteries to receive oxygen. The well saturated umbilical venous blood enters the inferior vena cava through the ductus venosus, bypassing, to a great extent, the liver. A simple diagram of Dawes shows the volume distribution of blood through the various compartments, assuming a total output of both ventricles of 200 ml. per kilogram per minute (Fig. 242).

What happens at birth to rearrange this complicated setup into the well known circulatory pattern of extrauterine life? The two principal factors responsible are the decrease in pulmonary resistance due to the sudden expansion of the lungs associated with the onset of breathing (Fig. 243), and the increase in systemic resistance due to the collapse and cutting of the umbilical cord.

The first breath is probably stimulated through chemoreceptors by the drop in arterial oxygen saturation (compression of the cord, diminution of uterine blood flow and separation of the placenta) during delivery.

As the pulmonary resistance drops, with the first few breaths, blood

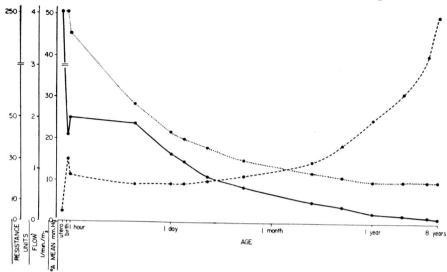

Figure 243. Changes in pulmonary arterial pressure, pulmonary blood flow and pulmonary vascular resistance with age. Note the precipitous drop in resistance within the first hour of life and the gradual drop through the first year. Pulmonary arterial pressure drops more gradually; pulmonary flow increases instantaneously in the first hour, and further later on. Dark line, resistance; dotted line PA pressure; interrupted line, PA flow.[598]

is diverted from the ductus arteriosus, and virtually the total right ventricular output is poured into the left atrium. This extra amount of blood in the left atrium, the sudden increase in resistance confronting the left ventricle, and, probably, the greatly increased systemic flow, raise left atrial pressure (Fig. 244) and result in closure of the flap of the foramen ovale. Thus the two circuits are separated; the foramen ovale is closed by the increased left atrial pressure, and the patent ductus arteriosus is bypassed by virtue of the sudden expansion of the pulmonary arterioles.

Although dramatic changes occur within a few minutes or hours, the changes are not *completed* for many days or even weeks. The pulmonary arterial mean pressure drops from about 50 mm. of mercury in intrauterine life to almost 25 within the first day, but a further gradual fall to about 15 mm. proceeds for at least another month. The calculated pulmonary vascular resistance drops precipitously with the first breath, paralleling the sudden increase in pulmonary flow, from about 250 units per square meter to about 40. A further decrease to about 10 units is accomplished within the first day, but probably normal adult values of 1 to 2 units are not reached until some time after the first year[598] (Fig. 243). Pathologic evidence supporting the concept of a gradual change in the pulmonary vascular tree after birth has been supplied by Adams and his associates.[451]

The ductus arteriosus constricts rapidly within minutes after the establishment of respiration, certainly as a result of an increase in arterial pO_2 and possibly because of other factors. Dawes demonstrated that in lambs some flow occurs through this constricted ductus, but from aorta to pulmonary artery, not in the usual "fetal" right-to-left direction, as a result of the change in resistance in the systemic and pulmonary circuits.

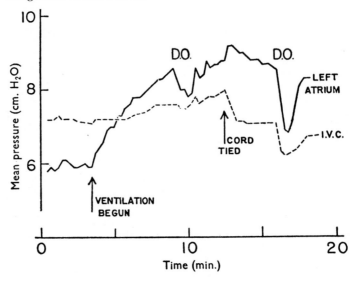

I.V.C.: inferior vena cava
D.O.: ductus arteriosus temporarily occluded

Figure 244. Closure of the foramen ovale. Note the increase in left atrial pressure with the onset of ventilation. Occlusion of the ductus diminishes left atrial pressure, and tying of the cord increases it.[190]

A left-to-right shunt through the ductus in human newborns under conditions of *respiratory distress* has been suspected by Burnard[112, 114, 115] and demonstrated at catheterization by Rudolph and his co-workers.[598] A left-to-right shunt through the ductus of *normal* newborns was suggested by Adams and his associates[5] with catheterization data, which, however, at least in the author's mind, may be subject to various interpretations. A right-to-left ductal shunt in the normal neonate was demonstrated by James[360] for a few hours after birth. The possibility of such a shunt for several days, with crying, has been demonstrated by Hultgren.[351]

It may be said, then, that partial closure of the normal ductus arteriosus, possibly by reversible, functional spasm, occurs within minutes. Crying, hypoxia and changes in pulmonary arterial and systemic arterial pressure may allow more or less flow of the blood through this vessel in a left-to-right or right-to-left direction. Nevertheless, within a few days, one to two weeks at the most, the normal ductus closes anatomically and no blood may flow through it. The exact mechanism of this closure is not known, but it certainly amounts to anatomic obliteration, perhaps due to thrombosis or even changes in the musculature of the wall of the ductus. I have always believed that the normal ductus is somewhat like placental tissue, having a certain life expectancy, and that at the end of nine months it undergoes involution. Support for this theory may be found in the fact that, occasionally, a premature baby may have a clearly open ductus for a month or two, a phenomenon almost never observed in normal full-term infants. These, then, would be the instances in which the first stage of the closing, the functional one, occurs as expected, but the permanent anatomic closure does not take place until the ductal tissue reaches its maturation. Further extension of this theory attempts to explain the patent ductus arteriosus as a congenital abnormality of the ductal tissue by suggesting that it does not undergo the anatomic involution at all.

Physiologic Consequences of Congenital Heart Disease

The clinical picture of individual congenital heart diseases, with the physiologic background, will be discussed in detail with the individual lesions. But certain general principles common to many forms of congenital cardiac malformation may be summarized here.

The physiologic consequences of the various congenital cardiac anomalies may be (1) arterial unsaturation, i.e. admixture of unoxygenated blood in the left side of the heart or the aorta, (2) overwork in terms of systolic or diastolic overloading of the ventricles, (3) inadequate systemic cardiac output, and (4) pulmonary arterial hypertension.

Arterial Unsaturation. Normally the blood in the pulmonary veins, the left side of the heart and the systemic arteries is more than 95 per cent saturated with oxygen. Consequently, if a blood sample obtained from a peripheral artery (femoral, brachial, and so forth) of the average person is analyzed by the Van Slyke method, its oxygen content should be at least 95 per cent of its capacity, i.e. 18 to 19 ml. of oxygen per 100 ml. of blood. Under certain circumstances, principally during crying or respiratory insufficiency of one sort or another, the oxygen saturation of the peripheral arterial blood may be as low as 92 per cent in apparently healthy people. If, however, the arterial oxygen saturation is 91 per cent or lower, arterial unsaturation is present.

CYANOSIS. Arterial unsaturation is not always accompanied by visible cyanosis, and cyanosis does not always mean arterial unsaturation. The bluish color of cyanosis is the result of an increased amount of reduced hemoglobin in the capillaries. Lundsgaard and Van Slyke[455] stated that at least 5.0 gm. of reduced hemoglobin must be present in the capillaries before clinical cyanosis is noted (Table 27, p. 793). Since the average person carries 15.0 gm. of hemoglobin per 100 ml. of blood, one-third unsaturation would have to exist at the capillary level before 5 gm. of reduced hemoglobin would be found. Since the capillary blood, according to Lundsgaard and Van Slyke, normally contains about 2.25 gm. of reduced hemoglobin, a drop in arterial saturation to 75 per cent will add the additional 3.0 gm. of reduced hemoglobin necessary for manifest cyanosis (Table 27). As a matter of fact, physicians who frequently see patients with cyanotic disease usually are able to recognize cyanosis in patients whose arterial oxygen saturation is 80 to 85 per cent.

One further point to be emphasized is that, according to this concept, the presence of cyanosis depends not only on the percentage of saturation of the arterial blood, but also on the absolute level of circulatory hemoglobin. Thus an 80 per cent saturation in a child who has 10 gm. of hemoglobin per 100 ml. of blood results in 2 gm. of reduced hemoglobin in the arterial blood, whereas the same percentage of saturation in a person with 15 gm. of hemoglobin is accompanied by 3 gm. of reduced hemoglobin and, thus, more definite cyanosis.

This, then, illustrates the point that definite arterial unsaturation may or may not be accompanied by cyanosis, depending on the degree of unsaturation and the absolute level of the hemoglobin.

On the other hand, definite, visible cyanosis may be present in patients whose arterial blood is fully saturated. These are persons in whom the extraction of oxygen is so complete that reduced hemoglobin is present at the capillary level in amounts greater than 5 gm., thus giving the clinical picture of cyanosis, with normal arterial oxygen saturation.

I am certain that, in a book written for pediatricians, the fact that "cyanosis" may indeed be imitated by methemoglobinemia or nitrite poisoning needs to be mentioned only briefly. Our more experienced, older teachers can remember the time when argyria, caused by prolonged administration of Argyrol, also had to be considered in the differential diagnosis.

These two types of cyanosis, the central (with arterial unsaturation) and peripheral (without arterial unsaturation), may be distinguished clinically by the fact that the former is much more generalized and severe, while the latter is usually milder, affecting only the tips of the fingers, toes and nose, and not the mucous membranes. Peripheral cyanosis is associated with evidences of a low cardiac output such as cold extremities, small pulse, and so forth. An easy and reliable method of distinguishing between the two types is by direct determination of the arterial oxygen content. Peripheral cyanosis may be seen in severe cases of mitral stenosis, pulmonary vascular obstruction, and pulmonary stenosis without right-to-left shunt, whereas central cyanosis is most likely to occur with intracardiac right-to-left shunts, although it may be caused by pulmonary disease as well.

In a patient with central cyanosis arterial unsaturation may occur either because the pulmonary veins themselves do not carry fully oxygenated blood, or because the fully saturated blood of the pulmonary veins becomes contaminated by reduced hemoglobin after it has been delivered to the left atrium. The first instance is an example of pulmonary cyanosis and can be identified in most instances if the inhalation of 100 per cent oxygen raises the arterial oxygen content to 100 per cent or more, with a corresponding increase in the plasma-dissolved oxygen. Patients with pulmonary cyanosis get pink when put in an oxygen tent or when they cry. On the other hand, if a right-to-left intracardiac shunt is responsible for the central cyanosis, the child will get much bluer when he cries and will not become completely pink in an oxygen tent. Although arterial samples from these patients may show a rise to normal oxygen level after inhalation of 100 per cent oxygen, this is accomplished at the expense of the dissolved oxygen, which in these cases stays at a low 0.5 to 1.0 volume per cent, instead of the 2 to 3 volumes per cent observed when patients with pulmonary cyanosis are given 100 per cent oxygen for 10 minutes. The clinical differential diagnosis of cyanosis is schematically presented in Figure 245.

Perhaps a few words could be spent here in explaining the physiology of central cyanosis. In the pulmonary type the hemoglobin does not become fully saturated with oxygen in the capillaries of the lung; whether the low pulmonary venous oxygen saturation resulting from this is due to the low oxygen tension of the alveolar air or to a barrier between the alveoli and

CYANOSIS

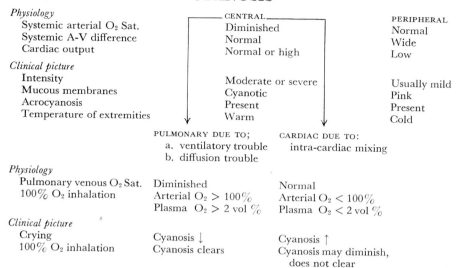

Figure 245. Schematic representation of the origins of cyanosis.

the capillaries, it can, at least theoretically, be corrected by increasing the oxygen tension in the alveolar air. This accounts for the good response to inhalation of 100 per cent oxygen in most of these cases. In other words, as the pO_2 of the alveolar air increases, the alveolar-capillary barrier is gradually overcome; consequently there is an increase in the oxyhemoglobin content of the blood, as well as in the dissolved nonhemoglobin-attached, oxygen content. Conversely, in instances of shunt cyanosis of the central variety, in which the hemoglobin in the lungs does become fully saturated, increasing the oxygen tension in the alveolar air results only in a lesser increase in the arterial oxygen content, which is due principally to the increased amount of dissolved oxygen in the plasma as it leaves the pulmonary veins. As the right-to-left shunt blood is added to this fully saturated hemoglobin and super-saturated plasma at, say, the ventricular level, the high-plasma oxygen is instantaneously transferred to the reduced hemoglobin in the shunt blood. Hence in these cases the plasma oxygen in the peripheral arterial blood may be below normal, and the arterial saturation is somewhat higher than it is with the inhalation of room air (Fig. 245). A further cause for improvement of shunt cyanosis when 100 per cent oxygen is inhaled may be due to changes in pulmonary vascular resistance.

Shunt cyanosis is always due to the addition of venous to arterial blood. For shunt cyanosis to occur, two things are necessary: (1) a communication between the two circuits, such as a septal defect or a patent ductus arteriosus, and (2) a resistance to flow of blood on the right side that is larger than the resistance to flow on the left side.

The size of the pulmonary blood flow bears on the question of cyanosis only in a quantitative sense; the smaller the pulmonary flow in relation to the systemic flow, the greater is the arterial unsaturation given the same amount of mixing. One may say that the color of the ink in the peripheral artery depends on the proportion of red ink (contributed by the pulmonary return) to the blue ink (furnished by the systemic return). These quantitative considerations are exemplified clearly in cases of single ventricle or persistent truncus arteriosus. Mixing here is essentially complete; still, a patient with a large pulmonary flow and a wide-open pulmonary vascular bed will have arterial oxygen saturation of 85 to 90 per cent. Another patient with the same intracardiac anatomy, but a constricted pulmonary vascular bed, will have a small pulmonary flow, a minor contribution of red ink to the common pool and, thus, arterial unsaturation of 50 to 60 per cent. But these are quantitative factors only, and *it should not be said that cyanosis is due to diminished pulmonary flow*. There are patients with severe pulmonic stenosis who have a considerably diminished pulmonary flow, with no trace of arterial unsaturation, as long as there is no communication between the pulmonary and systemic circuits.

The deep bluish color of cyanosis does not have to be illustrated by colored plates; it should be familiar to every physician. It is most obvious in the mucous membranes of the eyes and mouth, but occurs also in the fingers, toes and the glans penis. Less severe unsaturation may give rise to excessive redness of the lips, cheeks and finger tips; sometimes the parents of these children remark that this particular youngster has always had a "much better color" than the rest of the family.

CLUBBING. Under ordinary circumstances, then, the first result of arterial unsaturation is cyanosis. The second, slightly later, but almost as dramatic, consequence is the development of clubbing or hypertrophic osteoarthropathy (Fig. 2, p. 13). In its fully developed form this consists in a widening and thickening of the ends of the fingers and toes, accompanied by convex fingernails. Earlier forms of clubbing consist in shininess and tenseness of the terminal phalanges, obliterating the wrinkles usually present in this part of the skin. This incipient clubbing is usually accompanied by fiery red fingers, giving a characteristic picture of early, slight arterial unsaturation. I have seen full-blown clubbing in severely cyanotic children as young as two or three weeks old; ordinarily, however, it does not make its appearance until a child is one or two years old. For some reason it appears earliest and most pronounced on the thumbs. Physiologic and histologic studies of clubbing indicate that these fingers have an increased number of capillaries, with increased blood flow through myriads of arteriovenous aneurysms.[494] This is accompanied by an increase of connective tissue in the terminal phalanges.

Clubbing in children almost always indicates congenital heart disease of the cyanotic variety, although occasionally cirrhosis of the liver, subacute bacterial endocarditis, lung abscess or even a familial hereditary condition may be responsible for it.

POLYCYTHEMIA. Polycythemia, with increased hemoglobin content, is another consequence of arterial unsaturation. That a low arterial oxygen content acts as a stimulus to the bone marrow has been amply demonstrated, not only on patients with congenital malformation of the heart, but also in people living at high altitudes with low atmospheric oxygen tension.[353] The increased oxygen-carrying capacity achieved by this method is an extremely useful compensatory mechanism until the polycythemia reaches hematocrit levels of 80 per cent or more. At these levels, however, the benefits derived from the increase in available oxygen are probably outweighed by the disadvantages of the high viscosity. The therapeutic implications of these considerations will be discussed later (p. 651).

Dyspnea. Dyspnea on exertion is a characteristic feature of patients with arterial unsaturation. Exercise demands increased oxygen delivery to the tissues. In congenital heart disease with arterial unsaturation this is not possible. As a matter of fact, in many instances the amount of oxygen delivered may actually decrease on exertion because of the increased right-to-left shunt resulting from the decreased systemic resistance. Under these circumstances dyspnea and hyperpnea occur, possibly as a response to the stimulation of chemoreceptors.

Anoxia. Anoxic spells, consisting in an initial period of uncontrollable crying followed by paroxysms of dyspnea, cyanosis, unconsciousness and even convulsions, occur in certain types of cyanotic congenital heart disease, especially in tetralogy of Fallot. These alarming episodes are of utmost seriousness; they may even lead to the death of the patient. Usually they do not follow severe exertion, but, rather, occur early in the morning after a good night's sleep. Often they are associated with bowel movements or feeding; at other times they cannot be attributed to any single environmental factor. Their duration is from a few minutes to several hours. In mild cases they may occur once every two or three months, whereas in the severest instances a baby may have several of these episodes in one day. It is said that these attacks are an expression of cerebral anoxia due to a drop in arterial oxygen saturation. It has been suggested more recently[365] that this drop in arterial saturation is due to sudden spasm of the right ventricular infundibulum, resulting in a precipitous drop in the pulmonary flow. This may explain the beneficial effect of morphine and cyclopropane in these situations. Anoxic spells seldom make their appearance at birth; they usually start at three to four months of age and disappear before the fifth year of life.

Squatting. Squatting, described by Taussig,[682] is a characteristic posture assumed after exertion by patients with certain types of cyanotic congenital heart disease, specifically tetralogy of Fallot and, less commonly, pulmonary stenosis with an open foramen ovale (Fig. 1, p. 7). It first makes its appearance at about one and one-half years of age or when the child starts walking. Social pressure usually, though not invariably, abolishes it at eight to ten years of age. Detailed studies of our own and those of others[456] indicate that oxygen saturation, diminished by exercise, can be restored to normal more rapidly in a squatting than in a standing position (Fig. 246). This may be accomplished either by increasing systemic venous return or, possibly, by augmenting the peripheral resistance and thus diminishing the degree of right-to-left shunt. That the increased systemic venous return does indeed play a role in squatting is demonstrated by the fact that immediately after assumption of this characteristic posture a brief drop in oxygen saturation occurs, corresponding to the "dumping" of high unsaturated blood from the inferior vena cava into the common pool. This, then, is followed by the increase in peripheral saturation due to the increased pulmonary flow.

Overloading of the Ventricles. SYSTOLIC OVERLOADING. An increase in the resistance to outflow results in systolic overloading of the ventricles. In the left ventricle this occurs, for example, with aortic stenosis or coarctation of the aorta, whereas on the right side it may be the result of pul-

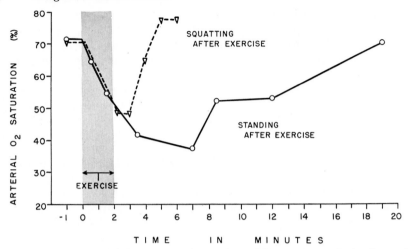

Figure 246. Effect of squatting on exercise-induced arterial oxygen unsaturation in a patient with cyanotic congenital heart disease.

monary stenosis or pulmonary vascular obstruction. The high pressure in the ventricle is usually best demonstrated clinically by the electrocardiogram. Striking changes such as increase in voltage, prolongation of ventricular activation time, depression of the S-T segment and inversion of the T wave allow an almost quantitative estimation of the height of pressure and the degree of hypertrophy in the appropriate ventricle. Indirect proof of systolic overloading of the ventricles can also be obtained from the evidences of atrial hypertrophy in the electrocardiogram. On the other hand, fluoroscopy is almost useless in detecting the presence of a small but concentrically hypertrophied ventricle. I have repeatedly encountered patients with maximal aortic stenosis, even leading to death, in whom the cardiac silhouette was essentially normal. This really is not surprising if one bears in mind the few millimeters or centimeters of thickening involved in maximal cardiac hypertrophy.

Chronic systolic overloading of the left ventricle is usually well tolerated without symptoms. The left ventricle is capable of performing many times its normal work load and thus ensures a normal cardiac output under a wide variety of circumstances. This great adaptability has the one disadvantage that it gives no warning to the patient that he is overtaxing his heart; hence the cases of sudden death, probably from ventricular fibrillation, in previously asymptomatic youngsters with aortic stenosis. At postmortem examination these patients may show tremendous cardiac hypertrophy with diffuse scarring as a result of ischemia. By the same token, congestive failure is a late manifestation of systolic overloading of the left ventricle; it occurs in the most advanced cases only, and usually at a time when treatment, medical or surgical, is not likely to restore the effectiveness of the circulation for any length of time.

Congestive failure may also be a late manifestation of systolic overloading of the right ventricle; in both instances it is a matter of utmost seriousness and often is beyond repair. But systolic overloading of the right side of the heart gives warnings sooner than its left-sided counterpart. If the obstruction is in the lung field, the pulmonary arterial hypertension resulting from this obstruction may cause dyspnea on exertion, and even at rest, possibly through stimulation of local pressure receptors. Whether the obstruction is at the pulmonary valvular or at the pulmonary arterial level, the right ventricle is frequently unable to exert the maximal effort that the left ventricle is capable of exerting under similar circumstances. Thus fatigue due to inadequate cardiac output becomes a prominent symptom. Finally, a right-to-left shunt may be established by forcing open a hitherto sealed or small foramen ovale, and symptoms referable to arterial unsaturation may appear. Thus systolic overloading of the right ventricle, in contrast to similar overloading of the left ventricle, gives a number of warning signs (dyspnea, fatigue, cyanosis) before congestive failure sets in.

DIASTOLIC OVERLOADING. Diastolic overloading of the ventricle in congenital heart disease is the result of an increased volume of blood being offered to it during diastole. Patent ductus arteriosus and aortic regurgitation are the commonest causes of diastolic overloading of the left ventricle, whereas pulmonary venous anomaly and atrial septal defect are the most frequent causes of pure diastolic overloading of the right ventricle. The increased volume of blood is handled by dilatation and hypertrophy of the ventricles and an increased stroke output. In contrast to the situation in systolic overloading, the radiologic picture is a much more sensitive index of this type of overwork than is the electrocardiogram. Radioscopy reveals a significantly enlarged heart, and the pulsations are vigorous under the fluoroscope even in moderate diastolic overloading, when the electrocardiogram may still be within relatively normal limits. Furthermore, striking radiologic evidence in this regard may be obtained, in all instances except aortic regurgitation, from the presence of pulmonary vascular engorgement. A note of caution should be sounded, however, by pointing out that pulmonary vascular engorgement, even with expansile pulsations, may not be the result of increased volume, but rather of increased pressure in the pulmonary arterial tree.

The physical examination is also extremely helpful in detecting diastolic overloading of the ventricles. One of the most sensitive indices is the presence of a diastolic rumble at the apex or the lower left sternal border which is common to all hearts with large diastolic volumes on the left or the right side. In free aortic regurgitation it is referred to as the Flint murmur; in septal defects it has no special name, but has been noted with large left-to-right shunts at any level. My impression is that the presence of a definite "shunt" diastolic murmur indicates a pulmonary-systemic flow ratio of at least 2:1. Another equally valuable sign of diastolic overloading of either ventricle is the presence of a hyperactive cardiac impulse, often accompanied by left chest prominence. Finally, infants with left-to-right shunts are more likely to have severe respiratory infections, even pneumonia.

Signs and symptoms of left-sided or right-sided congestive failure appear much earlier in patients with diastolic overloading, but represent therapeutically more approachable problems than the congestive failures resulting from systolic overloading. Medical or surgical treatment, or a combination of the two, may restore practically normal circulatory efficiency to these children with severe congestive failure.

Inadequate Cardiac Output and Underdevelopment. Inadequate cardiac output may be the result of a heart failing as a consequence of overloading; this is discussed in the section devoted to congestive failure (see p. 309).

Another type of maximal limitation of cardiac output is the one in which a congenital anomaly of the heart does not allow a left ventricular output under sufficient pressure and with adequate oxygen content to maintain life for any length of time. Prime examples of this are (1) complete transposition of the pulmonary veins or the great arteries and (2) the complete interruption of the circulation at the pulmonary, mitral or aortic valve level, or at the level of the aortic arch. In these cases death usually ensues within the first few weeks or months of life.

Varying degrees of physical underdevelopment are commonly found in patients with patent ductus arteriosus or atrial septal defect. Rarely, this may be the consequence of the somewhat decreased systemic output. More commonly it is secondary to the congestive heart failure inherent in the maximal diastolic overloading in these conditions. Occasionally a spectacular weight and lesser height spurt may be experienced by a child whose large patent ductus arteriosus or septal defect has been surgically corrected; this improvement is accompanied by improvement in the features of congestive heart failure without appreciable change in the resting systemic output. In an appreciable portion of the cases, however, particularly in instances in which physical underdevelopment is associated with only a small or moderate-sized left-to-right shunt, surgical correction of the defects leaves the growth and development of the patient largely uninfluenced. This leads to the concept that in many instances the underdevelopment represents a genetically determined abnormality and, thus, is influenced little by correction of the congenital cardiac defect. How much the frequent, severe respiratory infections contribute to the underdevelopment of children is hard to assess.

Although these views about the influence of moderately severe congenital heart disease on the physical development of children may not be uniformly accepted, the fact that the mental development of these youngsters is not influenced by their cardiac output finds universal agreement among workers in this field. Patients with severe congenital heart disease, cyanotic or not cyanotic, may be of normal or inferior intellect; most certainly there are more mentally retarded children among those with congenital heart disease than are seen in the general population. That these conditions are probably not causally linked to each other is proved by the fact that there is no direct correlation between the severity of the disease and the intelligence quotient and by the observation that corrective surgery has no influence at all on the mental development of these youngsters.

These two points should be stressed so as not to raise the hopes of parents who may expect miraculous improvement in physical or mental growth as a result of corrective surgery for congenital heart disease.

Pulmonary Arterial Hypertension. Probably no aspect of congenital heart disease has been discussed more thoroughly within the last twenty-five years than its association with pulmonary arterial hypertension. In 1927 Moschowitz[507] suggested that a correlation between the two may exist. Welch and Kinney[722] pointed to the association between left-to-right shunts and pulmonary vascular disease. Wood,[747] in 1952, and Swan,[677] in 1954, discussed the physiologic aspects of the problem. Cutler and his co-workers,[176] in the same year, pointed to the characteristic clinical picture of pulmonary vascular obstructive disease, irrespective of whether it is associated with congenital heart disease or is of the idiopathic variety. It was further emphasized that once pulmonary vascular obstruction supervenes, the clinical picture of the underlying congenital cardiac anomaly is obscured and the presenting signs and symptoms are those of pulmonary vascular obstructive disease. Paralleling these studies were the fundamental observations on functional pathology of the pulmonary vascular bed by Edwards, from 1950 on, brilliantly summarized in his Conner lecture in 1957.[212] The studies of Damman and Ferencz[182] also correlated the anatomy of the pulmonary vascular bed with physiologic observations on patients with congenital heart disease. More recently, data emphasizing the natural history of pulmonary vascular changes in children began to appear. Finally Berglund,[75] and then Rudolph and his associates,[599] brought into focus the physical factors governing the status of the pulmonary vascular bed. These are only a few of the many articles dealing with this topic. In the following paragraphs I shall attempt to summarize my own views on the matter, basing them on personal observation as well as on the references mentioned.[524]

It has been clearly established that congenital heart disease, specifically the lesions with a communication between the systemic and pulmonary circuits, is frequently associated with increased pulmonary arterial pressure. It is equally obvious, as will be discussed within the framework of the individual lesions, that children with simple secundum atrial septal defects rarely have pulmonary arterial hypertension, whereas it is common in persons with intraventricular communications. Our figures indicate, and this is supported by data from the literature, that during childhood less than 5 per cent of the patients with secundum atrial defects, about 10 per cent of the patients with endocardial cushion defects, and about 25 per cent of those with ventricular defects have pulmonary arterial mean pressure of more than 40 mm. of mercury. Since cardiac catheterization studies are not made on most patients with patent ductus arteriosus, no fully dependable figures relating to this lesion are available.

Since children with atrial septal defects have pulmonary flows just as large as, if not larger than, those with ventricular septal defects, it seems obvious that this factor, by itself, is not responsible for the increase in pulmonary arterial pressure. Indeed, it has been demonstrated repeatedly in animal experiments as well as in people who have undergone pneumonectomy that pulmonary flows three to four times larger than normal can be well accommodated within the normal pulmonary vascular bed without an increase in pulmonary arterial pressure, at least on a short-term basis.

It has been reasonably well proved that the transmission of high pressure from the left ventricle to the right ventricle or from the aorta to the pulmonary artery causes pulmonary arterial hypertension. In fact, it has been suggested that the basis of the pulmonary vascular obstruction in patients with ventricular defects is the persistence of the fetal pattern in the lung fields. Were this not to persist, in the face of a large ventricular defect, then all the blood from the left ventricle would go into the low-resistance right ventricle and pulmonary artery rather than into the relatively high-resistance systemic circuit. This would not be compatible with life. Thus normal involution of the pulmonary vascular bed does not take place in

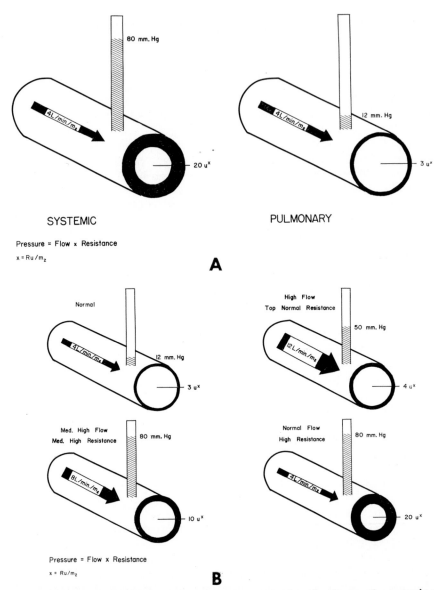

Figure 247. *A*, Normal circulatory dynamics. Note that the flow to the systemic and that to the pulmonary circuits are equal, but because of the low resistance (3 units) in the pulmonary circuit compared to the higher resistance in the systemic circuit (20 units), systemic pressure is considerably higher than pulmonary. *B*, Pulmonary hypertension and its relation to resistance and flow. Note the normal situation as in *A*. The high flow, top normal resistance is often seen in patients with patent ductus arteriosus. This is an exclusively hyperkinetic moderate hypertension. The lower left corner shows severe pulmonary artery hypertension which is partly hyperkinetic (large flow) and partly obstructive (high resistance). The lower right figure indicates the pure pulmonary vascular obstruction syndrome with normal pulmonary flow, but with pulmonary resistance at systemic level.

a patient with a ventricular defect, and the patient has approximately equal pressures in the systemic and pulmonary arteries from the time of birth. Obviously, this type of physiologic setup is seen only in patients with large ventricular septal defects, in which the size of the intraventricular communication is at least half the size of the aortic orifice. This same theory of the origin of pulmonary arterial hypertension also explains why patients with secundum atrial defects do not have high pulmonary arterial pressures; in these patients no pressure is transmitted from left to right, and, in fact, probably the flow itself is only minimal in early infancy (see p. 371).

This theory does not explain, however, why patients with ventricular defects of similar size may or may not have pulmonary arterial hypertension—why some small ventricular defects are associated with maximal pulmonary arterial pressures while other, considerably larger ones are associated with little pulmonary arterial hypertension. It also fails to explain why a patient with a large patent ductus arteriosus may not have pulmonary arterial hypertension and why patients with endocardial cushion defects (without ventricular septal defect) have more pulmonary arterial hypertension than those with secundum atrial septal defects.

These unanswered questions indicate that although the *persistence of the fetal pattern is unquestionably one factor,* and a major one, governing the association of pulmonary arterial hypertension with congenital heart disease, it is not the only one. I am sure that *individual susceptibility of the pulmonary arterioles,* as exemplified by the predominance of females in the group of patients having pulmonary vascular obstruction, has some bearing on the problem. Probably, *left atrial hypertension* (secondary to

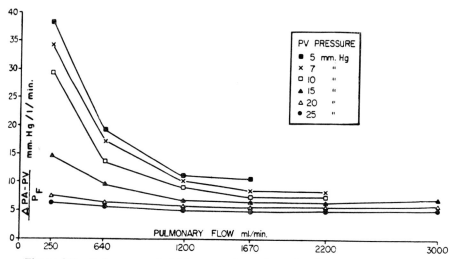

Figure 248. Pulmonary arterial hypertension; effects of pulmonary flow and pulmonary venous pressure. Note the effect of the flow and the pulmonary venous pressure on pulmonary vascular resistance, expressed as the gradient between pulmonary artery and pulmonary vein divided by pulmonary flow. It is clearly indicated that if the pulmonary flow is low and pulmonary venous pressure is low, as in the top line, then the resistance is high. As pulmonary flow increases, the resistance drops, presumably because of the distention of the pulmonary arterioles caused by the flow. Similarly, a distention occurs as the pulmonary venous pressure increases.[598]

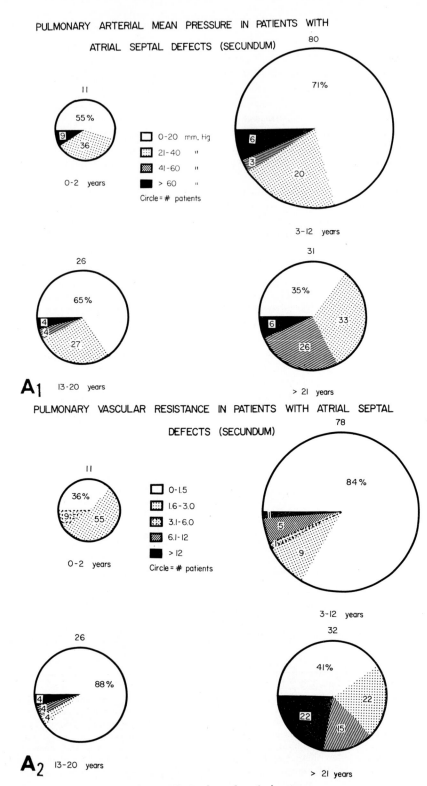

Figure 249. *See legend on facing page.*

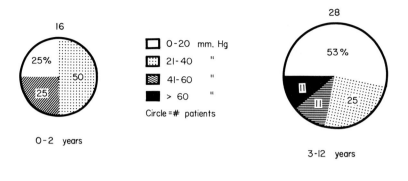

PULMONARY ARTERIAL MEAN PRESSURE IN PATIENTS
WITH ATRIAL SEPTAL DEFECTS (PRIMUM)

B₁

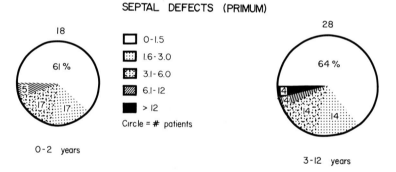

PULMONARY VASCULAR RESISTANCE IN PATIENTS WITH ATRIAL
SEPTAL DEFECTS (PRIMUM)

B₂

Figure 249. These figures represent pulmonary arterial mean pressures and resistances
in the four major left-to-right shunt groups. The patients are divided into 4 age groups: 0–2,
3–12, 13–20 and 21 years or more of age. The size of the circles is proportionate to the
number of patients in each group. In the figures relating to pressure the dark sectors imply
mean pressures of more than 60 mm. The shaded areas indicate mean pressures between 41
and 60 mm.; the stippled areas, 21 to 40 mm.; the white areas, 0 to 20 mm. In the resistance
graphs dark areas mean resistance units per square meter of more than 12; shaded areas,
between 6.1 and 12; closely stippled areas, 3.1 to 6; lightly stippled areas, 1.6 to 3; and white
areas 0 to 1.5.

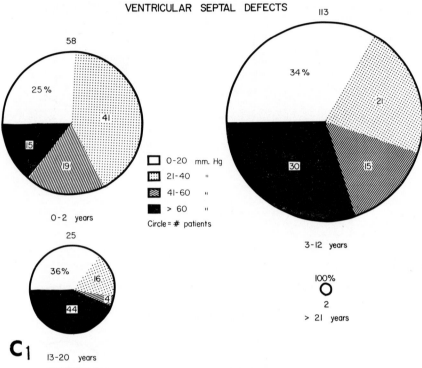

PULMONARY ARTERIAL MEAN PRESSURE IN PATIENTS WITH VENTRICULAR SEPTAL DEFECTS

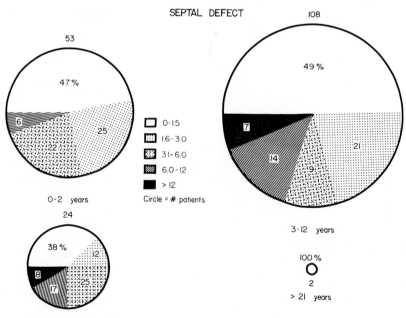

PULMONARY VASCULAR RESISTANCE IN PATIENTS WITH A VENTRICULAR SEPTAL DEFECT

Figure 249. *See page 361 for legend.*

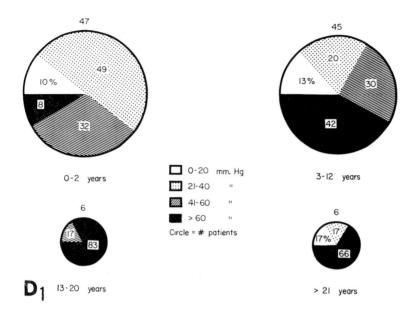

PULMONARY ARTERIAL MEAN PRESSURE IN PATIENTS WITH
PATENT DUCTUS ARTERIOSUS

47

49

10%

8

32

0-2 years

☐ 0-20 mm. Hg
▦ 21-40 "
▨ 41-60 "
■ > 60 "
Circle = # patients

45

20

13%

30

42

3-12 years

6

17

83

D₁ 13-20 years

6

17%

17

66

> 21 years

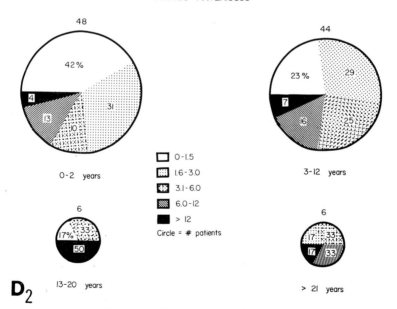

PULMONARY VASCULAR RESISTANCE IN PATIENTS WITH PATENT
DUCTUS ARTERIOSUS

48

42%

4

13

10

31

0-2 years

☐ 0-1.5
▦ 1.6-3.0
▩ 3.1-6.0
▨ 6.0-12
■ > 12
Circle = # patients

44

23%

29

7

16

25

3-12 years

6

17% 33

50

D₂ 13-20 years

6

17 33

17 33

> 21 years

Figure 249. *See page 361 for legend.*

mitral incompetence, such as is seen in endocardial cushion defect, or an incompetent left ventricle such as occurs in ventricular septal defect) also plays a role in the causation of pulmonary vascular disease.

After this discussion of the frequency and origin of pulmonary arterial hypertension in children with communications between the systemic and pulmonary circuits, a few words on the physiology may be in order. Basically, pulmonary arterial hypertension may originate from an increased pulmonary flow with normal pulmonary resistance (hyperkinetic) from normal pulmonary flow and increased pulmonary resistance (obstructive) or, most commonly, from a combination of increased resistance and increased flow ($P = R \times Q$) (Fig. 247).

Obstructive hypertension may be associated with normal pulmonary capillary pressure, in which case the site of pulmonary vascular obstruction is exclusively within the pulmonary arterioles. If increased pulmonary capillary pressure is associated with pulmonary vascular obstruction, then the primary obstruction is at the level of the pulmonary vein, the mitral valve or the left ventricle.

From the practical viewpoint it seems that hyperkinetic (flow) hypertension is a condition which can be corrected surgically with excellent results (patent ductus arteriosus) and in which elimination of the left-to-right shunt results in a drop in pressure to near normal values. If pulmonary vascular obstruction is secondary to pulmonary venous, left atrial or left ventricular disease, surgical correction of the obstruction on the left side may result in relief of the pulmonary vascular obstruction as well. Contrariwise, pure pulmonary vascular obstruction at the arteriolar level (some cases of atrial septal defect in adults and many cases of ventricular septal defect) with normal or diminished pulmonary flow is today an incurable disease. If surgical closure of the defect does not appreciably diminish pulmonary flow, the chances are that the patient will not long survive.

In situations in which pulmonary vascular obstruction is combined with hyperkinetic hypertension (most of the ventricular septal defects in children) the relative contributions of the two, among other things, will determine the efficacy of surgical treatment. Other factors, besides pulmonary flow and resistance, which influence the reaction of the pulmonary arterial tree are the absolute pressure levels in the pulmonary artery and in the left atrium (Fig. 248).

The histologic picture underlying the physiologic picture of pulmonary vascular obstruction will be discussed in detail later (see p. 420). Suffice it to say that intimal proliferation with thrombosis is the terminal, probably irreversible, lesion; it is seen only in adults and older children. On the other hand, the medial hypertrophy (persistence of the fetal pattern) seen uniformly in infants and younger children, and also encountered in some adults, is presumably reversible.

One further aspect to be touched on briefly is the course of the pulmonary arterial hypertension throughout the life cycle of patients with congenital heart disease. From the anatomic viewpoint there is no question that the most severe intimal changes are seen in widespread fashion only in adults; rarely they may occur in children beyond the age of ten, but to a much lesser extent. This indicates that long-standing hypertension results in intimal changes, as has been well documented for the systemic circuit in essential hypertension for many years. On the other hand, our own observations (Fig. 249), as well as the most careful studies in the literature, indicate that (1) if pulmonary arterial hypertension is not present in infancy or childhood, it is not likely to develop later and surely not before the third decade. (2) If pulmonary arterial hypertension is present in infancy, it is not likely to progress, either in terms of an increase in absolute pulmonary arterial pressure level or by conversion of hyperkinetic to obstructive pulmonary arterial hypertension, at least not within the first decade, and probably longer. Remember, however, that even though two catheterizations, several years apart, may reveal the same physiologic picture, the structural changes within the vessels may be totally different. (3) Finally, in rare instances, pulmonary arterial hypertension in infants may diminish or disappear for one reason or another within the first few years of life.

All this indicates that pulmonary arterial hypertension does not develop in children who have congenital heart disease; they may have it, indeed, but if so, they probably had it right from birth.

Existing pulmonary arterial hypertension rarely deteriorates during infancy and childhood in terms of physiologic observations. Anatomic deterioration in the form of development of intimal lesions is possible, but their widespread occurrence is not likely. In the group of patients having high pressure, deterioration during adolescence and beyond is possible, even probable.

Spontaneous improvement of existing pulmonary arterial hypertension in infants is possible, and surely no less likely than deterioration, within the first decade.

Classification

Table 28 (pp. 794–795) presents the classification which will form the framework for the presentation of the individual lesions. This schematic division is an attempt to present lesions in a logical sequence without being hindered by the artificial division of cyanotic or noncyanotic disease. It is hoped that this classification will make it easier for the reader to remember all the varieties of congenital heart disease.

15

COMMUNICATIONS BETWEEN SYSTEMIC AND PULMONARY CIRCUITS WITH PRE-DOMINANTLY LEFT-TO-RIGHT SHUNTS

INTERATRIAL COMMUNICATIONS

PATENT FORAMEN OVALE

The foramen ovale is a slitlike opening in the atrial septum at the site of the foramen secundum of the septum primum. As indicated in the discussion on embryology, the septum secundum, surrounding the foramen secundum in a crescent shape, leaves a slitlike opening which is covered in a valvelike manner by the free edge of the septum primum. The only important function of the foramen ovale is in intrauterine life, when it transmits inferior vena cava blood, which has a high oxygen content, to the left atrium. This is possible because in fetal life the high right atrial pressure keeps the valve of the foramen ovale open. Shortly after birth left atrial pressure rises and the flap is pushed tightly against the septum secundum, closing the foramen ovale functionally. Lind and Wigelius,[437] using angiocardiographic methods, could not demonstrate a functional opening in the foramen ovale at the end of the first week of life. Anatomic patency, however, may occur for several months, and even at the end of the first year of life approximately 50 per cent of all infants have a probe-patent foramen ovale. Probably, complete anatomic closure never occurs in 30 per cent of all persons.

The principal fact to remember about the foramen ovale is that it can allow only a right-to-left shunt because of the flap which covers it from the left side. Consequently, any functional communication between the two atria through this opening *must* go from right to left unless, of course, the foramen ovale is stretched by a distended left atrium to the extent that the flap no longer covers it completely. Such a situation may be seen in babies with a large patent ductus arteriosus. Preoperatively, a sizable left-to-right shunt may be demonstrated in these patients at cardiac catheterization. After division of the ductus, and corresponding diminution in left atrial size, the atrial shunt can no longer be detected.[603] Therefore, except in conditions associated with this "stretch phenomenon," a functional opening of the foramen ovale is possible only in situations in which the resistance to flow in the right side of the heart is higher than that in the systemic circuit, and therefore right atrial pressure is higher than left atrial pressure (Fig. 250). Thus the clinical picture of an open foramen ovale ordinarily consists in a right-to-left atrial shunt in cases of obstruction at the right ventricular, pulmonary valvular or pulmonary vascular level.

It should be mentioned, however, that fairly frequently at cardiac catheterization the left atrium may be entered through a functionally closed foramen ovale, thus pointing up the fact that passage through the atrial septum by the cardiac catheter does not, under all circumstances, indicate the presence of an atrial septal defect.

In summary, as a rule, the diagnosis of a functionally patent foramen ovale in extrauterine life should be made only in the presence of a right-to-left atrial shunt associated with right ventricular and right atrial hypertension.

ATRIAL SEPTAL DEFECT OF THE FORAMEN SECUNDUM TYPE

An atrial septal defect is any opening in the atrial septum not covered by a valve.

Incidence

In various authors' series atrial septal defect occurs with varying frequency; it ranked seventh among Abbott's[1] 1000 cases seen at postmortem examination, first among Wood's[748] 900 and fifth in our 3786 cases. In Keith's[380] series it also occupied fifth place. In approximately 15 per cent of all patients who have congenital heart disease and who live through infancy, an atrial septal defect is the principal lesion.

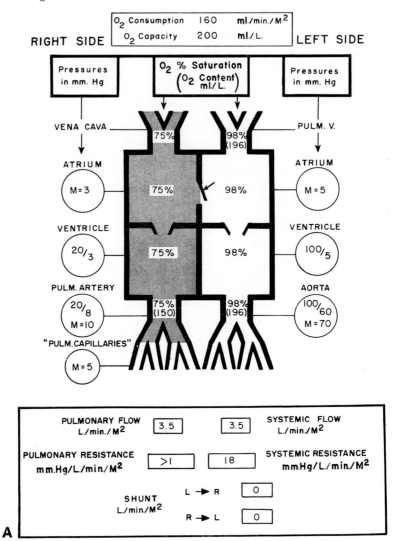

Figure 250. *See page 369 for legend.*

Anatomy

The foramen secundum lesion, high in the atrial septum, may be one large defect or may consist of several small, almost cribriform openings. It is the result of failure of the septum secundum to completely cover the foramen secundum. An associated anomaly of the pulmonary venous drainage is commonly present as well. A defect so high in the septum that the superior vena cava overrides it is referred to commonly, on embryologic grounds, as a sinus venosus defect. These are almost always associated with anomalous pulmonary venous drainage into the superior vena cava.[97, 327]

The size of atrial septal defects varies from at least 1 cm. in diameter, the smallest clinically significant opening, to virtual absence of the atrial septum. The average size is approximately 2 to 3 cm. in diameter.

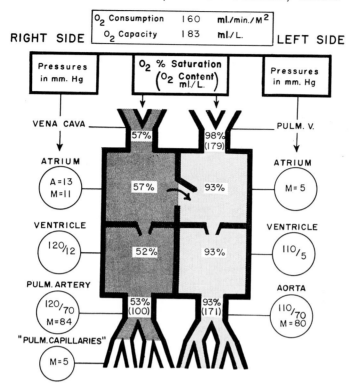

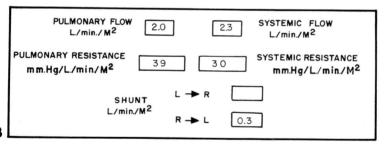

Figure 250. Schematic representation of the fact that the patent foramen ovale, because of its flap, allows a shunt only from right to left. The gradient favoring the left atrium in *A* does not allow a shunt, whereas the elevated right atrial pressure in *B* resulting from "primary" pulmonary vascular obstruction favors a right-to-left shunt.

The pulmonary arteries and the cavities of the right atrium and the right ventricle are large and often overshadow the left side of the heart and the aorta. The wall of the right atrium and the right ventricle is not grossly hypertrophied; dilatation dominates the picture.

Physiology

The flow of blood through an uncomplicated atrial septal defect, ranging from 1.0 to 20 liters per minute per square meter of body surface, is almost always exclusively from left to right by virtue of the fact that the pressure in the left atrium is higher than that in the right atrium through the entire cycle. This relative hypertension of the left atrium is dependent on the difference in the pressure-volume characteristics of the two ventricles.[204, 350, 439] Under normal circumstances the left ventricle, having to overcome the high-resistance peripheral circulation, is thicker and less distensible than the right ventricle, working against a low-resistance pulmonary circuit. Thus the left atrium must hypertrophy in order to fill this thick-walled chamber, and the left atrial pressure curve usually shows a taller A wave and a higher mean pressure than the right atrial pressure curve shows. Under ordinary circumstances, with an intact atrial septum, the left atrial mean pressure is approximately 8 to 10 mm. of mercury, whereas the right atrial mean pressure is only 4 to 5 mm. If a large defect (at least 2 by 2 cm.) is created in the atrial septum, the pressure in the two atria becomes equal, with the mean pressure about midway between normal right and left atrial mean pressures. At this level of common pressure in the two atria the right ventricle can be filled easily, but the left ventricle cannot. Consequently, all the caval blood entering the right atrium and much of the pulmonary venous blood entering the left atrium finds its way to the right ventricle and the pulmonary artery. The flow through this atrial defect probably occurs through the entire cardiac cycle. Dow[203] pointed to the teleological argument that the purpose of the entire circulation is to ensure an adequate systemic output. Consequently, if one assumes that a certain percentage of the pulmonary venous blood is shunted from the left to the right atrium, then the total pulmonary flow should be sufficient so that the percentage allotted from it to the left ventricle is compatible with life. Convincing proof of this hypothesis is afforded by figures which show widely varying pulmonary blood flows in cases of atrial defect in which systemic indices are within normal range.[82]

Certain anatomic variations of atrial septal defects may give rise to a small right-to-left, in addition to the sizable left-to-right, shunt. Most common among these are those defects which are so large and low that inferior vena cava blood is dumped directly into the left atrium, resulting in arterial oxygen saturation of $\pm$ 90 per cent.

Of course a change in resistance to outflow of the right ventricle, such as is seen in pulmonary vascular obstruction and pulmonary stenosis, changes the dynamics entirely and may result in a bidirectional or even an exclusively right-to-left shunt, through an ordinary secundum type of atrial septal defect. Pulmonary vascular obstruction is rare among children with ostium secundum atrial septal defects; certainly, it occurs in less than 5 per cent. As a matter of fact, often the pulmonary resistance is unusually low (less than 1 unit). In contrast, a high pulmonary vascular resistance (more than 3 units per square meter) is seen in approximately 25 per cent of the adults with atrial septal defects who are under our care. The latter figure obviously does not represent a random selection, but most cardiologists dealing with adults also describe a sizable portion of them as having pulmonary vascular disease.[55, 748] It also seems clear that in a number of cases the pulmonary vascular disease is relatively rapidly progressive. For this reason it has been assumed that the vascular disease in these patients, in contrast to that in children with ventricular septal defects, consists principally in intimal changes. Pathologic confirmation of this physiologic hypothesis is available (Fig. 251).

A further variant which should be mentioned is the association of atrial septal defect and a left-to-right shunt with mild pulmonary stenosis. The small gradient, usually less than 40 mm., across the pulmonary valve

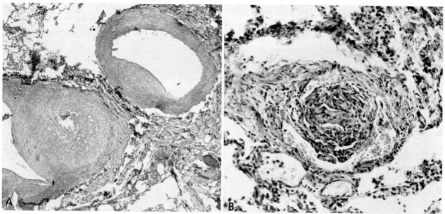

Figure 251. Severe pulmonary arteriolar changes in a patient with pulmonary vascular obstructive disease. Note the intimal and medial proliferation as well as the thrombotic changes. ($\times$ 65.)

in these instances is probably due to an unusually large amount of blood attempting to get through a normal pulmonary valve during systole, rather than to true anatomic stenosis. Additional anatomic reasons may be found in the hypertrophy of the right ventricular outflow tract with the creation of a real obstruction to flow and dilatation of the main pulmonary artery segment.

Clinical Picture

The most significant feature in the history of the majority of children with atrial septal defect is the discovery of a murmur. Usually this is not noted until the child is well past the neonatal period, and in some instances not until the patient is more than five years old. It has been proposed that the late discovery of the murmur may be due to the relatively small left-to-right shunt occurring through the defect in infancy. If the hypothesis, mentioned above, relative to the importance of the pressure-volume characteristic of the right ventricle in determining the size and magnitude of the atrial shunt is correct, one would not expect to encounter a large left-to-right shunt, as long as the right ventricle maintained its fetal characteristics. As indicated before (p. 347), since the complete changeover from fetal to adult circulation takes a matter of months and even years, the involution of the right ventricle cannot be expected to take place instantaneously either. The slow change in the electrocardiogram from the infant to the adult pattern attests to the validity of this statement. It follows, then, that large left-to-right shunts, for the reason stated, are rarely seen in infants, and even murmurs, depending on the size of the shunt, are not commonly encountered. One further reason for the late discovery of the murmur of atrial septal defect is that the ejection murmur is so similar to what used to be labeled a "functional" murmur that even if it is heard by the physician, it is probably not attributed to "organic" causes unless other evidences (cardiac enlargement) of heart disease are on hand.

The symptomatology of atrial septal defect in children varies. Some patients have no complaints at all, whereas in others varying degrees of

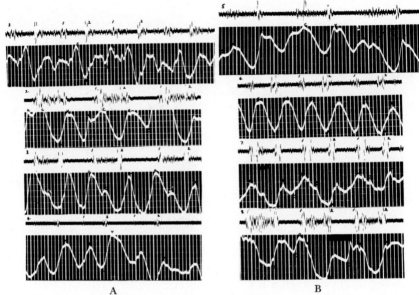

Figure 252. Phonocardiograms correlated with jugular venous pulse in eight cases of atrial septal defect. Note the systolic collapse in every instance and the tall V wave.[578]

exercise intolerance, episodes of right-sided congestive failure and frequent, severe respiratory infections are evident. As mentioned before, cyanosis is extremely rare beyond the newborn period, during which a transient right-to-left shunt, based on the relatively thick right ventricle, may indeed occur.

On physical examination these patients usually, though not invariably, appear thin and asthenic in build. The blood pressure is normal, with some tendency toward a narrow pulse pressure. The jugular venous pulse shows tall V waves preceded by a systolic collapse (Fig. 252). The liver may be palpable, but is not tender or pulsating. Left chest deformity is common. The cardiac impulse is hyperdynamic. It is maximal at the xiphoid process. A systolic thrill at the second left interspace indicates additional pulmonary stenosis. On auscultation, all patients with atrial septal defects have at least a systolic murmur, of ejection character, usually no more than grade 3 in intensity, and heard maximally at the second to third interspace, with poor transmission (Figs. 118, 137, pp. 116, 130). The origin of this systolic murmur is at the pulmonary valve, and it is due to the increased pulmonary flow. A harsh murmur at the lower left sternal border, sometimes increasing with inspiration, may be due to tricuspid regurgitation. If a secundum type of defect is associated with pulmonary stenosis, the typical stenotic murmur at the second left interspace will be the dominant feature.

Low-frequency diastolic murmurs (rumbles) are heard in all atrial septal defects in children with at least 2:1 pulmonary-systemic flow ratio. Usually these occur immediately beyond the second sound (Fig. 137, p. 130) and are best heard just at the lower left sternal border or near the apex. An early, high-frequency diastolic blow may be heard in patients who have an atrial defect associated with pulmonary vascular obstruction and pulmonary regurgitation (Fig. 135, p. 129).

The first heart sound is of average or high intensity, and is heard best at the apex. A variable click, common in patients with valvar pulmonic stenosis, is heard only rarely in uncomplicated secundum atrial septal defects. The second heart sound is always widely split (more than 0.05 second) at the second left interspace and is, as a rule, of normal intensity. Characteristically, the splitting does not increase with inspiration (Fig. 118). This "fixed" splitting of the second sound is one of the most important diagnostic clues of atrial septal defect. It distinguishes the murmur of atrial defect from a physiologic ejection murmur, and it also separates atrial septal defects with an appreciable flow from those in which the shunt is trivial. The splitting is due to delayed pulmonic closure, secondary either simply to the increased volume of blood the right ventricle has to eject or, as pro-

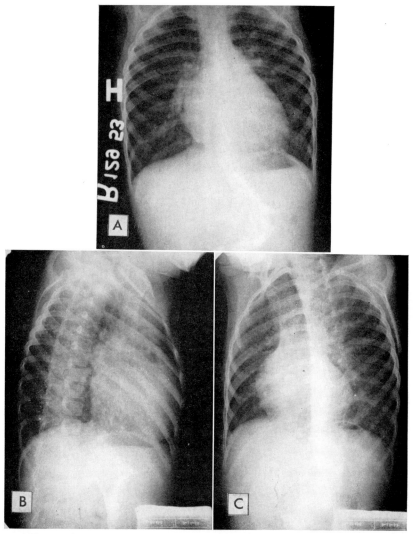

Figure 253. Typical atrial septal defect in posteroanterior, left anterior oblique and right anterior oblique views.

posed by Johnson,[364] to a specific delay in infundibular contraction. The "fixed" nature of the splitting is due to the single filling chamber with which both ventricles communicate; this common atrium responds to respiratory changes and influences systemic and pulmonary outputs in an identical fashion. A definitely accentuated second sound at the pulmonary area is heard only in children with pulmonary arterial hypertension. As previously mentioned, a third heart sound is heard commonly at the apex.

The roentgenologic findings are enlargement of the right side of the heart and enlargement and pulsation of the main stem and the small branches of the pulmonary artery (Fig. 253). The distribution of the pulmonary venous pattern, in contrast to normal, is such that the upper half carries as much blood as the lower half, or more.[364] The total cardiac size is in direct proportion to the size of the left-to-right shunt (Fig. 254), whereas the prominence and pulsations of the pulmonary vasculature do not have direct bearing on the size of the pulmonary blood flow. The enlargement of the right side of the heart involves the right atrium and the right ventricle to an equal degree. No isolated left atrial enlargement is present in uncomplicated atrial septal defect.

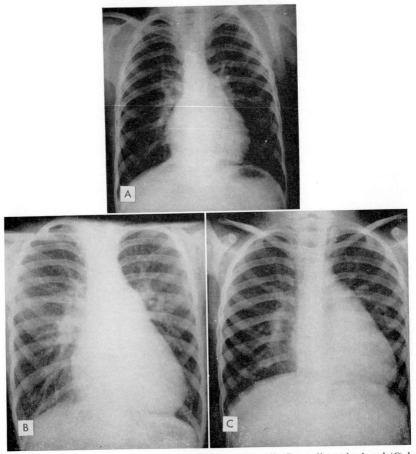

Figure 254. Posteroanterior views of patients with (*A*) small, (*B*) medium-sized and (*C*) large atrial septal defect.

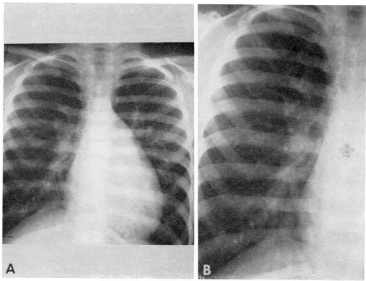

Figure 255. Typical roentgenogram of sinus venosus type of atrial septal defect. Note the characteristic right ventricular enlargement with pulmonary vascular engorgement seen in all atrial septal defects. Specific to this particular type is the absence of the shadow of the upper superior vena cava, the increase in the right hilar vessels (compared to the left), and, as is seen in the enlargement to the right, the horizontal pulmonary veins enter the upper cardiac shadow.

The sinus venosus defect may be recognized radiologically[202] (Fig. 255) by (1) the absence of the shadow of the superior vena cava high on the right side (the vessel being shifted to the left), (2) a localized bulge, indicating the entry of the right pulmonary vein into the superior vena cava, and (3) an apparent increase in the pulmonary vasculature of the right, as compared to the left, lung. This apparent increase in vasculature on the right side is due to the fact that the anomalous veins cross the pulmonary arterial pattern instead of running parallel to it.

The electrocardiogram shows an rsR′ pattern in aV_R and the right chest leads in practically all cases of atrial septal defect (Fig. 256). Prolonged P-R interval is noted in about 10 per cent of the children who have this anomaly. A significant degree of right ventricular hypertrophy with strain (indicating right ventricular hypertension) is an unusual feature of an uncomplicated foramen secundum defect, but may be encountered in cases complicated by pulmonary vascular obstruction or pulmonic stenosis.

The vectorcardiogram in ostium secundum atrial septal defect (Fig. 257) shows a clockwise rotation of the frontal plane with inferior orientation. The mean electrical axis is always between +30 and +170 degrees; in the majority of instances it is to the right of +90 degrees. The horizontal plane is usually anterior and inscribed clockwise. In most patients there is a terminal rightward and anterior force corresponding to the R′ inscription in the unipolar chest leads. A good correlation may be established between right and left ventricular work ratios and the dominance of the rightward and anterior forces.[431]

The findings at cardiac catheterization are as follows (Fig. 258):

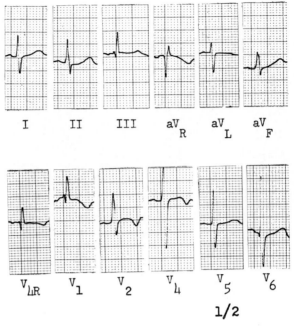

Figure 256.   Typical electrocardiogram of secundum atrial septal defect. Note the mean electrical axis of plus 105 degrees and the rsR′ pattern in aV_R, V_1 and V_2, and the deep S waves in V_5 and V_6.

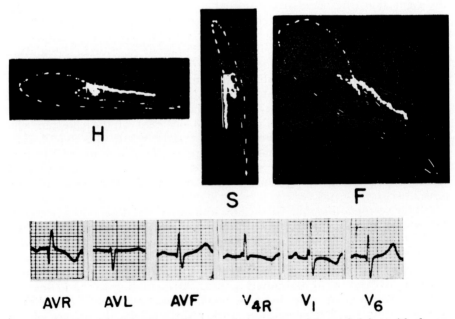

Figure 257.   Typical vectorcardiogram of secundum atrial septal defect with the corresponding unipolar leads below. Note the anterior rightward and inferiorly directed QRS loop, clockwise inscribed in the frontal plane and horizontal plane loop.

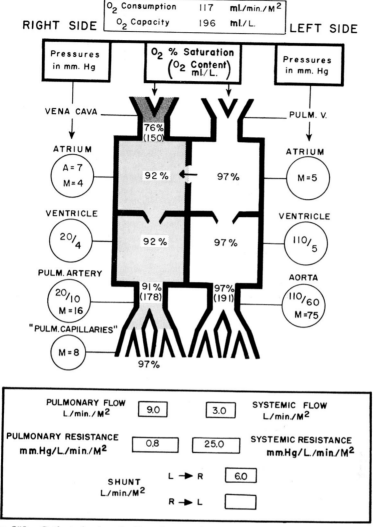

Figure 258. Catheterization findings in a patient with secundum atrial septal defect.

1. There is an increase in the oxygen content of the right atrium in the midlateral position over that of the superior vena cava. The magnitude of this jump in oxygen content is important. A 15 per cent increase, as a single observation, is significant; for a 10 per cent increase to be valid, I believe that at least 2 sets of observations may be necessary. It is almost completely useless to attempt to correlate the oxygen saturation of the inferior vena cava with that of the right atrium, because of the wide variety of values obtainable in the former location at varying times and at varying distances from the right atrium. In other words, in order to diagnose an atrial septal defect from oxygen saturation data, consecutive samples from the superior vena cava and the right atrium should be obtained. Difficulties may arise from pulmonary veins entering the superior vena cava and raising the saturation to a level indistinguishable from that

found in the right atrium (sinus venosus defect). Furthermore, occasionally, an excited adolescent with a high cardiac output, even without a pulmonary venous anomaly, may show superior vena cava saturation of 75 to 85 per cent. In these cases a shunt may be demonstrated only on exercise, when the superior vena cava saturation drops because of the widening of the arteriovenous difference, while pulmonary venous saturation is unchanged (see p. 155).

2. The pressures in the right side of the heart are usually within normal limits in children with ostium secundum defects, the chief abnormality being the frequent occurrence of tall V waves in the right atrium, giving rise to an M-shaped pattern with the A wave equal in height to the V wave, and an x and y depression (Fig. 259). Conversely, adults in their twenties or thirties may have more or less pulmonary arterial hypertension.

3. The pulmonary capillary pressure is normal.

4. Pulmonary resistance is low. There is no appreciable gradient between left atrial, or pulmonary capillary, and right atrial mean pressures if the defect is large (Fig. 160).

5. As a result of the large atrial shunt, the pulmonary blood flow becomes many times larger than the systemic flow; the smaller shunts have a pulmonary-systemic flow ratio of 2:1, whereas the larger ones may have a ratio of 4:1 or 5:1.

6. The peripheral arterial blood is usually more than 95 per cent saturated, except in patients with pulmonary vascular obstruction, pulmonic stenosis and low defects.

7. Occasionally the catheter may pass directly from the right atrium to the left atrium (Fig. 260), serving as presumptive evidence of an atrial septal defect. Usually this maneuver is easier to execute if the catheter is introduced through the inferior rather than the superior vena cava. It should also be reiterated that passage of the catheter through the atrial septum does not, by itself, indicate the presence of an atrial septal defect— it may simply demonstrate an anatomically, but not functionally, patent

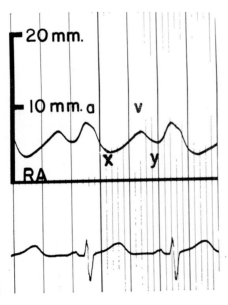

Figure 259. Characteristic right atrial tracing in patient with atrial septal defect. Note the M-shaped curve described by the A and V waves and the x and y depressions. The mean pressure in the right atrium is low.

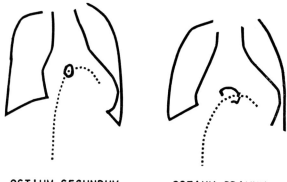

OSTIUM SECUNDUM   OSTIUM PRIMUM

Figure 260. The course of the catheter, schematically, through ostium secundum and ostium primum defects. Note the high crossing in the former and the low crossing in the latter. (M. H. Paul: Endocardial Cushion Defects. *Pediat. Clin. N. Amer.*, 5:1011, 1958.)

foramen ovale. The course of the catheter is relatively high across the atrial septum; this is of particular interest, in contrast with the low-lying endocardial cushion defect (Fig. 260).

8. Venous angiography, in our experience, is not a particularly useful tool in demonstrating the presence of an atrial defect; the dilution of the dye by the tremendous left-to-right shunt does not permit accurate visualization of the atria. Cine-angiography, with the catheter in the right atrium, also does not allow a right-to-left injection of the opaque medium. But contrast medium injected directly into the pulmonary artery will initially outline the left atrium and secondarily the right atrium through the atrial septal defect. In a second method the catheter is passed from the right to the left atrium with injection of the medium directly into the left atrium.

9. Indicator dilution curves clearly show a recirculation pattern, and a hydrogen electrode placed in the right atrium will register even minute left-to-right shunts. Injection of dye into the pulmonary veins, with sampling from the systemic artery, may uncover possible anomalous pulmonary venous connections.[85]

Course and Prognosis

The course of uncomplicated atrial septal defect depends on the size and the location of the opening. Apparently, small defects are tolerated without any difficulty for many years; as a matter of fact, they are compatible with normal life expectancy. Larger defects, with big left-to-right shunts, may cause trouble in two ways: (1) The large diastolic overloading may lead to congestive failure in early adulthood. (2) The persistently large pulmonary blood flow may lead to pulmonary vascular obstruction, in the late twenties or thirties. Once this appears, it is usually rapidly progressive and is accompanied by severe exertional dyspnea, diminution of the left-to-right shunt and the appearance of cyanosis.

As a rule, atrial defects are relatively well tolerated during infancy and childhood and almost never cause trouble. The average life expectancy of patients with atrial septal defects has been quoted as forty years,[82] but some live as long as seventy years. As a matter of fact, no statistically valid figures on the life expectancy of these patients is available at present. It is a fact that many asymptomatic patients in their fifties and sixties who have atrial septal defects are seen in the consultation rooms of my colleagues in internal medicine and cardiology.[384] Recently there have even been reports of surgery in these patients.[223]

Among the complications of atrial defect, rheumatic heart disease should be mentioned first. In our series it was present in sixteen of eighty cases seen at postmortem examination. Functionally significant mitral stenosis was present in seven (Lutembacher's syndrome). Bacterial endocarditis is unusually rare.[303] Atrial fibrillation does not occur in children with atrial septal defect, whereas Wood[746] found it in 10 to 20 per cent of his adult patients. The occurrence of pulmonary vascular obstruction in adults has already been discussed.

Differential Diagnosis

The following entities should be primarily considered in the differential diagnosis of atrial septal defect:

Rheumatic Heart Disease. Acquired mitral valve involvement and atrial septal defect may have several features in common. In both conditions, females are affected more frequently than males, the murmur is usually discovered late, systolic and diastolic murmurs are commonly heard at the apical or lower left sternal border, and the P-R interval may be prolonged. The presence of a basal systolic murmur, electrocardiographic evidence of an rsR' pattern, expansile pulsations of the hilar vessels on fluoroscopy and absence of isolated left atrial enlargement all point, however, toward an atrial septal defect. Often only cardiac catheterization can distinguish clearly between the two conditions.

Ventricular Septal Defect. A small ventricular septal defect with a harsh systolic murmur accompanied by a thrill at the lower left sternal border, together with electrocardiographic evidence of left ventricular dominance or hypertrophy and radiologic evidence of combined ventricular enlargement and a prominent left atrium, can easily be distinguished from an atrial septal defect. On the other hand, differentiation may be a great deal harder when there is a large ventricular septal defect with pulmonary arterial hypertension in which the systolic murmur is not so intense and the right ventricle dominates the picture in the electrocardiogram as well as in the roentgenogram. In this situation the evidence of pulmonary arterial hypertension, expressed in terms of a booming pulmonary closure, transient cyanosis and considerable right ventricular hypertrophy, as shown on the electrocardiogram, favors the diagnosis of a large ventricular septal defect.

Patent Ductus Arteriosus. The typical patent ductus arteriosus with its continuous machinery murmur, in which the electrocardiogram shows left ventricular dominance or hypertrophy and roentgenograms reveal left ventricular and left atrial enlargement, with a vigorously pulsating large aorta and pulmonary artery, is hard to confuse with an atrial septal defect. Conversely, an "atypical" patent ductus arteriosus, without a machinery murmur and with pulmonary hypertension, may present a difficult differential diagnostic problem which may be solved only by cardiac catheterization.

Transposition of the Pulmonary Veins. Complete transposition of the pulmonary veins commonly presents a picture readily distinguishable from atrial septal defect. These patients are prone to show congestive failure during infancy, and mild cyanosis is the rule. If, as is commonly the case, the veins enter the superior vena cava, the radiologic picture is pathognomonic as well.

Partial transposition of the pulmonary veins, on the other hand, may be indistinguishable from an atrial septal defect, even with the use of techniques such as cardiac catheterization and dye-dilution curves (see p. 736).

Trivial Pulmonic Stenosis. Pulmonary valve obstruction mild enough not to give rise to severe right ventricular hypertrophy or definitely ischemic lung fields may easily be confused with a small to moderately sized atrial septal defect. Occasionally the difference may be distinguished only at cardiac catheterization. Clinically, the heaving right ventricular impulse, the almost invariable presence of a systolic click, the relatively narrowly split second sound, which moves with respirations, and the harsher ejection murmur accompanied by a thrill all favor the diagnosis of pulmonic stenosis.

Treatment

One purpose of medical treatment of atrial septal defect is to bring congestive failure under control. The indication for anticongestive treatment is simply the presence of cardiac failure. Vigorous treatment along the lines previously indicated may often result in sustained improvement for several years.

In addition, it is important to try to prevent rheumatic fever in this group of patients. In view of their susceptibility to rheumatic infections, their respiratory diseases should be treated promptly and vigorously with antibiotics. Many cardiologists believe that continuous chemoprophylaxis should be recommended, similar to the regimen for patients with known rheumatic heart disease. I do not subscribe to this thesis.

The surgical closure of atrial septal defect was first proposed by Murray.[515] Other techniques have been successfully worked out by Bailey,[33] Gross,[313] Swan,[68] Brock,[92] Björk,[60] and others. In the Bailey technique, and its modifications, the defect is closed by suturing its lower edge to the top of the right atrium. In the Gross procedure, if the defect is small enough, it is sutured directly or through an atrial well; the larger ones are closed with a plastic sheet. The Swan operation is performed under direct vision in a bloodless field, under hypothermia. In Brock's technique, hypothermia is used only if the defect proves to the exploring finger to be too large to be sutured by one of the simpler techniques. In the Björk procedure the atrial defect is closed by a purse-string suture applied to the interatrial groove.

Within the last three or four years in our institution total cardiopulmonary bypass has been used for the correction of this defect. Our mortality rate, like that of other reputable clinics using a variety of techniques, has been in the neighborhood of 1 to 2 per cent. Obviously, the advantages of using the pump oxygenator for this purpose are (1) ample time to repair the defect and any complications and (2) good visualization. The disadvantages are (1) the difficulty of blood procurement and (2) the inherent dangers of bypass, with opportunities for bleeding, inadequate output, overtransfusion, and damage to the central nervous system. With all these pros and cons, I think that, in an institution with a good blood program, where cardiopulmonary bypass is used daily for a number of purposes, this is probably the ideal mode of repair. Contrariwise, in another center where the pump oxygenator is not used with the same frequency, and where difficulties may be encountered with the blood bank, probably hypothermia is the best approach to the problem.

The best operative risk today is a patient in his early teens or twenties who has a large foramen secundum defect with no complications; patients in congestive heart failure and those with high pulmonary resistance present higher than average risks. At present pulmonary vascular obstruction leading to a right-to-left shunt probably indicates an inoperable situation. Arterial unsaturation without pulmonary vascular obstruction, based on the anatomy of the defect, does not significantly increase the operative risk.

On the basis of these considerations, patients with an uncomplicated

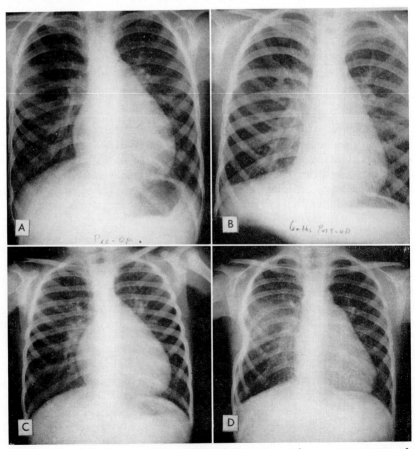

Figure 261. *A* and *C,* Preoperative and, *B* and *D,* postoperative roentgenograms of two patients with closure of atrial septal defect.[82]

Pre-Operative

Apex
2 LIS

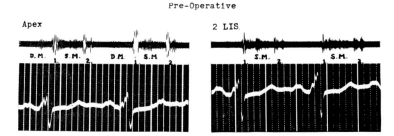

Post-Operative

Apex
2 LIS

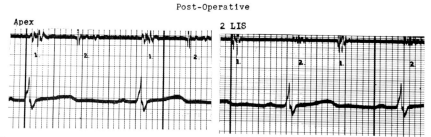

Figure 262. Preoperative and postoperative phonocardiograms in patient with closure of atrial septal defect.

secundum defect and a large (at least 2:1) left-to-right shunt should be considered candidates for operation. Surgery for a patient who has an atrial septal defect with pulmonary vascular obstruction should be undertaken only with full cognizance of the high risks, which, however, may not be insurmountable.[49] Patients with a net right-to-left shunt, however, should not be subjected to surgery. For the time being, a patient who has less than a 2:1 pulmonary systemic ratio, with or without pulmonary arterial hypertension, is not considered a suitable candidate for operation.

The results of successful surgical closure of an atrial septal defect are gratifying, indeed. The heart diminishes in size (Fig. 261), exercise tolerance increases, and congestive failure is no longer present. Systolic and diastolic murmurs diminish or even completely disappear (Fig. 262). The second sound is now normally split and moves with respirations, unless complete right bundle branch block develops postoperatively. At postoperative cardiac catheterization the pulmonary flow equals the systemic flow. In some cases, however, fluoroscopy reveals a persistent hilar dance for some months, and the electrocardiogram may remain unaltered.

The postoperative course of these children is usually uneventful. Atrial fibrillation may develop in older patients; usually it responds well to digitalis and quinidine within a few days or a week. Occasionally after operation the arrhythmia of a patient cannot be converted to sinus rhythm immediately. Fortunately, as a rule, after a six-week period of digitalis treatment at home, such patients are found to have regular sinus rhythm. The incidence of the postpericardiotomy syndrome among our patients is between 10 and 15 per cent.

We have seen three patients in whom closure of a secundum atrial septal defect resulted in the enclosure of the inferior vena cava in the left atrium and the consequent development of cyanosis, postoperatively. Re-operation within a week or two is indicated.

Summary

Atrial septal defect should be considered in the diagnosis of all patients with a left-to-right shunt and an rsR' pattern in the electrocardiogram. Auscultatory, electrocardiographic and radiologic data may distinguish between ostium secundum and ostium primum defects. Cardiac catheterization reveals a significant increase in oxygen content in the right atrium, normal right ventricular pressure and large pulmonary blood flow. Patients with an uncomplicated ostium secundum lesion, with a large shunt, should be considered candidates for operation. In carefully selected cases the mortality rate is less than 2 per cent.

ENDOCARDIAL CUSHION DEFECTS (OSTIUM PRIMUM ATRIAL SEPTAL DEFECTS)

Congenital cardiac abnormalities resulting from defective fusion of the endocardial cushions and the interatrial and interventricular septums are referred to as "endocardial cushion defects." Depending on the severity of the abnormality, I shall distinguish between complete and incomplete endocardial cushion defects. In the former no separation of the tricuspid and mitral rings exists, whereas in the latter group two separate valve rings are found.

Anatomy

The most common manifestation of the *complete* endocardial cushion defect is the so-called common atrioventricular canal, in which a large, low atrial defect lies directly, without a lower rim, over the common atrio-ventricular valve ring and is contiguous with a ventricular defect of variable size. There is a large cleft in the anterior leaflet of the mitral valve and in the septal leaflet of the tricuspid valve, so that common anterior and posterior atrioventricular cusps serve both ventricles.

The *partial* endocardial cushion defect is known as an ostium primum defect and consists of the characteristically situated large atrial septal defect almost always with a mitral cleft and more or less involvement of the tricuspid valve. Two separate valve rings may be identified, and the ventricular septum is intact.

Two other variations of partial endocardial cushion defect will be discussed elsewhere (see p. 415). One is a ventricular septal defect in the endocardial cushion defect position (posterior and not extending beyond the papillary muscle of the conus, with the superior edge behind the septal leaflet of the tricuspid valve). Viewed from the left ventricle, these defects do not lie directly beneath the aortic valve leaflet.[533] The second is congenital mitral regurgitation secondary to a cleft mitral valve without a septal defect.[679] Edwards[214] described an interesting and surgically important attribute of the cleft mitral valve within this syndrome: namely, short chordae tendineae connecting the cleft valve to the interventricular septum and, thus, contributing further to the degree of mitral regurgitation.

Among Evans's fifty patients there were twenty-seven with incomplete and twenty-three with complete atrioventricular canals.[232] Among the twenty-seven patients in whom the endocardial cushion defect was of the incomplete variety, three had no atrioventricular clefts, fifteen had mitral clefts only, six had mitral and tricuspid clefts, and in three there was a common atrium with a mitral cleft.

In both the complete and incomplete types the atrioventricular node and the bundle of His may be interrupted, either congenitally or by progressive fibrosis.

The enlargement of the right ventricle, right atrium and pulmonary artery in patients with these defects is accompanied by left ventricular and left atrial enlargement, probably secondary to the mitral regurgitation. As a rule, the aorta is small.

Physiology

A patient with a partial endocardial cushion defect may show physiologic characteristics indistinguishable from those seen in patients with a large secundum atrial septal defect: namely, a sizable left-to-right shunt with normal pulmonary arterial pressure. More often, however, mitral regurgitation is present as well, contributing left ventricular volume work to the physiologic profile. Patients with the complete form of endocardial cushion defect combine the features of left-to-right shunt at the ventricular and atrial levels with those of atrioventricular valve regurgitation and, commonly, pulmonary vascular obstruction. Because of the latter phenomenon, the atrial and ventricular shunts are usually bidirectional.

Clinical Picture

The association of mongolism with endocardial cushion defects is well known. From the cardiac viewpoint, depending on the severity of the anatomic and physiologic derangements, a variety of clinical profiles may be encountered. We have seen strapping, athletic adolescent boys, who were essentially asymptomatic, with a good-sized ostium primum defect and trivial mitral regurgitation. At the other end of the spectrum is the maximally underdeveloped young infant with a common atrioventricular canal, in chronic congestive heart failure, with early cyanosis. Surely, on the whole, the patients with endocardial cushion defects show signs and symptoms of heart disease much earlier than those who have a simple secundum atrial septal defect. It is probably the murmur of mitral regurgitation that draws the attention of the pediatrician to the heart, even in infants with relatively innocuous defects. The infantile pressure-volume characteristics of the right ventricle, so effective in masking secundum atrial septal defects, cannot obviate mitral regurgitation.

On physical examination, tricuspid regurgitation may be discovered by inspecting the jugular venous pulse. Here, instead of the M-shaped pattern seen with secundum atrial septal defects, the A wave is considerably overshadowed by the V wave. The cardiac impulse encompasses the right and the left ventricle, the former dominating in patients with pulmonary vascular obstruction and the latter in those with mitral regurgitation. There is left chest deformity. The size of the liver and its pulsatile nature depend on the presence or absence of congestive heart failure and the involvement of the tricuspid valve. The peripheral pulses are not remarkable.

On auscultation (Fig. 263) the first sound at the apex may be loud. The second sound is well split, and if the left-to-right atrial shunt is sizable, the splitting is "fixed." The pulmonic closure may be accentuated if pulmonary vascular obstruction is present; clearly, this will occur in patients in whom the splitting is relatively narrow. A loud third sound is heard at the apex. In addition to the pulmonic ejection murmur, secondary to the large pulmonary flow, a loud murmur of mitral regurgitation is also heard at the apex. It is hard to distinguish the murmur of tricuspid regurgitation in these cases, but occasionally a pansystolic murmur at the lower left sternal border, increasing in intensity with inspiration, suggests the presence of tricuspid incompetence. An early and mid-diastolic rumble heard at the lower left sternal border and the apex originates at the mitral or the tricuspid valve. In contrast to children with pure secundum atrial septal defects, systolic and diastolic thrills may be felt at the apex and the lower left sternal border in more than half of these patients.

In the roentgenograms, in addition to enlargement of the right ventricle and the right atrium, left ventricular and left atrial enlargement is present in varying degrees, depending on the anatomic situation. The degree of pulmonary vascular engorgement depends on the size of the left-to-right shunt (Fig. 264). *Severe and progressive cardiomegaly may be seen with this defect at an early age* (Fig. 265).

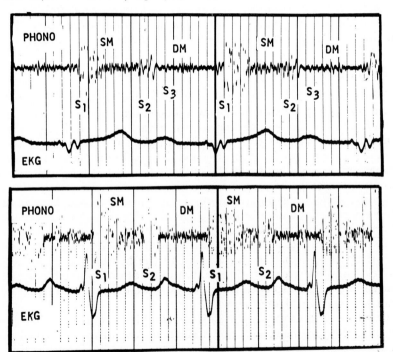

Figure 263. Phonocardiogram in patient with endocardial cushion defect. The upper tracing is obtained at the second left interspace, and the lower at the apex. Note the low frequency, low intensity systolic murmur at the second left interspace with the widely split second sound, third sound and diastolic murmur. In the lower tracing note the murmur of mitral regurgitation and a diastolic flow murmur.

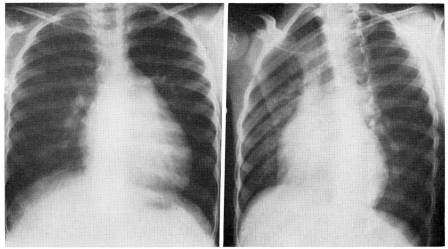

Figure 264. Posteroanterior and left anterior oblique views of the heart of a patient with a sizable endocardial cushion defect. Note the cardiac enlargement involving both ventricles, the prominent pulmonary artery segment, the narrow aorta and pulmonary vascular engorgement.

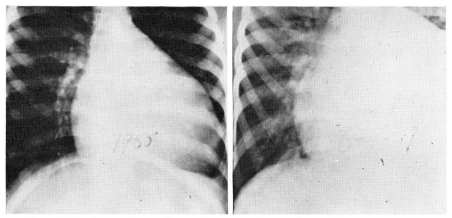

Figure 265. Progressive cardiac enlargement in a patient with endocardial cushion defect. The posteroanterior film on the left was obtained in 1955, and the film on the right in 1957. Shortly after the latter film had been taken the child died in congestive failure.

The electrocardiogram is one of the most important diagnostic clues to the abnormality. A mean electrical axis superior to 0 degrees, and most of the time to the left of —30 degrees, is a sine qua non of the diagnosis. An rsR' pattern with a relatively taller R than occurs in a secundum atrial septal defect is present in aV_R and the right chest leads. In addition, evidences of left ventricular hypertrophy may be obtained from aV_L and the left chest leads. The P-R interval is prolonged in more than 50 per cent of the patients, and the P waves often indicate atrial hypertrophy. It may be emphasized that patients with the *complete* form of endocardial cushion defect are more likely to have mean axes to the right of —90 degrees and also to have taller R waves in the right chest leads, as an expression of pulmonary arterial hypertension (Fig. 266).

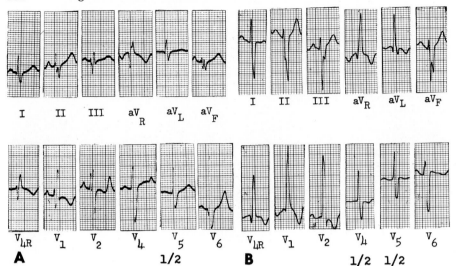

Figure 266. The electrocardiogram in endocardial cushion defect. *A,* Axis minus 45 degrees and rsR' pattern in V_{4R} and V_1. This is characteristic of the incomplete form of the disease without pulmonary vascular obstruction. *B,* Axis minus 105 degrees and chest leads show right ventricular hypertrophy. This tracing is from a patient with a complete form of endocardial cushion defect, with pulmonary vascular obstruction. Note that in both instances the frontal plane loop is counterclockwise.

In the vectorcardiogram the frontal plane is inscribed in a counterclockwise direction. The forces are principally superiorly and anteriorly directed. Usually, but not invariably, the horizontal plane is inscribed clockwise, and a terminal rightward and anterior force is noted (R') (Fig. 267). The vectorcardiogram here, as in the secundum atrial defects, correlates well with the right and left ventricular work ratios.

It may be stated without much hesitation that the left axis deviation and the counterclockwise frontal plane loop do not depend on the presence or absence of mitral regurgitation, but rather on a conduction defect.[697, 698]

Cardiac catheterization reveals the following (Fig. 268): (1) There is an increase in oxygen content at the right atrial and right ventricular levels. The size of the oxygen jump in percentiles may not be used as an index of the relative size of the shunt at the atrial and ventricular levels. To begin with, an increase from 80 to 85 per cent is much more significant than an increase from 70 to 75 per cent. Also, tricuspid regurgitation, as well as streaming, may confuse the issue. Consequently it is best to calculate the size of the total shunt on the basis of the difference between the oxygen content of the superior vena cava and that of the pulmonary artery and to attempt to localize the dominant element by other methods (cineangiography, dye dilution curves). (2) If the atrial defect is of appreciable size, left atrial or pulmonary capillary mean pressures are identical with right atrial pressures. On the whole, these pressures are higher than they are in children with secundum defects, probably because of the mitral regurgitation. Also, the V waves may be more dominant for the same reason. Pulmonary arterial and right ventricular pressures are significantly elevated in patients with the *complete* form of endocardial cushion defect. (3) Pulmonary capillary and left atrial pressure pulses (Fig. 269), as well

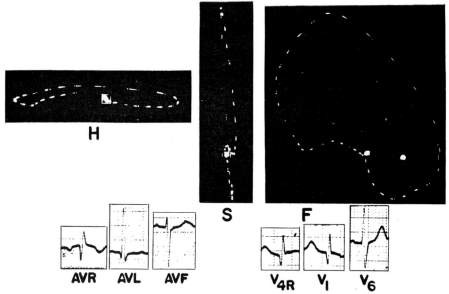

Figure 267. Typical vectorcardiogram of incomplete form of endocardial cushion defect. Note the superiorly directed loop in the sagittal plane and the counterclockwise loop in the horizontal and frontal planes. Note also that the areas to the left and the right are about equal in the horizontal plane loop.

as left ventricular tracings, may show evidences of mitral regurgitation. (4) Usually the pulmonary resistance is normal in patients with simple ostium primum defects. In contrast, those with the *complete* atrioventricular canal almost invariably show evidences of pulmonary vascular obstruction. About 20 per cent of the children who have endocardial cushion defects have pulmonary resistances higher than 3 units. (5) Maximal pulmonary flows, resulting in pulmonary systemic flow ratios of 4:1 or more, are not commonly seen in patients with endocardial cushion defects. The involvement of the left ventricle and the mitral valve and the pathophysiology of the defect, as well as the increased pulmonary resistance, contribute to this fact. Even with severe cardiac enlargement the pulmonary flow usually is not much larger than three times the systemic flow. (6) The arterial oxygen saturation in patients with a *complete* atrioventricular canal is usually less than 90 per cent. This, of course, parallels the arterial oxygen saturation in the presence of a ventricular defect and pulmonary vascular obstruction. As a rule, the arterial blood of children with simple ostium primum abnormalities is fully saturated. Infants with severe forms of endocardial cushion defects, in cardiac failure, may have pulmonary venous unsaturation, which, in turn, contributes to the low saturation of the arterial blood as well. (7) The passage of the catheter through the atrial septal defect characteristically takes a low course in these patients (Fig. 260). Frequently a direct communication between the right atrium and the left ventricle may be demonstrated. Withdrawal of the catheter from the left ventricle to the right ventricle, without an intervening atrial tracing, does not prove the presence of a complete canal. (8) Selective cine-angiography, using pulmonary arterial, left atrial or left ventricular injection, is useful in demonstrating the left-to-right atrial or ventricular shunt. Left

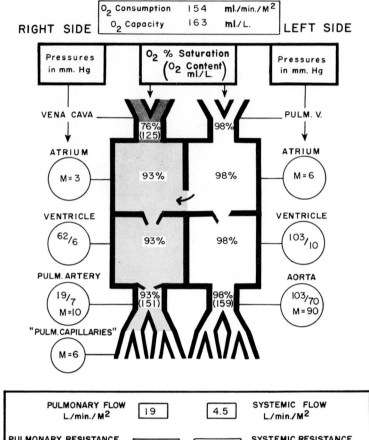

Figure 268. Catheterization findings in a patient with endocardial cushion defect.

ventricular injection of a radiopaque medium is a good method for demonstrating the presence of mitral regurgitation. (9) Dye dilution curves, with injection into the superior vena cava or right atrium and sampling from the systemic artery, show evidences of recirculation. It is interesting that, in contrast to secundum atrial septal defects, there is no preferential left-to-right shunting from the right pulmonary veins, since the ostium primum defect is situated low in the atrial septum.

A right-to-left shunt at the atrial or ventricular level may also be demonstrated by dye dilution methods in most patients with a complete atrioventricular canal.

Finally, mitral regurgitation may be assessed, but probably not quantitatively, by injecting cardio-green into the left ventricle and sampling from the left atrium.

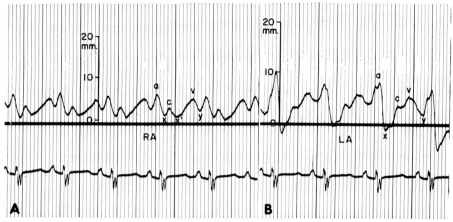

Figure 269.   Pressure tracings in a patient with endocardial cushion defect.

Course and Prognosis

No accurate information is available as to the life expectancy of pa-tients with endocardial cushion defects. As a matter of fact, probably no accurate estimation is ever possible about an abnormality covering the wide spectrum from ostium primum to complete atrioventricular canal. Yet certain generalizations may be safely made. (1) On the whole, the life expectancy of these patients is definitely shorter than that of those with a secundum atrial septal defect. Although occasionally a patient with an endocardial cushion defect may live to be thirty or forty years old, this is rare. Children with the complete form of endocardial cushion defect usually show evidences of congestive heart failure in infancy and may die within the first few years of life; even those with the most favorable course show fatigue, dyspnea, underdevelopment and some cyanosis by the time they enter their teens. At the other end of the spectrum are those with the simple primum defects, with only minimal mitral regurgitation; such a patient may be completely asymptomatic through puberty, although the heart is big. Even these patients almost invariably have symptoms when they reach their twenties. Between these two extremes are the patients with a sizable ostium primum defect and significant mitral regurgitation. (2) Once congestive heart failure and progressive cardiomegaly are noted, the course may be rapidly downhill. I have seen deterioration in the clini-cal condition of patients between the ages of five and ten years (Fig. 265). (3) As mentioned earlier, pulmonary vascular disease is two to three times as frequent in this group as it is in children with secundum atrial septal defect. This, in addition to the right and left ventricular volume work, contributes to the early appearance of cardiac failure in these patients. Atrial fibrillation is common in patients beyond their teens.

Differential Diagnosis

Rheumatic Heart Disease.   This may be confused even more easily with endocardial cushion defects than with secundum atrial septal defects because of the almost invariable presence of the murmur of mitral regurgitation. Nevertheless the electrocardiographic features of the disease, together with the characteristics of the second sound and the early appearance of the murmur, usually enable the physician to make the diagnosis on clinical grounds alone.

Secundum Atrial Septal Defect. Secundum atrial defects may be differentiated from endocardial cushion defects on the basis of the electrocardiographic findings, the murmur of mitral regurgitation, and the manifestation of left ventricular involvement in the physical examination and the roentgenograms. It should be mentioned that, occasionally in a child with a secundum atrial septal defect and a stocky build, a mean electrical axis of —15 and even —30 degrees (but with a clockwise frontal plane loop) may be seen. The early appearance of evidences of heart disease, as well as the severity of the manifestations, tends to favor the diagnosis of endocardial cushion defect. Finally, pulmonary vascular obstruction is much more common in children with endocardial cushion defects than in patients with secundum atrial septal defects. The differences at cardiac catheterization have been discussed in detail (see p. 388).

Ventricular Septal Defect. Although a mean electrical axis of 0 to —30 degrees may be found in approximately 10 per cent of the patients with ventricular septal defect, an axis to the left of —30 degrees should raise a strong suspicion of an endocardial cushion defect. The murmur of mitral regurgitation favors the diagnosis of endocardial cushion defect, though it may be observed in patients with large ventricular septal defects, as well. Absence of a significant apical systolic murmur makes the diagnosis of endocardial cushion defect rather unlikely. At catheterization the oxygen data are perhaps the least helpful in the differential diagnosis; dye dilution curves, cine-angiograms and the demonstration of a significant pressure gradient from left atrium to right atrium provide the most helpful physiologic data.

Complete Transposition of the Pulmonary Veins. The clinical picture of complete transposition of the pulmonary veins may imitate that of endocardial cushion defect, but the electrocardiogram in the former is invariably one of right axis deviation with a clockwise frontal plane loop.

Complete Transposition of the Great Arteries. A patient with complete transposition of the great arteries and a large pulmonary flow may have congestive heart failure in infancy and only moderate arterial unsaturation. The electrocardiogram also may be similar to that seen in endocardial cushion defect, with left axis deviation and a counterclockwise frontal plane loop. Occasionally, only the arterial saturation data or angiography, demonstrating the abnormal relation of the great arteries, can reveal the correct diagnosis.

Treatment

Surgical treatment of endocardial cushion defect has been possible only since the advent of total cardiopulmonary bypass. Our own experience indicates that the immediate surgical mortality rate is approximately 10 per cent in patients with the *incomplete* form of the anomaly.[624] In contrast, surgical repair of the *complete* form of endocardial cushion defect carries a risk of about 50 per cent at present.

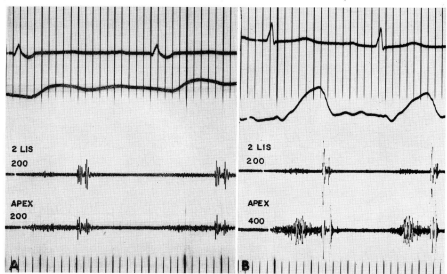

Figure 270. Postoperative phonocardiograms in patients with endocardial cushion defect. *A,* Note the absence of any significant murmur. The second sound is still split, but it moved with respirations. *B,* Persistent apical systolic murmur and variable split of second sound.

Among the survivors, the septal defect is closed with a high degree of accuracy. Residual mitral regurgitation, evidenced by the persistence of an apical systolic murmur, is found in most (Fig. 270). Hemodynamically significant mitral regurgitation, characterized by left atrial enlargement in the roentgenogram and P mitrale in the electrocardiogram, could be found in only 20 per cent of those with apical systolic murmurs.

Preoperative factors contributing significantly to the mortality seem to be (*a*) congestive heart failure, (*b*) increased pulmonary resistance, and (*c*) cardiac enlargement. Preoperative and postoperative anticongestive measures are indicated for most of these patients. Heart block may occur in the postoperative course, and it carries an ominous prognostic significance. Avoidance of heart block is mandatory for successful repair of endocardial cushion defect. Patients whose mitral regurgitation has not been alleviated by surgery, but whose atrial septal defect has been closed, may also have a stormy postoperative course. It is assumed that the blood, regurgitating through the incompetent mitral valve, now has to be accommodated in a relatively smaller left atrial chamber; this may lead to increased left atrial pressure, pulmonary edema and death. It is the possibility of this complication that should lead the surgeon to be particularly meticulous about the closure of the cleft mitral valve and the repair of the accessory chordae attaching the mitral valve to the ventricular septum.

Successful repair of endocardial cushion defect leads to considerable symptomatic improvement, diminished heart size (Fig. 271) and increase in weight. The electrocardiogram may not change significantly, though complete right bundle branch block is commonly observed. The mean electrical axis is not changed postoperatively, proving that this represents a conduction disturbance, rather than the results of mitral regurgitation.

I believe that all patients with endocardial cushion defects should be

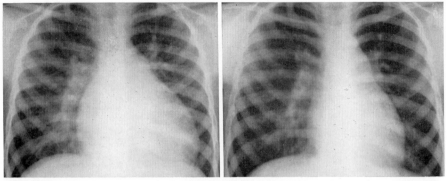

Figure 271. Postoperative improvement in the roentgenogram of a patient with endocardial cushion defect.

treated surgically, preferably between the ages of five and ten years. The
hemodynamic abnormality is severe enough and the downhill course often
precipitous enough to warrant early intervention. Surgery early in infancy
may be unavoidable in patients with a particularly severe variety of complete endocardial cushion defect.

Summary

Endocardial cushion defect should be considered the first diagnostic
probability in patients with a left-to-right shunt, severe left axis deviation
with a counterclockwise frontal plane loop, and an rsR' pattern in the
chest leads. Clinically, in addition to a left-to-right atrial shunt, there are
almost always evidences of mitral regurgitation. Infants with the *complete*
form of endocardial cushion defect are often cyanotic, have severe congestive heart failure and are underdeveloped. In contrast, in patients with
a *simple ostium primum* lesion, the symptoms may be all but indistinguishable from those of a secundum atrial septal defect. Many patients are
between these two extremes. Surgery, by means of cardiopulmonary bypass,
is recommended for patients between the ages of five and ten years, or
earlier if signs and symptoms warrant it.

SINGLE ATRIUM

This is a rare anomaly. Only about half a dozen cases have been encountered through the years in our institution. At the Mayo Clinic five cases
were encountered in a three-year period;[224] an additional eight cases have
been collected from the literature. It is the anomaly most commonly seen
with the Ellis van Creveld syndrome. Taussig[683] mentioned that it is frequently associated with isolated dextrocardia and levocardia with abdominal situs inversus.

Anatomy

This has been referred to as cor triloculare biventriculare, a heart
without a vestige of an atrial septum, but with two atrial appendages.
Associated clefts may be present in the atrioventricular valves, or a com-

mon atrioventricular canal may even be seen. In rare instances both the atrial and the ventricular septa are absent (cor biloculare; see Single Ventricle, p. 401).

Physiology

Usually the shunt in the common atrium is dominantly left to right, but a simultaneous right-to-left shunt exists also. The relative magnitude of the shunt depends mostly on the relation of the pulmonary to the systemic resistance. Irrespective of the size of the left-to-right and right-to-left shunts, the oxygen saturations in the two atria, ventricles, the aorta and the pulmonary artery are almost identical. It is important, however, to emphasize that, in contrast to complete transposition of the pulmonary veins, pulmonary arterial saturation here is *almost never higher* than systemic arterial saturation.

Clinical Picture

Some of these patients, like infants with complete endocardial cushion defects, have evidences of severe congestive heart failure early. Others gradually show dyspnea on exertion, fatigue, and some cyanosis. The symptomatology is similar to the spectrum seen in endocardial cushion defects and complete transposition of the pulmonary veins.

On physical examination these children usually have evidences of a large left-to-right shunt. The cardiac impulse is hyperkinetic, and there is left-sided (or in dextrocardia, right-sided) chest deformity. The cardiac impulse is most powerful at the xiphoid process, though an apical impulse may also be present. Cyanosis is noted, but is usually mild. The liver may be enlarged and pulsatile. A thrill at the apex is common. On auscultation

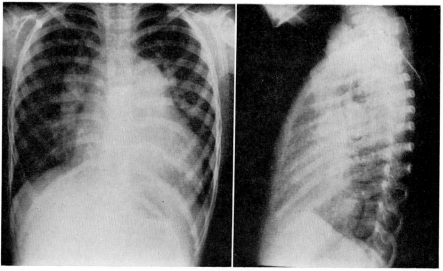

Figure 272. Posteroanterior and lateral films of a patient with a single atrium. Note the combined ventricular enlargement, pulmonary vascular engorgement and prominent main pulmonary artery segment.

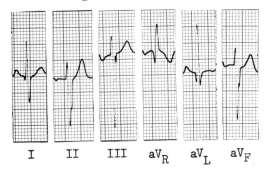

I   II   III   aV$_R$ aV$_L$ aV$_F$

Figure 273. Electrocardiogram of a patient with a single atrium and pulmonary arterial hypertension. Note the mean electrical axis at plus or minus 180, with a counterclockwise frontal plane loop, and the right ventricular hypertrophy in the chest leads.

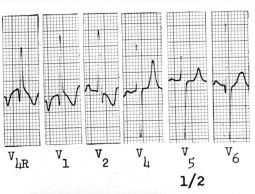

V$_{4R}$ V$_1$ V$_2$ V$_4$ V$_5$ V$_6$

1/2

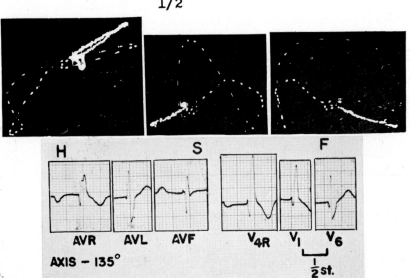

H   S   F

AVR   AVL   AVF   V$_{4R}$ V$_1$ V$_6$

AXIS – 135° $\frac{1}{2}$ st.

Figure 274. Vectorcardiogram of a patient with a single atrium and mitral and tricuspid regurgitation. Note the close similarity of the vector loops as well as of the unipolar electrocardiograms in this defect and endocardial cushion defect.

the first sound is usually loud; the pulmonary closure may or may not be accentuated, depending on the state of the pulmonary vasculature. The second sound shows fixed splitting, though on the whole this is less obvious than it is in patients with simple secundum atrial septal defects. A third sound is heard at the apex. In addition to the pulmonic ejection murmur of a large atrial septal defect, apical murmurs of mitral regurgitation may also be noted, as well as an early or mid-diastolic flow rumble. Roentgenologic examination reveals right atrial and right ventricular enlargement (Fig. 272) with pulmonary vascular engorgement. Dextrocardia or abdominal situs inversus may be noted. The main pulmonary artery may be prominent.

The electrocardiogram is similar to that seen in endocardial cushion defect, with left axis deviation, a counterclockwise loop in the frontal plane, and a rsR' pattern in the right chest leads and aV_R (Figs. 273, 274).

At *cardiac catheterization* the following observations may be made (Fig. 275). (1) There is a large increase in oxygen saturation at the right atrial level, resulting in practically complete mixing of the blood at this point. All four chambers of the heart and the two great arteries have about an equal

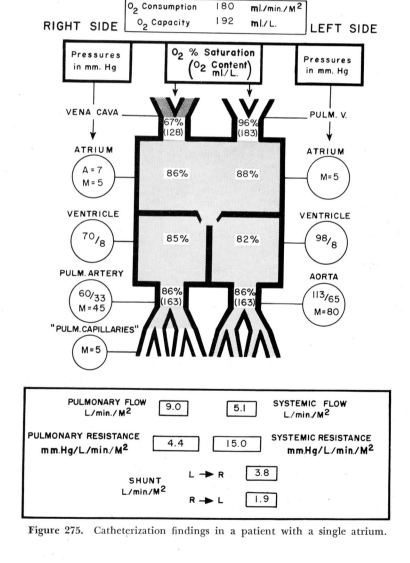

Figure 275. Catheterization findings in a patient with a single atrium.

percentage of oxygen saturation. As mentioned earlier, pulmonary arterial saturation is never higher than systemic arterial saturation (80 to 90 per cent). (2) There is slight elevation of atrial pressures, without an appreciable gradient between right and left atrial or pulmonary capillary pressures. Right ventricular and pulmonary arterial pressures may or may not be elevated. Systemic arterial pressures are normal. (3) Pulmonary resistance may or may not be elevated, but the pulmonary capillary pressure is usually normal. (4) Pulmonary flow is large, three to four times the systemic flow. (5) The course of the catheter across the atrial septum is similar to that seen in patients with endocardial cushion defect. (6) Cine-angiograms demonstrate the large pulmonary artery in the normal position. The left-to-right shunt at the atrial level may be seen best with injection into the pulmonary artery or left atrium. Left ventricular injection may reveal mitral regurgitation. On the whole, neither angiography nor dye dilution curves are particularly helpful in differentiating a common atrium from a large endocardial cushion defect. Identical contours of dye curves may be obtained with injection into the right and left heart chambers, the pulmonary artery and the pulmonary vein, but the appearance time is appreciably shorter with injection into the right atrium than into the right ventricle.

Course and Prognosis

The life expectancy of these patients depends less on the nature of the atrial septal defect than on the status of the pulmonary vasculature and the associated anomalies of the atrioventricular valve. Thus the general rules discussed in the section on endocardial cushion defects (see p. 391) hold for these patients as well. Because of the associated anomalies and the relatively frequent occurrence of pulmonary vascular obstruction in these patients, the outlook is appreciably poorer than it is for children with secundum atrial septal defects.

Differential Diagnosis

The conditions discussed in connection with endocardial cushion defects should be considered in the diagnosis of single atrium, also, with the exception that rheumatic heart disease and simple secundum defects usually are not considered seriously, because of the cyanosis. On the other hand, ventricular septal defect, complete transposition of pulmonary veins, complete transposition of the great arteries, mitral or tricuspid atresia and endocardial cushion defect should be excluded in every instance. The discussion of ventricular septal defect in the differential diagnosis of endocardial cushion defect is completely valid here (see p. 392).

Complete transposition of pulmonary veins should be excluded electrocardiographically by right axis deviation, though the presence of dextrocardia may render this rather difficult. Complete transposition of the arteries should be excluded angiographically and by establishing the fact that the oxygen saturation of the pulmonary arteries is never higher than that of the systemic arteries.

Finally, when a patient with endocardial cushion defect has, physiologically, a single atrium, differentiation is almost a matter of semantics.

If the oxygen saturation in all four chambers of the heart and the great arteries is essentially the same, I usually assume, for practical purposes, that no atrial septum is present.

Treatment

Successful surgical treatment of common atrium has been described. A new polyvinyl septum is created and inserted. Of five patients operated on for this condition, Ellis[224] reported four survivors. Indications for surgery are the same as those outlined for cushion defects. Operation, by means of the pump oxygenator, should be contemplated when the patient is between five and ten years of age, or sooner if the signs and symptoms warrant it. I would like to stress, however, that in spite of the encouraging results reported by the Mayo group, not enough patients have been operated on so far to render mortality statistics meaningful. For this reason, in addition to the complex associated anomalies and the probable presence of pulmonary vascular obstructive disease, I believe that at present probably a mortality rate of 50 per cent or more should be quoted.

Summary

Patients with a large bidirectional atrial shunt resulting in identical oxygen saturations in all four chambers and both great arteries may have, physiologically and anatomically, a single atrium. The endocardial cushion defect type of electrocardiogram differentiates this anatomic entity from complete transposition of the pulmonary veins, which may give rise to a similar physiologic picture. Surgery is indicated as long as a dominant left-to-right shunt is present, but the risks are probably high.

INTERVENTRICULAR COMMUNICATIONS

Incidence

On the basis of clinical observations, ventricular septal defect was always thought to be the most frequent type of congenital heart disease. This is not true in all series. Ventricular septal defect was fifth in frequency in Paul Wood's series.[745] On the other hand, Keith did find this to be the most frequent single lesion in his series, occurring in 22 per cent of the children with congenital heart disease. In our clinic this is the commonest lesion, amounting to almost 20 per cent. If, however, complications of ventricular septal defect, with pulmonary stenosis as well as pulmonary vascular obstruction (tetralogy of Fallot and Eisenmenger's disease), are grouped together, then it is indeed the most common congenital malformation, not only in Keith's[380] and our series, but also in Wood's[745] and Abbott's.[1]

Anatomy

The defects of the ventricular septum vary in size from 0.5 to 3.0 cm. in diameter.

The development of the ventricular septum has already been discussed briefly. Most of the defects are probably due to a developmental anomaly of the bulbus cordis rather than of the septum inferius. This theory finds good substantiation in the frequent association of these lesions with another defect of the bulbus, namely, infundibular pulmonary stenosis (see Tetralogy of Fallot).

A great deal of confusion and innumerable classifications often make the nature of ventricular defects hard to understand. One of the many obstacles is the difficulty in determining clinically the site of the opening in the ventricular septum and thus identifying the lesion as high or low, membranous or muscular in type. In fact, as was pointed out by Selzer,[627] the majority of the defects observed at postmortem examination are high and anterior in the membranous septum connecting the subaortic portion of the left ventricle with the tricuspid portion of the right ventricle; most of these defects include, by definition, a certain degree of overriding of the aorta. In a minority of cases postmortem examination reveals the opening to be low in the muscular septum, and in a still smaller number the ventricular septum is entirely absent (single ventricle).

Edwards, in his excellent chapter on congenital heart disease in Gould's *Pathology of the Heart*,[212] divided ventricular septal defects into four types, according to position: (1) outflow, (2) inflow, (3) both outflow and inflow, and (4) left ventricular-right atrial communications.

The *outflow* defects (Fig. 276) lie between the pulmonary valve above and the septal leaflet of the tricuspid valve below when looked at from the right ventricle, and immediately below the aortic valve if inspected from the left side. These are the most common locations, probably representing four out of five ventricular defects. Most of these outflow defects lie inferoposterior to the crista supraventricularis on the right side and below the right aortic cusp on the left (Fig. 276 (*2*)). A minority of the outflow defects are anterosuperior to the crista, some almost below the pulmonic valve on the right (Fig. 276 (*1*)),and below the junction of the left and right aortic cusps on the left side. These "outflow defects" of Edwards were referred to previously as "high" defects and include all the "membranous" defects of previous classifications. Nevertheless *only the ones posteroinferior to the crista may involve the membranous part*. The ones above the crista never involve the pars membranacea. It should also be stressed that, although many of these "high" or "outflow" defects are large, one cannot equate high defect with large defect, under any circumstances.

The *inflow* defects of Edwards are always posterior to the papillary muscle of the conus and are situated exclusively in the posterior muscular septum. The most common location is beneath the septal leaflet of the tricuspid valve on the right (Fig. 276 (*3*)) and anterior to the posteromedial commissure of the mitral valve on the left. Rarely, "inflow" defects may be located near the apex of the heart and may be multiple (Fig. 276 (*4*)). These "inflow" defects were referred to in the past as "low" or "muscular" defects and always were thought to be small. We know today that this also is not invariably true.

Combined inflow and outflow defects are rare. They occupy a large portion of the muscular and membranous septum, not extending anterior to the crista, but going back posteriorly beneath the tricuspid valve. Viewed

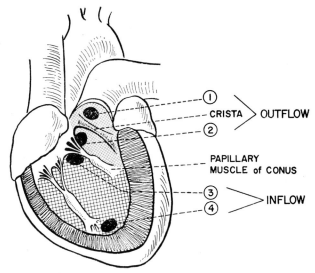

Figure 276. Schematic representation of the most common locations of ventricular septal defect, seen through the right ventricle. Inflow portion is cross-hatched, outflow shaded.

from the left side, they are usually not immediately beneath the aortic cusps, but are separated from them either by part of the membranous septum or by muscle fibers. These defects closely resemble the lesions seen with the endocardial cushion defect complex.

The *left ventricular-right atrial communications* may be summarized best by referring to Figure 277, from Edward's paper.[214, 558] The possibility of left ventricular-right atrial communications is based on the anatomic fact that the tricuspid valve is lower than the mitral valve, and thus part of the left ventricle is at the level of the right atrium in the vertical axis. In the most common variety of this entity, a deficiency of the membranous septum is associated with a cleft in the septal leaflet of the tricuspid valve.

There may, indeed, be a close correlation between physiology and anatomic location of the ventricular septal defect, as Becu and his associates maintained.[50] But I am unable at present to confirm or deny an exact correlation of this sort.

It may be well to discuss here briefly the anatomy of *single ventricle,* in which there is complete absence of the ventricular septum. Usually the atria are normal (cor triloculare biatriatum), but occasionally there is only one atrium (cor biloculare). The great arteries are commonly, but not invariably, transposed; they may even be in a corrected transposition relation. The outflow portion of the right ventricle may or may not be obstructed. Valvar pulmonic stenosis is rare. Abnormalities of the atrioventricular valves may be present. Rarely is single ventricle an anatomically uncomplicated defect.

One word about *overriding aorta.* This concept (that in certain types of ventricular septal defects, specifically in those seen with the tetralogy of Fallot or Eisenmenger's complex, the aorta abnormally communicates with the right ventricle) is not accepted by most observers today.[628] Rather, it is believed that under *normal* circumstances the ventricular septum prevents the subvalvar orifice of the aorta from freely communicating with

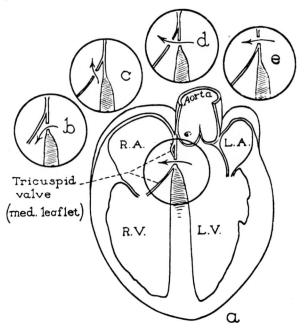

Figure 277. Locations of left ventricular-right atrial shunts. Note the fact that in the frontal plane the tricuspid valve is lower than the mitral valve. As a consequence, part of the right atrium is in the same plane as the left ventricle. Thus, direct communication between left ventricle and right atrium is possible without any defect in the tricuspid valve. This is the type A variation of left ventricular-right atrial shunt. In type B the communication is from left ventricle to right ventricle, and tricuspid regurgitation produces the shunt into the right atrium. In type C there is an opening in the medial leaflet of the tricuspid valve. Type D is a combination of types B and C and is the most common form of left ventricular-right atrial shunt.[214]

the right ventricle. If, experimentally, a ventricular defect is created at the junction of the right and the posterior aortic cusps, then, in a sagittal section, the aorta will indeed "override" the septum. Of course this physiologic overriding, inherent in the presence of an outflow ventricular septal defect, is accentuated by the distortion of the crista, secondary to the hemodynamic consequences of a large ventricular septal defect or the tetralogy of Fallot.

Finally, one ought to mention the surgically important fact that the bundle of His usually skirts the lower edge of the ventricular defect.

Physiology

The timing, direction and size of a shunt through a ventricular septal defect are determined by well known physical laws; the principal governing factors are the size of the defect and the pressure gradient between the two ventricles. Because, under ordinary circumstances, the pressure in the left ventricle is higher, through the entire cardiac cycle, than it is in the right ventricle, an opening in the ventricular septum results in a shunting of blood from left to right, principally during systole. The height of the systolic pressure in the two ventricles is largely determined by the respective resistances confronting them. Minor alterations in the resistances of the two circuits may result in a radical change in the ventricular shunt. Similarly, a relatively small change in the size of the opening can increase or decrease the flow through the septal defect.

In addition to these two main factors, the degree of overriding of the aorta also plays a part in determining the dynamics of ventricular septal defect. It is debatable how great actually is the role of overriding. It seems clear that the greater the degree of overriding (everything else being equal), the greater is the cyanosis. At the same time, *this factor is probably not as important as was thought in the past, and a certain amount of overriding is inherent in any sizable ventricular defect high in the septum.*

One final, and almost completely unanalyzed, factor in determining the dynamics of ventricular septal defect is the effect of the muscular contraction of the septum on the size of the opening during systole.

The lesions to be discussed in this section are those with predominantly left-to-right shunts; those associated with predominantly right-to-left shunts will be discussed in the chapter on valvular and vascular lesions (see p. 600).

If the ventricular septal defect is small, a considerable systolic gradient with a relatively small shunt may exist between the two ventricles. Conversely, if the ventricular defect is large (at least 1.0 cm. in diameter or at least half the size of the aortic orifice), no significant gradient between the two ventricles can exist; thus the right ventricular pressure will be equal or close to that of the left ventricle. Depending on the status of the pulmonary vasculature, this right ventricular hypertension may be the result either of a tremendous flow through the ventricular septum or of an increase in the resistance in the pulmonary circuit. This concept, that increased pressure may be the result of large flow, increased resistance, or a combination of the two, is clearly expressed in Ohm's Law—Pressure = Flow × Resistance.

If the ventricular septal defect is associated with pulmonary stenosis, usually infundibular, a moderate degree of left-to-right shunt may persist in the face of elevation of right ventricular pressure and in association with normal pulmonary arterial pressure.

If the ventricular septal defect involves a deformity of the aortic valve as well, a combination of ventricular septal defect with aortic regurgitation results. Other associated malformations to be discussed are ventricular septal defect with atrial septal defect, ventricular septal defect with patent ductus arteriosus, and ventricular septal defect with coarctation of the aorta.

Complete absence of the ventricular septum results functionally, as well as anatomically, in a single ventricular chamber, with a uniform oxygen content in the right ventricle, aorta and pulmonary artery and identical pressures in the right ventricle and the aorta. If the defect in the membranous part of the septum, posterior and inferior to the crista, communicates with the right atrium directly or through a cleft in the septal leaflet of the tricuspid valve, a jet of blood is directed into the right atrium, the right ventricular pressure is usually below systemic level, and the left-to-right shunt is moderate only.

A classification of interventricular communications, based on the principles outlined, is presented in Table 28, (p. 794).

SIMPLE VENTRICULAR SEPTAL DEFECT

Small to Moderate Ventricular Septal Defect

Roger,[589] in 1879, described 2 completely asymptomatic patients with identical cardiac findings; in one of these, postmortem examination revealed a small ventricular septal defect. Since that time all asymptomatic small ventricular septal defects have been called Roger's disease. Further important contributions to the definition of the syndrome have been made by Taussig,[682] Selzer[627] and Wood.[752]

With the introduction of cardiac catheterization a new physiologic definition of small ventricular septal defect was sought, to supplement the historical one based on anatomy and symptomatology. In our clinic small ventricular septal defect is defined as a "ventricular defect with a small to moderate left-to-right shunt, but *without* significant right ventricular hypertension." By Gorlin's orifice formula,[292] these defects are calculated to be less than 1.0 cm. in diameter.

Within this framework, then, one can talk about the trivial ventricular defects and designate these as "Roger's disease" if one is particularly fond of eponyms. These are the lesions with a pulmonary-systemic flow ratio of less than 1.5:1.0, no pulmonary arterial hypertension, and a defect probably less than 0.5 cm. in diameter. They blend almost imperceptibly into the moderate-sized ventricular defects, also without pulmonary arterial hypertension, but with a 2:1 left-to-right shunt. These probably correspond to defects of 0.5 to 1.0 cm. in diameter.

The incidence of small defects within the large group of ventricular septal defects is hard to determine with any accuracy, since the clinical criteria are unreliable, cardiac catheterization may not reveal the smallest left-to-right shunts, except by means of very sensitive techniques, and they may be missed even at postmortem examination. Yet it may be fair to say that about 25 per cent of all ventricular septal defects in the pediatric age group can be classified as small. Among ninety-eight patients studied by our group, approximately twenty-five could be classified in this category.[264]

Clinical Picture

The outstanding clinical feature is the discovery of a heart murmur, usually within the first weeks. of life, but seldom, if ever, at birth. As a matter of fact, with only few exceptions, the murmur makes its appearance within the first two or three weeks after birth. Symptoms are more common than was hitherto believed, at least in the group of patients we have had the opportunity to study. Mild exercise intolerance, fatigue, dyspnea on exertion and repeated severe respiratory infections were noted in at least two thirds of our patients. Symptoms usually do not begin until after the second year of age. On the other hand, there is a group of patients, with the classic profile of a small ventricular septal defect in childhood, who early in infancy have been extremely sick with congestive heart failure.

On the whole, at physical examination these children are average in development. Cyanosis, clubbing and redness of the fingers and toes are uniformly absent. A mild degree of left chest prominence is common.

The cardiac impulse is moderately forceful and usually involves the apex. A systolic thrill at the lower left sternal border (but not at the suprasternal notch) is almost always present. The blood pressure is normal, the jugular venous pulse is not unusual, and there is no evidence of congestive failure.

On auscultation both the first and second heart sounds are within normal limits. More commonly than not, an appreciable splitting of the second sound, changing with respiration, can be heard at the second left interspace (Fig. 278).[705] A third heart sound is commonly noted at the apex. A harsh systolic murmur (grade 3 to 6) (Fig. 133, p. 127) is present in all patients and is heard maximally at the lower left sternal border, particularly over the xiphoid process. This murmur, although loud and harsh, does not transmit as well to the neck and the back as the murmur of semilunar stenosis. Transmission to the lower right sternal border may be good.

Phonocardiographically, the murmur varies between the classic pansystolic murmur (Fig. 279), a diamond-shaped murmur indistinguishable from that of infundibular pulmonic stenosis (Fig. 278), and an early decrescendo systolic murmur (Fig. 280), not lasting beyond the first half of systole.

Low-frequency, rumbling murmurs are heard at the apex during mid-diastole or presystole in about two thirds of the patients (Fig. 138, p. 130).

Roentgenologic examination reveals the heart to be normal or slightly enlarged (Fig. 281). The enlargement involves mainly the right ventricle, with or without simultaneous left ventricular and left atrial involvement. The main pulmonary artery is normal or only slightly enlarged, and the pulmonary vasculature shows slight engorgement, usually without a hilar dance.

The electrocardiogram is within normal limits in most instances. The unipolar chest leads show left ventricular dominance, with variable increases in voltages over the left ventricle. Significant degrees of right ventricular hypertrophy and P pulmonale are absent. A significant degree of incomplete right bundle branch block is relatively rare. The P-R interval is usually normal.

Figure 278. Phonocardiogram of a patient with small ventricular septal defect without pulmonic stenosis. Note the diamond-shaped murmur and the well split second sound.[705]

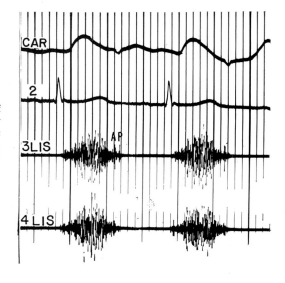

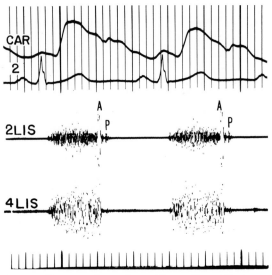

Figure 279. Phonocardiogram of a patient with small ventricular septal defect. Again, note the well split second sound, this time with a holosystolic plateau-shaped murmur at the fourth left interspace.[705]

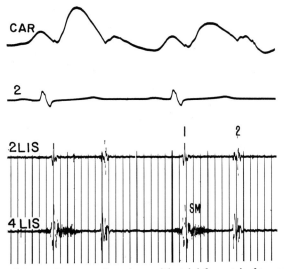

Figure 280. Phonocardiogram of patient with trivial ventricular septal defect. Note the short, early decrescendo systolic murmur. This is the kind of murmur that is likely to disappear entirely, indicating closure of the ventricular defect.[705]

At cardiac catheterization (Fig. 282) the distinguishing features are as follows: (1) The oxygen content of the blood in the right ventricle is higher than that of the right atrium. In order for the increased oxygen content to be significant, there should be either a 10 per cent jump on one set of samples or a 5 per cent increase on at least 2 occasions. It should be reiterated, however, that the smallest ventricular septal defects, the most classic examples of Roger's disease, may not show any significant increase in oxygen saturation at the ventricular level. Systemic arterial

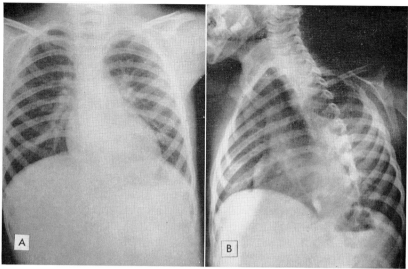

Figure 281. Roentgenograms in (*A*) posteroanterior and (*B*) left anterior oblique views of patient with small ventricular septal defect.

saturation is usually normal. (2) Pressures and pressure pulses are normal on both sides of the heart. (3) The resistance in the pulmonary circuit is usually normal or low. (4) The pulmonary flow is 1.5 to two times the systemic output. (5) Occasionally the catheter enters the left ventricle or the aorta through the defect. (6) Cine-angiograms, with injection of contrast material into the left ventricle, may demonstrate a left-to-right shunt which is too small to change the oxygen saturation of the right ventricle. (7) Dye curves, with injection into the right atrium or right ventricle and sampling from the systemic artery, may show a recirculation curve with prolonged disappearance time if the shunt is sizable enough. A more sensitive method for the demonstration of a left-to-right ventricular shunt is to introduce a hydrogen electrode into the right ventricle and to allow the patient to inhale hydrogen. (8) Finally, occasionally, an intracardiac phonocatheter may demonstrate a loud murmur in the right ventricle which disappears on withdrawal of the catheter into the right atrium and diminishes when the catheter enters the pulmonary artery (Fig. 148).

Course and Prognosis

Small ventricular septal defects are thought to be benign lesions. Roger's[589] original description implies the innocuousness of this condition. Taussig[682] stated that the condition is compatible with long and active life. Whether the optimistic view of these and other authors is fully justified is hard to tell, since their prognostication is based primarily on clinical diagnosis and rarely on postmortem findings. No accurate long-term evaluation of these patients will be possible until some of the children in whom this diagnosis was established early, at cardiac catheterization, can be followed up through several decades.

From the viewpoint of the pediatrician, however, it can be stated with confidence that, at least during childhood, these patients do ex-

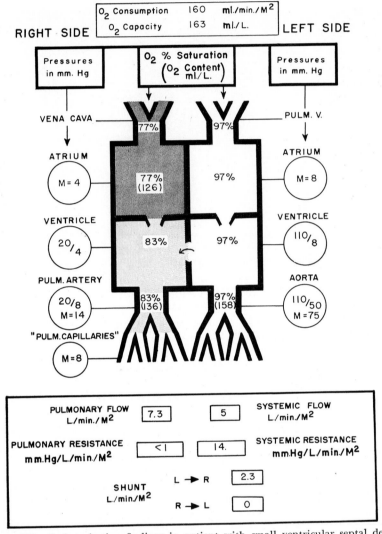

Figure 282. Catheterization findings in patient with small ventricular septal defect.

tremely well. Although many of them show minimal symptoms, these tend not to progress and may even improve. We have noted, as have others,[717] that harsh systolic murmurs (grade 4 to 5 in intensity) may disappear throughout childhood. We have assumed, as others have, that this represented spontaneous closure of a ventricular septal defect. Within recent years we,[529] as well as Evans,[231] have been able to prove that this, indeed, occurs in some instances.

One further interesting point to be stressed is that, whereas adults in their thirties, forties and even sixties who have atrial septal defects frequently are seen in the offices of cardiologists, few older patients with asymptomatic ventricular septal defects are followed up in a similar fashion. This contrasts markedly with the high incidence of this lesion in children. A number of explanations for this discrepancy may be suggested. (1) A large number of the defects may close spontaneously. (2) The increase in chest diameter may mask the auscultatory findings. (3) The patients may die early in adulthood. (4) The condition may assume the profile of more serious disease (tetralogy of Fallot, Eisenmenger's complex, and so forth). At present there are no statistically valid figures to indicate a preference among these possibilities; my own impression is that many more may close spontaneously than was hitherto believed.

One of the complications of ventricular septal defect is bacterial endocarditis. The infective process may affect the margins of the defect or the right ventricular wall opposite the septal opening. The incidence of this disease, as quoted by various authors, ranges from 25 to 51 per cent. At present, however, in my estimation, with the widespread use of chemotherapy and chemoprophylaxis, considerably less than 15 per cent of the children with ventricular septal defect are likely to contract bacterial endocarditis. It should be stressed, however, that hemodynamically insignificant lesions may also predispose to endocarditis.

Although rheumatic fever is not a common complication of ventricular defect, the two conditions certainly may coexist. The sudden development of congestive failure in a patient with hitherto asymptomatic ventricular septal defect ought to raise the suspicion of rheumatic carditis. Recognition of this combination is becoming increasingly important, since evidence of congestive failure may well be considered an indication for closure of the ventricular septal opening. Certainly one's enthusiasm for cardiac surgery would decrease considerably if it could be proved that the patient's symptoms were not due to the presence of the defect, but rather were caused by an associated inflammatory lesion.

Differential Diagnosis

The differential diagnosis of small ventricular defects may be difficult. Several possibilities must be considered.

Left-to-Right Shunts. DEFECTS OF THE FORAMEN PRIMUM. Atrial septal defects of the foramen primum type are difficult—almost impossible—to distinguish from small ventricular defects on auscultation alone. The rsR' pattern with left axis deviation and a counterclockwise frontal plane loop, usually present with ostium primum, may be the most reliable feature in the clinical differential diagnosis. Cardiac catheterization may be helpful, but often the answer is equivocal.

DEFECTS OF THE FORAMEN SECUNDUM. A foramen secundum defect is relatively easy to differentiate from a small ventricular septal defect. The soft, blowing systolic murmur at the second left interspace, the absence of a thrill, the widely split fixed second sound, the exclusively right-sided cardiac enlargement and the considerable degree of incomplete right bundle branch block, all rather sharply separate foramen secundum defects from the small Roger type of ventricular septal defect. Results of cardiac catheterization are usually diagnostic.

LARGE VENTRICULAR SEPTAL DEFECTS. Large ventricular septal defects can be distinguished from smaller ones by the severity of the symptoms, the frequently booming pulmonary closure, the relatively softer systolic murmur, the suspicion of cyanosis, the cardiac enlargement involving both ventricles and the pulmonary artery, and the right ventricular hypertrophy, shown in the electrocardiogram. The two entities can be distinguished easily at cardiac catheterization on the basis of the right ventricular pressure level.

PATENT DUCTUS ARTERIOSUS. If accompanied by the characteristic machinery murmur, typical patent ductus arteriosus cannot be confused with a small ventricular defect. The so-called atypical patent ductus arteriosus resembles a large ventricular septal defect; hence it too should present little difficulty in the differential diagnosis of a small ventricular defect.

Infundibular Pulmonary Stenosis. Infundibular pulmonary stenosis not severe enough to give rise to right ventricular hypertension of more than 60 mm. of mercury, and thus not producing a right ventricular hypertrophy type of electrocardiogram, is extremely difficult to differentiate from a small ventricular septal defect. It may be helpful to remember, however, that isolated infundibular pulmonic stenosis is a rare condition. Thus the problem, if presented, more often takes the form of whether a ventricular septal defect is present with or without pulmonic stenosis. The two conditions have in common a rough systolic murmur and a thrill at the lower left sternal border, but the murmur of pulmonary stenosis is somewhat rougher, is more diamond-shaped, and transmits better to the neck and back than the characteristic murmur of a ventricular defect. As mentioned earlier, fairly frequently the two conditions are indistinguishable phonocardiographically.[705] Also, in pulmonary stenosis, low-frequency diastolic murmurs are absent, and the pulmonary second sound is usually diminished. The clinical differential diagnosis is often unsatisfactory, however, and if an accurate diagnosis is desired, cardiac catheterization must be resorted to.

Infundibular pulmonary stenosis with right ventricular pressure in the systemic range usually, though not invariably, is associated with tetralogy of Fallot, and thus is sharply separated from the acyanotic small ventricular defect. But there is a small group of patients who have infundibular stenosis, significant right ventricular hypertension and a ventricular septal defect who do not exhibit cyanosis at rest (acyanotic tetralogy of Fallot). This syndrome still can be distinguished from Roger's disease on the basis of cyanosis on exercise and the right ventricular hypertrophy shown in the electrocardiogram in almost every instance of tetralogy of Fallot.

Rheumatic Mitral Regurgitation. The systolic murmur of rheumatic mitral regurgitation may resemble rather closely that of a small ventricular defect, and both may exhibit apical diastolic murmurs. The electrocardiographic and the x-ray examinations may be essentially normal in both conditions.

A history of rheumatic fever, the relatively late discovery of the murmur, and its localization to the apex and transmission toward the posterior axilla and the left lung base usually, but not invariably, suggest the diagnosis of mitral regurgitation, even without cardiac catheterization.

Mild Congenital Aortic Stenosis. Aortic stenosis without significant left ventricular hypertrophy may resemble a small ventricular defect. In both conditions there may be a rough systolic murmur with a thrill, discovered in early infancy, a normal-sized heart without symptoms, and a normal electrocardiogram.

The stenotic nature of the murmur, heard maximally at the aortic area, usually makes the differential diagnosis possible even without cardiac catheterization.

Endocardial Fibroelastosis.   It may be hard to distinguish subendo-cardial sclerosis with mitral or aortic valvular involvement, or both, from a ventricular septal defect; as pointed out previously, the murmur of both mitral and aortic valvular lesions may closely resemble the one associated with a ventricular defect. In subendocardial sclerosis the heart is diffusely enlarged, the pulmonary vasculature is relatively normal, and the electro-cardiogram may show significant left ventricular hypertrophy. Right heart catheterization may reveal no abnormalities or may demonstrate an ele-vation of right atrial mean, right ventricular end-diastolic, pulmonary arterial mean and "pulmonary capillary" mean pressures. Some of these patients have complete atrioventricular block; they may easily be the group responsible for the legend that complete heart block is common in patients with a small ventricular septal defect.

Murmurs at the Lower Left Sternal Border.   Whether harsh murmurs at the lower left sternal border without any other abnormality of the heart, revealed clinically or at catheterization, are small ventricular septal defects, not giving rise to a detectable left-to-right shunt, cannot always be decided. These murmurs may well represent ventricular defects; on the other hand, they may originate from an entirely normal heart. I prefer to say that patients with this syndrome have no significant heart disease. With the newer ancillary techniques of cardiac catheterization (cine-angiography, dye curves, hydrogen electrode) usually even the most minute defects may be detected.

Treatment

On the whole, patients with a trivial ventricular septal defect do not require treatment. Surgical closure by means of the pump oxygenator is feasible, but, in our experience, it does not represent a completely innocu-ous procedure. Until it may be demonstrated that operative correction of these defects presents a less than 1 per cent mortality risk, approximately that of surgery for patent ductus arterious, I cannot, with a clear conscience, suggest surgery in an asymptomatic patient who has only a minimal (less than 1.5:1.0 pulmonary-systemic flow ratio) left-to-right shunt and no elec-trocardiographic or roentgenologic abnormalities. In my opinion, surgery on these patients will be justifiable only if either the surgical mortality inher-ent in the cardiopulmonary bypass and ventriculotomy reaches the ideal level indicated, or statistically meaningful data on a shortened life ex-pectancy of these patients become available. At present, to the best of my knowledge, neither of these conditions is fulfilled; thus I would not advise operation on such patients.

Patients with moderate-sized ventricular septal defects, i.e. patients who have some symptoms, slight cardiac enlargement, a normal or moderate degree of left ventricular hypertrophy in the electrocardiogram and a 2:1 left-to-right shunt without pulmonary arterial hypertension, are ideal can-didates for operation if they are between five and fifteen years of age. The probability that these patients will eventually suffer ill effects from their cardiovascular anomaly if it is not corrected is good; the operative risks should not be greater than 5 per cent.

Short of operation, these children should be allowed to lead normal, active lives. Protection against bacterial endocarditis is mandatory. Reexamination with roentgenologic and electrocardiographic documentation at two- to three-year intervals is desirable.

Summary

The diagnosis of a small ventricular septal defect should be considered in patients with congenital heart disease who have slight symptoms and in whom a harsh systolic murmur with a thrill at the lower left sternal border is the only definitely abnormal clinical cardiac finding. Cardiac catheterization may provide a definite diagnosis. Normal findings at right heart catheterization, however, do not definitely exclude the presence of a trivial ventricular defect. Patients with this condition should be allowed to lead a normal life. Surgery is indicated only for the hemodynamically significant lesions.

Large Ventricular Septal Defect

For the purposes of this classification, a large ventricular septal defect is defined as one in which there is a close approximation of right ventricular to systemic arterial pressure across the ventricular septum. Usually, though not invariably, the shunt across this defect is large, resulting in a pulmonary flow that is more than twice the systemic flow. The defect is at least 1 cm. in diameter. Selzer[627] estimated that the size of the opening is at least half the size of the aortic orifice.

Taussig[682] first focused attention on high and large ventricular septal defects in contrast to the small and low ones first described by Roger.[589] Selzer[627] emphasized the fact that the size, rather than the location, of the defect constitutes the principal difference between the two conditions. Other authors, particularly Wood,[752] Keith[378] and Fyler and his associates,[264] have since described the clinical and physiologic findings in this condition.

The incidence of these lesions is probably exaggerated because patients with large defects have more severe symptoms and thus are more likely to seek medical care than are patients with smaller defects. Among Wood's sixty cases, twenty-five probably should be considered to have large ventricular defects. In our series of ninety-eight patients, more than half, fell into this category.

Clinical Picture

In contrast to Roger's disease, patients with a large ventricular septal defect appear sick. Usually, though not invariably, these children have severe symptoms early, sometimes even preceding the discovery of the murmur and the underlying heart disease. All but one of our patients had symptoms by the time they were one year old, and more than 20 per cent of them were sick within the first few weeks of life. It is worth emphasizing that, whereas in patients with semilunar stenosis heart murmurs are noticed within the first day or two of life, in patients having ventricular septal defects the murmurs often are not discovered until the end of the first week or two of life. Of course this may be further juxtaposed to the even later discovery of murmurs with atrial septal defect of the secundum type. An adequate physiologic explanation for these time relations may be found in the sequence of changes in right ventricular pressure. In semilunar stenosis a pressure gradient exists as soon as the appropriate flows across the pulmonic or aortic valves are established, irrespective of the levels of the vascular resistance. No appreciable flow across the ventricular septum is possible until right ventricular pressure drops appreciably below that of the left ventricle. Finally, no sizable shunt across the atrial septum is likely until the appropriate long-term regression in the pressure-volume characteristics of the right ventricle occurs.

The symptoms may be the same as those in Roger's disease, but they tend to be more severe. Dyspnea, exercise intolerance, fatigue and repeated attacks of pneumonia are almost invariably present; in addition, episodes of congestive failure and cyanosis occur in about one third of the patients. Hemoptysis, an almost pathognomonic sign of pulmonary arterial hypertension, may occur in older children and of course is a common cause of death in adults.

At physical examination these children are poorly developed; only rarely does their development place them above the twenty-fifth percentile line, and most of the time they fall below the third percentile line of a standard developmental chart. Slight cyanosis, or redness of the fingers, is noted in as many as half of the patients. Some chest deformity is almost invariably present. A strong, even visible, xiphoid impulse often accompanied by an apical thrust is usually observed. Pulmonary valve closure is commonly palpable, as is an ejection click. A thrill is palpable in only about half of these patients; this is in contrast with cases of small ventricular septal defects, in which a thrill is present almost without exception. The systemic blood pressure is normal. When congestive failure is present, the liver is enlarged, the neck veins are distended and pulsatile, with prominent A and V waves, and pulmonary rales are heard. The first heart sound is usually accentuated, and the second sound is booming at the pulmonary area and narrowly split. The split changes with respirations. An ejection click is present in the pulmonic area of the patients with pulmonary vascular obstruction and a dilated main pulmonary artery. A third sound may be present at the apex. A systolic murmur, usually plateau-shaped and holosystolic, but occasionally short and decrescendic (in patients with small pulmonary flows and very high resistance), is heard at the lower left sternal border. The loudest murmurs are heard in patients with large flows; patients with high pulmonary resistance usually have somewhat less intense systolic murmurs. Although the murmur does not transmit as well to the neck and the great vessels as does the murmur of semilunar stenosis, it may be heard well throughout the chest, anteriorly and posteriorly, and it transmits very well to the apex. At the latter position it may be hard to differentiate the murmur of ventricular septal defect from that of mitral regurgitation. Low-frequency, low-intensity, rumbling, mid-diastolic or presystolic murmurs are heard well at the apex and the lower left sternal border in the majority of these children (Fig. 138). *This flow murmur usually occurs later in diastole than that associated with a secundum type of atrial septal defect* (Fig. 137). As mentioned previously, in the latter group the rumble is protodiastolic in timing.

Protodiastolic, high-frequency, blowing murmurs of pulmonary regurgitation are heard in approximately a third of these patients with increased pulmonary arterial mean pressure. This murmur should be clearly differentiated from the diastolic murmur of aortic regurgitation; in the latter group the systemic blood pressure is wide, the pulmonary arterial mean pressure is relatively low, and there is no conspicuous dilatation of the main pulmonary artery.

Roentgenologic examination reveals considerable cardiac enlargement, involving both ventricles and the left atrium. The main pulmonary artery segment is prominent, and the pulmonary vasculature is engorged. The aorta is of average size (Fig. 283) and the arch is on the left side in more

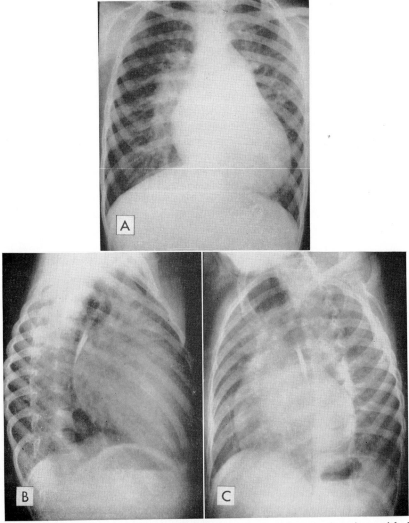

Figure 283. Roentgenograms (posteroanterior and both obliques) of patient with large ventricular septal defect.

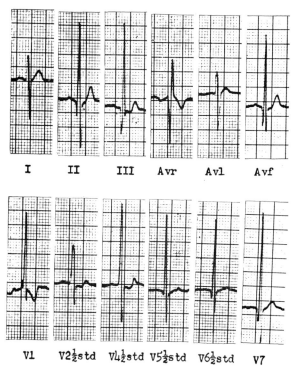

Figure 284. Electrocardiogram of patient with large ventricular septal defect and combined ventricular hypertrophy. This is the tracing that is thought to be characteristic of a ventricular defect with hyperkinetic pulmonary arterial hypertension.

than 95 per cent of the patients. At fluoroscopy the pulsations of the cardiac border are intense; the pulmonary artery pulsation is usually stronger than that of the aorta. The pulmonary vasculature almost invariably shows intrinsic pulsations.

The electrocardiogram shows right ventricular hypertrophy, alone or in combination with left ventricular hypertrophy, in practically all instances (Figs. 284, 285). Right bundle branch block may be present in less than half of the patients. Many show evidences of combined atrial hypertrophy. Although complete heart block is rare, first- or second-degree atrioventricular block is present in about 10 per cent of the cases. The mean electrical axis is usually between +90 and +150 degrees, with a clockwise frontal plane loop. Occasionally a patient, presumably with a ventricular septal defect in the endocardial cushion position, shows left axis deviation (beyond —30 degrees) and a counterclockwise frontal plane loop. Finally, a few patients with large left-to-right shunts and moderate elevation of the pulmonary arterial pressure show mean electrical axes between —30 and +90 degrees.

Electrocardiographic and hemodynamic correlations have been emphasized by our group[264] and even more so by DuShane and his co-workers[209] and by Keith,[708] particularly in relation to the question of operability in patients with ventricular septal defect. Adams and Anderson[6] have been unable to find a close correlation between the electrocardiogram and the hemodynamics. Suffice it to say here that, though the electrocardiogram

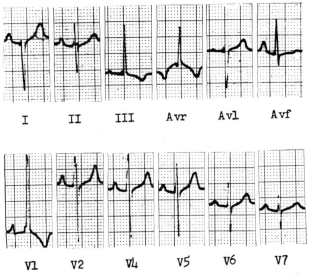

I   II   III   Avr   Avl   Avf

V1   V2   V4   V5   V6   V7

Figure 285. Electrocardiogram of a patient with ventricular septal defect and obstructive pulmonary arterial hypertension. Note the pure right ventricular hypertrophy.

is an excellent tool in the clinical evaluation of ventricular septal defect, I do not believe that this *alone* should be used as a magic formula in the clinical assessment of children with defects of the ventricular septum. Furthermore, I am certain that the very same people who propose so fervently the use of the electrocardiogram as *the* touchstone for evaluation of ventricular septal defect use first and foremost their superb clinical acumen, based on many years of experience with the clinical and laboratory aspects of congenital heart disease, to render a judgment about the operability of every one of their patients. Why imply, then, that the electrocardiogram decides and that the physician is, in effect, a rather primitive computer into which we feed a few figures in relation to mean electrical axes, q waves, R waves, and so forth, and come out with an opinion? It is vastly more subtle and exciting than all that.

With all these qualifications, certain simple statements may be made in relation to the electrocardiogram in the diagnosis of ventricular septal defects. (1) For all practical purposes, a normal electrocardiogram is seen only in patients with uncomplicated small to moderate ventricular septal defect, without right ventricular hypertension. (2) Pure right ventricular hypertrophy with a mean electrical axis to the right of +150 degrees and a clockwise loop in the frontal plane means pulmonary vascular obstruction. (3) The rare instance of pure left ventricular hypertrophy with a mean electrical axis to the left of +90 degrees and a counterclockwise frontal plane loop means a large flow with essentially normal resistance and right ventricular pressure well below systemic range. (4) Combined ventricular hypertrophy with a mean electrical axis of —30 to ±180 degrees may represent any pressure-flow relation within the pulmonary arterial hypertension group.

At cardiac catheterization there are significant and severe deviations from normal (Fig. 286). The principal abnormalities are as follows: (1) There is an increase in the oxygen content at the right ventricular, probably high outflow, level of at least 10 per cent on one set of samples or 5 per cent on 2 sets. Systemic arterial saturation may be normal or somewhat decreased. In the latter situation, particularly in infants, left atrial or pulmonary venous saturation should also be determined, to ascertain whether the systemic arterial unsaturation is due to a true right-to-left shunt or to pulmonary factors. (2) Right atrial pressure is usually normal; it may be elevated with prominent V waves in cases of congestive heart failure. Left atrial or pulmonary capillary pressure is appreciably higher than right atrial pressure, as much as 15 to 20 mm. of mercury (mean), particularly in patients who have large flows. Pulmonary arterial pressure approximates systemic arterial pressure, by definition. Systemic arterial pressure is normal. The pressure contour of the right ventricle closely approximates that of the left ventricle. (3) Pulmonary resistance is less than 3 units per square meter in approximately 35 to 40 per cent of children. Most of those who have elevated resistances have calculated figures of only 3 to 6 units, but a third of those with higher than normal resistance already have maximal obstruction (more than 9 units per square meter) in childhood. (4) Pulmonary-to-systemic flow ratios are more than 2:1 in most instances. Very large shunts (more than 4:1) were seen in only about 25 per cent of our patients. (5) If the catheter traverses the ventricular septum, it usually passes to the left of the crista supraventricularis into the aorta, or less frequently into the left ventricle (see Fig. 325, p. 472). This maneuver is possible in at least 25 per cent of these patients in our laboratory. This is the only *certain* method of demonstrating the presence of a ventricular septal defect. Of course it is possible, much more frequently, particularly in infants, to enter the left atrium and even the left ventricle across a foramen ovale. (6) Cine-angiography, with injection of contrast material into the left ventricle, is a most graphic way of demonstrating the size and location of a ventricular septal defect. A somewhat less satisfactory, but still reasonably adequate, demonstration may be accomplished by injection into the left atrium or the distal portion of the pulmonary artery. Right ventricular injection with a high pressure injector, reversing the physiologic left-to-right shunt, may also help in visualizing the septal defect. In our hands this latter method has not been too satisfactory. Furthermore, I cannot even be absolutely certain whether the dye really passes across the ventricular septum or through the atrial septum via tricuspid regurgitation. (7) Dye dilution studies, with injection of the dye proximal to the pulmonary valve and sampling from a systemic artery, show the expected recirculation pattern. Left ventricular injection with sampling from the right ventricle or pulmonary artery shows only an early appearance time.

If the pulmonary resistance is higher than the systemic resistance, the shunt through the ventricular defect is entirely right to left, and no significant increase in oxygen at the right ventricular level occurs. These patients, usually, though not exclusively, adolescents or adults, will be discussed with those having pulmonary vascular obstruction, even though in certain respects they belong in this group of ventricular septal defects.

If the pulmonary resistance, though significantly higher than the top normal of 3 units per square meter, is lower than or equal to the systemic resistance, left-to-right or bidirectional shunting occurs through a large,

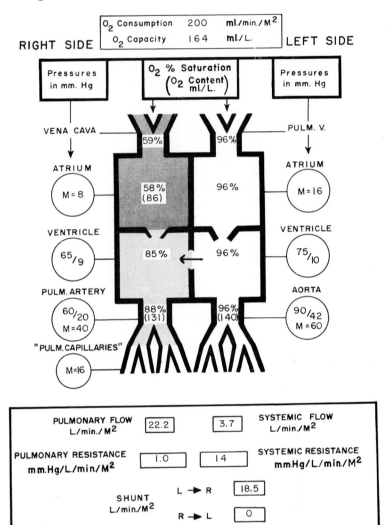

Figure 286. Catheterization findings of patient with large ventricular septal defect.

high ventricular septal defect. The left-to-right shunt may vary from 1.5 to 10 liters per square meter per minute. The right-to-left shunt, if present, amounts to between 1 and 4 liters per square meter per minute when the patient is at rest. All in all, the anatomic differences between the heart of a patient with pulmonary vascular obstruction and a ventricular septal defect, the heart of another with "Eisenmenger's syndrome" and that of a third with a large ventricular septal defect may be slight, indeed. The principal difference is in the status of the pulmonary vasculature; the role of overriding of the aorta, although real, is probably of secondary importance. "Eisenmenger's syndrome" is nothing but a large ventricular septal defect with a significant and progressive increase in pulmonary resistance.

Course and Prognosis

As pointed out previously, patients who have large ventricular septal defects are likely to have severe symptoms, and may even die from infection or congestive failure in early infancy. No statistically accurate figures on the mortality rate are available.

It is interesting to note the wide swings the opinions of the medical profession have undergone in estimating the prognosis of children with ventricular septal defect. Until ten to fifteen years ago it was assumed that ventricular defect was an innocuous lesion; it was referred to as Roger's disease, and everybody thought that it was compatible with relatively normal life expectancy. In the 1947 edition of his text White[727] stated: "There are no symptoms of ventricular septal defect unless complications develop." With the rapidly increasing interest in congenital heart disease and the introduction of cardiac catheterization techniques, but inadequate understanding of the medical treatment of these children, ventricular septal defect suddenly became a condition with a high mortality rate in infancy, a most malignant disease, and the dangers of progressive pulmonary vascular obstruction were emphasized.[225, 488] Then, with a broader view of the problem and the introduction of vigorous anticongestive measures, the pendulum swung back, and it was recognized that most infants with large ventricular septal defect may indeed be salvaged.[205, 459] It is clear that if death occurs in patients with ventricular septal defect during the first fifteen years of life, it is almost certain to happen within the first six to twelve months. But surely, on the whole, under adequate medical management, the mortality rate should be about 5 per cent.

Those who survive the first one or two years of life may improve remarkably. This improvement may be due to a diminution of the left-to right shunt across the ventricular septum, secondary to one of three mechanisms: (1) diminution of the size of the defect itself, (2) development of pulmonary infundibular obstruction,[268] and (3) development of pulmonary vascular obstruction.[209]

It is also possible for a patient to improve without a change in the size of the shunt; I would assume that this is secondary to the development of left ventricular hypertrophy, diminished left atrial and pulmonary capillary pressures and a secondary drop in pulmonary arterial pressure.

Obviously not all infants with ventricular septal defects who reach their first birthday improve rapidly thereafter. A certain proportion stay in chronic congestive heart failure, never gaining weight and being generally miserable.

Of all these possible courses that an infant with a large ventricular septal defect may take, the most unfavorable ones include the estimated 5 per cent in whom there is progressive pulmonary vascular obstruction and the 5 per cent who die at an early age. The other possibilities (closure, development of infundibular pulmonic stenosis, development of left ventricular hypertrophy and even continued congestive heart failure) do not all represent irremediable losses; obviously, some of them represent tremendous gains.

It is my impression that, under adequate medical management, an infant with a ventricular septal defect is more likely to improve than to take an unfavorable downhill course. Obviously, every infant must be judged on his own merit. But were one to prognosticate the outcome of 100 infants with large ventricular septal defects, I would guess that 90 per cent of them would be as well on their fourth or fifth birthday as they were on their first, and many of them better.

It may be said, then, with reasonable certainty, that most infants with large ventricular septal defects may be successfully carried through infancy and early childhood by skillful medical management. Survival beyond the age of forty is rare, however.[101] Difficulties arise principally from two sources.

First, pathologically, there is good evidence that the pulmonary vascular changes seen in older children and adults with ventricular septal defect are considerably different from those seen in infants. Understandably, the data do not represent repeated lung biopsies on the same patient, but rather single observations on a large number of patients with ventricular septal defect at different ages.[212] The muscular pulmonary arteries of infants with large ventricular septal defect closely resemble the fetal arterioles. They are characterized by a thick muscular media and, occasionally, a thickened adventitia. Intimal changes are seldom, if ever, seen in this age group. In contrast, in older children and adults, occlusive intimal lesions may be seen in the muscular arteries. Of course not all patients more than two years old have intimal changes, but these changes *never* occur in patients less than two. Furthermore, with increasing age, particularly after the age of ten years, these intimal changes seem to become more numerous. Similar trends have been described in terms of wall-to-lumen ratios by Damman and Ferencz.[182]

In addition to the changes in the muscular arteries, there are also differences in the small arterioles of infants and adults. In infants the arterioles have thick walls with small lumen; in adults, thin walls with wide lumen. Occasionally the thin-walled arterioles may rupture into the adjoining space.

There is, then, presumptive pathologic evidence that pulmonary vascular obstruction is a progressive disease in *some* patients with large ventricular septal defect. I would like to stress that since this theory is not based on repeated observations on the same patient, it is *presumptive* evidence. Surely it does not happen in *all* patients, and certainly *not* in those with *small* defects. Furthermore, it should be restated that even pathologically, the most severe vascular lesions are seldom seen in patients less than ten to twelve years of age.

Physiologic confirmation of this progression of pulmonary vascular obstructive disease in childhood is lacking. Most of the good evidence[460, 523, 663] in this regard points to the basic stability of the pressure-flow relations throughout childhood in 90 per cent of the patients with ventricular septal defect. Published observations to the contrary do not seem convincing to me.[720]

In trying to reconcile the pathologic with the physiologic observations, putting the whole picture in its proper perspective, the following thoughts are presented. Unquestionably, pulmonary vascular obstruction may or may not exist in infants. When it exists, it probably is based pathologically on reversible medial changes. At the other end of the spectrum is the adult with a large ventricular septal defect and pulmonary arterial hypertension, in whom pulmonary vascular obstruction is likely to be more severe than it is in infants and is much more likely, but not certain, to be based on irreversible intimal changes. These two extremes of the pathologic spectrum are probably distinguishable by physiologic methods in that the calculated pulmonary vascular resistance is likely to be much higher in the older patients than in the infants. Also, oxygen and other pulmonary vasodilators (acetylcholine) may be more effective in infants than in adults.

It is much more difficult to demonstrate physiologic differences between the pulmonary vasculature of a young child (two to five years old) and an adolescent, though pathologically the adolescent may already show some intimal changes. But these are probably scattered enough and mild enough not to affect the physiologic picture significantly.

Unquestionably, then, I would say that a large percentage (more than 50 per cent) of the patients who have large ventricular septal defects will eventually have progressive pulmonary vascular obstruction, leading to diminished pulmonary flow, cyanosis, hemoptysis and death. Death due to pulmonary vascular disease usually occurs in the twenties and thirties. There is no evidence, clinically or pathologically, that widespread irreversible pulmonary vascular changes are likely to occur before the late teens.

The second source of difficulties affecting patients with large ventricular septal defect is congestive heart failure. This may appear in children who, for some reason, do not respond with pulmonary vascular obstruction to the presence of a large defect. These are the patients whose congestive failure may never be properly controlled; the left ventricle never hypertrophies enough to be able to cope adequately with the tremendous volume of worked imposed upon it. These are the infants and young children with chronic congestive heart failure who are terribly underdeveloped and suffer repeatedly from pneumonia.

Another group of patients who may go into congestive failure are adults whose ventricular defect has been relatively well compensated throughout childhood and adolescence, but whose reserve has gradually become exhausted. Atrial fibrillation supervenes, evidences of mitral and tricuspid regurgitation appear, and the patients die of chronic congestive heart failure.

These, then, are the two principal modes of death of patients with large ventricular septal defect: namely, pulmonary vascular obstruction and congestive heart failure. Congestive heart failure may cause death in approximately 5 per cent of the *infants* with large ventricular septal defects, but almost never in *children*. Irreversible pulmonary vascular changes are extremely unlikely in infancy and rare throughout childhood. Pulmonary vascular obstruction becomes more and more probable after adolescence.

The complication of ventricular septal defects by associated bacterial endocarditis or rheumatic carditis has already been discussed (see p. 409).

Differential Diagnosis

The problems of differential diagnosis in cases of large ventricular defect concern primarily the other defects in which there is a left-to-right shunt.

Endocardial Cushion Defect. A defect of the foramen primum, especially if it involves a small portion of the ventricular septum as well, may be mistaken for a large ventricular septal defect. The most important distinguishing feature is the electrocardiogram (see p. 387).

Foramen Secundum. A lesion of the foramen secundum is different from a large ventricular septal defect. In addition to the distinctive features enumerated in the discussion of Roger's disease, there is the added distinction that an uncomplicated defect of the foramen secundum is almost never accompanied by significant pulmonary arterial hypertension in children.

Small Ventricular Septal Defect. See page 409.

Patent Ductus Arteriosus. Atypical patent ductus arteriosus, or aorto-pulmonary fenestration, cannot with certainty be distinguished by clinical means from a large ventricular septal defect. The more evidence of left ventricular enlargement there is in the roentgenogram and left ventricular hypertrophy in the electrocardiogram, the wider the pulse pressure, and the higher at the left sternal border the murmur is located, the more a patent ductus arteriosus should be suspected. Also the second sound in a patient who has a patent ductus arteriosus with pulmonary arterial hypertension may show more splitting than occurs with a corresponding ventricular septal defect and pulmonary arterial hypertension. The similarities are so striking that I believe, for practical purposes, that a patent ductus arteriosus should be considered seriously in the differential diagnosis of every severely sick infant with a ventricular septal defect. Cardiac catheterization should be contemplated in every such case.

Single Ventricle. A single ventricle is only quantitatively different from a large ventricular septal defect; the symptoms and signs are more severe. At catheterization the pressures and oxygen contents in the systemic artery and the pulmonary artery are essentially identical. Transposition and common truncus arteriosus are commonly demonstrable at angiocardiography.

Truncus Arteriosus. Truncus arteriosus with large pulmonary arteries may be considered in the differential diagnosis. Ordinarily, the characteristic shape on the roentgenogram, the presence of a diastolic murmur, in addition to the murmur of aortic stenosis, and the usually more severe course make the distinction possible on clinical grounds alone. If, in the face of obvious pulmonary arterial hypertension, the electrocardiogram shows pure left ventricular hypertrophy, truncus arteriosus alone or in combination with a single ventricle may be suspected. Angiocardiography usually establishes the diagnosis.

Treatment

The surgical treatment of ventricular septal defect has been one of the principal accomplishments in pediatric cardiology during the past five years. As indicated in the previous edition of this volume, Murray,[515] Mustard,[516] Lillehei[435] and Kirklin[210, 391] pioneered in this field. Since then we have successfully closed many ventricular septal defects at our own institution, as have others in this country and abroad.

All ventricular septal defects are closed by means of some type of pump oxygenator. The approach to the defect is conventionally through a ventriculotomy, through the right ventricular outflow tract, or more recently through an atriotomy, approaching the ventricular septum through the tricuspid valve. Cardioplegia, through hypothermia or anoxia, is used to allow proper visualization and a quiet field.

A number of surgeons, using different techniques and different types of pump oxygenators, operating in different patients with different defects, at different ages, have reported variable results at medical meetings. For some reason, the number of reports in medical journals is much smaller. A compilation and comparison of these results have been referred to by a number of cynics (all medical men) as the "numbers game."

Because of the multiplicity of the factors involved, it is extremely hard for anyone to appreciate the mortality pertaining to any one patient, at any one age, at any one center. The only thing one really knows in this confused field is the experience at one's own institution.

In terms of large ventricular septal defects, i.e. patients whose pulmonary arterial pressure approximates systemic arterial pressure, a risk of between 10 and 25 per cent should be assumed at present. Factors tending to place a patient in the lower ranges of this wide spectrum are (1) weight more than 30 pounds, (2) absence of congestive heart failure, (3) large pulmonary flow, (4) calculated resistance of less than 5 units per square meter, (5) relatively low left atrial or pulmonary capillary pressure, and (6) age less than 20 years. Of course the opposites of these increase the mortality.

Any one of the following factors serves as a contraindication to total repair in our institution at present: (1) age less than one year, (2) a pulmonary arterial pressure of systemic range with less than a 2:1 pulmonary-to-systemic flow ratio, and (3) a net right-to-left shunt. From these thoughts the following indications for surgery on a large ventricular septal defect are given: (1) A patient with a large (more than 2:1), pure, left-to-right shunt, with pulmonary capillary or left atrial pressure of less than 15 mm. of mercury, with a pulmonary resistance of less than 5 units and without congestive heart failure is an ideal candidate. We prefer to operate on these children when they are between the ages of 5 and 15 years; a mortality rate of 10 per cent or less may be expected. (2) These same patients may have to be operated on sooner if they have evidences of congestive heart failure or progressive cardiac enlargement. The risk in patients between the ages of 2 to 5 years, under these circumstances, may be estimated at 10 to 15 per cent. (3) Children with large, pure left-to-right shunts, but with left atrial and pulmonary capillary pressures greater than 15 mm. of mercury, or those with pulmonary resistances between 5 and 10 units, fall into a high-risk category at any age. The risk here may be quoted as 15 to 20 per cent. We propose surgery for these patients as soon as possible after they reach the weight of 30 pounds because we feel that it is among these patients that the earliest irreversible pulmonary vascular changes may occur. The operative risks in such patients beyond puberty may well be in the 20 to 25 per cent range. (4) Patients with a bidirectional, though small net left-to-right, shunt at the ventricular level and a pulmonary resistance of more than 10 units are not being operated on at our institution at present.

These indications are based on our present concept of the relative stability of the clinical and physiologic status of patients with ventricular septal defect from infancy through early childhood and on the preference of our surgical colleagues, for technical reasons, to deal with larger patients.

These are our thoughts in August, 1961; they may well have changed by the time this book is published.

If the operation is successful and the ventricular defect is closed, notable changes occur in the patient. The murmur disappears (Fig. 287), pulmonic closure is less loud, and the heart is less active. Roentgenograms show a decrease in heart size (Fig. 288). In approximately 80 per cent of the patients the electrocardiogram shows complete right bundle branch block (Fig. 289); hence the persistent splitting of the second sound. At catheterization no shunt is demonstrable, and the pulmonary arterial pressure drops. How near to normal the pulmonary arterial pressure returns in these patients is a matter of controversy. Our experience, supported by data from Adams,[6] indicates that usually the drop in pressure is commensurate with the elimination of the left-to-right shunt (Fig. 290). The resistance is usually not changed; it may even increase slightly. There are only a few patients in whom an actual drop in resistance and flow occurs. Paralleling these changes in the heart and circulation are an increase in appetite, a gain in weight, and the disappearance of fatigue.

Complications may occur in the postoperative course. No exhaustive discussion of these will be attempted here; the various items will be described only briefly.

1. *Complete heart block.* This is a highly dangerous and often fatal byproduct of surgery for a ventricular septal defect. Fortunately its incidence, as the skill of the surgeons improves, is much less than it used to be. Most centers encounter less than 10 per cent block, postoperatively. If block is present at the end of the operation, insertion of wires for eventual attachment to a pacemaker is mandatory. It is our custom to "drive" these

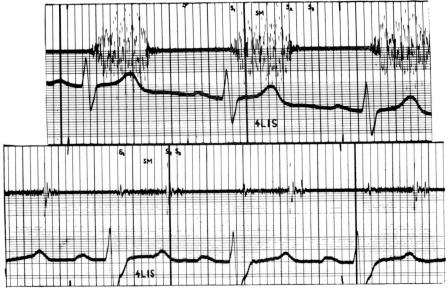

Figure 287. Preoperative and postoperative tracings of patient with ventricular septal defect. Note the high-intensity, high-frequency, plateau-shaped murmur on the top, preoperatively, and the minimal, low-frequency, low-intensity murmur, postoperatively, at the bottom. Note also the widely split second sound in the postoperative tracing, corresponding to the widened QRS complex, secondary to surgery.

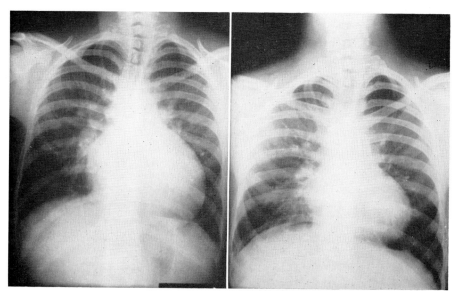

Figure 288.   Preoperative and postoperative roentgenograms in patient with large ventricular septal defect. Note the considerable diminution in heart size in the postoperative film.

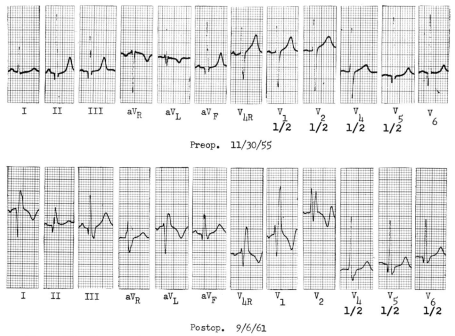

Figure 289.   Preoperative and postoperative electrocardiograms in a child with ventricular septal defect. Note the considerable diminution in heart size in the postoperative lower tracing.

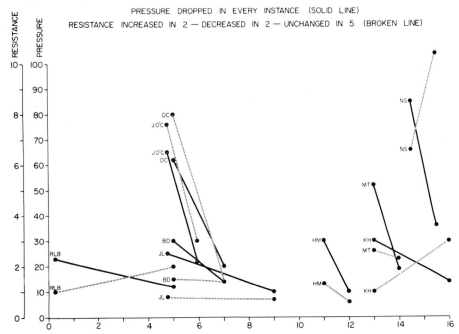

Figure 290.   Preoperative and postoperative catheterization studies in nine patients with ventricular septal defect. The solid lines indicate pressure changes, and the interrupted lines, changes in resistance. It may be seen that the pressures in all patients have dropped. The resistance stayed about the same in five patients: M.T., H.M., B.D., J.L. and R.L.B. It dropped significantly in two patients: D.C. and J.O'C. It increased significantly in two others: K.H. and N.S.

patients with the pacemaker, constantly for 2 to 4 days, at the rate of ±100 beats per minute. In this way the probability of permanent heart block may be lessened.

If the block does not disappear, Isuprel, administered by mouth or by rectum, perhaps supplemented with Diuril to lower the serum potassium level, may be used to establish a rate between 50 and 60 beats per minute. Digitalis should not be given to these patients routinely. If this treatment is not successful, a battery-driven, permanent pacemaker may have to be installed. In spite of all these remedies, complete heart block is still a devastating complication of ventricular septal defect surgery.

2. *Congestive heart failure.* Because, at present, the development of heart failure is comparatively common, most patients with large left-to-right shunts should be digitalized postoperatively. Ventricular function curves from dogs, after ventriculotomy, indicate that digitalization improves the performance of the damaged heart muscle. Gerbode and his associates[274] implied that the technique of ventriculotomy may influence the development of congestive heart failure.

3. *Hemorrhage.* Probably the diagnosis and treatment of hemorrhage should be discussed within the general aspects of pump surgery.

4. *Hypotension.* Hypotension may be secondary to hemorrhage, congestive heart failure or pulmonary factors. The last may be the consequence of increased resistance or of left ventricular failure. Postoperative acidosis

also predisposes to hypotension, and vasopressors are ineffective if the pH is low.

5. *Tamponade.* If tamponade occurs, it is due to hemorrhage into the pericardial sac.

6. *Metabolic acidosis.* This, like hemorrhage, represents a general problem of the postoperative course when pump oxygenators are used.

7. *Pulmonary changes.* These may occur because of hemorrhage, atelectasis or increased tracheobronchial secretions.

8. *Arrhythmias.* Arrhythmias, other than complete block, consist of supraventricular premature beats, an occasional atrioventricular dissociation, and rarely, atrial fibrillation. Obviously, fibrillation should be treated as outlined in the section on atrial defects (see p. 383). Ordinarily the former conditions should not alarm the cardiologist; they may not need treatment at all.

9. *Disturbances of the central nervous system.* These are usually due to poor perfusion of the brain or to prolonged hypothermia. Increased intracranial pressure can be treated with urea, and the metabolism may be lowered by placing the anesthetized patient on an ice mattress.

10. *Tricuspid regurgitation.* Transient tricuspid regurgitation after ventriculotomy, manifested by the characteristic murmur and the prominent V wave of the jugular venous pulse, is seen fairly frequently after closure of the ventricular septal defect. The differentiation of these phenomena from a residual leak across the ventricular septum may be extremely difficult. I would like to emphasize once more, however, that on the whole, if a ventricular defect has been successfully closed, no murmurs are audible over the heart. *In nine out of ten cases a residual murmur of more than grade 2 in intensity means that there is a residual shunt.*

A palliative operation for patients with ventricular septal defect has been proposed by Muller and Dammann.[512, 513] The technique consists in the creation of pulmonic stenosis by constricting the pulmonary artery immediately above the valve. This would result in (*a*) an increase in resistance at the pulmonary arterial level, (*b*) a diminution in the size of the left-to-right shunt across the ventricular septal defect and, thus, secondarily, in diminution of left ventricular flow work and left atrial pressure, (*c*) no increase in right ventricular pressure work, since with a large ventricular defect right ventricular pressure would be at systemic level anyhow, (*d*) a drop in pulmonary arterial pressure beyond the constriction, and (*e*) slight arterial unsaturation because of the right-to-left shunt secondary to the increased resistance to right ventricular outflow.

In other words, by means of this operation an "acyanotic tetralogy of Fallot" would, in effect, be created. This ingenious and physiologically sound procedure proves beneficial in that (1) it improves congestive heart failure, (2) it protects the patients from the effects of pulmonary arterial hypertension, and (3) it allows improved growth and development. Unfortunately, most of the published mortality risks are sufficiently high (25 to 50 per cent) that the procedure should not be taken lightly.[690] Also, complete repair of ventricular septal defects, even in young children, should be practical soon enough that one hesitates to subject them to another thoracotomy unless it is absolutely necessary.[392] On the other hand, reports from the West Coast indicate that patients with ventricular septal defect in whom pulmonary arteries have been "banded" in the past may later undergo complete surgical correction.[497]

At present, on the basis of these considerations, we recommend banding of the pulmonary artery when there are (1) anatomically incorrectible lesions with large pulmonary flow and pulmonary arterial hypertension (truncus arteriosus, transposition of the great arteries with ventricular septal defect and increased pulmonary flow) or (2) anatomically correctible ventricular septal defects with increased pulmonary flow and pulmonary arterial hypertension in patients whose size and level of pulmonary resistance (with the present amount of surgical skill) makes definitive correction highly dangerous. Within this group, in our institution, only small babies (weighing less than 15 pounds) with chronic congestive heart failure, recurrent pulmonary edema and practically no weight gain since birth, are considered for operation.

Summary

Patients with large ventricular septal defects are seriously ill. Symptoms of congestive failure, underdevelopment and severe respiratory infections usually begin in infancy. The diagnosis is based on the presence of a rough systolic murmur at the lower left sternal border, accompanied by clinical, electrocardiographic and roentgenologic evidences of pulmonary arterial hypertension. If a child survives the first two or three years, he usually gets better and may lead a relatively normal life for one to two decades. Cardiac catheterization is indicated to provide an understanding of the physiologic mechanism and to differentiate these patients from those with atypical patent ductus arteriosus. Operation, at a time acceptable to the surgeon and at a risk honestly stated and acceptable to the parents, is indicated in all patients with a left-to-right shunt at least equal to the systemic flow. The risks of such an operation vary tremendously, depending on the skill of the surgeon, the condition of the patient and the nature of the defect.

COMPLICATED VENTRICULAR SEPTAL DEFECT

Ventricular Septal Defect with Mild Pulmonic Stenosis

Ventricular septal defect with pulmonary stenosis, depending on the relation between systemic and pulmonary resistance, includes a number of clinical entities, ranging all the way from the exclusively left-to-right shunt group[89, 596, 602] to the tetralogy of Fallot. The condition to be discussed here is one in which the shunt through the ventricular defect is exclusively or predominantly left to right because of the relative mildness of the pulmonary stenosis; the other entities will be discussed in the section on Pulmonary Stenosis.

Incidence

Ventricular septal defect with pulmonic stenosis is a relatively common defect; there were twenty such instances in our ninety-eight cases of ventricular defect. Wood[752] found it in 1.3 per cent in his series of 900 patients.[264]

Anatomy

The majority of these defects lie posterior to the crista supraventricularis and somewhat more superior than the usual ventricular septal defect. Their size varies greatly, but probably most of them are large (0.5 to 1.5 cm.). The obstruction to right ventricular outflow is usually at the infundibular level.

Physiology

The degree of pulmonic stenosis may be relatively slight. It is not always clearly demonstrable anatomically, but it is always present in a physiologic sense; a significant pressure gradient (more than 25 mm. of mercury) between the right ventricle and pulmonary artery is always found at cardiac catheterization. In spite of the increase in resistance at the right ventricular outflow tract, the total systemic resistance is still higher than the total pulmonary resistance; thus the left-to-right shunt through the ventricular septal defect.

Clinical Picture

Perhaps the clinical picture resembles that of Roger's disease more than that of a large ventricular septal defect. A murmur was the only complaint in a third of our patients; the others had various degrees of dyspnea and fatigue and had frequent respiratory infections. Episodic cyanosis is a relatively common presenting symptom in this group.

The murmur is usually discovered early; in all our cases it was present before the child was one year old, and often it was noted at birth. The age at which symptoms begin varies from birth to eight years.

At physical examination many of these children are well developed and proportionately nourished. More than half of the patients in our group ranked at or above the twenty-fifth percentile line on our standard development charts. Frank cyanosis is rare. Left chest deformity is the rule, with few exceptions. The cardiac impulse is maximal at the xiphoid process, with an occasional left ventricular type of impulse as well. A pronounced thrill is always present at the left sternal border; in most cases this is maximal at the lower left sternal border, but in some instances it appears to be stronger at the upper left sternal border. Rales and hepatomegaly are noted in the few patients who have congestive failure. Blood pressure is usually normal.

At auscultation the heart sounds are usually not remarkable, although the second sound is usually well split with a diminished pulmonary component (Fig. 291). Seldom is there a systolic click. A harsh, stenotic systolic murmur is noted at the midsternal or lower left sternal border in every instance. Although in many cases it is impossible to distinguish this "stenotic" murmur from the murmur of a ventricular defect without pulmonic stenosis, differentiation may be attempted on the basis of criteria enumerated previously (p. 410). Occasionally one has the distinct impression that a ventricular septal defect type of systolic murmur, heard over the xiphoid process, can be differentiated from a stenotic murmur noted at the mid-left sternal border; such a fine differentiation between two similar systolic murmurs, occurring simultaneously, may be impressive to an audience of medical students, but is of little practical value and is full of pitfalls. Low-frequency, early or mid-diastolic murmurs are present at the lower left sternal border and the apex in about half of the cases; early blowing diastolic murmurs are rare and may indicate pulmonary arterial hypertension, occasionally, absence of the pulmonary valve (see p. 441), or even aortic regurgitation.

Roentgenologic examination reveals cardiac enlargement involving both ventricles (Fig. 292). The main pulmonary artery is usually normal or diminished in size, and pulmonary vascular engorgement without hilar dance is present. In at least 25 per cent of our cases there was a right aortic arch. Occasionally the left atrium seems prominent in the right anterior oblique view.

The electrocardiogram showed right ventricular hypertrophy or combined ventricular hypertrophy in twelve of our twenty cases. Left ventricular dominance was present in eight. Incomplete right bundle branch block is commonly observed. P pulmonale is relatively rare (occurring in four of our twenty cases).

Cardiac catheterization (Fig. 293) reveals the following: (1) There is an appropriate oxygen increase at the right ventricular level, as outlined in the data on simple ventricular septal defect (see p. 406). Mild systemic arterial unsaturation due to a right-to-left shunt may be present; this is commonly noted on exercise and occasionally even at rest. (2) Right ven-

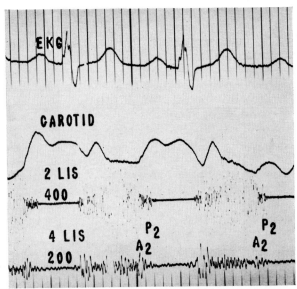

Figure 291. Phonocardiogram of patient with ventricular septal defect and pulmonic stenosis. Note the high-intensity, high-frequency, plateau-shaped murmur with widely split second sound.

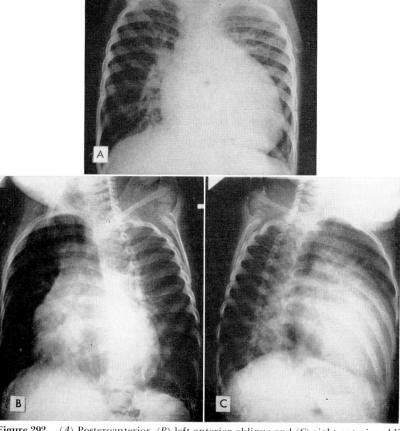

Figure 292.   (*A*) Posteroanterior, (*B*) left anterior oblique and (*C*) right anterior oblique roentgenograms of a patient with ventricular septal defect and pulmonary stenosis with a left-to-right shunt.

tricular pressure is usually at systemic level, with an infundibular gradient between the right ventricle and the pulmonary artery. Pulmonary arterial systolic pressure, if the right ventricular pressure is at systemic level, is greater than 40 mm. of mercury (differentiating this lesion from tetralogy of Fallot). Left atrial and systemic arterial pressures are normal. (3) Pulmonary resistance is usually normal. (4) Pulmonary-to-systemic flow ratios vary from 2:1 to 4:1. A simultaneous small right-to-left shunt may also be calculated at rest; on exercise this may increase considerably. (5) The course of the catheter across the ventricular septum is similar to that described in the section on Ventricular Septal Defect (see p. 407). (6) Selective angiography into the right ventricle may demonstrate the anatomy of the infundibular stenosis. Left ventricular injection outlines the ventricular septal defect. (7) Dye dilution curves with injection into the right heart chambers show the characteristic recirculation pattern, and if the catheter is located proximal to the pulmonary valve, an early appearance time indicates a minimal right-to-left shunt.

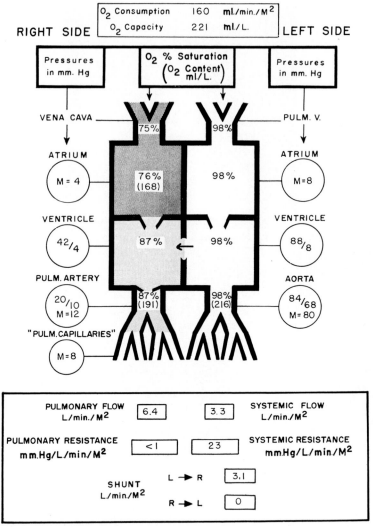

Figure 293. Catheterization findings in patient with small ventricular defect, pulmonic stenosis and a left-to-right shunt.

Course and Prognosis

The course of a patient with ventricular septal defect and pulmonic stenosis is a fascinating one. Most of these patients have little trouble during infancy and early childhood; in this respect they resemble patients who have Roger's disease. A few of them, however, are severely ill and have signs and symptoms identical to those seen in children with large ventricular defects.

As time goes on, usually by the time they are four to six years of age, evidences of left-to-right shunt diminish, pulmonary vascular engorgement becomes less definite, and the apical diastolic rumble disappears. Coincidentally, pulmonic stenosis increases, sometimes to the point at which the picture becomes similar to that of tetralogy of Fallot. At other times a salutary balance is established between the left-to-right shunt and the pulmonic stenosis, resulting in complete freedom from symptoms and normal pulmonary vasculature.[268, 529]

The incidence of complicating subacute bacterial endocarditis and rheumatic fever is about the same as in straightforward ventricular septal defect.

Differential Diagnosis

The differential diagnosis of ventricular septal defect with pulmonic stenosis is essentially the differential diagnosis of its component parts (see appropriate paragraphs in the sections on small and large ventricular septal defects and pulmonary stenosis). Special emphasis should be placed on the following entities:

Small Ventricular Septal Defect. Sometimes it is impossible to differentiate a small ventricular septal defect from a ventricular defect with pulmonic stenosis without resorting to cardiac catheterization. The distinguishing points have already been discussed (see p. 410).

Large Ventricular Septal Defect. Large ventricular defects should not present any real problem in the differential diagnosis because of the evidences of pulmonary arterial hypertension commonly inherent in this lesion.

Infundibular Pulmonary Stenosis. Infundibular pulmonic stenosis with definite diminution of the pulmonary vasculature and absence of an apical diastolic rumble is usually hard to distinguish from the combination of ventricular defect and pulmonic stenosis. *Isolated infundibular stenosis is a rare condition,* however. Thus this diagnosis should be made cautiously.

Patent Ductus Arteriosus. Seldom is ventricular septal defect with pulmonic stenosis confused with typical patent ductus arteriosus. But an atypical patent ductus arteriosus may sometimes be thought of in patients in whom the ventricular defect and the left-to-right shunt occur beyond the point of maximal stenosis at the infundibular level. The reason for this is that, in these instances, the right ventricle is excluded from the flow-work inherent in the ventricular defect, and the left ventricle carries the entire shunt work load, much as it does in patent ductus arteriosus; therefore left ventricular dominance, or even left ventricular hypertrophy, may be manifest in the electrocardiogram in spite of moderate but definite pulmonic stenosis.

Treatment

In certain fortunate instances treatment may not be necessary at all; the two lesions may act on each other in a compensatory fashion.

If, however, the left-to-right shunt through the ventricular septal defect seems large, or if the right-to-left shunt becomes bothersome on exercise or crying, complete repair, by means of cardiopulmonary bypass, should be contemplated.

Surgery consists in closure of the defect. Whether simultaneous infundibular resection is indicated, as in patients with true tetralogy of

Fallot, depends on the pressure gradient between the right ventricle and the pulmonary artery and on the size of the pulmonary flow. If the flow is tremendous and the gradient small, only closure of the ventricular septal defect is necessary. Conversely, with a moderate shunt and appreciable right ventricular obstruction, a combined procedure is recommended. Furthermore, if relief of the infundibular stenosis is indicated, this may be accomplished in certain instances by resection of the infundibulum alone, whereas in other patients insertion of a prosthesis to enlarge the outflow tract is necessary. It should be obvious that careful, on-the-spot evaluation of the patient on the operating table is necessary before the proper steps can be taken. Surgical experience should not be substituted for, but should be augmented by, the use of pressure transducers.

Operative mortality rate is relatively low, 5 to 10 per cent in the patients 5 to 15 years of age. Indications for operation are essentially the same as those given for ventricular septal defect, except that the dangers of pulmonary vascular obstruction should not be feared. March and his associates[478] emphasized the danger of reopening of the ventricular defect after complete repair of ventricular defect with pulmonic stenosis. They believed that this is more likely to happen when these lesions are combined than in pure ventricular defect and suggested immediate reoperation.

Medical management includes allowing these patients full range of activities, using chemotherapy and chemoprophylaxis as indicated, and treating manifestations of congestive failure if they occur.

Summary

Ventricular septal defect with pulmonic stenosis should be suspected from the clinical features characteristic of both lesions—a stenotic systolic murmur accompanied by an apical diastolic rumble, pulmonary vascular engorgement and right or left ventricular hypertrophy, as revealed by the electrocardiogram. Cardiac catheterization establishes the diagnosis. Surgical repair, if required, is successful in most instances.

Ventricular Septal Defect with Aortic Regurgitation

Ventricular septal defect with aortic regurgitation is a distinct clinical syndrome which gains significance by its close resemblance to a large patent ductus arteriosus by the high incidence of bacterial endocarditis and by the rapid progression of the disease.

Incidence

This anomaly was probably first mentioned by Laubry and Pezzi in 1921.[410] More recently Wood and his associates[752] reviewed the literature briefly and discussed the two cases which they encountered within the group of sixty ventricular septal defects studied. At The Children's Hospital Medical Center in Boston we have had four patients with this condition among our ninety-eight patients with ventricular defects. More recently, another twenty patients with this diagnosis have been studied. Scott and his co-workers[626] reported seven cases of their own and reviewed twenty-two from the literature in which the diagnosis was proved at post-mortem examination. Collins and his associates[155] reported three cases studied clinically.

Anatomy

Anatomically, the lesion consists of a small to moderate defect, immediately beneath the aortic valve, which is usually situated between the right and the posterior cusps if looked at from the left side, and is anterior and superior to the crista if viewed from the right side. The thickened, prolapsed right coronary cusp frequently herniates through the ventricular septal defect, obstructing it, at least in part, and also, not too infrequently, presenting an obstruction to right ventricular outflow. Occasionally the posterior, but never the left, cusp may be involved.

Physiology

The load is carried principally by the left ventricle and the left atrium. The left ventricular stroke volume must provide for the needs of the peripheral circulation, the regurgitant volume into the left ventricle through the aortic valve, and the left-to-right shunt. In addition to the increased left ventricular volume work inherent in the lesion, increased left ventricular pressure work is also often required by the elevation of the systemic systolic pressure. The ventricular septal defect, as well as the frequently associated mild to moderate pulmonic stenosis, may result in elevation of the right ventricular pressure work.

Clinical Picture

Clinically, this lesion resembles a large patent ductus arteriosus. A murmur is usually discovered in the neonatal period. In at least three instances in our experience, the murmur when first heard was purely systolic and was compatible with that heard in patients with simple ventricular septal defect. It was not until some years later, at the age of two to five years, that the presence of the protodiastolic blow was appreciated. Symptoms of dyspnea, fatigue and frequent severe respiratory infections manifest themselves early. On physical examination these patients are usually stunted and frail, considerable left chest deformity is present, and the cardiac impulse is maximal at the apex, and rocking. A thrill is palpable along the entire left sternal border. Evidences of right-sided and left-sided failure are common. The pulse pressure is wide, with diastolic readings close to zero.

At auscultation one is impressed with the loud (grade 5 to 6) systolic and grade 3 diastolic murmurs, audible along the entire precordium. By careful analysis and phonocardiography the murmurs can usually be separated into a grade 3 systolic component, maximal at the xiphoid process, and a grade 3 to 4 systolic-diastolic, usually to-and-fro, but rarely continuous murmur at the mid and upper left sternal borders. These murmurs, as expected from their maximal intensity, transmit well throughout the precordium, neck and back. In addition, apical, low-frequency mid-diastolic and presystolic murmurs also can be heard. The first heart sound is moderately accentuated, and the pulmonary second sound is loud and moderately well split, if it can be distinguished at all from the extremely loud systolic-diastolic murmur (Fig. 294).

In patients with full-blown aortic regurgitation, roentgenologic examination shows maximal cardiac enlargement involving both the left and the right ventricles, though the former usually predominates (Fig. 295). Left atrial enlargement is the rule. The main pulmonary artery and the aorta are both prominent, and the pulmonary vasculature is engorged and shows expansile pulsations.

Moderate degrees of cardiac enlargement are seen in patients in whom the aortic insufficiency is only slight (Fig. 296). In still others a distinct progression of cardiomegaly may be noted through the years (Fig. 297). Characteristically, in the patients with full-blown disease, the heart is much larger than one would expect, either from the degree of pulmonary vascular engorgement or from the calculated pulmonary flow. Also, the pulmonary vascular engorgement does not account for the widening of the pulse pressure obtained on physical examination. It may be speculated on the basis of these discrepancies that the left-to-right ventricular shunt cannot

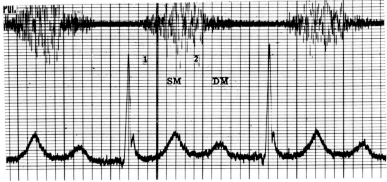

Figure 294. Phonocardiogram of patient with ventricular septal defect and aortic regurgitation.

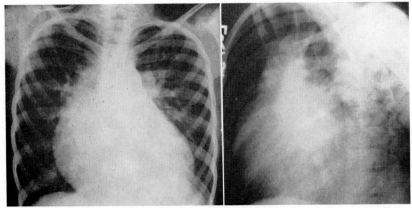

Figure 295. Posteroanterior and oblique views of patient with ventricular septal defect and aortic regurgitation.

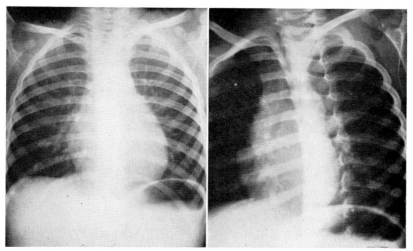

Figure 296. Roentgenogram of patient with ventricular defect and slight aortic regurgitation. Note that there is only a moderate degree of left ventricular enlargement and minimal pulmonary vascular engorgement.

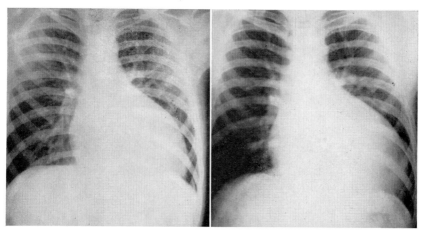

Figure 297. Progressive cardiac enlargement throughout a two-year period in a patient with ventricular defect and aortic regurgitation.

well explain the severity of the lesion, nor is it likely that the "aortic runoff" occurs into the pulmonary vascular bed.

The electrocardiogram reveals left ventricular hypertrophy, with strain and little, if any, evidence of right ventricular hypertrophy (Fig. 298) in severe cases.

Cardiac catheterization (Fig. 299) reveals the following data: (1) Oxygen saturation data indicate a moderate or even small left-to-right shunt at the level of the right ventricular outflow tract. A slight additional increase in oxygen saturation, usually less than 5 per cent, may be noted at the pulmonary arterial level. Systemic arterial saturation is usually normal. (2) Right ventricular pressure is high, approximating systemic levels. Frequently there is a gradient between the right ventricle and the

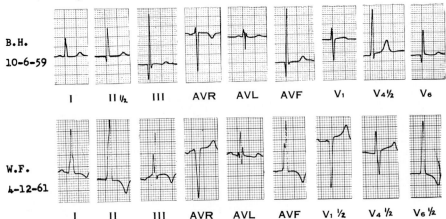

B.H.
10-6-59

I   II ½   III   AVR   AVL   AVF   V₁   V₄½   V₆

W.F.
4-12-61

I   II   III   AVR   AVL   AVF   V₁ ½   V₄ ½   V₆ ½

Figure 298. Electrocardiograms of two patients with ventricular defect and aortic regurgitation. Upper tracing from patient with mild aortic regurgitation. Note the mean electrical axis of plus 75 degrees and the tall left ventricular voltages with deep Q waves. Contrast this with the lower tracing from a patient with a severe form of the disease. Note the mean electrical axis of plus 45 degrees, tall voltages and S–T and T wave changes throughout the standard limb leads, aV$_F$ and V$_6$. These two tracings may serve as another illustration that the strict differentiation between "systolic" and "diastolic" overloading is untenable.

pulmonary artery at the infundibular or, less commonly, at the valvar level. Left atrial or pulmonary capillary pressure is elevated. Left ventricular systolic and end-diastolic pressures may be high also. The systemic artery shows a wide pulse pressure, commensurate with the degree of aortic regurgitation. The upstroke time of the systemic arterial pressure pulse is rapid. (3) Pulmonary resistance is usually normal. (4) Pulmonary-to-systemic flow ratios are relatively low, particularly in view of the large heart. It is assumed that the prolapsing cusp actually represents a resistance to the flow from the left to the right ventricle. (5) The course of the catheter is the same as that encountered during the study of patients with ventricular septal defect. (6) Retrograde aortography, with the catheter placed immediately above the aortic valve, is indispensable for the diagnosis. A quantitative assessment of the degree of aortic regurgitation is not possible in this fashion, but the anatomic details are most helpful to the surgeon. (7) Dye dilution curves are used in the differential diagnosis as well as for the quantitative estimation of aortic incompetence. The intracardiac phonocatheter, by registering the continuous murmur in the right ventricle rather than in the pulmonary artery, is helpful in differentiating this lesion from a patent ductus arteriosus.

Course and Prognosis

These patients usually have increasing disability, with development of congestive failure, and death occurs before the end of the second decade. Like patients with aortic regurgitation of other etiologies, once these patients show evidences of congestive heart failure or angina, the prognosis is very poor and the downhill course, rapid. On the other hand, many of the adolescents with cardiac enlargement may be able to perform

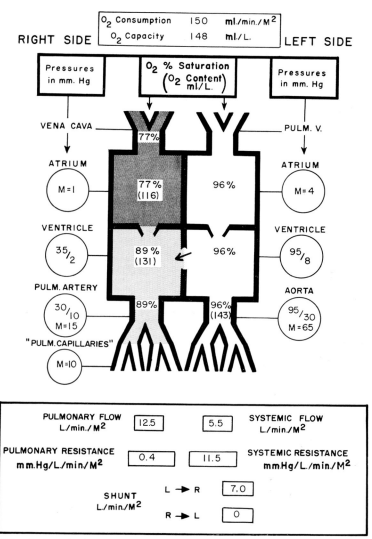

Figure 299. Catheterization findings in patient with ventricular defect and aortic regurgitation.

strenuous physical activities without any obvious difficulty. The incidence of bacterial endocarditis is high.

Differential Diagnosis

Patent Ductus Arteriosus. This is the most common differential diagnostic problem. Most of these patients do not have the characteristic, continuous machinery type of Gibson murmur; the murmur rarely may be continuous (though most often it is to and fro), but it lacks the late systolic crescendo typical of that heard with patent ductus arteriosus. Furthermore, the point of maximal intensity is usually at the third to fourth left interspace rather than at the second to third. Further clinical clues pointing away from a patent ductus arteriosus and toward ventricular septal defect with aortic regurgitation are the presence of an additional murmur of pulmonic stenosis and the aforementioned discrepancy between heart size and pulmonary vascular engorgement. If at cardiac catheterization the increase in oxygen content is relatively small and occurs principally, even exclusively, at the ventricular level, the diagnosis of patent ductus arteriosus is rather unlikely. The passage of the catheter from the right ventricle to the ascending aorta, rather than from the pulmonary artery to the descending aorta, also excludes patent ductus arteriosus as the only defect. The presence, at catheterization, of an appreciable gradient across the right ventricular outflow tract also militates somewhat against the presence of a patent ductus arteriosus. The usefulness of the intracardiac phonocatheter in the differential diagnosis has already been mentioned.

Aortopulmonary Septal Defect. Usually, though by all means not invariably, aortopulmonary septal defect presents the clinical picture of a large left-to-right shunt at the main pulmonary artery level. Thus differentiation should not be directed toward ventricular septal defect with aortic regurgitation, but rather toward patent ductus arteriosus (see p. 474). Furthermore, aortopulmonary septal defects seldom are associated with a ventricular defect.

Ruptured Sinus of Valsalva. This may be easily differentiated from the entity under discussion if the leakage occurs suddenly as a catastrophic event. If, however, there is a small congenital fistula in the sinus of Valsalva, then clinical differentiation is possible only by means of first-rate angiograms. Often only surgical exploration, under cardiopulmonary bypass, reveals the correct diagnosis. One further confusing feature of this particular aspect of the differential diagnosis is that, as mentioned before, ventricular defect with aortic regurgitation may also be a progressive disease in which the patient, when first seen, is thought to have only a simple ventricular defect, and in which the features of aortic regurgitation manifest themselves only later, because of the progressively more severe prolapse of the aortic cusp. It should be clear, then, that frequently a ruptured aneurysm of the sinus of Valsalva is almost impossible to differentiate from a ventricular septal defect with aortic regurgitation.

Coronary Arteriovenous Fistula. Coronary arteriovenous fistula should also be considered in the differential diagnosis of patients with loud continuous murmurs at the lower left sternal border. Commonly, these patients have no gross hemodynamic abnormalities, only a loud murmur. Depending on the chamber which receives the coronary arterial blood, the murmur may be systolic and diastolic (right ventricle and atria) or only diastolic (left ventricle). The site of the aneurysm may be seen on plane films, but is best outlined by retrograde angiograms.

Common Truncus Arteriosus. Common truncus arteriosus with a large pulmonary flow may give rise to a clinical picture simulating ventricular septal defect with aortic regurgitation. In truncus arteriosus, however, there is pulmonary vascular engorgement, and the main pulmonary artery cannot be seen at its usual position. At catheterization the pulmonary artery may be extremely difficult to enter from the conventional position in the right ventricle. If it is entered at all, the oxygen saturation is found to be identical with that in the aorta.

Absence of the Pulmonary Valve with Ventricular Septal Defect.   See below.

Treatment

Ventricular septal defect with aortic regurgitation is a surgically correctible condition today. In view of the complex anatomic situation, the relatively small experience any one center can accumulate with this rare condition, the poor state of the left ventricular myocardium in the advanced cases and the gross scarring and deformity of the prolapsed aortic cusp, a mortality rate no lower than 30 per cent should be quoted for this operation. Even if the patient survives operation, it is questionable how complete and how permanent will be the repair of the aortic valve. Nevertheless, because of the serious prognosis of the condition, surgery is advisable, preferably before late adolescence, to prevent development of cardiac enlargement and left ventricular fibrosis.

Surgery, using the pump oxygenator and deep hypothermia, consists first in exploration and repair of the aortic valve from above, and then of closure of the ventricular septal defect by direct suture and support of the aortic valve from below through a ventriculotomy. These repairs, if successful, have most gratifying results.[659]

Summary

Ventricular septal defect with aortic regurgitation is similar to large patent ductus arteriosus. The to-and-fro nature of the murmur, coupled with its localization at the lower left sternal border, should make the cardiologist suspect this lesion instead of a large ductus. Cardiac catheterization, or even thoracotomy, may be necessary to confirm the diagnosis. Retrograde aortography may likewise be necessary. Surgery, with relatively high risks, is recommended.

Ventricular Septal Defect with Absence of the Pulmonary Valve

Incidence

The syndrome of ventricular septal defect with absence of the pulmonary valve was first reported by Lavenne[411] and later by Campeau and his co-workers.[137] Miller and his associates[496] reported cases simulating tetralogy of Fallot, and finally Onesti and his associates[541] described a case with postmortem findings. We have seen four such cases during the past ten years. Its incidence cannot be accurately stated, but it must be extremely rare.

Anatomy

The ventricular defect is usually large and is in its conventional position in the outflow tract of the right ventricle, below the aortic orifice. The pulmonary valves are replaced by fibrous tissue or are represented only by a small "nubbin" of valvar tissue. A subvalvar obstruction of the right ventricular outflow tract may also be present.

Physiology

The hemodynamic effects of the abnormality depend on the severity of the three components of the lesion. The ventricular septal defect imposes a strain on the left ventricle, whereas the pulmonary regurgitation, inherent in the absent valve, places a burden on the right ventricle. The infundibular stenosis, if present, also increases right ventricular work, but may compensate for the pulmonary regurgitation and may actually diminish the left-to-right shunt, as well. Thus the clinical profile depends on the interplay of these three factors.

Clinical Picture

Depending on the underlying physiologic abnormality, the patients may present the clinical profile of a large ventricular septal defect or of tetralogy of Fallot. In the former instance, infundibular stenosis is minimal; in the latter it dominates the picture. In both situations the long, loud, protodiastolic murmur in the pulmonic area dominates the auscultatory findings. In addition, no pulmonic closure may be heard (Fig. 300). Finally, the main pulmonary artery is aneurysmally dilated and vigorously pulsatile (Fig. 301), and the electrocardiogram shows right ventricular hypertrophy. These findings are characteristic of both varieties of absence of the pulmonary valve with ventricular septal defect. Within this general group, the patients without a significant degree of infundibular stenosis show no cyanosis and have hyperactive left and right ventricles with left chest deformity, congestive heart failure and all the other evidences of a large ventricular septal defect. In contrast, those with significant infundibular stenosis are cyanotic; the murmur of infundibular stenosis can be heard, and the left ventricle is not hyperactive. In brief, these patients present the clinical picture of tetralogy of Fallot, but with a large, pulsatile main pulmonary artery and a loud, early diastolic blow.

At *cardiac catheterization* (Fig. 302) the following observations may be made: (1) A left-to-right shunt is observed at the ventricular level. Arterial unsaturation may be present, depending on the degree of infundibular stenosis and the state of the pulmonary vasculature. (2) Characteristically, the pressure tracings reveal pulmonic insufficiency, with pulmonary arterial diastolic pressure close to, if not identical with, right ventricular diastolic pressure (Fig. 303). Usually there is a systolic gradient across the right ventricular infundibulum. The levels of the right atrial mean and right ventricular end-diastolic pressures depend on the state of the myocardium and the severity of the lesion. (3) In none of our patients was the pulmonary resistance significantly elevated, but Campeau's patients[137] showed pulmonary vascular obstruction. (4) The pulmonary-to-systemic flow ratio varies from a large left-to-right to a net right-to-left shunt. (5) There is nothing unusual about the passage of the catheter, except that the pulmonary artery may be difficult to enter because of the strong valvar incompetence. It may be possible to traverse the ventricular septum in the con-

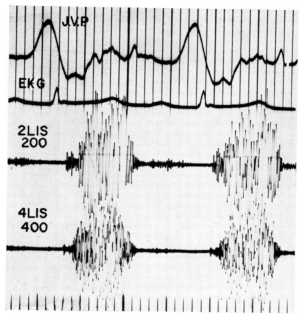

Figure 300. Phonocardiogram of patient with absence of the pulmonary valve. Note the high-frequency, high-intensity stenotic murmur and the low-frequency, low-intensity diastolic murmur at the second left interspace, occupying most of diastole.

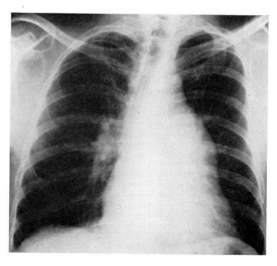

Figure 301. Posteroanterior film of patient with left ventricular septal defect, pulmonic stenosis and absence of the pulmonary valve. Note the prominent main pulmonary arterial segment with only a moderate increase of the pulmonary vasculature.

ventional position. (6) Cine-angiograms, with injection into the pulmonary artery, demonstrate pulmonary regurgitation. (7) Dye dilution studies reveal the magnitude of the left-to-right and right-to-left shunts and may show curves characteristic of pulmonary regurgitation.

Course and Prognosis

Not enough cases have been described in the literature to warrant even an approximation of the life expectancy of these patients. One of our patients was an asymptomatic worker in his mid-thirties. The others were children and adolescents. Onesti's[541] patient died in infancy; others lived to their forties.[411] I suspect that the course depends on the actual physiology in the individual patient. In patients who have infundibular stenosis the course is more or less like that of patients with tetralogy of Fallot, whereas in those without infundibular stenosis the course is the same as that with severe, large ventricular septal defect, with eventual development of pulmonary vascular obstruction and congestive heart failure.

In the differential diagnosis the only important entity to be mentioned is ventricular septal defect with aortic regurgitation. The protodiastolic murmur of pulmonary regurgitation may be easily confused with that originating from the aortic valve unless one searches carefully for peripheral evidences of aortic regurgitation. The large and vigorously pulsating pul-

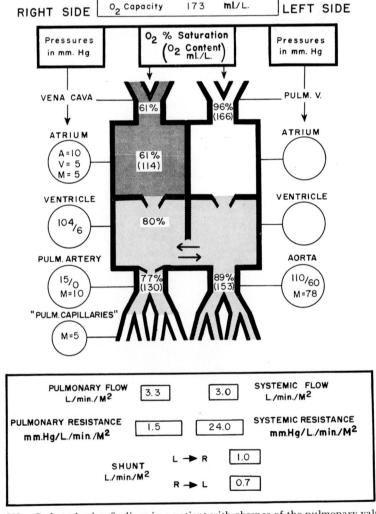

Figure 302.   Catheterization findings in a patient with absence of the pulmonary valve, ventricular septal defect and infundibular pulmonic stenosis.

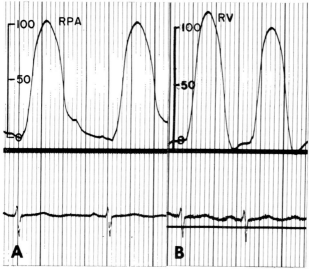

Figure 303. Pressure tracing from the pulmonary artery and the right ventricle of a patient with absence of the pulmonary valve. Note the practically identical pressure pulses in the two chambers.

monary arteries and, of course, the angiograms are the best means of differentiation. Positive identification of a loud pulmonic closure excludes the diagnosis of absence of the pulmonary valve and should raise the suspicion of pulmonary vascular obstruction with secondary pulmonary regurgitation.

Treatment

Until adequate replacement for the absent pulmonary valve is found, complete correction of the defect is not feasible. We have not operated on patients of this type yet, but it may be possible to close the ventricular defect, relieve the infundibular stenosis and leave the patient with some pulmonary regurgitation. The long-term prognosis of pulmonary regurgitation as a solitary lesion is not known, but there is some evidence that moderate degrees may be tolerated well for many years. The many patients with postoperative pulmonary regurgitation after Brock procedures and the large number of asymptomatic patients with idiopathic pulmonary regurgitation attest to the validity of this hypothesis. On the other hand, Kay and Thomas[375] found that in dogs whose pulmonic valves were completely excised, systolic and diastolic pulmonary hypertension developed, and some died in congestive failure.

Therefore I would not subject patients with this syndrome to surgery at present unless they show symptoms of a sizable right-to-left shunt or congestive heart failure. Under such circumstances closure of the ventricular septal defect and relief of the pulmonic stenosis are indicated.

Summary

In patients with ventricular septal defect who have a loud, long pulmonary regurgitant murmur and large, pulsating pulmonary arteries with no pulmonic closure, absence of the pulmonary valve may be suspected. These patients may present either the picture of a large ventricular septal defect or that of tetralogy of Fallot. Surgery is not recommended, except for patients with moderate or severe symptoms.

Ventricular Septal Defect with Atrial Septal Defect

This is not too rare a combination. Five to ten per cent of the ventricular defects are associated with an additional atrial septal defect. I am not including in this category patients with endocardial cushion defects in

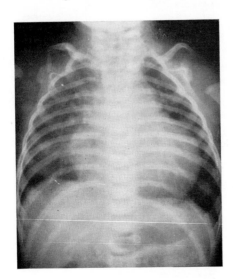

Figure 304.   Posteroanterior roentgenogram of infant with combined ventricular and atrial septal defects. This child was in severe congestive heart failure. Note the cardiac enlargement involving principally the right ventricle, right atrium and pulmonary artery. Note also the pulmonary vascular engorgement.

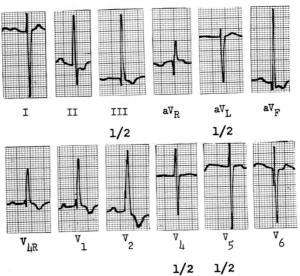

Figure 305. Electrocardiogram of patient with ventricular defect and atrial defect. Note the mean electrical axis of plus 135 degrees, right ventricular hypertrophy, and questionable left ventricular hypertrophy on the basis of aV_F.

whom the two lesions are contiguous; rather I am discussing a separate ventricular and a separate atrial opening. No long discussion of this combination of anomalies is necessary. It should suffice to point out that these patients present the clinical picture of a large ventricular septal defect (Figs. 304, 305). But at catheterization a significant increase in oxygen content occurs at the atrial and the ventricular levels (Fig. 306). Furthermore, the catheter may be passed easily from the right atrium to the left atrium. As mentioned earlier, this latter point does not necessarily indicate the presence of anything more than a patent foramen ovale, particularly in infants and small children. In patients with combined ventricular and atrial defects, however, the mean pressure in the right atrium and that in the left atrium and/or pulmonary capillaries is closely similar. This feature tends to separate ventricular septal and atrial septal defect from

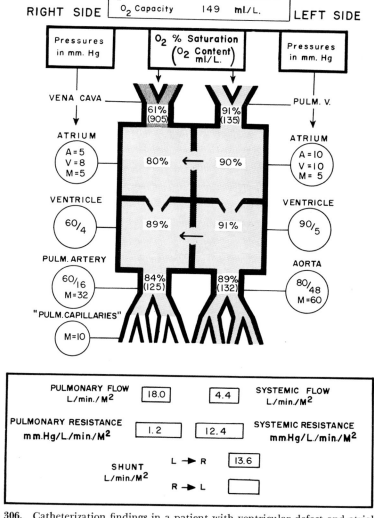

Figure 306. Catheterization findings in a patient with ventricular defect and atrial defect.

ventricular septal defect with tricuspid regurgitation and left ventricular-right atrial shunts. Of course the electrocardiogram sets aside the group with endocardial cushion defects rather sharply. From all other clinical and physiologic viewpoints this combination of lesions is practically identical to a large ventricular septal defect. If anything, these patients may be somewhat sicker, earlier, than the average patient who has a ventricular septal defect, and surgery, preferably through a right atrial approach, may be indicated relatively early.

Large Ventricular Septal Defect with Patent Ductus Arteriosus

The combination of these two anomalies occurs fairly frequently. The incidence is hard to assess accurately, but in a three-year period eighteen such patients were encountered in our institution.[612]

Anatomy

There is nothing unusual about the anatomy of these patients except that both the ductus arteriosus and the ventricular septal defect are usually large.

Physiology

A left-to-right shunt, at both the ventricular and pulmonary arterial levels, and pulmonary arterial hypertension are the physiologic consequences of the anomalies. The latter phenomenon places the burden on the right ventricle, whereas the shunt affects principally the left ventricle and the left atrium. In many instances pulmonary vascular obstruction contributes to the pulmonary arterial hypertension.

Clinical Picture

Most of these patients show congestive failure, underdevelopment and severe dyspnea early in infancy. As a matter of fact, of the children with large ventricular septal defect, those who also have a sizable patent ductus arteriosus are among the sickest.

On physical examination, underdevelopment is striking (Fig. 307), and the pulse pressure is wide (more than 50 mm. of mercury) in almost every instance. The rest of the observations made at physical examination (Fig. 308) are indistinguishable from those characteristic of a large ventricular septal defect, except that the systolic murmur is often heard as well, if not better, at the second to third left interspace as at the third to fourth. A characteristic Gibson murmur is heard only rarely in these infants.

At roentgenologic examination one is impressed by the cardiac enlargement involving the left ventricle and the left atrium, with pulmonary vascular engorgement and a prominent main pulmonary artery. In addition to the active engorgement of the pulmonary artery, pulmonary venous congestion is frequently noted. All these features are indistinguishable from those associated with a large ventricular septal defect; they are helpful

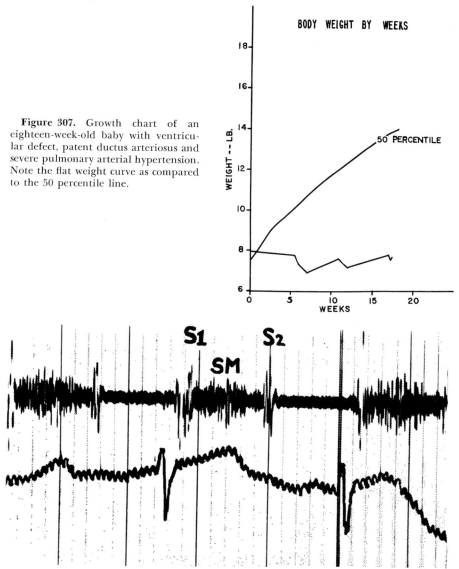

Figure 307. Growth chart of an eighteen-week-old baby with ventricular defect, patent ductus arteriosus and severe pulmonary arterial hypertension. Note the flat weight curve as compared to the 50 percentile line.

Figure 308. Phonocardiogram of patient with ventricular defect and patent ductus arteriosus. Note the low-frequency, low-intensity ejection type of systolic murmur without any indication of a continuous component.

only in the sense that if the left atrium and the pulmonary artery are *not* enlarged, the diagnosis of ventricular septal defect and patent ductus arteriosus seems unlikely.

The electrocardiogram is indistinguishable from that seen in patients with a large ventricular septal defect. It almost always reveals right ventricular hypertrophy, alone or in combination with left ventricular hypertrophy. Pure left ventricular hypertrophy is seen in only about 10 per cent of the patients.

Cardiac catheterization reveals the following (Fig. 309): (1) In more than 75 per cent of the patients there is at least a 10 per cent increase in the oxygen content of the right ventricle (particularly in the outflow tract) over that of the right atrium. In contrast, the oxygen saturation data suggest patent ductus arteriosus in only a minority (25 per cent) of the patients. Most of them have arterial unsaturation. In some this is due to congestive heart failure, causing pulmonary venous unsaturation. An increase of more than 5 per cent in the oxygen saturation at the pulmonary arterial level is rarely seen, according to our experience. (2) Pulmonary arterial hypertension is the rule. Moderate to severe left atrial or pulmonary capillary hypertension is present in all patients. Systemic arterial pressure is often elevated, with a wide pulse pressure, a rapid upstroke and a low dicrotic notch. (3) Almost one third of the patients have high pulmonary resistance. Occasionally, pulmonary vascular obstruction may be severe

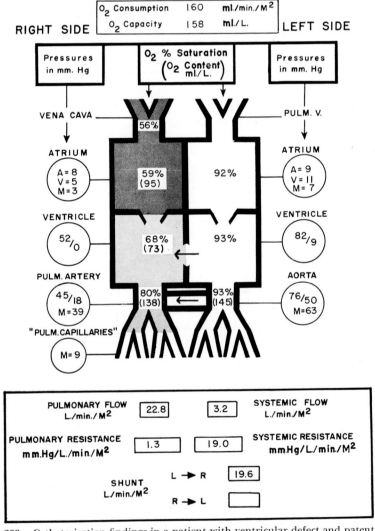

Figure 309. Catheterization findings in a patient with ventricular defect and patent ductus arteriosus.

even in infants. In some patients an unexpected increase in pulmonary resistance has been noted after division of the patent ductus arteriosus. (4) The pulmonary-to-systemic flow ratio usually reveals a large (more than 3:1) left-to-right shunt. It is extremely difficult to assess what proportion of this shunt occurs at the ventricular and at the ductal levels, but in most instances the ventricular shunt seems to dominate. (5) The passage of the catheter from the pulmonary artery to the aorta furnishes the principal evidence for the presence of a patent ductus arteriosus in the majority of instances. In contrast, the catheter crosses the ventricular septum in only a minority of the cases. Thus it may be stated that, whereas oxygen data are most helpful in diagnosing the ventricular defect, the course of the catheter enables the cardiologist to document the presence of a patent ductus arteriosus. (6) Cine-angiograms with injection into the aortic arch and the left ventricle may be helpful in outlining the site of the left-to-right shunt. (7) Dye dilution curves, with injection into the left ventricle and the ascending aorta and with sampling from the pulmonary artery, may give not only qualitative, but also quantitative, estimates of the respective left-to-right shunts.

Course and Prognosis

As indicated previously, these infants are usually very sick. Often, vigorous anti-congestive measures are not effective in combating left-sided failure; repeated attacks of pneumonia plague these miserable-looking babies, who often do not weigh any more at four months than they did at birth. They depend on an oxygen tent to the extent that they can barely survive outside the hospital.

With patience, perseverance and vigorous medical treatment, however, one may enable a significant proportion of these to live beyond their first birthday. After that they usually start improving gradually, though I have not had a large enough number of them followed up to know what their ultimate prognosis is without surgery. Nevertheless I have seen some patients in whom the size of the ductus as well as of the ventricular shunt diminished markedly in time. The course of other patients, who obviously have a *large* patent ductus arteriosus with a typical Gibson murmur, is clearly a different matter. These behave much more like patients with a patent ductus arteriosus, and most of them are treated early by surgery; thus no follow-up under a medical regimen is available.

Differential Diagnosis

Large Ventricular Septal Defect. Unless the catheter clearly passes from the pulmonary artery to the aorta, beyond the left subclavian, or unless a clear-cut left-to-right shunt, by means of oxygen saturation or dye methods, is demonstrated, this group of patients cannot be distinguished from patients with a large ventricular septal defect. A wide pulse pressure, a large left atrium and a prominent main pulmonary artery in a patient with evidences of maximal left-to-right shunt at the ventricular level may focus attention on this combination of anomalies.

Patent Ductus Arteriosus. The absence of the characteristic Gibson murmur and the presence of a significant degree of right ventricular hypertrophy in the electrocardiogram separate these patients, clinically, from those having a simple patent ductus arteriosus. Some of the children with a patent ductus may have small ventricular septal defects, but this is a different situation clinically, hemodynamically and prognostically.

Truncus Arteriosus. That truncus arteriosus may be indistinguishable, clinically, from the combination of ventricular septal defect and patent ductus arteriosus should be evident from the fact that the physiologic situations are identical. In both instances a large ventricular septal defect is associated with an additional large communication at the level of the great arteries.

In the physical examination the presence of definite cyanosis may tend to favor truncus arteriosus, as does the absence of a main pulmonary artery at its usual place in the roentgenogram.

Cine-angiograms, by outlining the origin of the pulmonary artery, are most helpful in the differential diagnosis. Additional evidence may be obtained by a critical consideration of the oxygen saturations in the systemic and pulmonary arteries; if these are identical, the diagnosis of truncus arteriosus is more likely.

Aortopulmonary Fenestration. Physiologically, and even embrylogically, this anomaly is so similar to a common truncus arteriosus that it must be considered in the differential diagnosis. Clinically, differentiation may be impossible. At catheterization, however, the catheter, after leaving the pulmonary artery, characteristically enters the ascending aorta to the right of the innominate artery, establishing the diagnosis (see p. 498). Angiographic confirmation may also be obtained.

Treatment

Of course the optimal treatment for patients with large ventricular septal defect and patent ductus arteriosus consists of surgical closure of the ventricular defect with simultaneous division, or ligation, of the ductus. This is a difficult surgical feat in a small infant, weighing barely more than birth weight, in chronic congestive failure.

The next seemingly logical approach, then, is to take care of the patent ductus arteriosus only and hope that by this simple operation the situation may improve to the extent that surgery for the ventricular septal defect may be postponed. We have tried this approach in at least ten patients and found appreciable improvement in only two. Three of the remaining died, and the clinical status of the others was unchanged. In some of the survivors, catheterization showed an increased pulmonary resistance; in others, a left-to-right shunt of preoperative magnitude persists, now exclusively through the ventricular septal defect.

Our present policy is to treat both defects simultaneously by surgery, if the surgeon thinks this is technically feasible. If the risks of repairing the ventricular septal defect seem prohibitive, medical measures are pursued vigorously. Only with extreme reluctance, if the situation is clearly untenable, do we recommend division of the patent ductus arteriosus with simultaneous banding of the pulmonary artery. This latter maneuver, without an additional thoracotomy, should diminish the ventricular left-to-right shunt as well as serve to protect the pulmonary vasculature.

I would like to re-emphasize that these therapeutic principles relate only to patients with large ventricular septal defect and patent ductus arteriosus, in whom the shunt through the ventricular defect is clearly of major, and probably of dominant, significance. Patients with a clear-cut clinical and hemodynamic picture of patent ductus arteriosus with trivial ventricular defect should be treated promptly by division of the ductus arteriosus.

Summary

Patients with large ventricular septal defect and patent ductus arteriosus cannot be distinguished clinically from those with large ventricular defect alone. A wide pulse pressure, an enlarged left atrium and a prominent main pulmonary artery in a very sick youngster should raise the suspicion of this combination of anomalies. At catheterization a left-to-right shunt is usually clearly demonstrable at the ventricular level, and the catheter passes with ease through the patent ductus arteriosus. Ideally, both defects should be treated simultaneously by surgery. In view of the high risks of this operation in young infants, conservative treatment is recommended. Only as a last resort should division of the ductus arteriosus with simultaneous banding of the main pulmonary artery be considered.

Ventricular Septal Defect and Coarctation of the Aorta

This anomaly, occurring in probably less than 5 per cent of the patients with ventricular septal defect, will be discussed in detail in the section on Coarctation of the Aorta (see p. 521), since most of the patients are admitted with this diagnosis. In effect, this represents only a large shunt at the ventricular level, usually associated with pulmonary hypertension. The size of the shunt is due, not only to the size of the defect, but also to the relatively higher than normal left ventricular pressure.

SINGLE VENTRICLE

From the physiologic viewpoint the complete absence of a ventricular septum should not be regarded as a situation basically different from a large ventricular septal defect. Often, after a thorough study, using all the available clinical and laboratory methods, the question of whether one is dealing with a single ventricle or a large ventricular defect becomes one of semantics alone.

Because of the rather distinctive anatomic situation and the relatively poor prognosis, however, it may be worth while to discuss this anomaly under a separate heading, but within the group of defects of the ventricular septum.

Incidence

This is a rare anomaly. It was present in only 10 of our 577 cases of proved congenital heart disease. Abbott[1] reported 13 in her series of 1000 cases observed at postmortem examination. Keith[380] encountered the anomaly in 2 per cent of the children in his series who had congenital heart disease. Edwards[214] quoted its frequency as about 3 per cent.

Anatomy

The typical case is distinguished by relatively normal atrioventricular valves opening into the inflow portion of a single ventricular chamber; separated from this common ventricle by a muscular ridge is a rudimentary outflow chamber, the remainder of the bulbus cordis, giving rise to one or both great vessels. In more than 75 per cent of the patients the vessels are either completely transposed or are in the corrected transposition relation to each other. Dextrocardia may be present also. There may be obstruction of the subpulmonic tract or the subaortic tract, or, in still other situations, both great arteries may communicate freely with the common ventricle. In most patients an atrial septum is present, but in about 25 per cent a so-called cor biloculare is encountered. Among these patients mitral or tricuspid atresia is common.

Physiology

From the aforementioned considerations it must be clear that anatomically, as well as physiologically, this is an extremely heterogeneous group. The pressure in all portions of the single ventricular chamber and the oxygen saturation in the ventricle and both great arteries are *approximately* the same. One has to say "approximately" because streaming may bring about some modification even of this basic criterion. Depending on the size of the pulmonary flow, the patient may or may not be cyanotic. *The probability that a single ventricle is a solitary lesion not associated with any other serious* (and often incorrectible) *anomaly is rare.*

The physiologic criteria of identical saturation in both great arteries and identical pressures in "both" ventricles do not necessarily indicate an anatomically single ventricle; these may simply be due to a *physiologically* single ventricle, i.e. a large ventricular septal defect. Usually the difference is that in patients with only a physiologically single ventricle associated anomalies may not be present, whereas with an anatomically single ventricle, other serious defects are almost invariably encountered.

Clinical Picture

In view of the varieties of the anatomic and physiologic situations, the clinical picture will be sketched only briefly by alluding to the possible profiles a single ventricle may present: (1) large ventricular septal defect. This, without other anomalies, is rare. (2) Transposition of the great arteries, with ventricular septal defect (see p. 699), (3) corrected transposition with ventricular septal defect (see p. 713), (4) tetralogy of Fallot (see p. 638), (5) tricuspid atresia (see p. 678), (6) mitral atresia (see p. 581), (7) endocardial cushion defect, complete (see p. 384), (8) single atrium (see p. 394), (9) dextrocardia with tetralogy of Fallot (see p. 741), (10) truncus arteriosus (see p. 505).

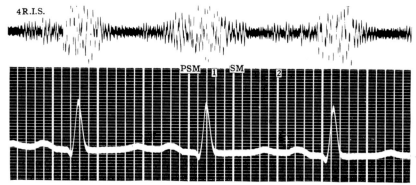

Figure 310. Phonocardiogram of patient with single ventricle. Note the loud presystolic and systolic murmur at the fourth right interspace.

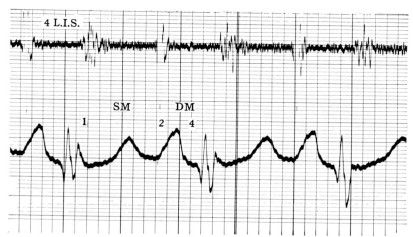

Figure 311. Phonocardiogram of patient with single ventricle. Note the faint systolic and diastolic murmur at the fourth left interspace.

The history, physical findings (Figs. 310, 311), electrocardiograms (Fig. 312) and roentgenograms (Figs. 313, 314) vary tremendously according to the anatomy and physiology. It seems absurd to me to discuss "characteristic" electrocardiographic patterns or x-ray configurations for such a variety of clinical pictures. I have emphasized before that the "expected" single electrocardiographic pattern (Fig. 312) across the chest leads occurs only rarely. The only general statement that may be made about the clinical picture of this entity is that it represents severe and complex disease.

At catheterization one finds a single pressure pulse within the ventricle and nearly identical saturations in the great arteries. Within the past few years, if we have encountered these findings on routine catheterization, it has been our policy to take all possible measures to elaborate on (*a*) the position of the great arteries, (*b*) the gradient between the ventricle and both great vessels, and (*c*) the gradient across both atrioventricular valves. It is assumed that if the single ventricle is the only abnormality found, we are, in effect, dealing with a large ventricular septal defect only.

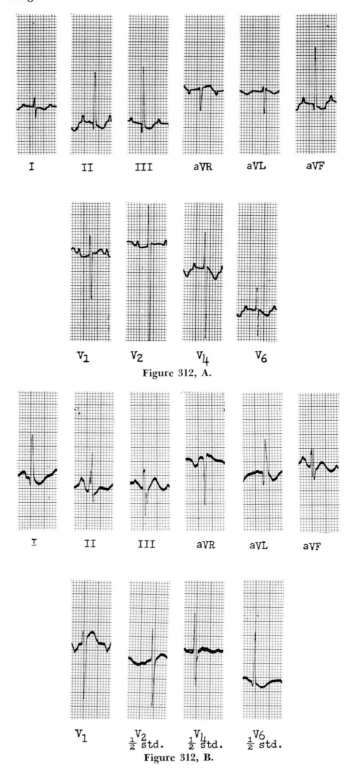

I   II   III   aVR   aVL   aVF

V₁   V₂   V₄   V₆

Figure 312, A.

I   II   III   aVR   aVL   aVF

V₁   ½ V₂ std.   ½ V₄ std.   ½ V₆ std.

Figure 312, B.

Course and Prognosis

Of eighty-five patients reviewed by Campbell and his associates,[136] half died at less than one year of age, but eighteen lived to be twenty. To a large extent, the associated anomalies seem to determine the outlook for these patients.

Differential Diagnosis

Differential diagnosis should be directed toward the specific entities within the framework of which single ventricle is presented.

Treatment

Treatment should be directed toward the associated anomalies. If, after careful search, no complicating lesions are found, the assumption can be made that this is a large ventricular septal defect, and it should be treated accordingly, by insertion of a prosthesis in place of the ventricular septum. We have never had the opportunity to treat an *anatomically* single ventricle surgically.

I cannot emphasize strongly enough that the finding of a *physiologi-*

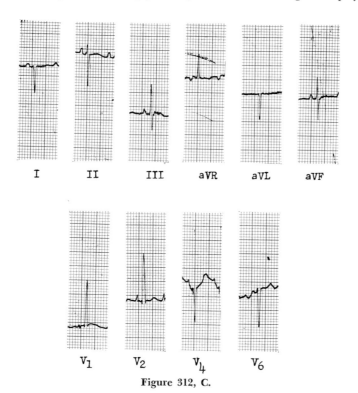

Figure 312, C.

Figure 312. Electrocardiograms of patients with single ventricle. *A,* Note the suggestion of left ventricular hypertrophy in the standard and unipolar limb leads and the single pattern rS in the four chest leads. *B,* Left ventricular hypertrophy. *C,* Right ventricular hypertrophy.

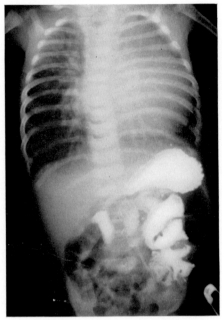

Figure 313. Posteroanterior roentgenogram of patient with single ventricle and pulmonary plethora.

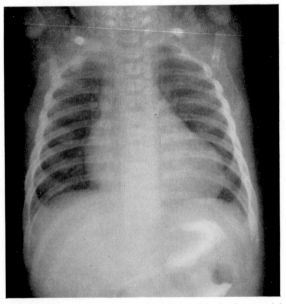

Figure 314. Posteroanterior roentgenogram of patient with single ventricle and pulmonary ischemia.

cally single ventricle should not imply that surgical correction is impossible. It should serve only as an impetus toward more careful search for associated anomalies. If none are found, surgery should be attempted, though, admittedly, the risks are high.

Summary

Physiologically, single ventricle without any other anatomic defect gives the clinical and physiologic image of a large ventricular septal defect and ought to be treated accordingly. A physiologically single ventricle with associated anomalies may present a spectrum of clinical profiles from dextrocardia, through transposition with ventricular septal defect, to tetralogy of Fallot. Treatment should depend on the nature of the associated anomalies.

LEFT VENTRICULAR-RIGHT ATRIAL SHUNTS

A special type of ventricular septal defect, resulting in a direct communication between the left ventricle and the right atrium, has been described by Gerbode and his co-workers[273] and by Perry and his associates.[558] Altogether, approximately twenty cases have been described in the literature.[84] We have encountered seven patients with this clinical diagnosis.

Anatomy

The possible anatomic variations giving rise to shunts from the left ventricle to the right atrium have been discussed (Fig. 277). The most common situation is the one in which the ventricular defect, in the outflow region, communicates with the right atrium through a defect in the medial leaflet of the tricuspid valve. Less commonly, the tricuspid valve is intact, and direct communication between the left ventricle and right atrium is possible through a high ventricular septal defect by virtue of the fact that the tricuspid valve is lower in the sagittal plane than is the mitral valve.

Physiology

In general terms, the physiologic abnormality consists in a left-to-right shunt into the right atrium, giving rise to increased volume work of the right ventricle, as seen in atrial septal defect. On the other hand, the regurgitation from the left ventricle into the right atrium, similar to that of mitral regurgitation or ventricular septal defect, implies increased left ventricular volume work as well. Usually the shunts are not maximal, and the pulmonary arterial pressure is elevated only moderately, or not at all.

Clinical Picture

A heart murmur is usually discovered in these patients within the first few months of life. Symptoms of underdevelopment, shortness of breath and an increased number of respiratory infections are, on the whole, mild.

On physical examination the findings cannot be distinguished from those encountered in patients with ventricular septal defect, including the characteristic murmur and the variability of the second sound with respirations.

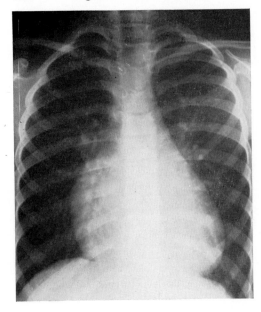

Figure 315. Posteroanterior roentgenogram of patient with left ventricular–right atrial shunt. Note the right atrial enlargement in a heart whose over-all dimensions are not very big. Also note that the pulmonary vasculature is not as engorged as one would expect from the size of the right atrium, were this an atrial septal defect.

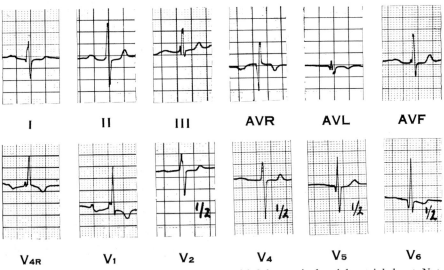

Figure 316. Electrocardiogram of patient with left ventricular-right atrial shunt. Note the right ventricular hypertrophy, the mean axis of plus 75 degrees, the prolonged P–R interval, and the flat-topped P_1 and P_2.

The roentgenograms usually show significant cardiac enlargement, involving particularly the right atrium, but also, to a lesser degree, the right and left ventricles (Fig. 315). *The cardiac enlargement is more significant than would be expected from the size of the left-to-right shunt.*

The mean electrical axis varies from +100 to −45 degrees. Evidences of right atrial hypertrophy with a prolonged P-R interval are prevalent.

In the chest leads there is usually combined ventricular hypertrophy with a V_{4R}' and QTC pattern over the right side of the precordium (Fig. 316).

At *cardiac catheterization* (Fig. 317) the following information may be obtained: (1) A significant increase in oxygen saturation occurs at the right atrial level. A second, and apparently smaller, increase may or may not occur at the right ventricular level. The systemic arterial blood is fully saturated. (2) The right atrial pressure is relatively low, appreciably lower than left atrial or pulmonary capillary pressure. In spite of the regurgitant jet, known to be present, there are no significant V waves because of the large right atrial reservoir. Right ventricular and pulmonary arterial pressures may be only slightly elevated, and the systemic arterial pulse pressure is normal. (3) Pulmonary resistance is low normal. (4) Pulmonary-to-systemic flow ratios are 2:1 or more, but maximal ranges

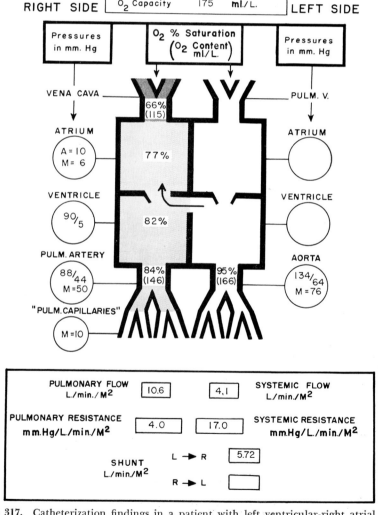

Figure 317. Catheterization findings in a patient with left ventricular-right atrial shunt.

are seldom encountered. (5) The course of the catheter is of considerable interest. In spite of the sizable "atrial" shunt, it may not be possible to pass the catheter from the right atrium to the left atrium even though the saphenous route is used. On the other hand, occasionally, the left ventricle may be entered from the right atrium with an approach from an antecubital vein. (6) At cine-angiography, with selective left ventricular injection, immediate opacification of the right atrium may be visualized, and dye enters the right ventricle only through the right atrium. (7) Dye dilution curves, with injection into the left ventricle and sampling from the right atrium and the right ventricle, show earlier appearance in the right atrium. Phonocatheters show a holosystolic murmur within the right atrium and, to a lesser extent, in the right ventricle.

Course and Prognosis

One of Gerbode's[273] patients with this defect lived to be forty-two years old, but most of the patients described in the literature are in their teens. Obviously, one cannot even guess at the average life expectancy of these patients, since few cases have been published and since the size and location of the opening are variable. It seems logical to assume, however, that since there is no direct communication between the right ventricle and the left ventricle, pulmonary arterial hypertension is not a limiting factor in the survival of these patients. Incidentally, this is a good argument supporting Dammann's[182] thesis of the role of the "common ejectile force" in the origin of pulmonary vascular obstruction. From this point of view, the prognosis for these patients may be better than that for patients with large ventricular septal defect. If the physiologic consequences of this lesion are compared with those of a secundum type of atrial septal defect, it is apparent that the addition of left ventricular flow work and the secondary left atrial hypertension may render the left ventricular-right atrial shunt the more serious defect; therefore the long-term outlook may be somewhere between the relatively benign secundum atrial defect and the severe, large ventricular septal defect.

Differential Diagnosis

Large Ventricular Septal Defect. The catheterization data indicating a shunt principally at the atrial level exclude large ventricular defect as an uncomplicated lesion. Although the clinical picture alone strongly suggests ventricular septal defect, the large right atrium without corresponding left atrial enlargement, the P pulmonale and prolonged P-R interval and, finally, the relatively moderate degree of pulmonary vascular engorgement with a large heart, may raise the suspicion of left ventricular-right atrial shunt even before cardiac catheterization.

Secundum Atrial Septal Defect. This diagnosis is immediately suggested at cardiac catheterization by the oxygen saturation data, but it cannot be accepted in the face of the clinical picture described. Furthermore, there is no equalization of right atrial and left atrial or pulmonary capillary pressures, and the atrial septum cannot be traversed with the catheter.

Endocardial Cushion Defect. Endocardial cushion defect presents the most difficult differential diagnostic problem if the mean electrical axis is to the left of —30 degrees. As a matter of fact, I believe that a left ventricular-right atrial shunt with this type of electrocardiogram corresponds embryologically, as well as anatomically, to an endocardial cushion defect with a ventricular septal defect and a cleft in the tricuspid valve.

Treatment

Surgical repair of the lesion is eminently practical, by means of the pump oxygenator, through a right atrial approach. Gerbode[273] reported five successful closures, Braunwald and Morrow one.[84] In our Institution, six patients with this defect underwent surgery, with five survivors. The optimal age of the patient for surgery is between five and fifteen years.

Summary

Patients in whom the clinical picture suggests a large ventricular septal defect, but who, at catheterization, seem to have evidences of an atrial left-to-right shunt, probably have a left ventricular-right atrial shunt. The diagnosis may be strongly suspected on the basis of the gradient between right atrial and left atrial pressures, the course of the catheter, and the registration of the murmur of ventricular septal defect within the right atrium; it may be proved at angiography. Surgery is recommended.

COMMUNICATIONS BETWEEN GREAT ARTERIES

A communication between the great arteries, in extrauterine life, may be either the result of persistence of a normal fetal structure (such as patent ductus arteriosus) or the outcome of a profound developmental anomaly (such as aortopulmonary fenestration or truncus arteriosus). These defects are totally different in terms of statistical significance as well as in their influence on cardiodynamics; they are grouped together for discussion only to preserve the anatomic framework of the presentation.

PATENT DUCTUS ARTERIOSUS

Incidence

Statistically, patent ductus arteriosus is a very important lesion. In Abbott's[1] series, as well as in Keith's[380] and Wood's,[748] it was the second most common deformity. In our own series it was the third most common lesion. (We have classified ventricular defect and tetralogy of Fallot separately.) The etiologic role of German measles and its particular predilection for the association of patent ductus arteriosus and pulmonic stenosis[333] have already been discussed. Alzamora-Castro[15] found positive correlation between high altitude living in Peru and patent ductus arteriosus. The familial evidence has been alluded to, and the dominance in females has been discussed (see p. 342).

Anatomy

The ductus arteriosus, much like the foramen ovale, is a structure necessary for maintenance of fetal circulation; it is through this channel that blood reaches the descending aorta from the pulmonary arterial system. The ductus connects the pulmonary artery, at its bifurcation, with the aorta, just beyond the origin of the left subclavian artery. Embryologically, it originates from the dorsal part of the sixth branchial arch. Patten[550] computed the cross section of the ductus at term to be about half that of the aorta.

Physiology

Some of the considerations to be discussed here have already been described in great detail in the section on the fetal circulation (see p. 344). A brief repetition does not seem out of order to conserve the integrity of the section.

In the fetus, because of the relative hypertension in the pulmonary circuit, the ductus carries blood from the pulmonary artery to the aorta. In the congenital anomaly to be discussed here the ductus arteriosus not only remains patent beyond the normal time limits, but is also considerably larger and thinner than the expected normal at birth. Whether the large size of the ductus is secondary to the fact that it has not closed at the normal time, or whether the size is the deciding factor in its patency, cannot be answered with certainty at present. How much of the right ventricular output actually is diverted through the ductus into the descending aorta at various stages of fetal life is a matter of lively controversy. It is likely, however, that in the last weeks of fetal existence more and more blood goes through the lungs and enters the pulmonary vascular system, thus reducing materially the flow through the ductus. Barcroft and his associates demonstrated the flow of blood through the ductus of a lamb for about five minutes after delivery; after that, "functional" closure occurred.[38] Dawes, also studying lambs, found that closure started within ten to fifteen minutes after birth, but he observed flow through a reduced lumen, with increased velocity and accompanied by a thrill, for several hours or days.[190]

In man, using angiocardiography, Lind[436] demonstrated anatomic patency for several months, and Hultgren[351] proved the presence of functional patency for several days after birth. Christie,[148] on the basis of postmortem examinations, demonstrated anatomic patency in 12 per cent of babies 2 months old and in 1 per cent of those one year old

On the basis of these data it seems increasingly clear that the anatomic closure of the ductus is not an instantaneous affair, but rather something that begins during the last weeks of intrauterine life and is not completed for several weeks after birth.

What are the factors which influence normal closure of the ductus arteriosus? There is no one answer to this important question. Kennedy[386] demonstrated conclusively that, in guinea pigs at least, increased oxygenation of the fetal blood causes a muscular constriction of the ductus. Lind[436] stated that interference with respiration in newborn infants causes a functionally closed ductus to reopen. Hultgren and his associates found evidence to suggest that breathing low oxygen mixtures may reopen the ductus in babies less than three days old.[351] In addition, it seems logical to assume that pulmonary vascular changes and pulmonary arterial pressure have an important effect on closure of the duct, although there are no conclusive studies proving this point. Finally, that factors other than those present at birth may profoundly affect the fate of the ductus arteriosus is proved by the observation that if the mother has German measles during the first trimester, a patent ductus arteriosus commonly occurs in the baby. The familial occurrence of the anomaly has also been described; I have seen siblings and a mother and daughter with patent ductus arteriosus.

The hemodynamic changes occurring at birth, specifically the lowering of the pulmonary arterial resistance due to respirations, and the increase in systemic resistance due to the occlusion of the umbilical cord, result in a reversal of the pressure relations between the aorta and the pulmonary artery. Thus a gradient exists across a patent ductus from the aorta to the pulmonary artery, resulting in a flow of blood from the systemic to the pulmonary circuit during systole as well as diastole, in typical cases. Under these circumstances the left atrium, the left ventricle and the pulmonary artery handle an appreciably larger volume of blood than do the right atrium and the right ventricle. In most instances the extra amount of blood may be accommodated within the pulmonary arterial bed without a significant increase in pressure. Because of the runoff from the aorta into the pulmonary artery, aortic diastolic pressure is low, and systemic pulse pressure widens. The large left ventricular stroke volume may result in "functional" aortic stenosis, disappearing with the closure of the ductus.

The hemodynamic considerations thus outlined are typical of most—probably 90 per cent—of the cases of patent ductus arteriosus. In a small number of instances, however, encompassing the largest patent ductus, pulmonary arterial hypertension with pulmonary vascular obstruction is present. In the moderate cases this may result in elimination of the diastolic gradient between the aorta and the pulmonary artery and, thus, in disappearance of the diastolic component of the continuous murmur. This may well be the case in early infancy when, with the persistence of a certain amount of the fetal structure of the pulmonary vasculature, only a systolic murmur may be heard. In patients with patent ductus arteriosus and severe pulmonary vascular obstruction, the pulmonary pressure may be higher than the aortic pressure through the entire cardiac cycle, resulting in a right-to-left shunt through the ductus and practically no murmur. This situation, as will be demonstrated later, changes the entire clinical and hemodynamic picture. In addition to, or even supplanting, the left ventricular flow-work, pulmonary arterial hypertension and right ventricular pressure-work come to the foreground, and the ductus becomes "atypical."

Simple Patent Ductus Arteriosus (Typical)

Clinical Picture

Many of these patients are asymptomatic, and only the discovery of a murmur leads them to the cardiologist. In others physical underde-velopment or an increased number of severe respiratory infections con-stitutes the chief complaint. On close questioning a history of easy fatig-ability and lack of stamina may be elicited.

At physical examination approximately 30 per cent of these children are short and slender. The underdevelopment is not due in all instances, however, to the hemodynamic effects of the cardiac abnormality. In many it represents an additional congenital anomaly. The infant born of a mother who had German measles during the first trimester of pregnancy certainly fits into this category. It is only in the patients with the largest ductus, carry-ing a large flow and resulting in some degree of congestive heart failure, that the hemodynamic effects may be responsible for underdevelopment. Even in these patients the retardation in weight is much more likely to result from the patent ductus than is the stunting in height.[700] Cyanosis or clubbing is never present. A thrill—systolic or systolic and diastolic—is often noted at the second left interspace and even at the suprasternal notch. Left chest prominence is common, and the cardiac impulse is hyperdynamic at the apex. The ductus with a large left-to-right shunt is characterized by bounding peripheral pulses and a wide pulse pressure.

At auscultation the continuous systolic-diastolic machinery murmur dominates the picture (Fig. 318). This murmur is usually loud (at least grade 3 in intensity) and is maximal at the upper left sternal border. It transmits well throughout the anterior part of the chest, but only mod-erately well to the neck and back. In contrast to other conditions giving rise to continuous murmurs, the ductus murmur is constant and varies little with respiration or position. Characteristically, the systolic com-ponent begins shortly after the first heart sound and proceeds in a cres-cendo configuration toward the second sound. The murmur usually reaches its peak at the time of the second sound and, thereafter, assumes a decrescendo configuration, trailing off and disappearing at various intervals before the first sound. In some patients the continuous murmur transmits better than average to the neck and back; in these patients the systolic part of the continuous murmur (by auscultation and phonocardiography) assumes a stenotic nature (Fig. 319). These patients may have stenosis of the pulmonary or aortic valve. A further variation of the typical murmur of patent ductus arteriosus is the one encountered in patients with a very small ductus. This murmur is faint, not completely constant, and blends almost imperceptibly into a venous hum.

In addition to the characteristic machinery murmur, an apical sys-tolic murmur (Fig. 320) may be heard. A low-frequency apical diastolic rumble is observed in all cases in which the flow through the lungs is at least twice the systemic flow.

The heart sounds may be completely obscured by this continuous roar-ing murmur, but occasionally a distinct, loud second sound may be heard at the pulmonary area. In patients with a large patent ductus arteriosus, careful auscultation and phonocardiography may reveal "paradoxical" splitting of the second sound, resulting from the increased duration of left ventricular ejection and the earlier closure of the pulmonic valve secondary to the increase in pulmonary arterial diastolic pressure and sometimes to left bundle branch block. The first heart sound is not re-

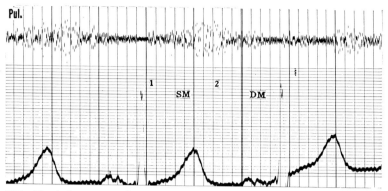

Figure 318.   Typical murmur of patent ductus arteriosus. Note the crescendic nature of the systolic element and the decrescendic nature of the diastolic portion.

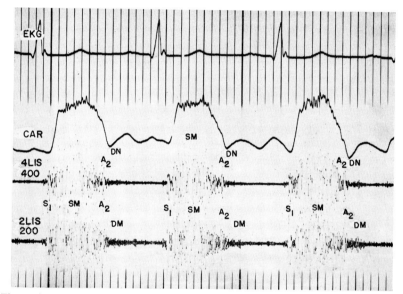

Figure 319.   Phonocardiogram of patient with patent ductus arteriosus and aortic stenosis. Note the continuous murmur from the first sound, through aortic closure, to the first half of diastole, seen best at 2LIS. In contrast to Figure 318, however, the peak of the systolic murmur is in midsystole rather than in late systole. This is the effect of aortic stenosis on the murmur, which also is pictured in the vibrations on the top of the carotid artery tracing.

markable. A third sound, as well as an aortic click, is commonly heard at the apex.

The results of radiologic examination depend a great deal on the magnitude of the flow through the ductus. Roentgenologically, patients with the smallest shunts have essentially normal hearts; those with larger shunts show features characteristic of the increased amount of blood in the left atrium, left ventricle and pulmonary artery: namely, (1) left ventricular and left atrial enlargement, (2) prominent pulmonary artery and large ascending aorta and aortic arch, and (3) pulmonary vascular engorgement[200] (Fig. 321). At fluoroscopy, if the ductus is of an appreciable size, the beat is hyperactive; the increased amplitude of pulsations involves to an equal degree the left ventricle, pulmonary artery and aorta. Expansile pulsations are frequently seen in the engorged pulmonary vessels.

The electrocardiogram, like the roentgenogram, may be almost entirely within normal limits in patients with a small ductus. If the shunt is large, the increased left ventricular flow-work is reflected in left ventricular hypertrophy (Fig. 322), with an occasional instance of P mitrale (Fig. 323). The mean electrical axis is normal; left axis deviation is present in about 10 per cent of the patients.

Cardiac catheterization (Fig. 324) is barely justifiable today in patients with typical patent ductus arteriosus. Nevertheless the following observations may be made: (1) There is at least a 6 per cent increase in the pulmonary arterial oxygen saturation as compared with that of the right ventricular outflow tract. The highest saturations may be found in the left rather than the main pulmonary artery. Very small patent ductus may not give rise to an increase in oxygen content sufficient to meet these criteria. Furthermore, as mentioned before, if the arterial oxygen saturation is increased greatly within the ventricle, because of a ventricular defect, then moderate increases due to a patent ductus arteriosus, at the pulmonary arterial level, may be hard to appreciate. The peripheral

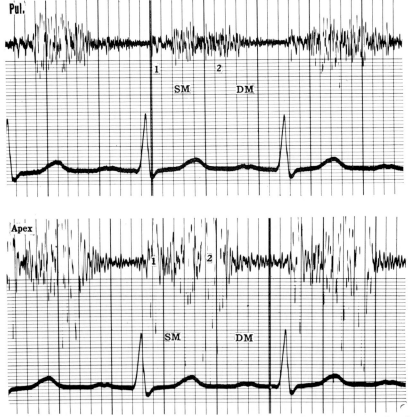

Figure 320.   Continuous machinery type of murmur at the pulmonary area and a loud systolic and low-frequency diastolic murmur at the apex.

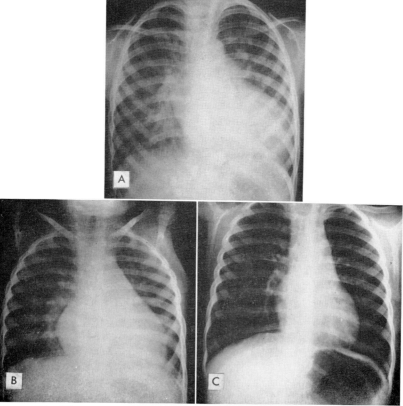

Figure 321. Three posteroanterior roentgenograms, one belonging to a patient with a small patent ductus arteriosus (*C*), the second to a patient with medium-sized (*A*) and the third one with a large patent ductus arteriosus (*B*).

arterial saturation is usually normal. (2) Pulmonary arterial and right ventricular pressures are normal in 50 to 75 per cent of the patients catheterized. This figure is probably lower than the real incidence of normal pulmonary arterial pressure, since, as mentioned, most of the patients with typical patent ductus arteriosus are not studied by cardiac catheterization. Left atrial or pulmonary capillary pressure, or both, may be slightly elevated (8 to 12 mm., mean), and the pulse pressure in the systemic artery is wide. The pressure pulse resembles closely that of aortic regurgitation. (3) Elevated pulmonary resistance is found in more than 30 per cent of all patients catheterized for a patent ductus arteriosus. Again, this is probably an unduly high figure, for the reasons given above; among all patients with typical patent ductus arteriosus it is probably less than 10 per cent. (4) The pulmonary-systemic flow ratio is certainly more than 1.5:1.0, and occasionally it may be closer to 4 or even 5:1. (5) In skillful hands the catheter may be manipulated across the patent ductus arteriosus in at least 50 per cent of the patients. A greater percentage than this may be quoted for young infants. On entering the pulmonary artery the tip should be pointed posteriorly and moved as far as the entrance into the left main pulmonary artery; on probing this area, the catheter suddenly takes a downward course into the descending aorta, passing beyond the left subclavian artery (Fig. 325). This course contrasts rather sharply with that encountered during passage across a ventricular septal defect or an aortopulmonary window. (6) Retrograde cine-angio-

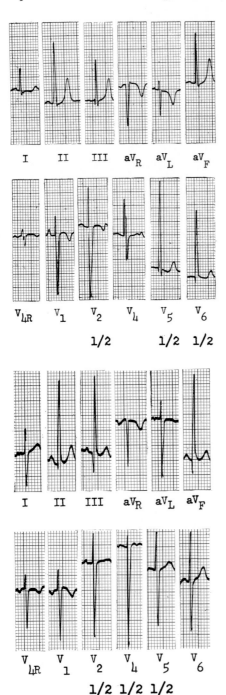

Figure 322. Electrocardiogram of patient with patent ductus arteriosus, indicating left ventricular hypertrophy. The axis is plus 75 degrees. Complexes are tall over the left chest leads. There is a Q wave in V_5 and V_6, and the T waves are symmetrical, tall and pointed in leads II and aV_F. There is sagging of the S-T segment in V_5 and V_6.

Figure 323. Electrocardiogram of patient with patent ductus arteriosus indicating left atrial hypertrophy, as seen in the notched P waves in lead I, the well marked P in aV_F, and the inverted P in V_{4R} and V_1.

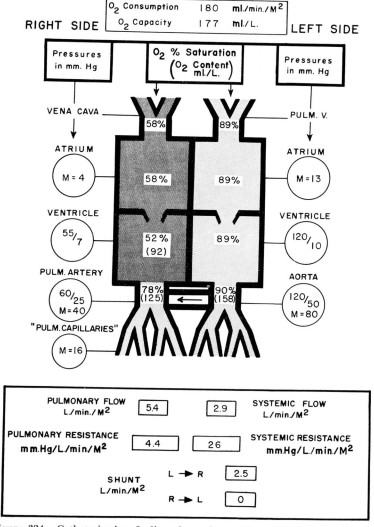

Figure 324. Catheterization findings in patient with patent ductus arteriosus.

grams, with injection into the ascending aorta, first reveal the aortic arch; then the pulmonary artery shows up below the aortic arch like a golfball. (7) Dye dilution curves, with injection into the aortic arch and sampling from the right ventricle and pulmonary artery, in succession, furnish clear proof of the aortopulmonary shunt, but do not enable differentiation between the various kinds of shunts at this level (aortopulmonary fenestration, truncus arteriosus, and so forth). The intracardiac phonocardiogram registers a clear-cut, continuous murmur in the pulmonary artery, but relatively little, if any, murmur within the right ventricle. It may be necessary to obtain intracardiac phonocardiograms and dye curves, or even to use a hydrogen electrode, to prove the presence of a trivial patent ductus arteriosus.

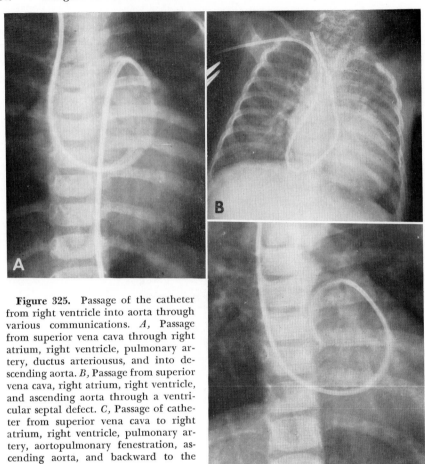

Figure 325. Passage of the catheter from right ventricle into aorta through various communications. *A,* Passage from superior vena cava through right atrium, right ventricle, pulmonary artery, ductus arteriousus, and into descending aorta. *B,* Passage from superior vena cava, right atrium, right ventricle, and ascending aorta through a ventricular septal defect. *C,* Passage of catheter from superior vena cava to right atrium, right ventricle, pulmonary artery, aortopulmonary fenestration, ascending aorta, and backward to the aortic valve.

Course and Prognosis

As mentioned earlier, only rarely is a typical patent ductus arteriosus diagnosed within the first few weeks of life, and practically never is the murmur recognized at birth. This statement, taken from the first edition, must be qualified to a certain extent in the light of newer knowledge. It is still true that a typical machinery murmur is heard within the first few days of life only in a rare instance of a premature infant with a patent ductus arteriosus. It is also true, however,[112] that by extremely careful auscultation a systolic, and even a systolic-diastolic, murmur may be heard transiently at the upper left sternal border within the first twenty-four to forty-eight hours of life in a sizable percentage of all newborns and in a high percentage of babies with the respiratory distress syndrome. These murmurs are recognized by only a few neonatologists at present, and they do not resemble by any means the typical machinery, train-in-the tunnel sound of a full-blown ductus murmur. As mentioned earlier (p. 464), these transient murmurs may be due to a transient left-to-right shunt through a partially functionally closed patent ductus arteriosus. They may have some bearing on the etiology of the respiratory distress syndrome. The rare presence of a typical continuous murmur at birth (except in premature infants) usually means another, probably more complex, anomaly.

Why a ductus arteriosus that presumably was present in intrauterine life, and will again show evidences of patency at one or two years of age, should not be detectable by auscultation at birth presents an interesting problem. The answer may lie in the absence of a significant pressure gradient between the systemic and pulmonary circuits; in other words, the ductus may be anatomically open, but there is no flow through it, because of persistence of the fetal type of pulmonary arterioles. In other cases the assumption has been made that a membrane obliterating the ductus has suddenly ruptured.[682] In addition to these anatomic and physiologic explanations, human factors, consisting in the sometimes exceedingly difficult auscultatory conditions in the newborn, may play some role in the late discovery of the typical murmur.

Even if a murmur is discovered within the first few weeks or months of life, it is seldom labeled as a continuous one. Most often only a systolic component is recognized, probably because only a systolic gradient between the two circuits exists. After six to twelve months of life, however, in most cases of typical patent ductus arteriosus, the characteristic murmur is noticeable. The average patient with this anomaly is nearly asymptomatic throughout childhood. As time goes on, in patients with a large ductus, fatigue and breathlessness become increasingly noticeable, and congestive failure may occur when he reaches the twenties or thirties. The occurrence of pulmonary arterial hypertension with pulmonary vascular obstruction is fairly common in these older patients. Shapiro and Keyes[635] found that a person with a patent ductus arteriosus who reaches his seventeenth birthday has only half the average life expectancy if the defect is not corrected by operation. Individual exceptions to this rule are numerous, and every cardiologist has seen patients with patent ductus arteriosus who, in their fifties and sixties, are completely asymptomatic.

I would like to re-emphasize the fact that fairly frequently spontaneous closure of a definitely patent ductus arteriosus may occur within the first few weeks or months of life in premature infants. There is some evidence that this may occur in children and even in adults, but it seems to be a rare phenomenon.

The great dangers for patients with patent ductus arteriosus are pulmonary vascular obstruction, congestive failure and bacterial endocarditis. It is possible that, with the decline in incidence of the last complication, the figures of Shapiro and Keyes may no longer be valid. No good statistical appraisal of the development of pulmonary vascular obstruction in these patients is available. As mentioned previously (p. 362), analysis of our own data from catheterized patients certainly indicates that, though significant pulmonary vascular obstruction is relatively rare in infants and children, it does become considerably more common in adults. Whether the adults in whom severe pulmonary vascular obstruction develops *ever* had a normal pulmonary vascular tree is difficult to know. My own conviction is that, probably, in most of these patients, some pulmonary arterial hypertension and pulmonary vascular obstruction were present from the start, but unquestionably the degree and the anatomic nature of the pulmonary vascular disease progress through the years.

Differential Diagnosis

The diagnosis of typical patent ductus arteriosus is simple. Gibson[275] stated that the clinical diagnosis of patent ductus arteriosus, based principally on the presence of the characteristic murmur, was correct in practically every instance of several thousand cases collected from all over the United States. Other conditions with systolic and diastolic murmurs to be considered are as follows:

Aortopulmonary Septal Defect. An aortopulmonary septal defect is practically indistinguishable from a patent ductus arteriosus, from the clinical viewpoint. In most instances the murmur is maximal on the lower left sternal border and is very loud. Cardiac catheterization or aortography, or both, may furnish the necessary clue, but exploratory thoracotomy should be performed if in doubt.

Coronary Arteriovenous Aneurysm. A coronary arteriovenous aneurysm may be suspected if high-frequency continuous murmurs are heard somewhere within the cardiac border, but not at the second left interspace. Cardiac catheterization and angiography may have to be performed to establish the diagnosis.

Pulmonary Arteriovenous Fistula. This may be recognized by the site of the continuous murmur over the back rather than at the second left interspace. Also, because of the veno-arterial (right-to-left) nature of the shunt, there is some cyanosis and clubbing if the communication is of any magnitude. Usually the heart is not enlarged on the roentgenogram, but the radiologist may recognize the aneurysm in the plane film.

Murmurs of Collaterals. Murmurs of collateral vessels may be heard in patients with coarctation of the aorta or tetralogy of Fallot, and may easily be identified by their location and nature and the presence of the underlying malformation. These murmurs are heard well throughout the back, and usually at the second right interspace, rather than being localized to the area of the ductus. Also, they lack the consistency of the patent ductus arteriosus murmur, and vary considerably with respirations. In patients with coarctation of the aorta, pressure applied with the stethoscope during auscultation causes the continuous murmur of collaterals to disappear.

Venous Hum. A venous hum is perhaps most frequently confused with a patent ductus arteriosus. Its evanescence, the accentuation of the diastolic component, its disappearance on compression of the ipsilateral jugular vein, its accentuation if the neck is extended and the patient sits up, and its virtual disappearance when he lies down usually allow an easy differential diagnosis.

Ventricular Septal Defect and Aortic Regurgitation. The murmur of ventricular septal defect with aortic regurgitation is more to-and-fro in nature, and its maximal intensity is at the lower left sternal border rather than at the second left interspace.

Aneurysm of the Sinus of Valsalva. If an aneurysm of the sinus of Valsalva ruptures into the right ventricle (ordinarily some time after puberty), the patient usually experiences the sudden appearance of congestive failure. Physical examination reveals for the first time signs suggestive of a patent ductus arteriosus in a person without known heart disease. This contrasts markedly with the slowly progressive course of patients with patent ductus arteriosus. An unruptured aneurysm or fistula of the sinus of Valsalva may open into the right ventricle and may give rise to a continuous murmur without significant symptoms for a long period. As a rule, the location and the sound of the murmur are sufficiently unusual that these patients are studied preoperatively at cardiac catheterization, and cine-angiograms usually reveal the diagnosis.

Truncus Arteriosus. The presence of arterial unsaturation usually makes the distinction between truncus arteriosus and patent ductus arteriosus fairly easy. Also, the systolic-diastolic murmur is seldom localized to the second left interspace, but may be heard with equal intensity at the second right interspace and over the back. Actually, whether these patients fit into the truncus arteriosus group, or whether they should be classified as extreme cases of tetralogy of Fallot is a matter of some controversy. My own experience indicates that, although systolic and diastolic (but mostly to-and-fro) murmurs may well be heard in patients with true truncus arteriosus of types I and II, the occurrence of a truly continuous machinery murmur is heard only in type IV, which, in my opinion, is indistinguishable from pulmonary atresia associated with a ventricular septal defect.

Peripheral Pulmonic Stenosis. Multiple "coarctations" of the peripheral pulmonary arteries may give rise to widespread continuous murmurs all over the thorax. This unusual distribution of the murmur, the absence of a late systolic crescendo, the presence of right ventricular hypertrophy and the absence of a hyperkinetic impulse are the clinical clues suggesting the diagnosis.

Treatment

The treatment of choice for typical patent ductus arteriosus is surgery. An operation is recommended for every child with this condition who is seen at The Children's Hospital Medical Center in Boston. This policy is based principally on two considerations: one is the unlikelihood that any patient with a patent ductus arteriosus will be able to live a symptom-free life for the average length of time, and the other is the fact that normal circulation is completely restored by this procedure, with a very low mortality rate.

It is easy to recommend surgery for patients who have symptoms. But recommending an operation, no matter how safe, for a child who, in the eyes of his parents, is completely healthy is difficult. The physician should be guided by his judgment of the individual situation. He should try to assess the size of the ductus on the basis of heart size, pulse pressure and presence or absence of an apical diastolic murmur. Consideration should be given to the parents' psychological make-up. Are they able to withstand the emotional strain of an operation better than living with the threat of bacterial endocarditis for many years? A final, most important consideration is the amount of surgical experience with this procedure in the community. I believe that, if one rationally examines all these factors and has a capable surgical team at one's disposal, operation will be recommended for most asymptomatic children as well as for those who have symptoms.

The question—fortunately seldom confronting the pediatrician—of what to advise an adult with an asymptomatic ductus is an even more difficult problem. I believe that not every one of these adults should be operated on; the smallest ductus may perhaps be left undisturbed as long as the patient is asymptomatic. This difference in attitude toward adults is explained by the slightly higher surgical risk and the increased postoperative morbidity in these patients, the sociologic implications of losing the head of the family, and finally by the fact that the benign nature of the lesion has already been demonstrated to a certain extent by freedom from symptoms for several decades.

Great technical strides have been made in the performance of this operation since the first successful ligation of a patent ductus arteriosus in 1939 by Gross.[310] At present the members of our surgical service at The Children's Hospital Medical Center believe that division of the ductus is more satisfactory than ligation and is equally safe. The principal advantage of dividing the ductus is the complete assurance against recanalization and subsequent development of bacterial endocarditis; at least eight cases of recanalization of ligated ductus were reported by Gibson.[275] The mortality rate of division of patent ductus arteriosus is quoted by Gross and Longino[311] as being less than 0.5 per cent in the asymptomatic group and 2.1 per cent in their entire group of 412 patients. The optimal age for surgery is between three and fifteen years, but patients ranging in age from two months to sixty years have been successfully operated upon. Within recent years we have operated on infants one year of age and less with success equal to that achieved in older children. As a consequence, we are no longer postponing surgery to an older age even in infants who are relatively asymptomatic; in patients who are sick, early operation is mandatory, of course. This policy of treating patent ductus arteriosus surgically when it is first encountered is possible only in centers where the personnel are well acquainted with cardiac surgery in infants. In institutions where they are not thoroughly familiar with these infants who have patent ductus arteriosus, operation between five and fifteen years may be much safer. *Even at these ages surgery at a large medical center is considerably safer.* Statistically significant proof of this thesis has been furnished in the literature, with mortality rates approximating 5 per cent in smaller hospitals as compared with 1 per cent or less in the large centers.[345]

If bacterial endocarditis occurs, it is preferable to eradicate the infection medically first and to operate about six months after complete bacteriologic cure. If the infection cannot be controlled by the most skillful use of antibiotics, surgery may bring about the desired cure of the endocarditis.

If the patient shows evidences of congestive failure, obviously this should be brought under control before operation.

The technical details of the operation and the preoperative and postoperative care are adequately covered in the appropriate surgical texts.[309] On the whole, the course of these patients after operation is remarkably smooth. The average stay in the hospital is two weeks or less.

Postoperatively, the heart diminishes in size, pulse pressure becomes normal, electrocardiographic and radiologic evidences of left ventricular hypertrophy disappear, and pulmonary vasculature becomes normal (Figs.

326, 327). In the majority of instances no murmur is heard by the time the patient is discharged. from the hospital. Occasionally a child has a residual systolic murmur (grade 2 to 3) at the apex or the lower left sternal border; most of these disappear within two years. A stenotic (aortic or pulmonary) type of murmur may appear or, as pointed out previously, may, in fact, have been present even before division of the ductus. Approximately a third of the patients who are abnormally short and half of those with substandard weight show considerable improvement postoperatively.

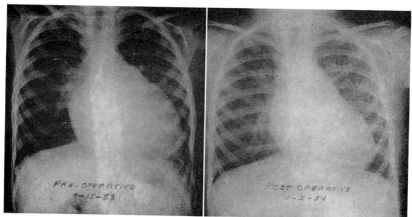

Fig. 326, A.

PRE-OPERATIVE ECG--Sept. 14, 1953

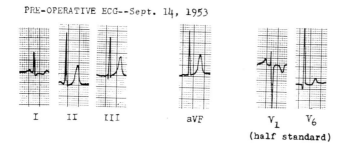

POST-OPERATIVE ECG--Jan. 5, 1954

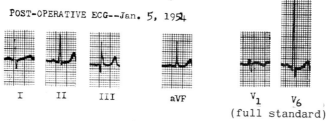

Fig. 326, B.

Figure 326. *A,* Preoperative and postoperative roentgenograms in a child with division of patent ductus arteriosus. *B,* The electrocardiographic changes following division of patent ductus arteriosus in the same patient.

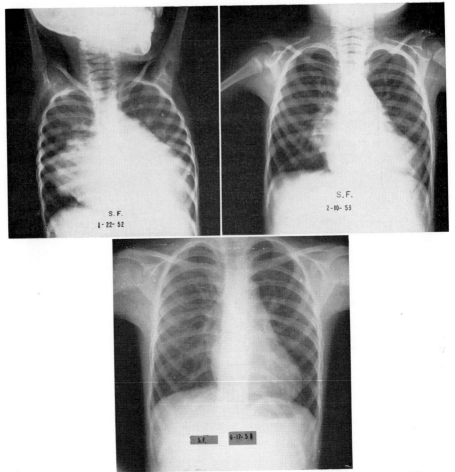

Figure 327. Preoperative and postoperative roentgenograms of patient with large patent ductus arteriosus. The film in 1952 is preoperative, showing maximal left atrial enlargement. The upper right quadrant is a film taken one year after division of a huge patent ductus arteriosus. Note the over-all diminution of heart size and the diminution of the size of the left atrium. The lower film, six years after operation, shows only slight cardiac enlargement and no left atrial enlargement. At this point the child has no murmur, and her blood pressure is normal.

For practical purposes, only patients with a large shunt and significant cardiac enlargement preoperatively, and not even all of these, show a satisfactory growth spurt after surgery. The timing of the operation has no influence whatsoever on the postoperative weight and height status.

Summary

Typical patent ductus arteriosus can be diagnosed in most instances by the presence of a continuous murmur at the second left interspace. Ancillary findings include radiologic and electrocardiographic evidences of a left-to-right shunt with increased left ventricular flow-work. Most patients are asymptomatic throughout childhood, but with increasing years they may become incapacitated and may die in congestive failure or with bacterial endocarditis. Surgical division, a safe and successful procedure, is recommended for all children with this anomaly.

Complicated Patent Ductus Arteriosus

PATENT DUCTUS ARTERIOSUS WITH PULMONARY HYPERTENSION ("ATYPICAL" PATENT DUCTUS ARTERIOSUS)

Clinical Picture

The majority of these patients have moderate or severe symptoms. Most of them are poorly developed and undernourished and are subject to frequent attacks of severe respiratory infection. Spells of cyanosis are commonly noted, and respirations are often rapid and labored. A murmur has been noted in all of them, but this is by no means the principal reason for their being brought to a cardiologist; most of them are sick children, indeed.

The typical history of an infant with a large left-to-right shunt reveals a baby who has not gained weight well at all, who breathes rapidly, has had severe respiratory infections and bouts of pneumonia and in whom congestive heart failure is developing. This picture contrasts markedly with that encountered in older children and adults who have maximal pulmonary vascular obstruction and a dominant right-to-left shunt; in these patients a heart murmur may have been noted some time in early childhood, but underdevelopment, dyspnea and respiratory infections have not been a dominant feature. Limitation of exercise tolerance and transient, slowly progressive cyanosis are the presenting symptoms. Patients who show the transition from the first to the second syndrome are seldom seen.

As a rule, at physical examination these patients are thin and scrawny; seldom do they rank above the tenth percentile on our standard developmental charts. Redness of the fingers and toes is common. Frank cyanosis and clubbing is present in less than 10 per cent of the cases; if such is noted, it may be either generalized or localized to the left hand and the lower half of the body. The neck veins may be distended; left chest deformity of moderate or severe degree is the rule. The cardiac impulse is rocking and palpable at the xiphoid process as well as at the apex. A thrill may be present at the upper left sternal border. The systolic pressure is usually elevated, with a widening of the pulse pressure. In the occasional patient with congestive failure, pulmonary rales are heard, and the liver is enlarged, but not pulsatile.

At auscultation the dominant feature is the booming, narrowly split second sound at the second left interspace. The first and third heart sounds are not remarkable. Systolic clicks, sometimes both at the apex (aortic) and at the second left interspace(pulmonic), may be heard. A grade 3 to 4 systolic murmur, mostly crescendic in configuration, is heard best at the second to third left interspace and transmits well throughout the precordium, but not too clearly to the neck and the back. An early diastolic murmur is heard in about two thirds of the cases. Commonly, the systolic and diastolic elements do not form a continuous murmur; a hiatus exists between the systolic murmur and the second sound, giving it a to-and-fro nature rather than a continuous one (Fig. 328). Even if the systolic murmur does continue through the second sound, the diastolic murmur may be short, and thus, again, the criteria for a truly "continuous" murmur are not completely fulfilled (Fig. 329). The administration of epinephrine, by raising the systemic pressure, without appreciably affecting the pulmonary vasculature, may bring out the continuous murmur. In a minority of cases only a systolic murmur at the second left interspace is heard (Fig. 330). In addition to the murmur at the second left interspace, apical systolic and mid-diastolic murmurs, and even a good apical presystolic crescendo murmur, reflecting

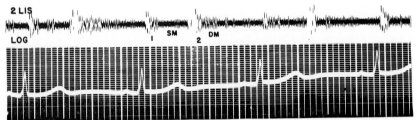

Figure 328.   Phonocardiogram of patient with atypical patent ductus arteriosus. Note the to-and-fro rather than continuous nature of the murmur. Also the crescendic nature of the systolic component is missing.

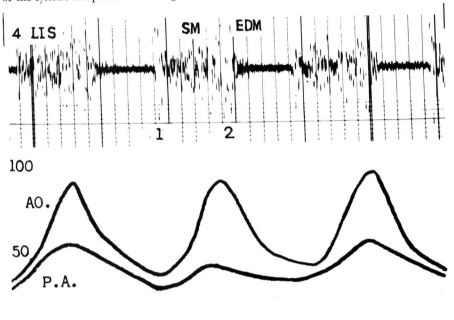

Figure 329.   Phonocardiogram of patient with atypical patent ductus arteriosus and pulmonary arterial hypertension. Note the simultaneous aortic and pulmonary arterial pressure tracings in the lower panel. The systolic murmur is maximal at the time of the second sound, which is the point when the pressure gradient between aorta and pulmonary artery is maximal. As the gradient between aorta and pulmonary artery decreases in diastole, because of the elevated pulmonary arterial diastolic pressure, the murmur becomes fainter, and even disappears.

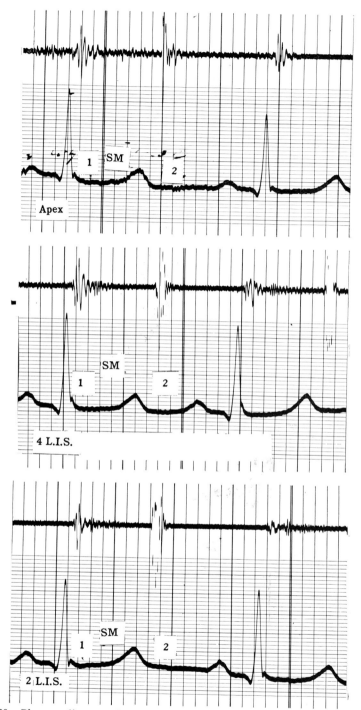

Figure 330. Phonocardiogram of patient with atypical patent ductus arteriosus. Note the faint systolic murmur. No definite diastolic murmur is noted.

the tremendous mitral valve flow, may be noted. The appearance of these babies is so characteristic that often simple inspection and palpation suggest the diagnosis. To begin with, many times they are "German measles" babies; thus the cataracts and mental retardation are noted at once. Furthermore, they are small and thin. As one's hand is placed on the thin chest, the powerful combined ventricular impulse hits the fingers, but the apical impulse is still maximal. The strong thrill, coupled with bounding radial and femoral pulses, makes one think immediately of a large patent ductus arteriosus with pulmonary arterial hypertension.

Roentgenologic examination always reveals a grossly abnormal cardiac silhouette. In addition to the enlargement of the left ventricle, left atrium and pulmonary artery, there is definite and even dominant right ventricular enlargement (Fig. 331). Frequently, in addition to the active pulmonary vascular engorgement inherent in a left-to-right shunt of some magnitude, there may be evidences of passive congestion. In the most

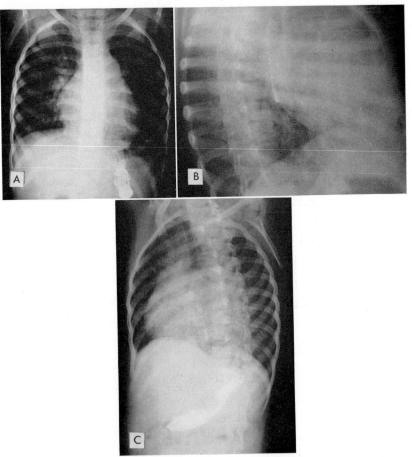

Figure 331. Posteroanterior and oblique roentgenograms of patient with atypical patent ductus arteriosus. Note the prominent main pulmonary artery, the absence of pulmonary plethora and the evidence of right ventricular enlargement in the left anterior oblique view.

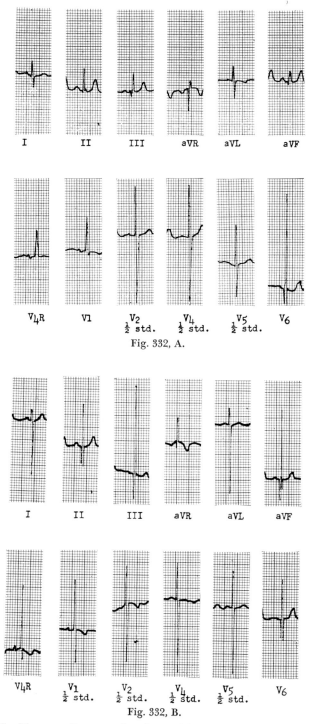

Fig. 332, A.

Fig. 332, B.

Figure 332. Electrocardiograms of patients with atypical patent ductus arteriosus. *A*, Mild right ventricular hypertrophy with definite evidence of left ventricular hypertrophy. *B*, Exclusively right ventricular hypertrophy.

advanced cases with pulmonary vascular obstruction the contrast between engorged hilar vessels and ischemic peripheral lung fields can be seen.

The electrocardiogram frequently reflects the increased pressure-work of the right ventricle by showing the presence of combined or even pure right ventricular hypertrophy, with or without incomplete right bundle branch block (Fig. 332). There is good correlation between the electrocardiogram and the pulmonary arterial mean pressure (Fig. 333), indicating that, at least in infants, pure left ventricular hypertrophy is rarely associated with pulmonary arterial pressure greater than 50 mm. of mercury; figures higher than this level are usually reflected in the electrocardiogram by indications of right ventricular hypertrophy.

The clinical picture described thus far is typical, particularly of infants with pulmonary arterial hypertension and a large pulmonary flow. It is also compatible with this physiologic setup if encountered in older children. But this picture of "hyperkinetic pulmonary arterial hypertension" should be contrasted with the profile of dominant "pulmonary vascular obstruction" (reversed ductus), which is more common in older children and adults, but may be seen occasionally in infants as well. The historical differences have been noted earlier.

On physical examination these patients cannot be distinguished from those having pulmonary vascular obstructive disease associated with ventricular or atrial septal defect (see p. 600). The heart is usually quiet with a right ventricular impulse. Murmurs are trivial and nonspecific. The second sound is narrowly split, if at all, and the pulmonary component is booming. There is slight to moderate cyanosis, favoring the left hand and lower half of the body. Roentgenologic examination shows an almost normal-sized heart, a prominent main pulmonary artery, diminished pulmonary vasculature and right ventricular configuration. The electrocardiogram shows pure right ventricular hypertrophy.

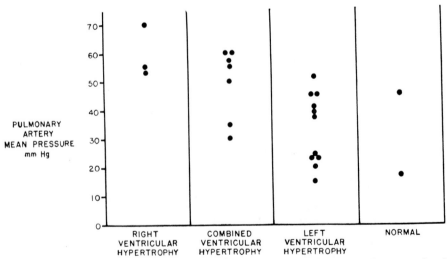

Figure 333. The electrocardiogram in infants with patent ductus arteriosus correlated with pulmonary arterial mean pressure. Note that patients with pure right ventricular hypertrophy always had mean pressures higher than 50 mm. of mercury. Conversely, infants with pure left ventricular hypertrophy never had pulmonary arterial mean pressures higher than 50 mm. of mercury.

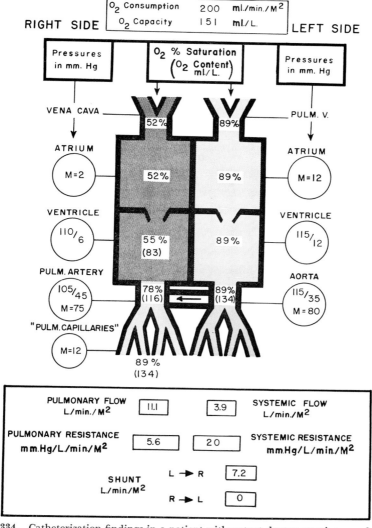

Figure 334.   Catheterization findings in a patient with patent ductus arteriosus and pulmonary arterial hypertension.

Cardiac catheterization (Fig. 334) reveals the following: (1) There is a significant increase (more than 6 per cent) in the oxygen saturation at the pulmonary arterial level in all the hyperkinetic types. But in patients with dominant pulmonary vascular obstruction this may not occur. Arterial oxygen saturation may be diminished either because of a right-to-left shunt through the "reversed ductus" or because of pulmonary factors secondary to left-sided failure. In the former situation the femoral arterial saturation is appreciably lower than the simultaneously obtained right brachial arterial sample, even though this also may be somewhat lower than normal. If the arterial unsaturation is due to pulmonary factors, the results of oxygen studies will be revealing (see p. 351), and, also, the saturation in the right brachial artery will be essentially the same as that in the femoral artery.

In addition to the increase in oxygen saturation at the pulmonary arterial level, definite evidence of a left-to-right shunt at the atrial level (see p. 377) may also be obtained in those infants with the largest shunts. In some cases this may be due to a complicating, true atrial septal defect; in other instances a sizable left-to-right shunt at the atrial level is probably due to an overstretched foramen ovale and may be eliminated by diminishing left atrial filling through division of the ductus.

There may also be an increase in oxygen saturation at the ventricular level in infants with "atypical" patent ductus arteriosus. In some instances this may, indeed, be due to an additional ventricular septal defect (see p. 448), but unless the increase in saturation at the ventricular level is at least 10 per cent, as compared to right atrial saturation, pulmonary regurgitation cannot be ruled out as the cause. (2) By definition, the pressures in the right ventricle and pulmonary artery are elevated and may reach systemic level. Right atrial pressure is usually normal, but left atrial or pulmonary capillary pressures are high (from 10 to 20 mm. of mercury, mean) in most of the hyperkinetic cases. Systemic arterial pressures show a rapid upstroke with wide pulse pressure. (3) Pulmonary arterial resistance may vary from normal, in patients with maximal pulmonary flow, to nearly systemic level in patients with obstructive hypertension. (4) Pulmonary-systemic flow ratios vary considerably, according to the type of hypertension present. In hyperkinetic infants maximal ratios (more than 5:1) may be encountered, whereas some adults may show a net right-to-left shunt. (5) The catheter can be passed through the large ductus in more than 75 per cent of the patients. Passage of the catheter, per se, does not prove the presence of a shunt. This depends on the pressure relation as well as on the size of the lumen. (6) Retrograde aortograms may be extremely useful in delineating a left-to-right shunt, whereas pulmonary arterial injections are used to demonstrate a dominant right-to-left shunt. (7) The use of dye dilution curves is essentially the same here as it is for patients with simple ductus arteriosus (see p. 471).

Course and Prognosis

Although, in later years, pulmonary arterial hypertension with pulmonary vascular obstruction may develop in patients with typical patent ductus arteriosus, on the whole this is a rather unusual happening. Probably all the patients being discussed here had had significant pulmonary hypertension in infancy. Whereas the late development of pulmonary vascular disease in the typical case of patent ductus arteriosus may be attributable to the prolonged effects of a large pulmonary blood flow,[181, 722] the presence of high pulmonary arterial pressure in infancy or early childhood must be explained on a different basis. Civin and Edwards[149] stated that in these cases the size of the ductus, for teleologic reasons, necessitates a narrowing of the pulmonary vascular bed in order to maintain an adequate pressure in the systemic circuit; as a matter of fact, they demonstrated the persistence of the fetal type of pulmonary arterioles, with narrow lumens, in some of their infants with the largest ductus. According to this theory, then, in patients with large aortopulmonary communications the pulmonary arterioles do not undergo the usual postnatal increase in the lumen; the increased pulmonary vascular resistance thus maintained helps to reduce the flow through the duct and to maintain an adequate systemic output.

Attractive as this hypothesis may be, I do not believe that it explains the pulmonary hypertension in all the patients in the group. Actually, in some instances a ductus of only moderate size is accompanied by significant pulmonary vascular obstruction, whereas in others, even though the ductus is very large, the pulmonary vasculature is entirely normal for the patient's age, both anatomically and physiologically.

Thus it seems that patients having an "atypical ductus" or a ductus with pulmonary hypertension do not represent a physiologically homogeneous group. Rather, there are two groups. The first group is made up of infants with large patent ductus, tremendously increased pulmonary blood flow and only slightly increased resistance; there is some evidence that after a few years, with only a moderate increase in the actual pulmonary arterial pressure, but with progression of the pulmonary vascular resistance, the left-to-right shunt may diminish, and pulmonary vascular obstruction may appear in some of these infants. These patients, like those with large ventricular septal defects, have a stormy infancy, replete with episodes of congestive failure, pulmonary edema and attacks of pneumonia. This difficult period is followed by a relatively symptom-free childhood; finally pulmonary vascular obstruction occurs, with cyanosis and death in adulthood. At one time or another these patients may present auscultatory phenomena typical of patent ductus arteriosus; electrocardiographic evidences of left ventricular hypertrophy may exist transiently, only to give way to evidences of combined ventricular hypertrophy. At cardiac catheterization the pressure in the pulmonary artery is significantly elevated, but not to the height of the systemic pressure; pulmonary resistance is usually only moderately elevated.

I believe that perhaps this progressive pulmonary vascular obstruction is more common in patients with large patent ductus arteriosus than it is in children with large ventricular septal defect, since the increased flow and pressure throughout the pulmonary bed are present during the entire cardiac cycle. I also have the impression that, for the reasons given, progression of already increased pulmonary resistance may occur earlier in patients with patent ductus arteriosus than in those with ventricular septal defect.

The second group is made up of patients who have a large or moderate-sized ductus with pulmonary vascular obstruction that may well be congenital. These people do not go through the same period of increased pulmonary blood flow as those in the first group; they are cyanotic from birth, and evidences of pulmonary vascular obstruction dominate their entire clinical picture. Strangely, their life expectancy may not be any shorter than that of the first group, but their symptoms are more uniform throughout life. These are the patients in whom the auscultatory findings are the least typical, in whom elecrocardiographic evidences of pure right ventricular hypertrophy are encountered, and in whom, at cardiac catheterization, the highest pulmonary arterial pressures associated with calculated pulmonary resistances equal to or higher than systemic resistance are encountered.

Differential Diagnosis

The differential diagnosis of "atypical" patent ductus arteriosus is one of the most difficult and most crucial encountered in pediatric cardiology. In my opinion, *an atypical patent ductus arteriosus should be excluded by cardiac catheterization in every case of a left-to-right shunt with pulmonary arterial hypertension if evidences of left ventricular hypertrophy are present, and particularly if the pulse pressure is wide.* If catheterization studies fail to furnish an unequivocal answer, surgical exploration should be contemplated.

If patent ductus arteriosus with pulmonary arterial hypertension is diagnosed on clinical grounds, often the abnormal auscultatory, roentgenographic or electrocardiographic features suggest the presence of an additional congenital malformation. Although accompanying congenital defects, notably atrial or ventricular septal defect, pulmonary stenosis, aortic stenosis, and so forth, have been described by several authors,[311, 352] the presence of such abnormalities should be diagnosed only after thorough studies. In my experience, most "atypical" features can be explained solely on the basis of the ductus with pulmonary arterial hypertension. Furthermore, for practical purposes, the presence of an additional congenital malformation should not make any difference from the therapeutic viewpoint, except in the extremely rare instance in which a tetralogy of Fallot is associated with a patent ductus arteriosus. The association of pure pulmonary stenosis or aortic stenosis with patent ductus arteriosus does not present a contraindication to operation; neither do septal defects. My thoughts on the therapeutic approach to ventricular septal defect associated with patent ductus arteriosus have been outlined earlier (see p. 448).

The principal lesions to be considered in the differential diagnosis are as follows:

Total Anomalous Pulmonary Venous Drainage.   The cardiac enlargement with congestive failure, the severe and pure right ventricular hypertrophy, and the characteristic roentgenogram usually enable the cardiologist to identify total anomalous pulmonary venous drainage. Occasionally, however, only the demonstration of systemic arterial blood in the right atrium at catheterization furnishes an unequivocal answer to the problem.

Atrial Septal Defect or Partial Pulmonary Venous Anomaly.   Atypical patent ductus arteriosus resembles atrial septal defect or partial pulmonary venous anomaly only from the radiologic viewpoint. The similarity of the two in terms of prominent main pulmonary artery with right ventricular hypertrophy and pulmonary vascular engorgement may be striking. Consideration of other factors, however, particularly the presence of a widely split, but not accentuated, fixed second sound, the selective right ventricular enlargement shown in the roentgenogram, and the incomplete right bundle branch block without evidences of left ventricular hypertrophy, as indicated by the electrocardiogram, usually enables the experienced observer to identify a communication at the atrial level.

Large Ventricular Septal Defect.   Large ventricular septal defect (with or without pulmonary stenosis or aortic regurgitation) may be impossible to separate from atypical patent ductus arteriosus without catheterization or even thoracotomy. Localization of the murmur at the lower left sternal border, the absence of the early diastolic components, and the presence of normal pulse pressure and of pure right ventricular hypertrophy all tend to favor a ventricular defect. But even the most experienced observers are likely to make serious mistakes. Hence it cannot be emphasized too often that if this particular point in differential diagnosis is seriously considered, catheterization should be carried out at the appropriate time, particularly if the patient is not doing well.

Truncus Arteriosus. In addition to the points enumerated on page 510, it should be mentioned that atypical ductus arteriosus, if accompanied by severe enough pulmonary arterial hypertension to give rise to cyanosis, usually is not accompanied by murmurs as loud and as ubiquitous as are seen with truncus arteriosus.

Aortopulmonary Fenestration. Aortopulmonary fenestration was discussed on page 498.

Aneurysm of the Sinus of Valsalva. See page 511.

Treatment

The treatment of patients with patent ductus arteriosus and pulmonary arterial hypertension cannot be summarized as easily as that of patients with typical patent ductus.

Patients who have large left-to-right shunts and only a slight to moderate increase in pulmonary resistance unquestionably should be subjected to operation; these patients may benefit tremendously from surgery, and the mortality rate for these small babies should not be high in *experienced hands.* Of twenty-one infants less than one year of age operated on at our institution, we have lost only one in the immediate postoperative period; two others died for other reasons, months later.[603] In view of the underdevelopment, the chronic congestive heart failure, the repeated bouts of pneumonia and even the possibility of progressive pulmonary vascular obstruction, operation is indicated as soon as the diagnosis is made. Usually this does not seem like a difficult decision, since, as mentioned earlier, these children are sick and need help.

The decision to operate on a patient belonging to the group in whom the pulmonary arterial hypertension is extremely severe and is principally due to pulmonary vascular obstruction without a significant left-to-right shunt is much more difficult to make. Without operation these patients cannot look forward to a normal life span. Death at an age appreciably younger than is expected for a normal person seems a foregone conclusion. On the other hand, many of these patients lead full and active lives into the fourth and fifth decades. Operation carries at least a 50 per cent risk. Furthermore, even if patients do survive the operation, the chances of reducing the established pulmonary vascular obstruction are remote.

The literature is filled with glowing reports of a postoperative decrease in pulmonary arterial pressure in patients operated on for patent ductus arteriosus, but careful study usually indicates clearly that the pulmonary arterial pressure drop paralleled the drop in pulmonary blood flow. I am not aware of any well substantiated case report in which an unequivocal return to normal of markedly elevated pulmonary arterial resistance was obtained by dividing the patent ductus arteriosus. So far, even though some of these patients with severe, even maxical, pulmonary vascular obstruction have survived the operation, improvement has not followed clearly. It is hoped that the vascular obstruction will not progress any further, but even this is more a matter of wishful thinking than proved fact. Actually, we have seen at least three patients in whom division of the ductus led

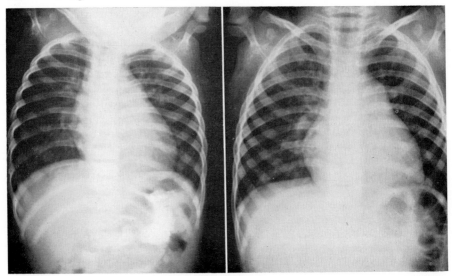

Figure 335. Roentgenogram of patient with patent ductus arteriosus, pulmonary arterial hypertension and pulmonary vascular obstructive disease. The film on the left was taken some weeks after successful division of the patent ductus arteriosus, with the persistence of pulmonary arterial hypertension due to pulmonary vascular disease. The film on the right shows the heart a year later, with progressive pulmonary vascular obstructive disease, maximal cardiac enlargement and a prominent main pulmonary artery.

to an increase of calculated resistance and in one case, even death (Figs. 335, 336). On the basis of these considerations our policy at present is to advise surgery if we can demonstrate a net left-to-right shunt resulting in a pulmonary flow at least 50 per cent greater than systemic flow. If the net shunt is right to left, surgery is contraindicated. In the No-Man's Land of a net left-to-right shunt less than 50 per cent of the systemic flow, the surgeon usually constricts the ductus on the operating table and watches the pressure in the pulmonary artery; if during a 10-minute constriction no appreciable drop (or even a rise) occurs, it may be wise to back out. Although the wise cardiologist deals with these problems with a great deal of trepidation, some of the most gratifying results may be obtained in these "borderline" patients (Fig. 337). Although the calculated resistance postoperatively is far from normal, it drops some; this, coupled with a low pulmonary flow, results in an appreciable lowering of the mean pulmonary arterial pressure and, thus, in a more hopeful long-term prognosis. I would like to emphasize that, at least at present, I am much more inclined to advise surgery in a patient with patent ductus arteriosus, pulmonary vascular obstruction and only a slight left-to-right shunt, than in a patient with a ventricular septal defect and similar physiologic data. I cannot help thinking that the rapidity of the procedure, the absence of a ventriculotomy and the fact that the pump oxygenator is not needed, all make ductus surgery, at present, an infinitely safer operation.

The medical support needed by these patients before, during and after operation is appreciable. Since congestive failure and pulmonary infections are common, the need for preoperative anticongestive measures and antibiotics is great. The use of spasmolytics, such as Priscoline, to reduce pulmonary obstruction has been tried. In our hands the results, on the whole, have been discouraging.

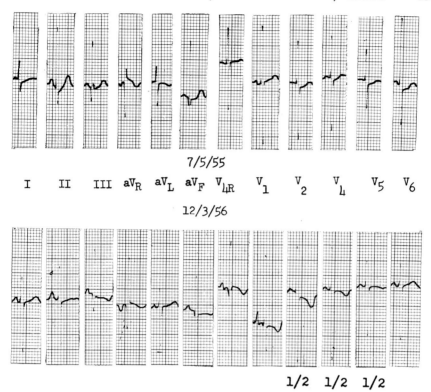

7/5/55

I   II   III   aV_R   aV_L   aV_F   V_{4R}   V_1   V_2   V_4   V_5   V_6

12/3/56

1/2 1/2 1/2

Figure 336. Electrocardiograms of patient with patent ductus arteriosus and pulmonary vascular obstruction. Tracing in 1955 shows an axis of plus 90 degrees and suggests combined ventricular hypertrophy. The lower tracing shows a mean axis of plus 135 degrees and right ventricular hypertrophy with P pulmonale. This tracing corresponds to the roentgenogram on the right in Figure 335, indicating progressive cardiac enlargement.

		O₂ Sat. %					Pressures in mm.Hg		Cardiac Index L/min./M²		Resistance u/M²	
		SVC	RA	RV	PA	Ao	PA (m)	SA (m)	P	S	P	S
C.I.	Preop.	67	66	66	83	96	88/43 (58)	120/75 (100)	9.1	4.1	5	20
	Postop.	69	67	66	63	100	100/55 (75)	103/60 (77)	3.1	3.1	21	25
M.R.	Preop.	80	77	75	86	96	90/55 (70)	90/40 (70)	6.8	4.1	7.6	16
	Postop.	76	68	75	75	96	70/20 (40)	95/58 (75)	5.7	5.7	6	12

Figure 337. *Top,* Preoperative and postoperative catheterization findings in a patient with progressive pulmonary vascular disease associated with patent ductus arteriosus, indicating the progression of pulmonary vascular resistance. *Bottom,* Preoperative and postoperative catheterization findings in another patient with patent ductus arteriosus and pulmonary vascular obstructive disease. Note that, in this instance, although the calculated resistance did not change much postoperatively, because of the diminution of pulmonary blood flow, the pulmonary arterial mean pressure dropped appreciably.

Summary

"Atypical" patent ductus arteriosus should be suspected in every patient who has evidences of a left-to-right shunt with pulmonary arterial hypertension. These patients are commonly subject to episodes of congestive failure and attacks of pneumonia; physically, they are greatly underdeveloped. At auscultation, in the great majority of instances, a systolic murmur is present at the upper left sternal border; early diastolic murmurs are also present in more than half of the patients. The pulse pressure may be widened. Electrocardiograms and roentgenograms show combined ventricular hypertrophy. Cardiac catheterization is indicated for every patient in whom such a lesion is seriously suspected.

PATENT DUCTUS ARTERIOSUS WITH AORTIC STENOSIS

In 1955 Bonam-Carter[73] focused attention on this combination of lesions, though earlier reports are available. More recently, Mark, Jacobson and Young[479] reported seven cases.

Incidence

This is probably a rare combination, although the exact percentage, for reasons to be given, may not be stated with accuracy. Bonam-Carter found it in 9 of 190 patients with patent ductus arteriosus.

Anatomy

Many times other complicating lesions are present (such as coarctation of the aorta or ventricular septal defect). The association with pulmonic stenosis should be mentioned, and also the extracardiac anomalies resulting from a "German measles" pregnancy.

Physiology

I cannot quote the incidence of this combination of lesions among our patients, since the exact definition is a difficult one depending on the physiologic criteria used. In a relatively high percentage of patients with patent ductus arteriosus there is a murmur at the second right interspace, and the electrocardiogram indicates moderate to severe left ventricular hypertension, both suggesting the presence of additional aortic stenosis. If, at catheterization, a gradient is found across the aortic valve, it must be decided how much of this gradient is due to the increased aortic flow and how much to an intrinsic defect of the aortic valve. As yet no accurate formula has been worked out for this correlation. Suffice it to say that slight gradients across a normal aortic valve are not at all uncommon in patients with large left-to-right ductal shunts. This, of course, adds left ventricular pressure-work to the flow-work inherent in the patent ductus arteriosus. Also, to a certain extent, it may distort the systemic arterial pressure pulse.

Clinical Picture

In most respects the history and physical examination cannot be distinguished from those of patients with simple patent ductus arteriosus. The associated intracardiac and extracardiac anomalies should be empha-

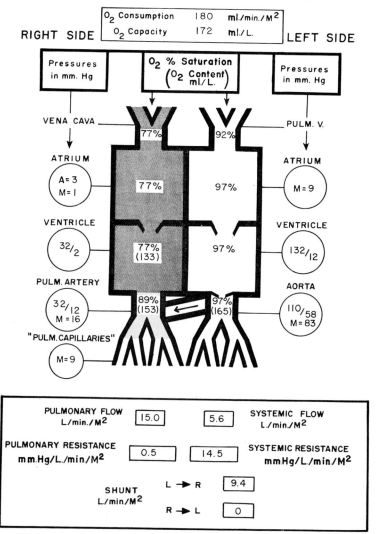

Figure 338.   Cardiac catheterization findings in a patient with patent ductus arteriosus and aortic stenosis.

sized, as well as the separate murmur of aortic stenosis heard at the second right interspace. This is accompanied by the characteristic thrill and transmits well to the neck vessels (Fig. 319). Paradoxical splitting of the second sound is sometimes noted, and the electrocardiogram shows left ventricular hypertrophy, and even strain, over and beyond what one would expect from the patent ductus arteriosus alone.

At *cardiac catheterization* (Fig. 338), the hemodynamic data are essentially similar to those described for patients with simple patent ductus arteriosus, except that a gradient across the aortic valve is found if looked for. Of course, most patients with patent ductus arteriosus are not catheterized at all, and catheterization of the left side of the heart is justifiable in an even smaller number.

Course and Prognosis

On the basis of information presently available, the natural history of this combination of defects seems to be practically identical with that of a large patent ductus arteriosus alone.

Differential Diagnosis

Sometimes the presence of a stenotic murmur, in addition to the Gibson murmur, draws the cardiologist's attention to the possible combination of ductus arteriosus with aortic or pulmonic stenosis. Which semilunar valve is involved may, of course, be difficult to determine. If the electrocardiogram shows right ventricular hypertrophy, pulmonic stenosis may be suspected. On the other hand, left ventricular hypertrophy may be compatible with mild aortic stenosis as well as mild pulmonic stenosis. Left ventricular hypertrophy with strain strongly suggests aortic stenosis. In addition, the localization of the murmur to the second right, rather than the second left, interspace implies an aortic lesion. Truncus arteriosus may also be present with evidences of a large left-to-right shunt, wide pulse pressure and a stenotic murmur at the second right interspace.

Treatment

It has been our policy to treat the patent ductus arteriosus first and to repair the aortic valve only as a second procedure if, without the ductal shunt, an appreciable gradient still persists across the aortic valve.

Summary

Patients with findings of patent ductus arteriosus, with the additional murmur of aortic stenosis, whose electrocardiograms indicate severe left ventricular hypertrophy, should be suspected of having aortic stenosis associated with the patent ductus. The ductus should be treated first; surgery for the aortic stenosis is indicated only if a residual gradient is demonstrable.

PATENT DUCTUS ARTERIOSUS WITH PULMONIC STENOSIS

Incidence

Six patients with this combination of anomalies had been seen at our institution before 1958.[333] Kjellberg and his associates[398] noted three among the forty-seven patients with patent ductus arteriosus in their series who underwent cardiac catheterization.

Anatomy

Associated noncardiac anomalies, particularly those suggesting that the mother had had German measles during pregnancy, are the rule rather than the exception. The ductus is usually large, and pulmonic stenosis is likely to be valvar.

Physiology

Unlike aortic stenosis, in pulmonic stenosis a gradient across the pulmonic valve may not be the consequence of the shunt. On the contrary, the left-to-right shunt, by raising pulmonary pressure, may possibly "mask" the presence of the pulmonic stenosis, which then becomes evident after ligation of the ductus.[398] More commonly this "masking" effect is auscultatory and electrocardiographic rather than physiologic. Pulmonic stenosis adds right ventricular pressure-work to the left ventricular flow-work inherent in the patent ductus arteriosus.

Clinical Picture

The associated noncardiac anomalies, the marked underdevelopment,

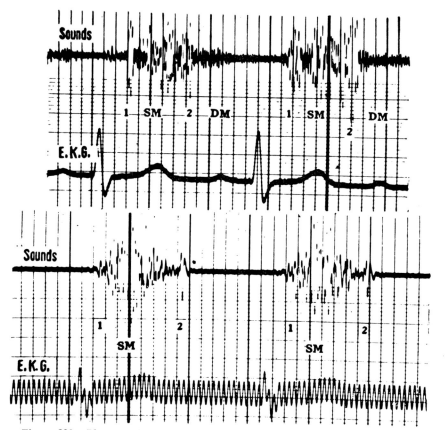

Figure 339. Phonocardiogram of patient with patent ductus arteriosus and pulmonic stenosis. Upper tracing shows the continuous murmur obtained before division of the ductus arteriosus. The lower panel shows the typical diamond-shaped murmur of pulmonic stenosis. Only the aortic closure is visible here. Pulmonic closure cannot be seen.

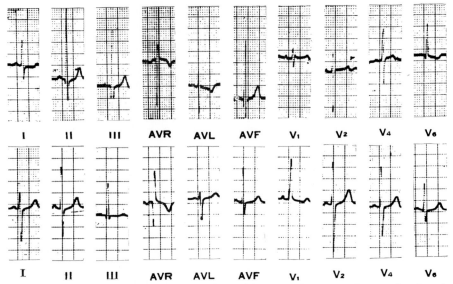

Figure 340. Electrocardiogram of patient with patent ductus arteriosus and pulmonic stenosis. Upper tracing is preoperative, with a mean electrical axis of plus 75 degrees and chest leads indicating left ventricular hypertrophy with strain. In contrast, in the lower panel the mean electrical axis is plus 120 degrees, and there is definite evidence of right ventricular hypertrophy in this postoperative tracing.

and the history of German measles in the first trimester of prenatal life are the most common features directing suspicion toward this combination. In addition, a stenotic murmur at the second left interspace (Fig. 339), super-imposed on the machinery murmur, may be noted by the careful observer. Pulmonic closure may not be particularly loud. Evidences of right ventricular involvement may be revealed by palpation, the roentgenogram and the electrocardiogram. Note that in some instances none of these features becomes obvious until after division of the patent ductus arteriosus (Fig. 340).

At *cardiac catheterization* (Fig. 341) the presence of a systolic gradient across the right ventricular outflow tract is the only feature distinguishing this entity from a simple patent ductus arteriosus.

Course and Prognosis

Frequently these patients present the clinical picture of a straightforward, large, simple patent ductus arteriosus, and only after division of the ductus is the pulmonic stenosis suggested. On the whole, these patients are sicker than the average youngster with a patent ductus arteriosus. How much this is due to the effect of widespread congenital anomalies and how much to the hemodynamic handicaps would be difficult to estimate.

Differential Diagnosis

Aside from consideration of a straightforward, large patent ductus arteriosus, patent ductus arteriosus with pulmonic stenosis needs to be

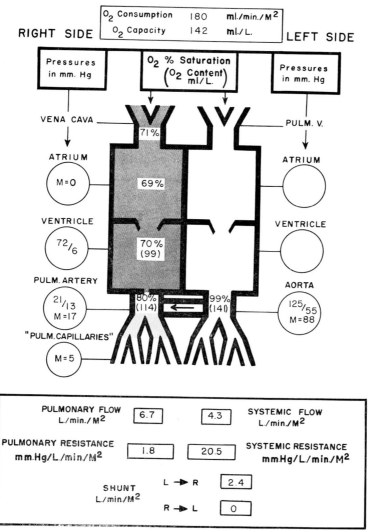

Figure 341.   Catheterization findings in patient with patent ductus arteriosus and pulmonic stenosis.

differentiated only from the combination of patent ductus with aortic stenosis (see p. 492).

Treatment

At present our policy is to study the patients with this clinical diagnosis at cardiac catheterization, preoperatively. Depending on the gradient found, the ductus is divided with or without simultaneous relief of the pulmonic obstruction. If the diagnosis is not made preoperatively, but becomes obvious on the operating table only after division of the ductus, a blind valvotomy from the pulmonary arterial side should be attempted.

This may well be curative; if not, a second operation, by means of cardio-pulmonary bypass, is still feasible.

Summary

Patients who are the known product of a "German measles" pregnancy as well as those who merely exhibit the characteristic extracardiac congenital anomalies should be suspected of having the combination of patent ductus arteriosus and pulmonic stenosis. Evidences of right ventricular hypertrophy, in addition to the left ventricular hypertrophy inherent in a patent ductus arteriosus, and a stenotic systolic murmur at the second left interspace are the distinguishing clinical features. Simultaneous surgery for both defects is indicated, if possible.

Patent Ductus Arteriosus and Coarctation of the Aorta

See Coarctation of the Aorta (p. 537).

Patent Ductus Arteriosus and Ventricular Septal Defect

See Ventricular Septal Defect (p. 448).

AORTOPULMONARY FENESTRATION

This is a rare anomaly. D'Heer and his associates[178] collected 34 cases from the literature in 1956. Skall-Jensen,[644] in a comprehensive report, described sixty-two cases; among these the diagnosis was made during life in thirty-five patients, and catheterization data were available for fifteen. We have had fifteen patients with this clinical diagnosis. Abbott[1] mentioned 10 cases in her series of 1000 postmortem examinations. The importance of the defect lies in its close clinical resemblance to patent ductus arteriosus.

Embryologically, this is the result of the incomplete development of the spiral ridges dividing the bulbus cordis; clearly this should result in a persistence of the fetal communication between the halves of the bulbus.

Anatomy

The defect, varying in diameter from 5 to 30 mm.,[308] is located just above the aortic valve in the anterior wall of the aorta. Sometimes it is practically inseparable from the coronary arteries; in other instances it is a few millimeters or even more than a centimeter above them. Almost without exception, the ventricular septum is intact.

Physiology

The physiologic effects of an aortopulmonary fenestration are identical with those of a patent ductus arteriosus; because of the gradient between systemic and pulmonary resistances, a shunt from the aortic to the pulmonary side occurs. The size of the defect and the ratio between the two resistances are the principal factors determining the magnitude of the left-to-right shunt.

It has been suggested[683] that in this malformation the volume-pressure relations between the aorta and the pulmonary artery are different enough from those encountered in patent ductus arteriosus to explain the more serious prognosis of aortic septal defect. From our experience with two patients who have small aortopulmonary windows, I would think that the prognosis may well depend principally on the size of the orifice.

Clinical Picture

For all practical purposes, the clinical picture cannot be distinguished from that of a large patent ductus. The only clue to the fact that this is not a clear-cut ductus arteriosus is that the murmur may be somewhat atypical and is situated lower and more medially than is customary.

The roentgenologic picture (Figs. 342, 343) and electrocardiographic findings (Fig. 344) are characteristic of a large patent ductus arteriosus, perhaps associated with pulmonary hypertension (Fig. 220).

At *cardiac catheterization* physiologic studies may yield information indistinguishable from that found for a patient having a large patent ductus arteriosus (Fig. 345). Pulmonary arterial hypertension of significant degree is the rule, with few exceptions (four of Skall-Jensen's[644] fifteen cases). D'Heer and Van Nelwenhizen[178] reported 2 cases in 1956 and described the characteristic course of the catheter in this condition. Catheterization is still the most useful method of differential diagnosis. These authors emphasized that (1) it is considerably more difficult to pass the catheter through an aortopulmonary window than through a patent ductus and that (2) if the catheter is passed into the aorta, it may be pointed in two directions, either backward through the ascending aorta to the aortic valve or forward into the right carotid or right subclavian artery (Figs. 346, 347). This contrasts sharply with the course of the catheter in patent ductus arteriosus (directly into the descending aorta and almost never to the right brachiocephalic trunk). If pulmonary vascular obstruction is associated with aortopulmonary fenestration, resulting in a right-to-left shunt (less than 25 per cent of the cases), right brachial arterial saturation is identical to femoral arterial saturation.

Gasul and his associates[267] reported a case in which differential diagnosis was possible by means of retrograde aortography. We have studied our patients at cine-angiography and found the characteristic visualization of the pulmonary artery from the ascending aorta, with a clear, sharp outline of the arch and the descending aorta.

Course and Prognosis

The natural history of the anomaly cannot be outlined with any certainty because of the paucity of reported cases. Survival varies, probably depending on the size of the opening (Fig. 348), from three days, reported by Hektoen,[334] to forty-eight years, reported by Moorhead and Smith.[500] Fewer than one sixth of the patients reviewed by Skall-Jensen[644] were more than fifteen years of age. Death usually occurs from congestive failure,

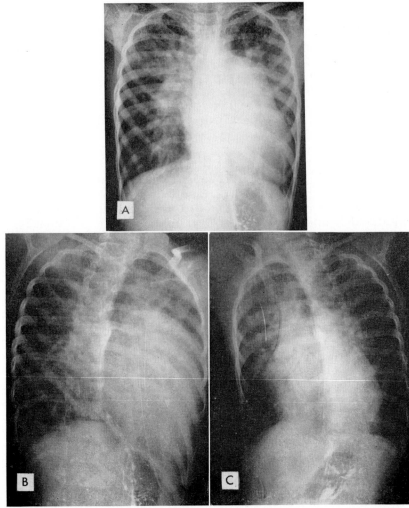

Figure 342. Posteroanterior and oblique roentgenograms of patient with aortopulmonary fenestration. Note the similarity between these films and those of patient with large patent ductus arteriosus.

probably associated with pulmonary vascular obstruction, although these patients should be equally susceptible to bacterial endocarditis as are patients with patent ductus arteriosus.

Differential Diagnosis

The differential diagnosis of aortopulmonary fenestration from large patent ductus arteriosus is practically impossible by clinical means and may be accomplished at cardiac catheterization only if the ascending aorta is entered from the pulmonary artery. Then the characteristic course (back to the aortic valve *and* forward into the right brachiocephalic trunk) establishes the diagnosis. Differentiation between this condition and *ventricular septal defect with aortic regurgitation* may be possible only by

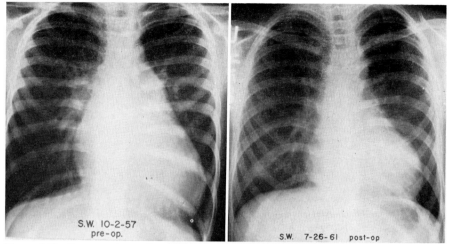

S.W. 10-2-57
pre-op.

S.W. 7-26-61 post-op

Figure 343. Preoperative and postoperative roentgenograms of patient with aortopulmonary fenestration. Operation was performed in 1960.

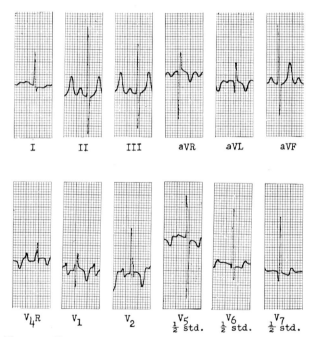

I   II   III   aVR   aVL   aVF

V_4R V_1 V_2 V_5 ½ std. V_6 ½ std. V_7 ½ std.

Figure 344. Electrocardiogram of patient with aortopulmonary fenestration. Note the presence of combined ventricular hypertrophy.

means of continuous pressure monitoring from the aorta into the right ventricle through the pulmonary artery. Because aortic and pulmonary arterial pressures may be practically identical, the presence of pulmonary arterial hypertension alone may not furnish sufficient evidence for differentiation. In such cases a phonocatheter may be helpful by demonstrating the maximal intensity of the murmur in the pulmonary artery rather than in the right ventricle.

Truncus arteriosus, particularly type I, may be indistinguishable from aortopulmonary septal defect by all methods except thoracotomy. The fact that the catheter can move in two possible directions, as indicated previously, may be the most helpful tool. In truncus arteriosus the tip of the catheter may be pointed forward only. Also, the identical oxygen saturations in the pulmonary artery and the aorta are more likely to occur in truncus arteriosus, though there is a great deal of overlapping in this regard. Finally, truncus arteriosus almost never occurs without an associated ventricular defect, whereas aortopulmonary fenestration is seldom seen with a ventricular septal defect.

Treatment

Surgical correction was first reported by Gross in 1952.[308] Since that time a number of patients have been treated successfully by a variety of

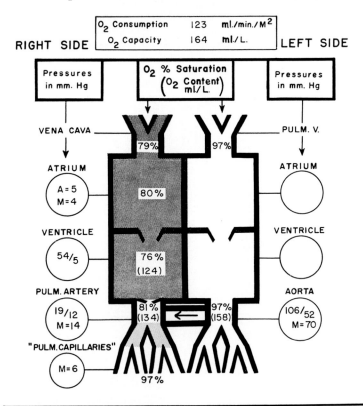

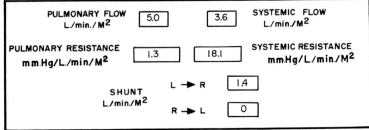

methods.[44, 163, 623] At present our surgeons use the pump oxygenator, with or without hypothermia, for closure of these defects. No valid figures of operative mortality are available, but I would think that 20 to 25 per cent may be a conservative estimate. Nevertheless all large defects with a sizable net left-to-right shunt should be treated surgically, preferably after the patients have reached a weight of 25 pounds.

Summary

Aortopulmonary fenestration is a communication between the two great arteries just above the semilunar valves. The diagnosis should be suspected in patients who have symptoms and signs of a somewhat atypical

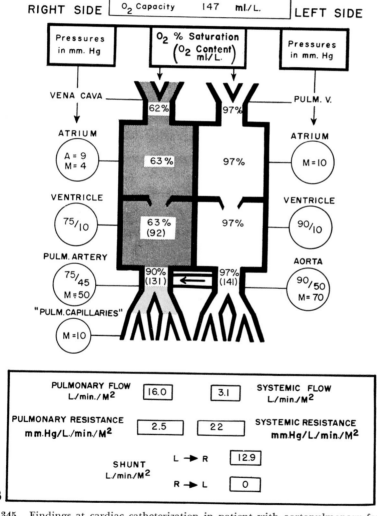

Figure 345. Findings at cardiac catheterization in patient with aortopulmonary fenestration. *A* indicates a small window with pulmonic stenosis. *B* shows the findings in a patient with a large fenestration.

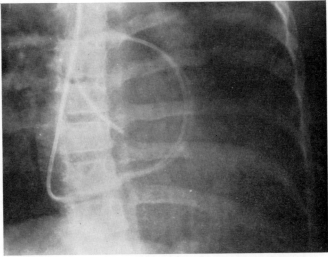

Figure 346. Catheter tip in ascending aorta, entered from the pulmonary artery through an aortopulmonary fenestration (see also Figure 325, *C*).

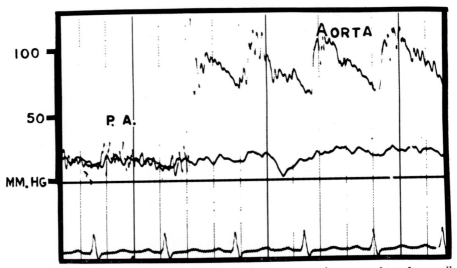

Figure 347. Withdrawal of catheter from pulmonary artery into aorta through a small aortopulmonary window. Note the pressure gradient between the two great arteries, indicating that this is, indeed, a small fenestration.

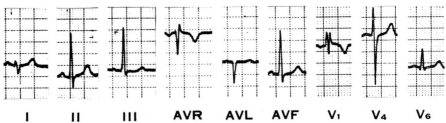

Figure 348. Electrocardiogram of patient with small aortopulmonary window. Note the mean electrical axis of plus 105 degrees and an rsR' pattern in V_1, without clear-cut evidence of either right or left ventricular hypertrophy.

ductus and is proved by passing the catheter from the pulmonary artery into the ascending aorta and into the right brachiocephalic trunk. Surgery, by means of cardiopulmonary bypass, is feasible at moderate risks.

PERSISTENT TRUNCUS ARTERIOSUS

Incidence

Truncus arteriosus is not a common lesion. Abbott[1] reported 21 cases in her series of 1000. Keith[380] reported nine children with this condition in his series. At The Children's Hospital Medical Center we have had fifteen patients in whom the diagnosis was proved at postmortem examination during the past twelve years and another five patients in whom the diagnosis was made clinically.

Anatomy

Complete failure of development of the bulbar ridges results in persistence of the fetal common arterial trunk. Since these ridges are also necessary to complete the development of the ventricular septum, persistent truncus arteriosus is always associated with a defect of the membranous septum and invariably communicates with both ventricles. Frequently the entire ventricular septum is absent. The number of semilunar valves varies from two to six. The ductus is absent in the majority of patients. The entire circulation, including the systemic arteries, the pulmonary arteries and the coronary arteries, is supplied from this common arterial trunk. The presence of the coronaries eliminates aortic atresia from the differential diagnosis.

Collett and Edwards[154] devised an anatomic classification consisting of four types of truncus arteriosus (Fig. 349). For practical, clinical purposes we have eliminated type 4 from consideration, since it cannot be distinguished from pulmonary atresia by any means short of a most careful postmortem examination. In these patients there are no visible pulmonary arteries, and the entire pulmonary circulation is through bronchial collaterals. This will be discussed in the paragraph on extreme tetralogy of Fallot (see p. 642).

In the other three types, pulmonary arteries originate (from the common trunk) proximal to the right brachiocephalic vessels. In type I (48 per cent of Collett and Edwards's cases) the takeoff of the single pulmonary artery is at the base of the trunk, and it runs parallel with the ascending aorta. Type II of our classification includes their types 2 and 3 (29 per cent and 11 per cent, respectively, in their series); it is characterized by a takeoff of one or both pulmonary arteries at right angles from the common trunk, at some distance above the semilunar valves. In type 2 of Collett and Edwards's classification both pulmonary arteries arise close together from the posterior wall of the trunk, whereas in type 3 one or both pulmonary arteries arise independently from either side of the truncus. Since we cannot distinguish type 2 from type 3, clinically, hemodynamically or angiographically, and yet are able in some instances to separate these two from type I, we find it more expedient simply to distinguish between types I and II, the latter including 2 and 3 of Edwards.

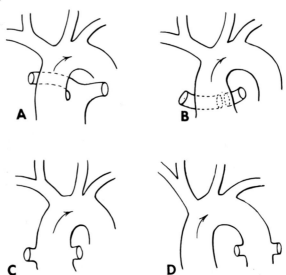

Figure 349. Schematic representation of the variations of common truncus arteriosus. *A*, Type I. *B*, and *C*, included in our classification as type II. *D*, not included by us in the definition of common truncus arteriosus; rather, we regard it as an extreme form of the tetralogy of Fallot syndrome.[214]

It should be mentioned that truncus arteriosus is associated with a right aortic arch in about 25 per cent of the patients and with a single ventricle in about the same proportion.

Whereas, in the majority of instances, the aorta, with its tributaries, and the coronary arteries are functionally adequate, the state of the pulmonary vessels may vary. The anatomic variations in the size of the pulmonary arteries are not extreme if we exclude type 4. In all the other types at least one moderately adequate-sized pulmonary artery is present and there is more or less pulmonary vascular obstruction.

Occasionally the right pulmonary artery may originate from the truncus, proximal to the innominate artery, whereas the left may take off directly from the right ventricle.

Physiology

Since blood leaving the heart through one common exit represents a practically complete mixture of the pulmonary (oxygenated) and systemic (unoxygenated) return, the arterial saturation of the truncus blood depends on the ratio of the systemic to the pulmonary flow. If the pulmonary arteries are adequate in size and the pulmonary circulation therefore large, the truncus blood will be relatively highly saturated. Conversely, if the pulmonary circulation is inadequate, either because of small pulmonary arteries or pulmonary vascular obstruction, the oxygen content of the blood in the common trunk will be nearly the same as that in the vena cava. The systolic pressure in the two ventricles is equal and identical with that obtained from the aorta. The pulmonary arterial pressure in most of our patients was at, or near, systemic arterial level. The oxygen content in the two ventricles, the aorta and the pulmonary arteries is almost always identical.

Clinical Picture

The clinical picture varies, depending on the status of the pulmonary arteries. A patient with two normal-sized pulmonary arteries and normal pulmonary resistance is practically acyanotic; the clinical picture resembles that of a large ventricular defect. On the other hand, a child with hypoplastic pulmonary arteries, a single pulmonary artery or pulmonary vascular obstruction may exhibit the worst degree of cyanotic congenital heart disease.

Most of the patients are known to have had heart disease since birth, and usually a murmur was noted within the first month of life. Their principal symptoms are dyspnea, fatigue and cyanosis, with or without evidences of congestive failure. At physical examination these children are poorly developed; most of them rank well below the third percentile on our development charts, and none of them ranks above the twenty-fifth percentile line. Prominence of the left side of the chest may be noted; a thrill is usually palpable at the second left, sometimes at the second right, interspace. Cyanosis varies considerably from patient to patient, but in rare instances it is completely absent. One infant was observed for almost two months in the wards at The Children's Hospital without definite evidence of cyanosis. The blood pressure is usually normal, although a person who has large pulmonary arteries may have a wide pulse pressure. Hepatomegaly and rales are noted in patients who have congestive heart failure.

The first heart sound is normal, but an aortic click is present in about half of the patients. Usually the second sound is accentuated or even booming. The expected narrowness of the second sound is not observed with any regularity. A loud pansystolic murmur is present at the lower left sternal border in most patients; a protodiastolic blow may be heard in about 50 per cent, but the 2 murmurs seem more to-and-fro than truly continuous (Fig. 350). A stenotic murmur may be heard at the second right interspace, and often an apical mid-diastolic rumble is present.

In the majority of patients the electrocardiogram shows left ventricular

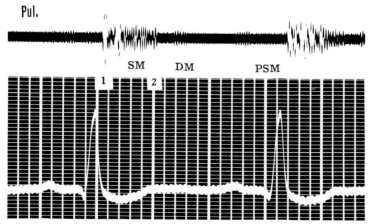

Figure 350. Systolic and diastolic murmurs in the pulmonary area in a patient with truncus arteriosus. Note the decrescendo shape of the systolic murmur, the faintness of the diastolic murmur and the presence of the presystolic murmur.

hypertrophy, alone or combined with right ventricular hypertrophy. Isolated right ventricular hypertrophy is rare. The mean electrical axis is
usually between +90 and +135 degrees; seldom is it to the left of +30
degrees.

The roentgenologic picture, in the "typical" case, shows absence of
the main pulmonary artery at its usual location, and pulmonary plethora
(Fig. 351). But the "typical" case is rather rare, and most often the roentgenologic image is nonspecific, with cardiac enlargement involving both
ventricles, and pulmonary vascular engorgement (Fig. 352). The main
pulmonary artery may be absent, as in the "typical" case, but more commonly it is normal or even increased in size. The "aorta" is large, and
in almost 25 per cent of the patients the arch is on the right side. Occasionally the left ventricle may form a bulge high on the left border of
the heart, at the place usually occupied by the pulmonary artery.

Cardiac catheterization (Fig. 353) reveals the following: (1) There is

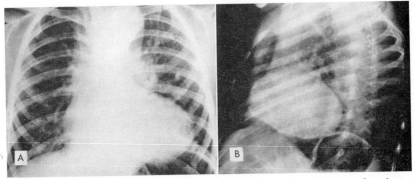

Figure 351. Posteroanterior and left anterior oblique roentgenograms of patient with
common truncus arteriosus. Note the absence of a main pulmonary artery, the large aorta,
left and right ventricular enlargement in the left anterior oblique view and the pulmonary
plethora in the posteroanterior view.

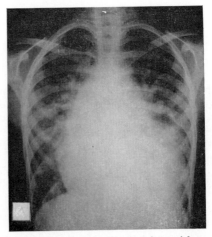

Figure 352. Posteroanterior roentgenogram of patient with common truncus arteriosus.
Note the pulmonary plethora, biventricular and right atrial enlargement and the broad
supracardiac shadow, where aorta and pulmonary artery cannot easily be differentiated.

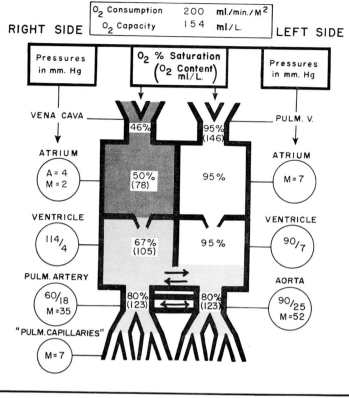

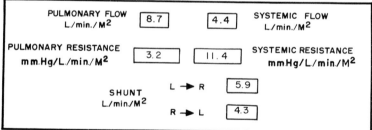

Figure 353. Catheterization findings in patient with common truncus arteriosus. Note the identical saturations in the great arteries with pulmonary artery pressure below systemic levels.

an increase in oxygen content at the right ventricular outflow level. Arterial unsaturation is always present, varying, among our patients, from 65 to 90 per cent; usually it is more than 84 per cent. The saturation in the systemic artery is usually, but not invariably, identical to that in the pulmonary artery. (2) Right atrial pressure may be slightly elevated, and the right ventricular pressure is almost always at systemic level. Left atrial or pulmonary capillary pressure may be normal or slightly increased. Systemic arterial pulse pressure is wide. Pulmonary arterial pressure is at, or slightly below, systemic level. (Note: Collett and Edwards's[154] type 4 is excluded from this discussion.) (3) Pulmonary resistance is high. (4) Pulmonic-systemic flow ratios depend on the size of the pulmonic flow and vary tremendously. (5) The course of the catheter is of interest, in that the pulmonary artery may sometimes be entered without much difficulty, particularly in type I. The course may be indistinguishable from that in patients with aortopulmonary fenestration or even ventricular septal defect (see p. 499). (6) Cine-angiography, with injection into the ascending aorta, may clearly outline the origin of the pulmonary artery, and particularly the high course of the left main pulmonary artery. (7) Dye-dilution curves are not particularly helpful in this situation.

Course and Prognosis

The natural history of the disease is variable. Many of the patients die before they are six months old. Keith[380] stated that approximately 15 per cent survive beyond the first year of life. I would place this figure nearer to 30 per cent, on the basis of our experience. Our oldest living patient at this time is seventeen years old. A few patients have been reported to live to the age of twenty or thirty years. The immediate cause of death is usually congestive failure, although pneumonia has contributed significantly to the death of our small infants. One of our patients was severely ill with bacterial endocarditis; another was successfully treated for a brain abscess.

Differential Diagnosis

Persistent truncus arteriosus may have to be distinguished from other types of cyanotic or acyanotic congenital heart disease, depending on the status of the pulmonary circulation.

In the absence of cyanosis large ventricular septal defect and patent ductus arteriosus should be considered in the differential diagnosis. A large ventricular septal defect is similar to truncus arteriosus in that both entail a communication at the ventricular level and are commonly associated with pulmonary arterial hypertension. The differences are discussed on page 422. The differential diagnosis of patent ductus arteriosus and persistent truncus arteriosus is discussed on page 475. That single ventricle may be associated with truncus arteriosus has already been discussed. For purposes of classification we would still regard this as truncus arteriosus. Other aortopulmonary communications and aortic runoffs to be considered in the differential diagnosis are (1) aortopulmonary fenestration (in which in addition to the characteristic course of the catheter the absence of a ventricular septal defect is a helpful diagnostic clue), (2) aneurysm of the sinus of Valsalva (the absence of cyanosis, the dramatic incidence of rupture and the site of the shunt—exclusively into the right ventricle—in addition to the characteristic anatomy outlined at cine-angiography, may all be useful diagnostic hints), and (3) coronary arteriovenous fistula (the absence of cyanosis, the characteristic murmur and the cine-angiograms are all helpful in the differential diagnosis).

Tricuspid atresia associated with transposition of the great arteries may also be confused with true truncus arteriosus. The question arises in a patient with cyanotic heart disease in whom the electrocardiogram reveals left ventricular hypertrophy. Clinical differentiation may be possible on the basis of the severe and exclusive left ventricular hypertrophy with left axis deviation usually noted in tricuspid atresia. In other instances only angiocardiography enables the cardiologist to make the diagnosis in vivo.

Treatment

Only medical therapy (antibiotics and anticongestive measures) is available at present. Cooley[161] reported repair of a type 1 defect by means of cardiopulmonary bypass, with survival for a few hours. Like others, we have tried banding the large pulmonary arteries which have an abnormal takeoff and tremendous pulmonary flow, with only moderate success. This approach may be used in patients with intractable congestive heart failure.

Summary

True truncus arteriosus is a large common vessel overriding both the left and the right ventricles. There may be severe or mild arterial unsaturation, depending partly on the size of the pulmonary artery originating from this common trunk and partly on the status of the pulmonary vasculature. A wide pulse pressure, a systolic and diastolic to-and-fro murmur, left ventricular hypertension, with or without associated right ventricular hypertrophy, and pulmonary plethora with abnormal origin of the great arteries characterize the clinical picture. Cardiac catheterization with angiography is necessary to confirm the diagnosis. In approximately two thirds of the patients life expectancy is limited to the first year of life. No definitive surgery is available; banding of the pulmonary artery may be attempted in infants having a very large pulmonary flow.

CONGENITAL ANEURYSM OF THE SINUS OF VALSALVA

Incidence

The incidence of this anomaly is low. Jones and Langley,[367] in their excellent review in 1949, reported 25 cases, three fourths of which, however, were acquired. Davidsen and his co-workers,[185] in 1958, reported 5 congenital cases and reviewed 17 from the literature. We have seen two patients with this anomaly within the past five years.

Anatomy

Aneurysmal dilation of the aortic sinus is a result of a congenitally imperfect fusion of the distal bulbar septum. It is a developmental disturbance only slightly less profound than that leading to a defect of the membranous ventricular septum. As a matter of fact, from my experience and according to reports, the two lesions frequently occur together, particularly if the right coronary sinus is involved.[109, 682] Apparently the aneurysmal dilatation seldom involves the left cusp. If the right coronary sinus is involved (as it is in three fourths of the cases), communication with the right ventricle occurs, whereas the posterior cusp (one fourth of the cases) usually ruptures into the right atrium.

Communication of an aneurysm of the aortic sinus with the cavities of the heart may take place either through a small congenital fistulous tract, boring through the myocardium into the right ventricle or right atrium, or by means of a sudden rupture. Again, this rupture may be either spontaneous or secondary to bacterial endocarditis. All these communications are based on a congenital anomaly of the aortic sinus and should be differentiated from acquired lesions (syphilis, arteriosclerosis, and so forth). Of course I have had no personal experience with the latter group, but drawing an analogy with other diseases (e.g. aortic stenosis), I wonder how many of these "acquired" lesions may also have congenital origins. One further thought relating to anatomy is that these may be progressive lesions; the underlying anomaly is, of course, congenital, but the condition develops and may indeed become noticeable only some time after birth.

Physiology

If the aneurysm of the sinus of Valsalva has no communication with intracardiac chambers, the physiologic results are negligible. The results of a sudden large rupture may be serious, although, since this is an *intracardiac* aneurysm, the results are almost never as immediately catastrophic as though the rupture were into the pleural or pericardial cavity. Small ruptures or small congenital fistulas may manifest themselves only as left-to-right shunts.

Clinical Picture

Basically, the clinical profile may assume one of two distinct patterns. One is that of a person who may or may not have been known to have

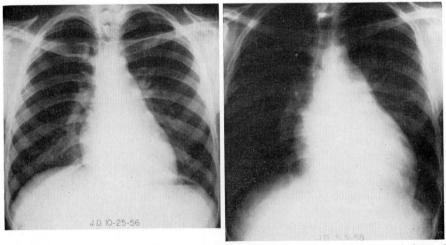

Figure 354. Two posteroanterior roentgenograms in a patient with ruptured sinus of Valsalva occurring after bacterial endocarditis. The film, taken in 1956, represents the cardiac silhouette before bacterial endocarditis when, on the basis of clinical and catheterization data, the patient was regarded as having a simple ventricular septal defect. The film taken in 1958, after the patient recovered from bacterial endocarditis, shows cardiac enlargement and congestive failure. A left sternal border diastolic murmur, indicated the rupture of the sinus of Valsalva. Shortly after this film had been taken the patient was operated upon, but did not survive.

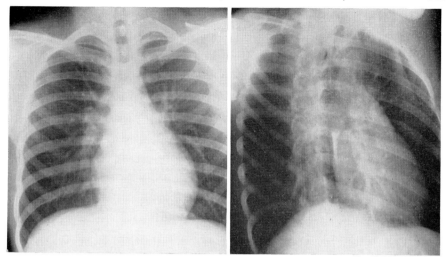

Figure 355. Posteroanterior and left lateral roentgenogram of patient with aneurysm of sinus of Valsalva, without congestive failure. The fistula here was congenital, not acquired. This patient was operated upon and did very well.

heart disease, but in whom evidences of aortic regurgitation, angina and left-sided failure suddenly develop (Fig. 354). If the patient was known to have heart disease, the chances are that he was classified as having a ventricular septal defect. After the development of the sudden episode of failure, the findings on clinical examination are those of a large patent ductus arteriosus. At first glance, the other pattern these patients may exhibit is indistinguishable from that of a simple patent ductus arteriosus, persisting without symptoms, for several years (Figs. 335, 356). This latter type of patient usually has a small to moderate-sized congenital fistula between the sinus of Valsalva and the right ventricle or right atrium, whereas in the former instance an aneurysm of the sinus of Valsalva ruptured suddenly into one of the right heart cavities.

It is the location of the murmur and its nature which, in addition to the acute onset in some of the patients, distinguish these patients at the bedside from children wih patent ductus arteriosus. The murmur is lower down on the left sternal border and is to-and-fro rather than continuous. The systolic murmur stops before the second sound, and the diastolic murmur, after a short crescendic phase, becomes decrescendic. It is interesting to note also that the diastolic component usually is the louder and may reach grade VI in intensity. In this respect it resembles coronary arteriovenous aneurysm.

The rest of the physical examination, the roentgenograms and the electrocardiograms are indistinguishable from those of a patient with patent ductus arteriosus. The aortic arch may be somewhat smaller than it is in patients with a truncus arteriosus, or even a large ductus.

The findings at *cardiac catheterization* are those of a left-to-right shunt at the atrial or ventricular level, depending on where the communication occurs. Cine-angiography is probably the most helpful tool in outlining the site of the aorto-cameral communication. The exclusion of the shunt at the pulmonary arterial level (patent ductus arteriosus) may, in itself, be a helpful result of right heart catheterization.

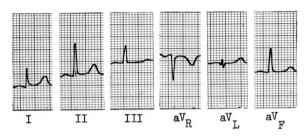

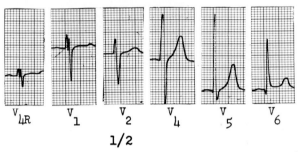

1/2

Figure 356. Electrocardiogram of patient with sinus of Valsalva fistula, without congestive heart failure. This is the cardiogram of the patient whose roentgenogram is shown in Figure 355.

Course and Prognosis

An aneurysm of the sinus of Valsalva which either has no communication with the chambers of the heart or is connected only through a small congenital fistula ought to be of no great significance and may even be compatible with normal life expectancy. Only the complications render this a serious condition. (1) Bacterial endocarditis is a real danger, affecting particularly the patient with coexisting ventricular septal defect. In addition to the obvious hazards of the endocarditis itself, there are the hemodynamic consequences of rupture even if bacteriologic cure is accomplished. (2) Rupture of the aneurysm, with or without bacterial endocarditis, is the most dreaded complication. If the opening in the aneurysm is large, death with congestive heart failure may occur in a matter of weeks or months. Smaller leaks may be compatible with survival for almost two years.[216] Rupture seldom occurs before puberty and may be precipitated by effort. (3) Coexisting deformities of the aortic valve may result in progressive aortic regurgitation. (4) Davidsen[185] mentioned compression of the bundle of His, with secondary complete atrioventricular block, as the cause of death in two patients.

It may be said then that, although the aneurysm itself, even with a small leak through a fistula, may have a relatively good prognosis, with survival to the fifth decade or even longer, the complications which may occur at any time make this a hazardous condition.

Differential Diagnosis

For practical purposes, *a history suggestive of sudden rupture excludes all the conditions to be discussed with the exception of ventricular septal defect and aortic regurgitation.*

Patent Ductus Arteriosus. Of course patent ductus arteriosus is the most important differential diagnostic problem. The abnormally loud murmur, with diastolic accentuation, located at the lower left sternal border, may suggest to the cardiologist that this may not be a simple patent ductus. Right heart catheterization studies which reveal no shunt at the pulmonary arterial level exclude this diagnosis.

Aortopulmonary Fenestration. The aortopulmonary window may also be excluded by the absence of a shunt at the pulmonary arterial level.

Common Truncus Arteriosus. The presence of equal oxygen saturations and pressures in the systemic and pulmonary arteries excludes an aneurysm of the sinus of Valsalva. In addition, the angiographic picture may be diagnostic.

Ventricular Septal Defect with Aortic Regurgitation, and Congenital Arteriovenous Fistula. Only first-rate angiograms, or even thoracotomy, permit differentiation between these conditions and congenital aneurysm of the sinus of Valsalva.

Treatment

Surgery, by means of cardiopulmonary bypass, is indicated some time after puberty to avoid complications. If rupture occurs, surgery is mandatory after brief, vigorous anticongestive measures have been carried out. The procedure involves closure of the aneurysm from the aortic side and obliteration of the fistula from the right side. We lost one patient after a rupture secondary to bacterial endocarditis, but operated successfully on a young man with a congenital, asymptomatic fistula opening into the right ventricle. In the American Heart Journal Evans and his associates[233] cited published reports of eleven surgical corrections to date. The need for prophylactic antibiotics to prevent bacterial endocarditis is particularly great in these patients.

Summary

Patients with a congenital aneurysm of the sinus of Valsalva are either completely asymptomatic or may appear to have a small patent ductus arteriosus. Severe complications, particularly rupture, usually occurring in young adults, may result in an alarming situation. Clinically, the loud diastolic murmur at an unusual location and, physiologically, the presence of a right atrial or right ventricular shunt suggest the diagnosis. Angiocardiograms are necessary to prove the diagnosis. Surgery is recommended.

CORONARY ARTERIOVENOUS FISTULA

Incidence

Coronary arteriovenous fistula is not a common anomaly. Gasul and his associates,[269] in their monograph in 1960, reported 52 cases, including 5 of their own. We have seen five patients with this condition at our institution.

Anatomy

Grant's[300] fundamental studies on the development of the coronary arteries furnish the embryologic explanation of this anomaly. In effect, one is dealing with a direct communication between a coronary artery and the pulmonary artery, or one of the cardiac chambers, without the interposition of a capillary system. The communication may consist of a single dilated coronary vessel or of numerous tortuous vermiform loops imbedded in the myocardium. The coronary ostium is large; the point of entrance into the cardiac chamber or the pulmonary artery is relatively small. Usually there are no associated anomalies. Either coronary artery may be involved, and the communication is most commonly with the right heart chambers or the pulmonary artery. Entrance into the chambers of the left side of the heart is rare, but one of our own most dramatic cases consisted of just such a communication between the left coronary artery and the left ventricle.

Physiology

Myocardial damage, secondary to the space-occupying properties of a tortuous aneurysm or to interference with effective coronary flow, is one possible physiologic consequence of the anomaly. The shunt itself may impose increased flow work on the right and, in rare instances, on the left side of the heart. In the majority of the cases reported, neither of these hazards seemed to be critical.

Clinical Picture

Most of the patients described in the literature, as well as those we have seen through the years, were asymptomatic. The discovery of a patent ductus type of murmur led to cardiac consultation. The pertinent finding on physical examination is the continuous murmur. The intensity and superficiality of this contrast markedly with the lack of symptoms and the absence of significant hemodynamic sequelae. This was certainly the case in four of our five patients and in most of the reported instances. In our fifth patient, with communication into the left ventricle, there were peripheral evidences of aortic regurgitation, such as wide pulse pressure, hyperdynamic left ventricle and cardiac enlargement.

Twenty-three patients studied by Gasul had continuous murmurs. He presented interesting thoughts on the nature of this murmur in relation to the point of entry of the fistula. He stated that if the point of entry is in either atrium, the systolic component is the dominant one, with midsystolic accentuation; if the fistula communicates with the left ventricle, the diastolic murmur is loud (Fig. 357), and with right ventricular entry the two phases of the murmur are of approximately equal intensity. A plausible explanation of these auscultatory phenomena may be found in the phasic pressure gradient between the aorta and the receiving chamber.

Roentgenologic examination may reveal a large ascending aorta and slight pulmonary vascular engorgement if the shunt flows into the right heart chambers. Right or left ventricular enlargement and atrial enlargement may be noted, depending on the anatomic situation. It is important

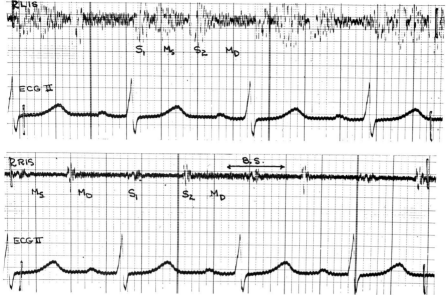

Figure 357. Short systolic and long, high-intensity diastolic murmur of patient with coronary arteriovenous fistula opening into the left ventricle. Note the loud murmurs at the second left interspace and faint ones at the second right interspace.

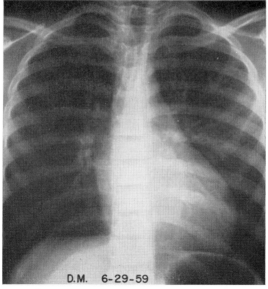

Figure 358. Posteroanterior roentgenogram of patient with coronary arteriovenous fistula opening into the right ventricle.

to stress again the innocuousness of the roentgenologic profile, in most instances, compared with the impressive murmur (Fig. 358). In one of our patients a localized bulge in the plane film at the left heart border proved to correspond to the aneurysm in the angiogram. The electrocardiogram usually reflects the degree of right or left ventricular involvement

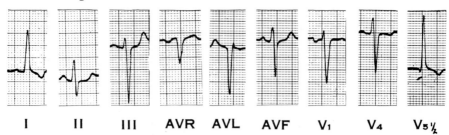

I   II   III   AVR   AVL   AVF   V₁   V₄   V₅½

Figure 359. Electrocardiogram of patient with coronary arteriovenous fistula opening into the right ventricle. Note the evidences of severe left ventricular hypertrophy and strain. These severe ischemic changes were present in a child with only moderate cardiac enlargement and with a relatively normal pulse pressure.

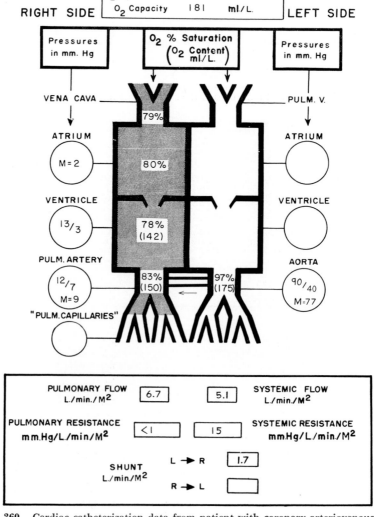

Figure 360. Cardiac catheterization data from patient with coronary arteriovenous fistula

in the process. As a rule, it is not grossly abnormal, though evidences of left or right ventricular hypertrophy may be present. In one of our patients evidences of left ventricular ischemia could be seen in the electrocardiogram (Fig. 359).

At *cardiac catheterization* (Fig. 360) evidence of a small left-to-right shunt (less than 2:1 in all but two of the cases reported) is noted if the entry is into the pulmonary artery or right heart chambers. With a left heart communication, catheterization of the right side of the heart is normal, but the peripheral arterial pulse pressure is wide. Cine-angiography, with injection into the ascending aorta, is the best diagnostic tool.

Course and Prognosis

Most patients with this anomaly live useful and active lives. Nine of thirteen patients studied by Taussig at postmortem examination had lived to be more than fifty-three years old. Gasul mentioned the dangers of bacterial endocarditis, pulmonary arterial hypertension, congestive failure and myocardial ischemia, but conceded that the lesion is compatible with longevity. The progressive cardiac enlargement in one of our patients bears evidence that not all these defects are innocuous (Figs. 361, 362).

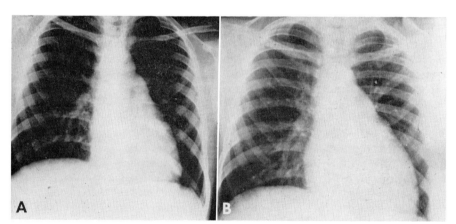

Figure 361. Progressive cardiac enlargement through a five-year period in patient with coronary arteriovenous fistula opening into the left ventricle.

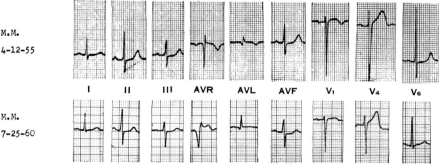

Figure 362. Progressive electrocardiographic changes in patient with coronary arteriovenous fistula opening into the left ventricle.

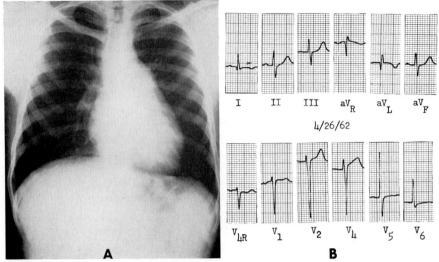

Figure 363. *A*, Posteroanterior roentgenogram after successful surgical repair of coronary arteriovenous fistula into the left ventricle. *B*, Postoperative electrocardiogram of the same patient.

Differential Diagnosis

Most of the entities to be considered have been discussed in detail: patent ductus arteriosus (p. 474), aortopulmonary fenestration (p. 498), truncus arteriosus (p. 510), aneurysm of the sinus of Valsalva (p. 515) and ventricular septal defect with aortic regurgitation (p. 434).

Treatment

Gasul recommended surgery, without necessary recourse to the pump oxygenator, as the choice of treatment. This approach was used successfully in four of his five patients. We have treated two patients successfully at surgery, one with and another without the pump oxygenator (Fig. 363). Operation consists in first obliterating the entry of the vessel into the heart and then ligating the coronary artery proximal to the fistula. I am not sure that all patients may be treated without using cardiopulmonary bypass, and I am also not quite certain of the innocuousness of the procedure. The tendency to longevity of these patients must be counterbalanced with the ease of the operation. I have no doubt in my mind that if evidences of cardiac enlargement, electrocardiographic changes and large shunts are present, surgery is indicated. I am not absolutely sure, however, that I would recommend surgery for a patient whose only sign and symptom is the presence of a murmur.

Summary

Patients with a loud, superficial continuous murmur who have no evidences of cardiac embarrassment may have a coronary arteriovenous fistula. Angiocardiography is the best diagnostic tool, and surgery is recommended in selected cases.

16

VALVULAR AND VASCULAR LESIONS WITH A RIGHT-TO-LEFT SHUNT OR NO SHUNT AT ALL

COARCTATION OF THE AORTA

Incidence

Coarctation of the aorta is a common congential anomaly. IIt is the third most common lesion in Abbott's[1] series, seventh in our own, sixth in Wood's[748] and seventh in Keith's[380] group. The sex ratio is approximately 2:1, males predominating. On the whole, this anomaly probably represents less than 10 per cent of all congenital cardiac abnormalities.

Anatomy

Coarctation is a narrowing of the lumen of the aorta, usually occurring in the area of the insertion of the ligamentum arteriosum. Depending on its relation to the ductus arteriosus, coarctation of the aorta is sometimes divided into long "preductal" (between the left subclavian and the ductus) and localized "postductal" (at or beyond the insertion) types. Rare instances of coarctation higher in the aortic arch (even proximal to the innominate artery)[467] or far along the descending aorta have also been described.[48]

The etiology of coarctation of the aorta was thought to depend on the closure of the ductus arteriosus and the constriction resulting therefrom.[682] Recent evidence points away from this explanation, however. Edwards[219] stated that the lesion is due to an intrinsic defect in the structure of the medial layer of the aortic wall consisting of a peculiar thickening of the media, projecting into the lumen of the vessel and rendering it narrow (less than 8 mm.) and eccentric.[219] It is my distinct impression that coarctation of the aorta is not of equal severity at birth in all patients, and that, in fact, in many instances it may be a gradually progressive lesion. Possibly the superimposition of intimal thickening, noted in adults, may be the anatomic basis of this progression. A biophysical explanation of this has been suggested by Rodbard.[588] Whether the collaterals necessary for maintenance of an adequate postnatal circulation are developed during intrauterine life or not is a matter of lively controversy; the available evidence favors the presence of these structures in the fetus. The collateral channels bring blood to the lower half of the body by bypassing the aortic block. In essence, both subclavian arteries are the principal sources of the collaterals. The right subclavian communicates to the intercostals via the vertebral arteries and the spinal artery on one hand and through the cervical and scapular branches on the other. The left subclavian artery, if proximal to the coarctation, feeds blood to the lower half of the body through the internal mammaries and the intercostals.

Associated vascular anomalies include atresia or stenosis of one or the other subclavian artery, anomalous origin of the right subclavian artery, bicuspid aortic valve, in rare instances a double aortic arch, and, of course, patent ductus arteriosus. Among the intracardiac abnormalities associated with coarctation of the aorta, ventricular septal defect and mitral regurgitation should be mentioned prominently.

Physiology

The principal physiologic problem in coarctation of the aorta is the maintenance of adequate blood flow and pressure in the lower half of the body in the face of severe narrowing of the lumen of the aorta. Apparently this is achieved by means of three adaptive mechanisms. One is the elevation of the systolic pressure in the proximal aortic segment. The second is vasoconstriction in the arterioles to maintain a high diastolic pressure. The third is the bypassing of the aortic block by means of collaterals or a ductus arteriosus opening distal to the coarctation. By utilizing one or more of these three mechanisms, the mean pressure in the lower extremities is maintained at a level of about 60 mm. of mercury, the minimal pressure needed for adequate kidney function. The pressure pulses in the arms reveal elevated systolic, diastolic and mean pressures, with a widened pulse pressure, whereas the tracings for the leg look damped with low systolic and elevated diastolic pressures (Fig. 364). If the block

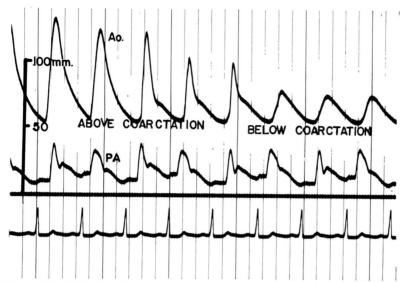

Figure 364. Withdrawal tracing through coarcted segment of the aorta. Note the rapid upstroke and high presssure above the coarctation and the damped tracing below the aortic obstruction. Note also the slight pulmonary arterial hypertension.

is complete and if the compensatory mechanisms are not sufficient, survival is not possible.

The role of renal factors in the production of the hypertension associated with coarctation of the aorta is questionable. My impression, based on the relatively prompt return of the blood pressure in the arms in most children, postoperatively, and supported by recent experimental evidence,[390, 725] is that renal influences in this respect are minimal, at least in the young.

The effect of exercise on the blood pressure and cardiac output of these patients should be mentioned briefly. Taylor and his associates[686] found that a resting high cardiac output, elevated systolic pressure in the arms and slightly raised pulmonary capillary mean pressure all increase significantly with exercise in patients with coarctation of the aorta.

A classification of coarctation of the aorta into "adult" and "infantile" types, based on the location and length of the coarcted segment, is meaningless in view of present-day physiologic and therapeutic concepts. The so-called adult type (a localized constriction just opposite the insertion of the ductus arteriosus) may be associated occasionally with a patent ductus supplying the lower half of the body with blood and may cause death in congestive failure in infancy. On the other hand, the so-called infantile type (a long narrow segment between the left subclavian and the ligamentum arteriosum) may be associated with relative longevity in some cases. Also, from the clinical viewpoint, the adult type may give rise to severe though reversible congestive failure in infants, whereas the infantile type can be completely asymptomatic for several decades. The terms "preductal" and "postductal" are anatomic counterparts of the historic "infantile" and "adult" types, and although they are of importance to the pathologist and the surgeon, they are of less significance to the physiologist and the clinician.

A physiologically, as well as clinically, more meaningful classification, to be followed in this text, divides coarctations of the aorta into those in which the left ventricle (directly or by means of collaterals) supplies the entire systemic circuit with blood (coarctation of the aorta with systemic left ventricle) and those in which the left ventricle supplies only the upper half of the body, while the parts below the coarctation are supplied with blood from the right ventricle through a ductus arteriosus (coarctation of the aorta with systemic left and right ventricles).

It should be understood that most, but surely not all, of the coarctations with systemic left ventricle represent "postductal," short segments. Similarly most, but not all, of the coarctations with systemic left and right ventricles are anatomically "preductal" and long. The ductus arteriosus in the latter group is always open and, by definition, carries blood from the pulmonary artery into the descending aorta. In the former group the ductus may or may not be patent; if open, it carries blood from the aorta to the pulmonary artery. It is important to emphasize that in some patients the ductus overrides the coarcted segment, allowing a bidirectional flow through the ductus; in still others, although the ductus opens below the coarctation, the flow of blood is still from the aorta to the pulmonary artery, and thus they correspond to the systemic left ventricle type.

COARCTATION OF THE AORTA WITH SYSTEMIC LEFT VENTRICLE

Simple Coarctation

Clinical Picture

Most children with coarctation of the aorta are asymptomatic; the condition is usually first recognized by the school physician or the pediatrician, when a routine examination reveals a murmur or the presence of arterial hypertension. Once in a while close questioning of the parents elicits complaints, consisting of pains in the calves on running, occasional fatigue, headaches and nosebleeds. It is interesting that asymptomatic coarctation of the aorta is rarely discovered in infants; it is usually diagnosed between the ages of four and five years, or even later.

At physical examination[576] these children (generally boys) are usually well developed and well nourished; some of them are quite athletic. Occasionally one is impressed by the broad shoulders and well developed arms, in contrast to the relatively narrow hips and thin legs. Cyanosis and clubbing are never present, and there are no evidences of congestive failure. Frequently a thrill is palpable at the suprasternal notch, where the carotid pulsations are unusually powerful. Mild left chest deformity may be present; the impulse is heaving and is maximal at the cardiac apex. In older children the dilated and tortuous intercostal arteries may be palpable over the back when the patient leans forward.[133] The radial arteries are powerful, especially on the right. The femoral pulses are either absent or weaker and later than the radial pulses. Blood pressure determinations (with proper-sized cuffs) show the systolic pressure of the arms to be higher than that of the legs, whereas the diastolic pressures are equal. This relative hypertension of the arms is the pathognomonic feature of coarctation of the aorta; the systolic pressure in the arms does not have to be significantly higher than the average in an absolute sense. The systolic pressure of one arm (usually the right) may be 20 to 30 mm. higher than that of the other arm without necessarily implying that an added anomaly of one of the subclavian arteries is present. In instances in which the difference in pressure between the 2 arms is more than 30 mm. of mercury, some added abnormality, such as stenosis, atresia or anomalous origin of one of the subclavians, must be assumed. The pulsations of the abdominal aorta are often absent. The feet may feel cooler to touch than the hands.

At auscultation the heart sounds are usually normal in intensity and splitting, although the second sound is often louder at the aortic area than at the second left interspace. A constant, apical ejection click is frequently observed. Systolic murmurs are noted in approximately 90 per cent of the patients. The pathognomonic murmur is the rough, stenotic systolic murmur over the back originating from the coarcted segment itself. Spencer and his co-workers[660] indicated that if the aortic block is severe (a lumen of less than 2.5 mm.), the murmur at the site of the coarctation becomes continuous. Of course if the block is complete, no murmur originates from this site. Systolic ejection murmurs, or continuous murmurs, may also be noted over the collaterals in the back; indeed, these may be obliterated easily by the pressure of the stethoscope on the intercostal arteries. A stenotic systolic murmur of aortic stenosis is present in 15 to 20 per cent of the patients, and a blowing murmur at the apex or lower left sternal border, suggesting mitral regurgitation, is heard with about equal frequency (Fig. 365).

In addition to the continuous murmur mentioned, protodiastolic murmurs, characteristic of aortic regurgitation, may be heard fairly frequently (in 15 per cent of the patients) and, like the murmur of aortic stenosis, are often attributed to the presence of a bicuspid aortic valve. Finally, apical mid-diastolic rumbles are heard in 10 per cent of the patients; the explanation of this may lie in the dilated left ventricle or in the encroachment of the hypertrophied septum on the mitral orifice.

The roentgenologic picture may be entirely normal in a few cases. In most instances, however, left ventricular enlargement is easily recognized (Fig. 366). Left atrial prominence is present in severe cases. The main pulmonary artery and pulmonary vasculature are normal in size and activity. The aorta is often hypoplastic, and the impression of the descending arch on the barium-filled esophagus often can be recognized by its E shape (Fig. 367). The first arc of the E is the impression of that part of the aorta which precedes the coarctation, the middle segment is the coarctation itself, and the second arc is caused by the poststenotic dilatation. In an overpenetrated film the aorta itself may be seen assuming a big three shape, consisting of the same components as the E, only in the reverse. "Scalloping" of the ribs, due to erosion of the inferior and ventral aspects of the main body of the ribs by the collaterals, is rarely seen in patients younger than eight years of age (Fig. 32, p. 42), but has been encountered in an infant as young as eight months. At fluoroscopy the powerfully contracting left ventricle may be noted.

The electrocardiographic pattern may vary from a normal tracing to one showing left ventricular hypertrophy, depending on the severity of the coarctation (Fig. 368). Evidences of severe left ventricular strain are rare in children with simple coarctation of the aorta; its presence, particularly if associated with a stenotic murmur at the second right interspace,

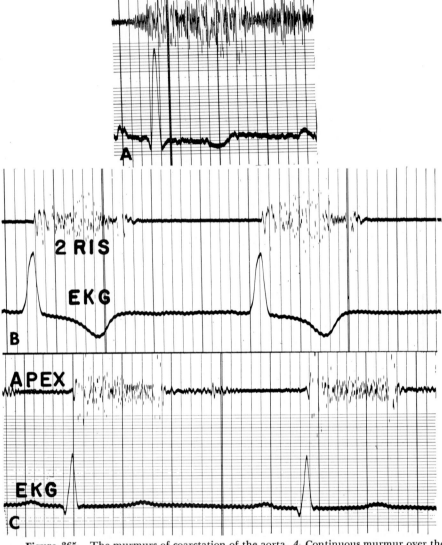

Figure 365. The murmurs of coarctation of the aorta. *A*, Continuous murmur over the back. *B*, Stenotic murmur at the second right interspace, with an early apex resulting from the aortic valve gradient associated with coarctation of the aorta. *C*, Apical systolic murmur and mid-diastolic rumble, characteristic of mitral regurgitation, associated with coarctation of the aorta.

should raise the suspicion of additional aortic stenosis. In our experience, pure right ventricular hypertrophy is never present in patients with uncomplicated coarctation of the aorta after the age of six months, but occasionally a child with otherwise typical simple coarctation of the aorta will have a terminal R′ in the right chest lead, or a mean electrical axis as far to the right as +120 degrees.

Cardiac catheterization (Fig. 369) is seldom performed now in patients with simple coarctation. The meager data available offer the following

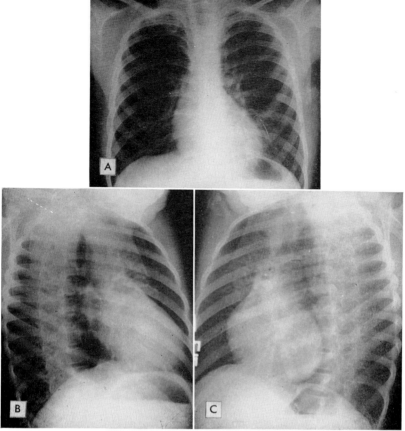

Figure 366. Posteroanterior and oblique roentgenograms of patient with moderately severe coarctation of the aorta. Note the small aortic knob and evidences of left ventricular enlargement.

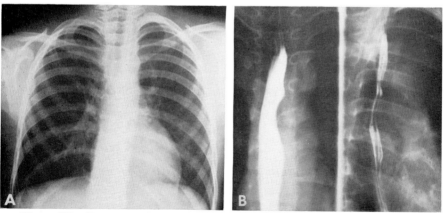

Figure 367. Posteroanterior and right anterior oblique roentgenograms of patient with coarctation of the aorta showing the impression of the coarcted segment on the barium-filled esophagus (E sign).

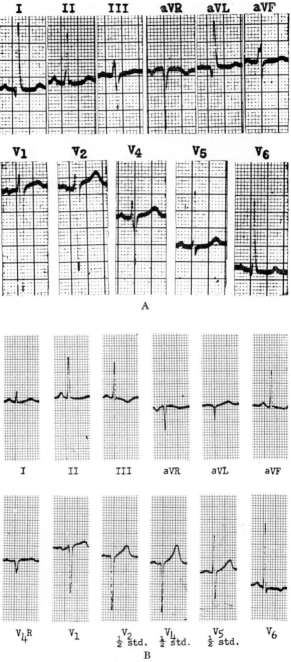

Figure 368. *A*, Electrocardiogram in mild coarctation of the aorta. Note the tall voltages representing left chest leads with good Q waves and deep S waves in aV_R and V_1 and V_2. *B*, Severe coarctation of the aorta with tall left ventricular voltages and inverted T waves in aV_F and V_6. This type of tracing is seldom seen in children with pure coarctation of the aorta, although it may be seen in adults. If it is encountered in a child with coarctation, the presence of a strain pattern should suggest associated aortic stenosis.

information:[58, 668] (1) There is no evidence of a shunt in either direction. The systemic arterial saturation is normal. (2) There may be mild elevation of pulmonary arterial and pulmonary capillary pressure which is increased on effort. Systemic arterial pressure is elevated in the arms, often with widening of the pulse pressure. The femoral arterial pressure pulses are low and damped. If there is any suspicion of aortic stenosis, the pressure gradient across the aortic valve should be determined. (3) Systemic resistance is high, and pulmonary resistance may be slightly elevated. (4) Systemic and pulmonary flows are equal and often large. (5) In mild to moderate coarctations the catheter may be passed, in a retrograde fashion, from the femoral artery across the narrowed segment. (6) Retrograde aortography is the ideal method for outlining the site and the length of the coarcted

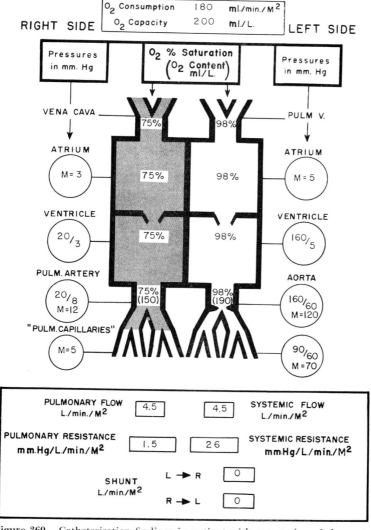

Figure 369.   Catheterization findings in patient with coarctation of the aorta.

segment; however, its use is recommended only in unusual cases. (7) Dye-dilution curves are not used routinely in these studies.

Course and Prognosis

The natural history of patients with simple coarctation of the aorta is rather uneventful, at least through childhood. If the dangers of bacterial endocarditis can be avoided by the judicious use of chemotherapy and chemoprophylaxis, these patients seldom have any serious difficulty during the first two decades. The only complications I have seen in this age group related to hypertensive encephalopathy or cerebrovascular accidents. These are obviously severe, even fatal complications, but certainly they occur in less than 5 per cent of the cases.

According to the data collected by Reifenstein and his co-workers[576] at postmortem examinations, only a quarter of these patients can be expected to live through the fourth decade, unless an operation is performed. The others die considerably earlier, as a result of bacterial endocarditis, ruptured aorta or hypertensive cardiovascular disease. Campbell and Baylis[129] indicated that most patients get along well for the first two decades, although systolic and diastolic hypertension increases through puberty. Five of thirty-seven patients followed up by him through their third decade, and two of the seventeen in their fourth decade died rather suddenly. The fact that there were only two patients in their fifth and sixth decades may be of considerable significance. *The statistical significance of these studies as related to the life expectancy of any single patient with coarctation of the aorta is questionable.*

Differential Diagnosis

The differential diagnosis of simple coarctation of the aorta should present no problem to the physician who, as part of his routine physical examination, palpates the femoral pulses and tries to compare the pressures in the arms and legs in patients with weak or late femoral pulses.

Treatment

The treatment of coarctation of the aorta is surgical. There are cogent reasons to suggest that all patients with coarctation of the aorta should be operated on to assure normal life expectancy and to eliminate the threat of bacterial endocarditis.[307]

Since the initial work by Crafoord and Gross hundreds of patients with coarctation of the aorta have been treated surgically.[172, 307] The optimal age of operation is between 7 and 20 years; the operative risk in asymptomatic patients of this age group is less than 5 per cent.[619] Operation can be performed in patients of practically all ages, although the mortality rate may be higher. Indications for early operation are (1) persistent hypertension of more than 180 mm. of mercury, (2) severe symptoms of fatigue, headache, chest pain and leg aches, (3) evidence of significant associated mitral regurgitation or of a sizable left-to-right shunt through a ventricular septal defect, and (4) persistent, significant cardiomegaly.

The operation consists in division of the ligamentum arteriosum and wide excision of the coarcted segment. Preferably, the two aortic segments are then sutured directly together. If the gap left by the excision is too large, if the upper aortic segment is of inadequate caliber, if an aneurysm is present, or if there are other technical reasons, an aortic graft may be inserted with success.[307]

In 60 per cent of the patients the blood pressure falls to normal levels (less than 130 mm. of mercury, systolic) after this procedure, and in only 2 per cent of the patients is it higher than 150 mm.; the femoral pulses can be easily palpated. It is interesting to note that the systemic systolic pressure drops significantly within the first postoperative day, but seldom returns to normal levels for two to three weeks after operation.

As a rule, at The Children's Hospital Medical Center in Boston, cardiac catheterization or aortography is not performed before operation in cases of simple coarctation of the aorta. The clinical profile is usually outlined clearly enough to make these procedures unnecessary in the ordinary case. The use of aortic grafts and the availability of a vessel bank make the accurate preoperative outline of the obstruction less important to the surgeon than it was formerly.

Of course, if the clinical picture is not a typical one, all available means of investigation should be pursued before proceeding with an operation. One should mention specifically, as an indication for preoperative study, the suspicion of an abdominal coarctation of the aorta. The possibility of this rare anomaly should come to mind if, in a patient with known coarctation, the abdominal aorta is easily palpable. Further evidence may be furnished by the paucity of the collaterals in the thoracic cage and the presence of the loud murmur of collaterals over the abdomen and the posterior lumbar region. Finally, the roentgenologic examination fails to show the characteristic **E** or 3 signs, and rib notchings are few and are restricted to the lower part of the thoracic cage.

Among the rare postoperative complications should be mentioned hemorrhage, damage to the central nervous system (cord or brain), renal damage, pulmonary emboli, mesenteric arteritis (with ileus), recurrent nerve injury and congestive heart failure.[619]

Indeed, postoperative hemorrhage may be severe enough to cause death if the aorta in an older person has atheromatous changes or if the bleeding leads to a false aneurysm and continues for days or even a week. If there is any suspicion of hemorrhage, exploration is mandatory.

Most of the patients with postoperative damage to the spinal cord have residuals ranging from mild paresis to paraplegia. Probably the youngest and oldest patients will be subject to this complication; therefore, for these patients, mild hypothermia is used on our surgical service. Although the patients with the longest period of aortic occlusion and the widest interruption of the collateral circulation are the ones in whom damage to the spinal cord is most likely to occur, individual susceptibility, partly due to age, plays a significant role.

Brain injuries frequently lead to death in the young. Sometimes the etiology may be found in the sudden increase in systolic pressure when the clamps are applied to the aorta. In other instances no good reason for the development of brain damage is apparent.

Mesenteric arteritis, manifesting itself by severe abdominal pain and ileus about one week postoperatively, should be treated conservatively for a few days. If no improvement occurs, exploration should be carried out; in one of our patients resection of a gangrenous segment of the bowel was necessary.[619]

Summary

Patients with a systolic pressure significantly higher over the arms than over the legs have coarctation of the aorta. There is no evidence of a shunt in either direction. Both the electrocardiogram and the roentgenogram show evidences of left ventricular hypertrophy. Elective surgery is recommended for patients between seven and twenty years of age. Operative relief of the coarctation at much younger or older ages is possible at higher risks, if indicated.

Coarctation of the Aorta with Congestive Failure in Infancy

Whereas the vast majority of patients with uncomplicated coarctation of the aorta associated with systemic left ventricle are asymptomatic throughout childhood, in a minority of these infants (certainly less than 10 per cent) severe congestive failure develops. Why these infants behave so differently from others with similar anomalies is not known with certainty. Hypotheses, based on the site of the ductal opening in the fetus and on the consequent differences in the development of collaterals, have been proposed repeatedly[30, 760] to explain the difference between the clinical course of the two groups. For reasons given elsewhere,[408] I am unable to accept these hypotheses as the sole or even dominant ones; rather, I believe that the infants in whom congestive failure develops have the severest degree of coarctation at birth, whereas, in the others, it develops progressively through the years.

Clinical Picture

The description that follows is based principally on 9 patients we observed before 1956 at The Children's Hospital Medical Center in Boston.[408] Patients seen since this time have confirmed this pattern in a consistent fashion. In these infants, symptoms usually begin within the first three months, often the first few weeks of life. Their weight gain is poor, they are irritable, and they have feeding problems, dyspnea, excessive perspiration and even occasional cyanosis.

At physical examination they look sick and have tachypnea, tachycardia and perioral cyanosis. As a rule, the liver is enlarged, and moist rales may be heard over the lungs. Peripheral edema is rare. On auscultation a gallop rhythm is frequently noted, and a systolic murmur is heard at the left sternal border in almost all instances. The femoral pulses are weak and late in comparison with the right radial pulse, or may be completely absent. "Flush" pressure over the arms is at least 20 mm. of mercury higher than over the legs; the flush pressure over the legs, however, is rarely less than 50 mm. of mercury.

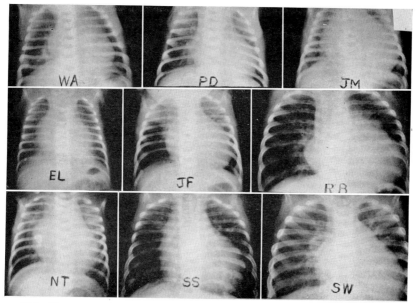

Figure 370. Posteroanterior roentgenograms of nine patients who went into congestive failure in infancy with coarctation of the aorta.[408]

The roentgenologic picture is dominated by the features of congestive failure. Cardiomegaly is maximal (Fig. 370), the heart is globular in shape, the beat is poor, and there is passive congestion of the lungs.

Electrocardiograms are always abnormal; an abnormal degree of either right or left ventricular hypertrophy, with or without changes in the T wave, is present.

In the patients studied at cardiac catheterization (Fig. 371), the only unusual finding was the increase in pulmonary arterial and pulmonary capillary pressures. The latter may approximate pulmonary edema levels, even at rest (20 to 30 mm. of mercury), and the former may be near systemic levels. Arterial unsaturation, probably due to pulmonary venous unsaturation secondary to congestive heart failure, may contribute to the elevation of the pulmonary arterial pressure. We have seen two infants with presumptive evidence of congestive heart failure in whom the pulmonary arterial pressure was near normal at rest, but increased precipitously on crying.

Course and Prognosis

If treated properly, the congestive failure in these desperately sick infants may disappear within a few days or weeks. A satisfactory weight gain is not observed for many weeks or even months, however. Eventually the infants start behaving normally and show no evidences of heart disease except the persistence of the murmur and the relative hypertension of the arms. The heart size diminishes slowly, but as the chest diameter grows, it does assume normal size within a few years (Fig. 372). The electrocardiographic changes are striking; eventually all patients have left ventricular hypertrophy regardless of whether they exhibited left, right or combined

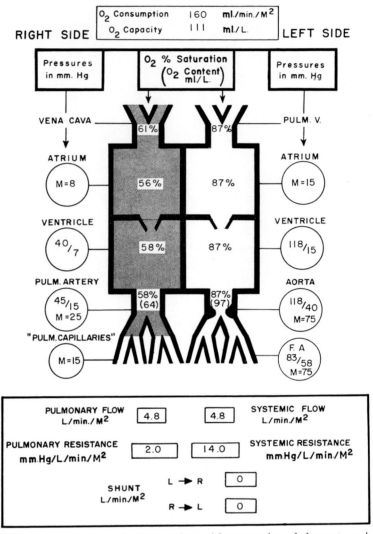

Figure 371. Catheterization findings in patient with coarctation of the aorta and congestive heart failure.

ventricular hypertrophy in early infancy (less than six months of age) (Fig. 373). On the basis of our present experience, we, at The Children's Hospital Medical Center, believe that if the pattern of left ventricular hypertrophy is not present by six months of age, the patient probably does not have an uncomplicated coarctation of the aorta. Repeat catheterization reveals a return of the pulmonary capillary and pulmonary arterial pressures toward normal.

Differential Diagnosis

As mentioned before, the differential diagnosis should not present any particular problem if one remembers to feel for the femoral pulses

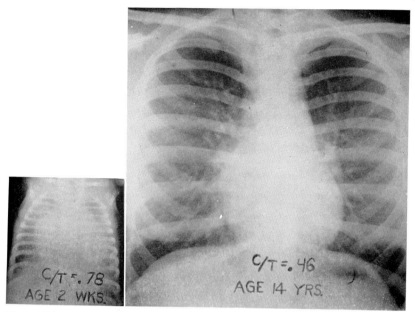

Figure 372. Posteroanterior roentgenograms taken 14 years apart. The small film on the left shows maximal cardiac enlargement at two weeks of age. The large picture on the right shows only slight cardiac enlargement at age of 14 years just before operation for coarctation of the aorta.[408]

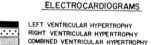

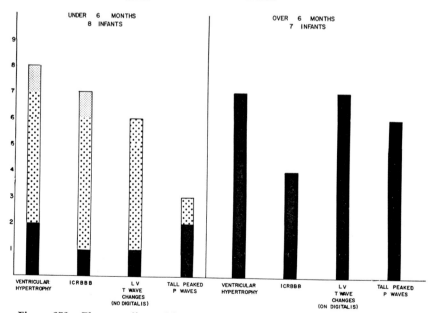

Figure 373. Electrocardiographic patterns in infants with coarctation of the aorta and congestive failure. A comparison of tracings in those less than six months and more than six months of age.[408]

of every patient and to measure both arm and leg pressures in all patients with weak or late femoral pulses.

The condition most commonly considered in the differential diagnosis of these youngsters is primary myocardial disease (see p. 257). Patients in both groups have in common severe cardiac enlargement without characteristic murmur, congestive failure in early infancy, and electrocardiographic evidences of left ventricular hypertrophy. Once congestive failure has been controlled, careful blood pressure measurements make the differential diagnosis easy. In patients with poor circulation, however, we have repeatedly been unable to obtain accurate readings.

Other lesions to be considered in the differential diagnosis are the entities grouped under the heading of the *hypoplastic left heart syndrome*.[536] in which coarctation of the aorta may be only one part of a most complex set of anomalies, including severe obstruction of the mitral and aortic valves. The maximal cardiac enlargement within the first few days of life, the severe and exclusive right ventricular hypertrophy, and the poor response to anticongestive measures, all direct attention to the hypoplastic left heart syndrome.

Finally, coarctation of the aorta accompanied by a *ventricular septal defect* or a *patent ductus arteriosus* may also have to be differentiated from the coarctation in infants with congestive failure. The hyperdynamic cardiac impulse, the mid-diastolic rumble and the active pulmonary vascular engorgement may become manifest only after adequate anticongestive measures have been undertaken. As a matter of fact, Keith and his associates[280] included patients with the hypoplastic left heart syndrome as well as those with a ventricular septal defect or patent ductus arteriosus in their discussion on coarctation of the aorta in infants. This grouping makes a valid comparison of his results with ours and those of Engle's difficult.[256]

Treatment

The treatment of infants with simple coarctation of the aorta and congestive failure should be attempted first by medical means. Vigorous treatment with digitalis, oxygen, morphine, antibiotics and diuretics has resulted in disappearance of symptoms in all our patients thus treated.[408] The changes in the radiologic and electrocardiographic pictures have already been discussed. By the use of this approach we are enabling these children to benefit from surgery at an optimal age, with minimal risk, instead of subjecting them to operation during infancy, when there is a mortality rate of 25 to 40 per cent, without a guarantee of satisfactory and permanent relief of the hypertension. Digitalization should be continued as long as necessary, usually for at least six months.

A similar therapeutic regimen has been used by Engle and her co-workers[256] with similar success. They reported that only eight of thirty infants with coarctation of the aorta and congestive heart failure proved to have uncomplicated lesions, and all these survived with only medical treatment. On the other hand, all who died in Engle's series, and half of those who survived, had complicated intracardiac defects in addition to the coarctation. Our experiences in the pathology laboratory support this thesis; not a single infant with uncomplicated coarctation of the aorta has been seen at postmortem examination within the past twelve years in our institution.

Keith and his associates[280] reported 108 cases, including all their infants with coarctation and congestive failure; they concluded that unless medical treatment of cardiac failure is eminently successful within 12 hours after admission to the hospital, surgery is indicated.[517] An operative mortality rate of 41 per cent was given for infants in the first month of life, and 29 per cent for those between one month and one year. In contrast, mortality under medical treatment in their series was 87 per cent for the first month and 50 per cent for the first year. Within the last year Keith[376] has recommended that in these critical situations only division of the ductus should be carried out, and that surgery for the coarctation should be postponed until later.

It may not be as difficult to reconcile the two viewpoints as it seems at first glance. To begin with the last point, there is no disagreement that patients with cardiac failure caused by a patent ductus arteriosus (with or without coarctation) should be treated surgically, promptly. But this is a ductus problem and not a coarctation problem.

Secondly, everybody agrees that when these patients are first seen, they should be given vigorous anticongestive measures. Thirdly, there is unanimity that if medical treatment is not effective, surgery ought to be attempted.

The disagreement, then, is limited to the period of time allotted to medical management. The Toronto group considers the first twelve hours after admission to be critical. We believe that five to seven days after the introduction of anticongestive measures may be nearer our own end-point. We also believe that if competent medical management is not effective, the chance of finding a surgically remediable lesion are slim indeed. Nevertheless we think it may be worth a trial.

Summary

In infants with the severest degrees of aortic block, congestive failure may develop. The diagnosis is based on the presence of relative hypertension of the arms. The electrocardiograms and roentgenograms are always grossly abnormal. Anticongestive measures are usually successful in tiding these patients over until operation can be easily performed at an appropriate age.

Coarctation of the Aorta with Left-to-Right Shunt

Whereas most patients with coarctation of the aorta have no communication between the systemic and pulmonary circuits, and the systolic overload is carried entirely by the left ventricle, a number of patients have been encountered in our clinic in whom coarctation of the aorta was accompanied by definite pulmonary plethora and right ventricular hypertrophy. The anatomic situation usually reveals a ventricular defect or a patent ductus arteriosus opening above, at or even below the site of the aortic block.

Clinical Picture

Symptoms of exertional dyspnea, fatigue, repeated severe respiratory infections and failure to thrive manifest themselves early in these patients. In terms of severity of symptoms, these children rank between the patients with simple coarctation and the infants who have congestive failure. On the whole, the presenting complaints are more characteristic of patients who have large left-to-right shunts than of those with coarctation of the aorta.

At physical examination the patients are usually poorly developed. Cyanosis and clubbing are absent, but the fingers and toes are commonly fiery red. Left chest deformity with a hyperdynamic combined ventricular impulse is the rule; a thrill is frequently present at the left sternal border. Evidences of mild left-sided or right-sided congestive failure may be noted. Relative hypertension of the arms is present.

The observations at auscultation vary, depending on the site of the communication between the systemic and pulmonary circulations. If the communication is through a large patent ductus arteriosus (which, incidentally, is the most frequent site) and the pulmonary vascular resistance

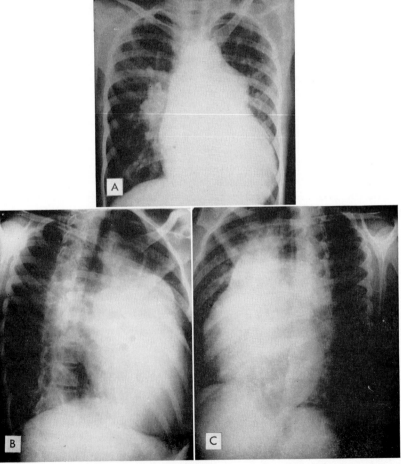

Figure 374.   Posteroanterior and oblique roentgenograms of patient with coarctation of the aorta, patent ductus arteriosus and a left-to-right shunt.

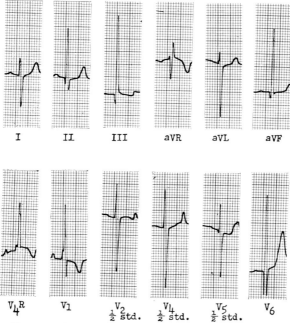

I   II   III   aVR   aVL   aVF

V_4R V_1 $\frac{1}{2}$std.V_2 $\frac{1}{2}$std.V_4 $\frac{1}{2}$std.V_5 V_6

Figure 375.   Electrocardiogram of patient with coarctation of the aorta, patent ductus arteriosus and a left-to-right shunt. Note right axis deviation and combined ventricular hypertrophy.

is relatively low, a typical machinery murmur may be heard. If the ductus is small or the pulmonary vascular resistance is near the systemic level, only a second left interspace systolic murmur is noted. If a ventricular defect forms the communication between the left and right sides, the murmur typical of ventricular defect may be heard if the shunt is sizable. If the opening is small, little if any murmur can be observed. The second sound at the pulmonary area is always booming, but may be narrowly split; a mid-diastolic rumble is present if the shunt is large.

The roentgenologic picture is characteristic of the large left-to-right shunt group (Fig. 374). A significant degree of cardiac enlargement, involving both ventricles and often the left atrium, is present. Pulmonary plethora with expansile pulsations is uniformly noted. The main pulmonary artery is usually large and active; the aorta varies considerably in size and activity.

Electrocardiographically, combined ventricular hypertrophy is noted without selective atrial hypertrophy. Intraventricular conduction disturbance is common (Fig. 375).

Cardiac catheterization (Fig. 376) reveals evidences of a left-to-right shunt at the appropriate level and pulmonary arterial and left atrial hypertension. Arterial unsaturation may be secondary to congestive heart failure. The catheter frequently enters the ductus arteriosus.

Course and Prognosis

The natural history of these patients is similar to that of others who have pulmonary hypertension associated with a communication between

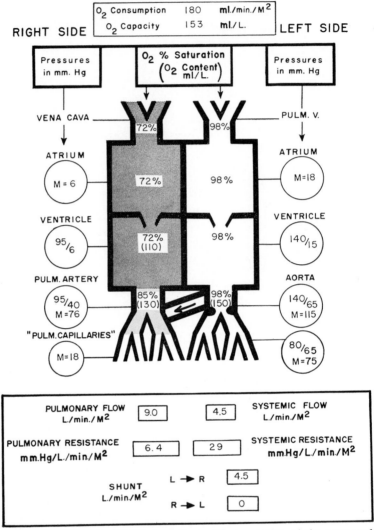

Figure 376. Catheterization findings in patient with coarctation of the aorta and patent ductus arteriosus.

the two circuits. The symptoms may be rather serious during infancy and early childhood. Improvement, perhaps secondary to the development of medial and intimal changes in the pulmonary arterioles, occurs by about four to five years of age and lasts through the first two decades of life. In early adulthood severe dyspnea on exertion develops; this is followed by cyanosis, congestive failure and death.

Differential Diagnosis

The differential diagnosis of this syndrome is particularly important in respect to coarctation of the aorta with a systemic right and left ventricle, i.e. a ductus carrying *pulmonary arterial blood* into the *distal* part of the *aorta*. The similarities between the two groups are striking. Patients in both groups have the typical blood pressure findings of coarctation of the aorta associated with some evidence of right ventricular hypertrophy, as shown on the roentgenogram and the electrocardiogram, in addition to pulmonary plethora. Identification of the patients with systemic right and left ventricle is often possible by (1) definite evidence of cyanosis, particularly over the left arm and the lower half of the body; (2) severe or exclusive right ventricular hypertrophy, according to the electrocardiogram; and (3) absence of a significant or typical murmur. At cardiac catheterization no evidence of a left-to-right shunt is found, and the pulmonary arterial pressure is higher than or identical with the pressure in the femoral artery. The catheter often enters the descending aorta.

Treatment

Medical management of infections and congestive failure, preoperatively and postoperatively, obviously is indicated. Surgical removal of the aortic block should be undertaken only if the parents are willing to assume the considerable risk inherent in the procedure. At the time of operation the ductus arteriosus should be divided. The purpose of surgical intervention, over and above the usual ones listed in the section on simple coarctation of the aorta, is to decrease the size of the left-to-right shunt by lowering systemic arterial pressure and to forestall progression of the pulmonary vascular disease. In my experience the more severe the pulmonary vascular obstruction, the more hazardous is the operation. If the pulmonary vascular resistance has reached a level at which the shunt is exclusively or predominantly from right to left, then the operative risk becomes prohibitive; as long as, at least part of the time, the shunt is from left to right, operation should probably be attempted. In some of our patients with ventricular septal defect or patent ductus arteriosus and coarctation of the aorta, spectacular improvement occurred after relief of the aortic obstruction. Simultaneous closure of the ventricular septal defect is not possible for technical reasons. If the two conditions coexist, it has been our practice to relieve the coarctation first.

Summary

The presence of right ventricular hypertrophy and pulmonary plethora in patients with coarctation of the aorta suggests pulmonary arterial hypertension and a communication between the systemic and pulmonary circuits. The most common site of such a communication is a patent ductus arteriosus, although ventricular defects are also seen. Surgery is indicated, as long as the shunt is predominantly left to right, although the mortality rate is relatively high.

COARCTATION OF THE AORTA AND AORTIC STENOSIS

See Aortic Stenosis (p. 564).

COARCTATION OF THE AORTA WITH SYSTEMIC RIGHT AND LEFT VENTRICLES

Incidence

This type of congenital heart disease is relatively rare in patients beyond the neonatal period. It is a common cause of death in early infancy, however.[538]

Anatomy

The principal circulatory abnormality in these patients is the presence of a large patent ductus arteriosus opening *below a coarctation* and *supplying the descending aorta with pulmonary arterial blood* (preductal coarctation). The coarcted segment may be short or may extend for several centimeters along the aortic arch, but is usually proximal to the origin of the left subclavian artery. More often than not this is a complex anomaly; it may be associated with congenital aortic or mitral valvular disease within the framework of the hypoplastic left heart syndrome, but it also may occur in conjunction with ventricular septal defects and with complete transposition of the great arteries. I believe that this is the anomaly formerly referred to rather loosely as "infantile" coarctation of the aorta.

Physiology

The physiologic effects of the malformation depend to a great extent on whether it is associated with other major cardiac anomalies. If the hypoplastic left heart syndrome or transposition of the great arteries is present, obviously there will be severe and early alterations in the hemodynamic picture. If coarctation of the aorta is the only anomaly present, then, during fetal life, the circulation will not deviate significantly from normal except for the probable presence of left ventricular hypertrophy; difficulties will arise, however, as soon as the shift toward extrauterine circulation begins. At this time the ductus arteriosus does not close normally, but, rather, furnishes the lower half of the body with blood. Thus right ventricular hypertension is maintained and the legs receive unoxygenated blood.

Clinical Picture

In the neonatal period there is severe left-sided and right-sided congestive failure; dyspnea, cyanosis and feeding difficulties dominate the picture. At physical examination the cyanosis is usually generalized. Occasionally differential cyanosis is noted, the upper half of the body, especially the right hand, being pink and the legs showing definite blueness. Chest deformity is common; most often it consists in a significant increase in the anteroposterior diameter of the chest. The cardiac impulse is usually hyperdynamic and is maximal at the xiphoid process.

Auscultation seldom contributes anything specific to the diagnosis. A blowing systolic murmur, and possibly a low-frequency diastolic murmur, is usually heard at the lower left sternal border, the systolic component transmitting well to the neck and the back. The second sound at the pulmonary area is usually accentuated. Rales are commonly heard over both lung fields, and the liver is enlarged, but not pulsating.

The femoral pulses are weak and late, but seldom absent. In the majority of instances the systolic pressure in the arms is definitely higher than in the legs; however, *there are infants with coarctation of the aorta and systemic right and left ventricle in whom no pressure gradient between the arms and legs exists because of the simultaneous presence of a large ventricular defect, resulting in equal systolic pressure in the two circuits.*

Roentgenologic examination reveals cardiac enlargement, involving all chambers, with pulmonary vascular engorgement (Fig. 377). At fluoroscopy the cardiac beat is poor, and expansile pulsations are rarely noticeable.

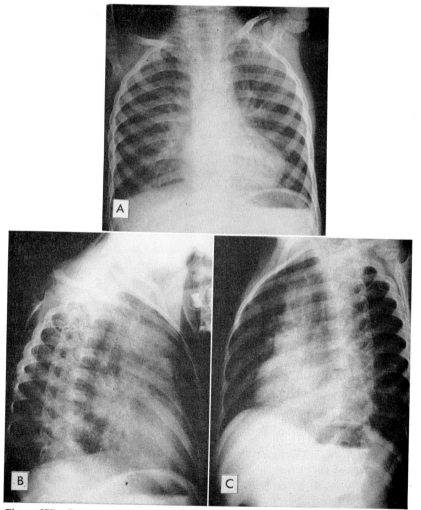

Figure 377. Posteroanterior and oblique roentgenograms of patient with coarctation of the aorta and systemic left and right ventricles. This patient was about nine years old when these films were taken.

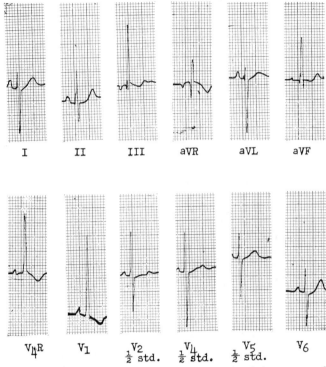

Figure 378. Electrocardiogram of patient with coarctation of the aorta and systemic left and right ventricles. Note the high degree of right ventricular hypertrophy.

None of the characteristic evidences of coarctation of the aorta on the esophagus, mentioned before, can be noted in these babies.

The electrocardiogram invariably reveals right ventricular hypertrophy of abnormal degree, with or without simultaneous evidences of left ventricular hypertrophy (Fig. 378).

Cardiac catheterization and angiographic studies reveal data similar to those encountered with a "reverse ductus." (1) Arterial oxygen saturation in the femoral artery, and possibly in the left brachial artery, is 5 to 10 per cent lower than in the right brachial artery. Usually there is no significant increase in oxygen saturation at the pulmonary arterial level. (2) Pulmonary arterial pressure equals levels obtained in the femoral artery, but is appreciably lower than that in the left ventricle and the right brachial artery. A pressure gradient may be demonstrated by passing the catheter in a retrograde fashion across the coarcted segment. Right atrial and left atrial hypertension may or may not be present. (3) Pulmonary resistance is elevated, usually to systemic levels. (4) Pulmonary-systemic flow ratios are between 0.8 and 0.5. (5) The catheter can be passed easily from the pulmonary artery through the ductus, into the descending aorta. Retrograde arterial catheterization from the femoral artery may demonstrate the site and length of the coarctation. (6) Cine-angiography, with injection into the pulmonary artery or right ventricle, outlines the ductus and the descending aorta, whereas the levogram reveals the ascending aorta with its tributaries. (7) Dye-dilution curves or intracardiac phonocardiograms have not been used with any frequency in our laboratory in the analysis of these cases.

Course and Prognosis

Most of these babies die within the first days or weeks of life in congestive failure. A minority may survive infancy and may reach adolescence or even the third decade of life, with cyanosis and exercise intolerance, but, on the whole, with remarkable adjustment to their disabilities.[218] In effect, these people behave like many other patients with pulmonary vascular obstructive disease and a right-to-left shunt. Why some patients die early in congestive heart failure and others may live for twenty years, I do not know. I would suspect, however, that the survivors represent relatively "pure" defects of coarctation with systemic right and left ventricles and pulmonary vascular obstruction, whereas the others have many other complicating lesions.

Differential Diagnosis

The differential diagnosis of coarctation of the aorta with systemic right and left ventricle may be approached from three aspects. 1. The differentiation of this specific type of coarctation of the aorta from all other types mentioned may be accomplished with certainty only if femoral arterial and right brachial arterial pressures and oxygen contents are measured simultaneously. The anomaly should be suspected, however, in any patient more than six months old with coarctation of the aorta in whom right ventricular hypertrophy is present in the electrocardiogram.

2. The second aspect of the differential diagnosis is the problem of newborn infants in severe congestive failure who may or may not have coarctation of the aorta. Obviously the discovery of relative hypertension in the arms establishes the diagnosis easily; however, sometimes in newborn infants it is difficult to determine the blood pressure and to interpret it correctly. As a rule, if some degree of cardiac compensation can be accomplished with vigorous anticongestive measures, the correct blood pressure values are much easier to determine. If compensation cannot be achieved and an accurate diagnosis is desired for these desperately sick infants, cardiac catheterization may be attempted, more to rule out other diagnoses than to establish the presence of a coarctation of the aorta.

3. The third aspect of the differential diagnostic problem is the one in which a "reverse ductus" is diagnosed clinically and at catheterization, but the question arises as to whether a coarctation of the aorta is present. The only way to solve this problem is to obtain simultaneous pressure measurements from the right brachial artery (if there is no anomalous right subclavian artery) and the femoral artery.

Treatment

Medical treatment may improve congestive failure to a considerable extent, but obviously it cannot postpone for many years the inevitable end.

In both children and adults operation carries a high mortality rate, the situation being identical to that in patent ductus arteriosus with pulmonary vascular obstruction.[675] In some of the younger infants, in whom, presumably, permanent organic pulmonary vascular obstruction has not yet developed, surgery has been successful.[165, 517, 760] I presume that it is this type of patient for whom Keith and his associates[280] recommend emergency surgery.

At The Children's Hospital Medical Center in Boston our policy is to treat all infants with coarctation of the aorta and congestive failure with anticongestive measures. If prompt and lasting improvement occurs, we assume that the patient has coarctation of the aorta, with systemic left ventricle and congestive failure. If the medical regimen is unsuccessful, operation, at high risk, is recommended, and the surgeon is warned of the possibility that a ductus arteriosus may open below the coarctation and may carry blood from the right to the left side of the circulation.

Summary

Coarctation of the aorta with systemic right and left ventricle should be suspected in every patient in whom there is relative hypertension of the arms and electrocardiographic evidence of right ventricular hypertrophy; in infants less than six months of age this represents only presumptive evidence, but in older children it is highly suggestive. The diagnosis may be confirmed by simultaneous right brachial and femoral arterial blood samples and pressure tracings. Medical management, at best, may prolong life for some years. In older patients surgery is difficult; in young infants good results have been reported in a few instances.

AORTIC STENOSIS

General Principles

Until recently aortic stenosis was exclusively an anatomic concept; a narrowing of the left ventricular outflow tract at postmortem examination was considered to indicate aortic obstruction. The clinical profile was based entirely on patients whose diagnosis was confirmed anatomically, a situation similar to that of pulmonary stenosis fifteen years ago, i.e. before the introduction of right heart catheterization. With the advent of left heart catheterization a physiologic definition, i.e. the presence of a gradient between the left ventricle and the aorta, has supplanted the old anatomic concept. At present, the diagnosis of aortic stenosis is made on the basis of the following clinical findings: (1) a second right interspace "stenotic" systolic murmur with good transmission to the neck and the back, (2) evidences of left ventricular hypertrophy or enlargement on the roentgenogram or electrocardiogram, (3) no evidence of a left-to-right or right-to-left shunt, and (4) a systolic gradient of more than 10 mm. of mercury across the aortic valve.

According to data on adults with aortic stenosis,[499] the principal etiologic factors causing this anomaly are rheumatic fever and arteriosclerosis. Since, for all practical purposes, arteriosclerosis does not occur in childhood, and since the development of rheumatic aortic stenosis in all well documented cases takes several years, presumably, all young children with aortic stenosis have a congenital lesion. One further point, first emphasized by Kiloh[389] and later mentioned by Levine,[499] is that a history of rheumatic fever is rare in pure aortic stenosis, whereas it is common in patients with combined aortic or multivalvular lesions. On this basis, then, all children in whom the murmur of aortic stenosis is discovered before the fourth year of age certainly have a congenital lesion. Most likely all those less than eight years old in whom such a defect is diagnosed and who have no history of rheumatic fever were born with the disease. A third category of patients is adults with pure aortic stenosis, with no history of rheumatic fever, in whom the presence of a congenital lesion cannot be proved, but should be suspected.[389]

Incidence

Congenital aortic stenosis is one of the more common congenital cardiac anomalies. Abbott[1] found 23 instances in 1000 postmortem examinations. Keith[380] quoted a 3 per cent incidence among his patients with congenital heart disease, and a similar figure is quoted by Campbell and Kauntze.[131] In our institution we have more than 250 cases with the clinical diagnosis of aortic stenosis on file; in half of these the diagnosis was confirmed by cardiac catheterization. This would amount to an incidence of approximately 5 per cent of our patients with congenital heart disease.

Anatomy

Congenital aortic stenosis may be divided anatomically into valvar, subvalvar and supravalvar types. In the valvar type, representing close to 75 per cent of all cases, the cusps are thickened and may be bicuspid or fused to form a dome-shaped diaphragm with a central opening and a post-stenotic dilatation of the ascending arch of the aorta. Whether congenital valvar stenosis is truly a developmental anomaly or is the result of endocardial fibroelastosis localized at the aortic valve is difficult to decide clinically, but both situations probably exist. It is interesting to note that the valve leaflets are almost invariably thick, uneven and abnormal-looking. Furthermore (fortunately, in only a small number of patients), the valve ring, as well as the ascending aorta, may be hypoplastic. Subvalvar or subaortic stenosis usually consists of a fibrous ring encircling the left ventricular outflow tract approximately 5 to 10 mm. below the aortic ring and often involving the anterior cusp of the mitral valve. This defect, in contrast to the valvar lesion, is probably always developmental in origin.

An entirely separate type of subvalvar stenosis is the one referred to as "muscular" or "functional" subaortic stenosis, which will be discussed separately and may be classified among the myopathies. Finally, the patients with supravalvar stenosis may have a fibrous ring, or even a diaphragm, at some distance above the aortic valve.[557]

Embryologically speaking, the valvar lesion probably occurs by about the seventh intrauterine week and, thus, later than the subvalvar. This may be the reason why valvar lesions are not commonly associated with septal defects, whereas, occasionally, subaortic stenosis does occur with a ventricular defect. Other lesions which may be associated with congenital aortic stenosis are coarctation of the aorta, patent ductus arteriosus, mitral stenosis and pulmonic stenosis.

Physiology

The principal physiologic burden of aortic stenosis is carried by the left ventricle. The problem is to maintain an adequate flow and pressure in the systemic circuit through an orifice which is reduced in size. Animal experiments[729] indicate that a reduction of the lumen of the aorta to at least 25 per cent of its original size is necessary before significant interference with blood pressure, pulse pressure or cardiac output occurs. Since the calculated area of the aortic orifice in adults is usually estimated to be 2.5 to 3.5 sq. cm., probably no significant interference with the circulation occurs, at least in the acute experiment, until it is reduced to less than 0.6 sq. cm.[294] Obviously, in children, who have a lower cardiac output, this figure is not valid. Thus in our formula for determining the size of the orifice, we have substituted the cardiac index for the cardiac output and have come to the conclusion that if the aortic valve area is less than 0.5 sq. cm. per square meter of body surface, probably critical obstruction exists. If the size of the aortic orifice is reduced below this critical level, compensatory mechanisms are called into action: the left ventricular diastolic volume and, considerably later, the end-diastolic pressure increase in order to elevate the left ventricular peak systolic pressure. Isometric contraction is slightly longer; ejection time and total systole become con-

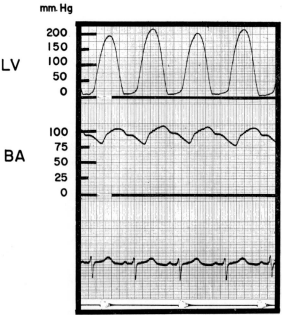

Figure 379. Pressure gradient in patient with critical aortic stenosis. Note the left ventricular pressure approximating 200 mm. of mercury, the brachial arterial pressure barely reaching more than 100 mm. of mercury. Note also the slow upstroke and the late peak on the brachial arterial pressure tracing.

siderably prolonged. The pressure within the left ventricle may rise as high as 200 to 250 mm. of mercury, but seldom higher. The aortic and peripheral arterial tracings show a slow rise with a low anacrotic notch or slur, a wide plateau with vibrations corresponding to the systolic murmur, and a slow descent often with an absent dicrotic notch (Fig. 379). As the left ventricle attempts to maintain the necessary systolic pressure it hypertrophies, and its oxygen needs increase. At the same time the coronary blood flow does not increase proportionately; it may even become smaller because of (1) involvement of the coronary ostia in the stenotic process, (2) shortening of diastole, the time when the coronary arteries fill, (3) the squeezing effect on the coronaries by the high left ventricular systolic pressure, and (4) possibly a suction effect on the coronary ostia by the high-velocity flow through the small aortic opening. As a result of all these factors and the increased oxygen requirement of the hypertrophied myocardium, relative coronary insufficiency exists in the severest cases of aortic stenosis.

Clinical Picture

There are about five times as many males as females in our series. Most of our patients were brought to the cardiologist because of the discovery of a heart murmur; in slightly less than half of the cases the murmur was discovered before the child was one year old; in a third of them the child was between one and four, and in the remainder between five and eight years of age. As mentioned earlier, the discovery of the murmur within the first twenty-four to forty-eight hours of life is characteristic for patients with semilunar stenosis.

Most of these youngsters are not sick at all. More than half of our patients had no symptoms whatsoever (Fig. 380); in the remainder careful questioning elicited symptoms of mild fatigue, dyspnea and abdominal

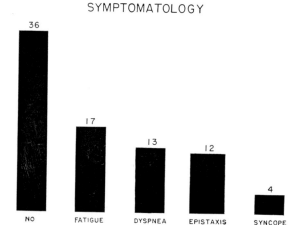

Figure 380. Symptomatology in 67 cases of congenital aortic stenosis.

or precordial pain. In contrast to adults with this disease, syncope was rare. Only four of sixty-seven patients had a history of fainting. Associated cardiac or extracardiac anomalies are rare.

The physical development of these children is usually excellent. More than half of our patients ranked above the fiftieth percentile on our development chart. In body build they resembled children with simple coarctation of the aorta. No cyanosis, clubbing or congestive failure was noted in any instance. The clinical diagnosis was based on the three criteria previously enumerated. Left chest deformity was rare, and the cardiac impulse was heaving and maximal at the apex in most cases. A systolic thrill was felt in all but one of our patients. In 80 per cent of them it was maximal at the second right interspace; in the others it was best felt at the lower left sternal border, or even at the apex. Often the thrill was transmitted to the suprasternal notch and the carotids, particularly in patients with valvar stenosis.

At auscultation a constant aortic click (Fig. 112) is present at the apex or the lower left sternal border in most of the patients with valvar stenosis.[577] In contrast, patients with subvalvar stenosis rarely have an ejection sound. The second sound in patients with severe stenosis (a gradient of more than 40 mm.), whatever its anatomy, is narrowly split, if at all. In children with maximal stenosis (a gradient of more than 100 mm. of mercury) paradoxical splitting may be noted (see p. 117). The intensity of pulmonic and aortic closures is normal except in supravalvar stenosis, in which aortic closure may be exceptionally loud. A third sound is present at the apex in more than half of the patients.

The characteristic stenotic murmur (Fig. 381), at least grade 3 in intensity, is heard maximally at the second right interspace and transmits well to the neck, the carotids, the back, and even to the antecubital fossa, via the brachial artery. There is some suggestion that the peak of the diamond-shaped murmur of aortic stenosis is earlier in the cardiac cycle than the murmur of pulmonic stenosis (Fig. 130). Furthermore, the more severe the stenosis, the later the apex of the diamond occurs. On the whole, patients with valvar stenosis have the loudest murmur. Rarely, in an older child or adolescent, the murmur may be maximal at the lower left sternal border and apex. A separate apical blowing murmur, indicating mitral regurgitation, may be heard in approximately 25 per cent of the patients. A protodiastolic blow (Fig. 382) is heard in all patients with true subvalvar stenosis and in about 50 per cent of those with valvar lesions. Interestingly enough, patients with "functional" subvalvar stenosis

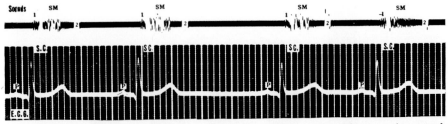

Figure 381. Phonocardiogram of patient with aortic stenosis without aortic regurgitation. Note the early apex of the diamond-shaped murmur, the systolic click and the single second sound.

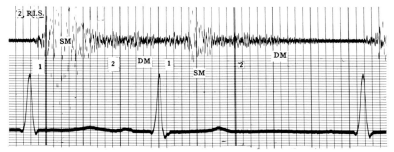

Figure 382. Phonocardiogram of a patient with aortic stenosis on a congenital basis associated with aortic regurgitation. Note the early diamond-shaped systolic murmur followed by the long diastolic murmur lasting throughout most of diastole.

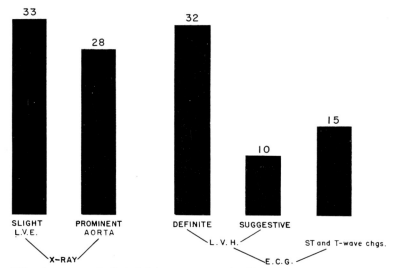

Figure 383. Summary of clinical laboratory tests in 67 patients with congenital aortic stenosis.

seldom, if ever, have protodiastolic blows. An apical mid-diastolic murmur is present in 15 per cent of the patients.

The systolic pressure over the arms and legs was within normal limits in most instances. The pulse pressure was normal in 54 of the 67 patients; in 8 instances it was less than 20, and in 5 it was more than 50. A difference in the blood pressure of the arms, favoring the right, may be noted.

Roentgenologic examination is not specific in most cases. Slight left ventricular enlargement was noted in about half of our patients; in twenty-eight, mostly those with valvar stenosis, the ascending aorta was prominent and showed increased pulsations (Fig. 383).

The electrocardiogram (Fig. 383) was within normal limits in less than 20 per cent of our patients; in the others left ventricular hypertrophy, of varying degree, was observed. Some of these completely asymptomatic patients showed the most severe, progressive, left ventricular hypertrophy, with evidences of strain (Fig. 384).

Among the clinical tools,[283] unquestionably the electrocardiogram is the most sensitive index of the severity of aortic stenosis. In 75 per cent

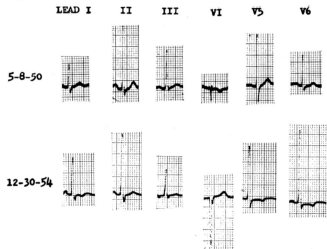

Figure 384. Severe left ventricular hypertrophy developing in a patient with congenital aortic stenosis in a four-year period. In the top tracing, in 1950, T waves in leads I and V_6 are upright, whereas in the bottom tracing, in 1954, T waves in these leads are inverted. Note also the increase in voltage in the chest leads in 1954.

of the patients with aortic valve gradients greater than 50 mm. of mercury, a left ventricular strain pattern is evident. Still, 25 per cent of the patients who have severe aortic stenosis have either normal electrocardiograms or tracings in which left ventricular hypertrophy may be diagnosed only by voltage criteria. Furthermore, about 10 per cent of our patients in whom there was electrocardiographic criteria of left ventricular hypertrophy without strain had only a slight gradient across the aortic valve. It follows, then, that although the scalar electrocardiogram is a good indicator of the severity of aortic stenosis, it is far from infallible.

Vectorcardiographic analysis of these patients seems somewhat more rewarding. Although at first glance we have obtained many false-positive diagnoses by this method, since most of our patients catheterized for aortic stenosis had significant left ventricular hypertrophy, still, measurements of the maximal QRS vector in the horizonal plane have a good quantitative indication of the severity of aortic stenosis (Fig. 385). Few patients with a maximal QRS vector of less than 1.0 mv. had significant left ventricular hypertension (Fig. 386).

Cardiac catheterization reveals the following (Fig. 387): (1) Oxygen saturations are normal in both sides of the heart and the great vessels. (2) Pressures throughout the right side of the heart and the pulmonary artery are normal at rest, though, in severe cases, pulmonary capillary and pulmonary arterial pressures may be slightly elevated. In critical situations with left ventricular failure, exercise may result in significantly elevated pulmonary wedge pressure. There is a systolic gradient across the aortic valve. Optimally, withdrawal tracings from the aorta to the left ventricle, or vice versa, are necessary for accurate estimation of the pressure gradient and localization of the obstruction (Fig. 388). Comparison of left ventricular and femoral arterial pressures may result in an underestimation of the gradient because of the standing wave effect in the femoral artery pulse pressure (see p. 17). Simultaneous cardiac output

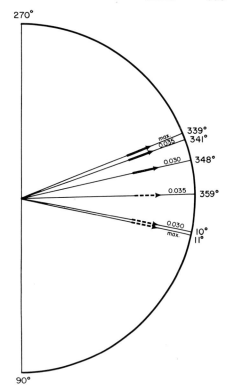

Figure 385. Direction of 0.030- and .035-second vector and maximum QRS vector (in degrees) in the horizontal plane in 45 controls and 40 patients with aortic stenosis. The controls are indicated by the arrows with the interrupted lines and the patients with aortic stenosis by the solid arrows. (From Hugenholtz and others. *Circulation.*)

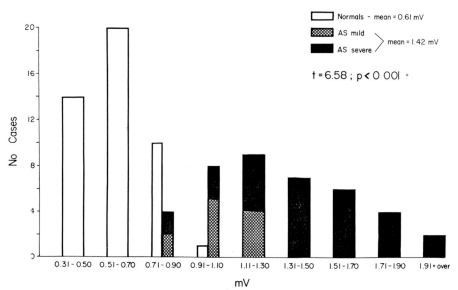

Figure 386. Distribution of magnitude of maximal QRS vectors (in millivolts) in the horizontal plane in forty-five normal children and forty patients with aortic stenosis. (From Hugenholtz and others. *Circulation.*)

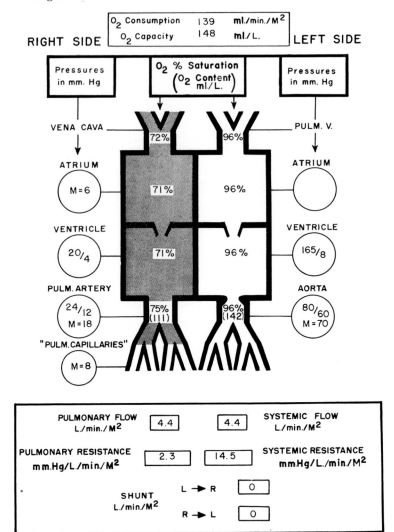

Figure 387. Catheterization data in patient with aortic stenosis.

determination is necessary for estimation of aortic valva area. Left ventricular end-diastolic and left atrial mean pressures may be elevated as much as 10 to 20 mm. of mercury in the patients with critical stenosis. Critical stenosis in our laboratory is defined as (a) a peak systolic gradient of more than 50 mm. of mercury, (b) a mean systolic ejection gradient of more than 40 mm. of mercury, and (c) an aortic valve area of less than 0.5 sq. cm. per square meter.[193, 506] Analysis of the brachial arterial or central aortic pressure pulses fails to give a quantitative estimate of the severity of the stenosis. Although most patients with severe stenosis have delayed upstroke time, or a prolonged rate of ascent, some of the patients with the most severe stenosis have the shortest upstroke time in the brachial artery or central aotric tracings.[414] (3) Systemic and pulmonary resistances are normal. (4) Systemic output, of course, equals pulmonary

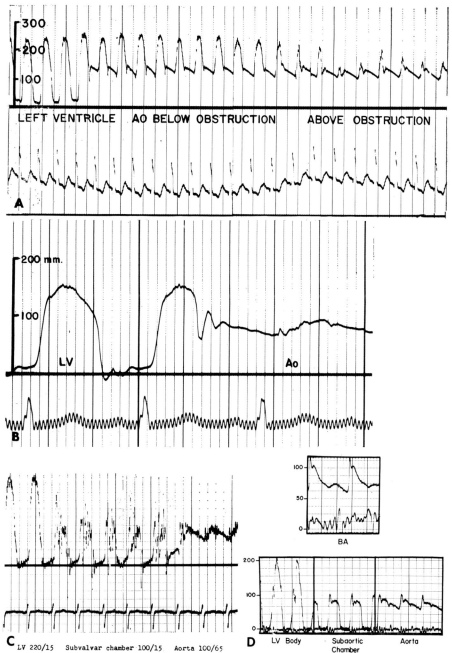

Figure 388. Withdrawal tracings in patients with aortic stenosis. *A*, From left ventricle in patient with supravalvar aortic stenosis. Note the abrupt change in the diastolic pressure when the aortic valve is traversed, without any significant change in the systolic pressure until the supravalvar obstruction is passed. *B*, Valvar aortic stenosis. Note the sudden change in systolic and diastolic pressures when the aortic valve is traversed. *C*, Localized aortic subvalvar stenosis. Note the sudden change in systolic pressure without change in diastolic pressure when the subvalvar chamber is entered, and the sudden rise in diastolic pressure when the aortic valve is traversed. *D*, Pressure pulses in patient with muscular subvalvar stenosis. Note the notch on the upstroke of the left ventricular pressure pulse, corresponding approximately to the level of the peak pressure of the subaortic chamber and of the aorta. Notice also the rapid upstroke in the aorta and in the brachial artery.

555

flow, but both may be on the high side. (5) The catheter may be passed across the aortic valve by one of the techniques of left heart catheterization described earlier (see p. 139). It is interesting to note that passage of a catheter even through a critically narrowed aortic valve is the rule rather than the exception in expert hands. (6) Cine-angiography, with left ventricular injection, is particularly helpful in localizing the area of stenosis and in identifying the muscular subaortic group. This technique may also be used to identify associated mitral regurgitation. (7) Dye-dilution curves and intracardiac phonocardiograms are not particularly useful tools at present in the study of patients with congenital aortic stenosis.

There is no certain way of differentiating valvar from subvalvar or supravalvar stenosis, but the most important differential diagnostic features of these three entities may be summarized as follows:

In *valvar stenosis* the systolic murmur is very loud at the second right interspace and transmits particularly well to the neck vessels. A protodiastolic blow is present in only 50 per cent of the patients, but a constant ejection click is noted almost invariably. A large ascending aorta is visible on the roentgenogram in about 50 per cent. A withdrawal tracing shows a sudden transition (within one beat) from a typical aortic to a left ventricular pressure pulse (Fig. 388, *B*). Among the associated anomalies, coarctation of the aorta and patent ductus arteriosus may be mentioned, but intracardiac anomalies are extremely rare.

In *subvalvar stenosis* the systolic murmur is slightly less intense and is heard maximally a little lower down, with poorer, but still good, transmission to the neck. There is no ejection click, but a protodiastolic murmur is almost invariably present. Dilatation of the aortic arch is rare. The withdrawal tracing reveals the characteristic infundibular chamber between the aorta and the left ventricle (Fig. 388, *C*). Associated anomalies, both intracardiac (ventricular septal defect, mitral valve disease and pulmonic stenosis) and vascular (coarctation and patent ductus arteriosus), are appreciably more common than in the valvar group.

Supravalvar stenosis may be identified with certainty only at left heart catheterization, with good withdrawal tracings (Fig. 388, *A*) and angiograms. Clinical clues supporting its presence may be a loud aortic closure sound, a small ascending aorta and relatively normal electrocardiograms in the face of severe left ventricular hypertension. Many of these patients are mentally retarded and have a peculiar facies.

Unfortunately, the clinical and hemodynamic profile of patients with a *hypoplastic aortic valve ring* (currently an uncorrectible lesion) closely resembles that of simple valvar stenosis. The small aortic arch may alert the cardiologist, and, theoretically at least, angiograms should reveal the exact anatomic situation.

Course and Prognosis

Although most children with aortic stenosis have few if any symptoms and lead entirely normal lives through childhood and adolescence, we (and others)[86, 482, 506] estimate the incidence of sudden death in these children at about 7.5 per cent (Table 29, p. 796). On the other hand, we know, from recent studies on a large number of patients with pure aortic stenosis, that their average life expectancy is more than sixty years.[499]

Therefore the question confronting the pediatric cardiologist is: Which patient will die of coronary disease and congestive failure at the age of sixty and which will drop dead suddenly in early adolescence, after minimal physical exertion, such as riding a bicycle? Obviously there is no simple answer. The most obvious clinical hint as to the severity of the disease is furnished by the electrocardiogram. It is my opinion that, although one cannot be certain that an aortic or subclavian aneurysm may not rupture in a child with a normal electrocardiogram, the presence of severe and progressive left ventricular hypertrophy with strain increases significantly the danger of sudden death. It has become obvious, however, within recent years[580] that children with critical aortic stenosis may present normal electrocardiograms or tracings, with only mild left ventricular hypertrophy and without strain. In these patients, as mentioned, the vectorcardiogram may furnish more conclusive evidence of severe left ventricular hypertrophy. Finally, the presence of even mild symptoms referable to aortic stenosis (chest pain, abdominal pain, fatigue and syncope), even in the face of normal electrocardiograms or vectorcardiograms, should serve as an indication for left heart catheterization, the only definite way of assessing aortic stenosis at present.

One further note of caution should be sounded. Although we have no information at present about the future course of children with mild aortic stenosis, it is possible that the mild stenosis may become critical during the adolescent growth spurt, paralleling the increase in resting output and the advent of strenuous athletic activities. Furthermore, even the mild aortic stenosis of adolescence may develop into severe obstruction in the fourth or fifth decade, as a congenitally thickened valve exposed to a jet effect becomes sclerosed and calcified.

Briefly, then, the assessment of congenital aortic stenosis should be made with great circumspection. Opinions as to severity should be expressed with certainty only in terms of the time of the examination; prognosis for the years and decades to come is a matter of speculation based on the reflections in a crystal ball rather than prediction based on statistically meaningful data. Special attention should be paid to symptoms, electrocardiograms and vectorcardiograms, and patients should be followed up particularly carefully during adolescence. If there is any indication of progression in severity, left heart catheterization should be repeated.

Death from aortic stenosis in children is almost never due to congestive failure; probably ischemic heart disease with ventricular fibrillation is the most common cause of death. Death in congestive failure may occur in infants with severe aortic stenosis.

Differential Diagnosis

The differential diagnosis of simple congenital aortic stenosis usually does not offer any great difficulties.

Muscular or "Functional" Aortic Stenosis. It should be possible to differentiate this entity, which will be discussed later (see p. 565), preoperatively from simple organic valvular and subvalvar stenosis. The late discovery of the systolic murmur, its localization at the apex, the rather loud mid-diastolic rumble and the absence of a protodiastolic blow are the auscultatory hallmarks of functional aortic stenosis. Although the pulse pressures are similar to those encountered in patients with simple aortic stenosis, the carotids are unusually vigorously pulsatile, with a rapid upstroke, particularly when considered in the light of evidences of severe aortic obstruction (on the electrocardiogram or at catheterization). On the roentgenogram the aorta is small, and the electrocardiogram shows a late ventricular activation time and deep Q waves over the left chest lead in some patients. At catheterization the behavior of the pressure pulses in the left ventricle and the aorta after ectopic beats and the angiograms of the left ventricle are diagnostic.

Rheumatic Aortic Stenosis.   Usually, rheumatic aortic stenosis can be excluded easily on the basis of the age of the patient, the absence of aortic regurgitation or multivalvular involvement, and the absence of a history of rheumatic fever.

Aortic Regurgitation.   Pure or dominant aortic regurgitation of a congenital nature is rare.[728] Obviously the etiologic evidence in these cases is purely circumstantial. The murmur and pulse pressure should make it easy to distinguish free aortic regurgitation with a slight stenotic murmur from dominant aortic stenosis associated with the slight murmur of aortic regurgitation.

Aortic Stenosis with Patent Ductus Arteriosus.   See page 492.

Aortic Stenosis with Coarctation of the Aorta.   The relative hypertension of the arms in patients with clinical features of simple aortic stenosis distinguishes it from this combination of anomalies (see p. 564).

Aortic Stenosis with Pulmonic Stenosis.   See Pulmonic Stenosis (p. 614). Any evidence of pulmonic stenosis (in terms of an additional stenotic murmur at the second left interspace, of right ventricular hypertrophy, or of a xiphoid impulse) in a patient with presumable aortic stenosis should draw attention to this combination of anomalies. The presence of corrected transposition of the great arteries may predispose to this combination.

Pulmonic Stenosis.   In its mildest form pulmonic stenosis without right-to-left shunt may be difficult to differentiate from mild aortic stenosis. Both conditions are characterized by a "stenotic" systolic murmur, and, in both, electrocardiograms and roentgenograms are normal. The three most useful clues in the differential diagnosis are the cardiac impulse, the site of maximal intensity of the murmur and the relative intensity of the second sound in the aortic and pulmonary areas. Occasionally no accurate decision can be made on the basis of these criteria, however. Under these circumstances cardiac catheterization may prove or disprove the presence of pulmonic stenosis. The more conservative cardiologist probably will do nothing about these children, since whichever disease they have is mild enough not to cause any significant change in the electrocardiogram, and therefore the differential diagnosis is of no real prognostic or therapeutic importance.

Small Ventricular Septal Defect.   The differences between aortic stenosis and a small ventricular septal defect of the Roger type are discussed on page 410.

Treatment

Children with severe simple congenital aortic stenosis should be treated surgically[482] by means of the pump oxygenator. This procedure (in our institution,[414] as well as in others[279, 393]) carries approximately a 10 per cent mortality risk at present. Most of the deaths are due to complicating factors (hypoplastic valve ring, parietal endocardial disease and severe congestive heart failure in infants less than six months of age). Actually, we have lost only 2 of 54 patients with simple aortic stenosis who were operated on between August, 1957, and February, 1961.[414] Operative indications are based on the finding at left heart catheterization of one or more of the following: (1) aortic valve area of less than 0.5 sq. cm. per square meter, (2) a mean systolic ejection gradient of more than 40 mm. of mercury or (3) a peak systolic gradient of more than 50 mm. of mercury.

Obviously, the first two criteria are more accurate, since aortic valve flow is included in the calculation. Nevertheless my own personal feeling is that *anybody with a peak gradient of 50 mm. of mercury or more, under any circumstances, probably needs surgery, and the flow calculations become important only when a peak gradient of less than this value is founds, in which case one ought to be very certain that an unusually low cardiac output, at the time of the catheterization, was not responsible for the low gradient.* One further situation (see p. 166) that may produce a falsely low gradient is the use of femoral arterial systolic pressure rather than central aortic pressure in the gradient calculations.

If one assumes that only left heart catheterization may serve as an indication for surgery, then the indications for left heart catheterization in children with congenital aortic stenosis should be defined also. At present I think that one or more of the following criteria should serve as an indication for study of the left side of the heart in patients with the clinical diagnosis of aortic stenosis: (1) electrocardiographic evidences of left heart strain, (2) vectorcardiograms indicating severe left ventricular hypertrophy, (3) symptoms attributable to aortic stenosis or (4) strong athletic tendencies in an adolescent with the clinical picture of aortic stenosis.

Perhaps, for practical purposes, children with the classic picture of simple congenital aortic stenosis whose electrocardiograms show left ventricular strain may be operated on without determination of the gradient, though the surgeon then would have no clear idea of the anatomic situation to be encountered at operation.

The results of surgery in the survivors are good. The aortic gradient was either abolished or significantly reduced in nine of thirteen patients in our series in whom preoperative and postoperative left heart catheterization was carried out (Fig. 389). Among the patients with only clinical postoperative evaluation, symptomatic improvement occurred in all, and electrocardiographic improvement, in half.

The postoperative electrocardiographic changes are interesting. In only one of our patients with subvalvar obstruction, thus far, have we noticed significant electrocardiographic improvement (thirty months postoperatively), even though the gradient was totally abolished in four. In contrast, the electrocardiogram mirrored accurately the hemodynamic improvement of all the patients with valvar stenosis (Table 30, p. 797). In other words, the electrocardiogram may be used as an accurate tool for postoperative evaluation only in the valvar group (Fig. 390). Consequently, among the patients with only clinical postoperative evaluation, the 50 per cent whose electrocardiograms returned to normal may be assumed to have obtained considerable benefit from surgery. On the other hand, among the

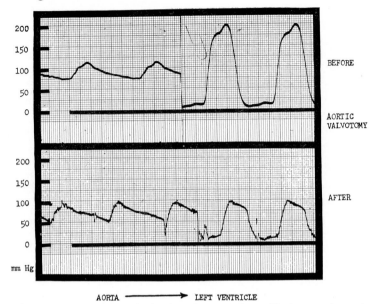

Figure 389. Pressure pulses obtained at the operating table in a patient who underwent successful aortic valvotomy. Top tracing, before operation, with a 100-mm. gradient. There is no appreciable gradient postoperatively.

Valvar Aortic Stenosis

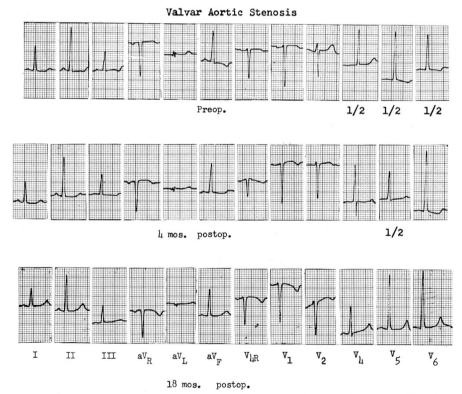

Figure 390. Postoperative improvement in the electrocardiogram of patient with valvar aortic stenosis.

50 per cent who failed to show electrocardiographic improvement, only those with valvar stenosis are likely to have significant residual obstruction; the ones with subvalvar stenosis may or may not have obtained relief.

The matter of postoperative aortic regurgitation should be discussed briefly. As mentioned earlier, all the patients with subvalvar stenosis had a protodiastolic blow preoperatively; in some, this disappeared after operation. Among the patients with valvar stenosis, aortic regurgitation was present postoperatively in all those who had it before surgery and in a few others. In only one patient was the postoperative murmur of aortic regurgitation accompanied by a widened pulse pressure, indicating a hemodynamically significant defect. Whether significant aortic regurgitation will eventually develop in the others, who now have only a short protodiastolic blow of no obvious hemodynamic significance, it is too early to tell.

The optimal age for operation is between five and fifteen years. Because of the slow reversal of the electrocardiographic changes in the subvalvar lesions, these may have to be operated on relatively early (five to ten years). Probably patients with moderate stenosis who are not candidates for operation, or those waiting for surgery, should abstain from competitive exercise.

Summary.

Children with aortic stenosis probably have congenital disease. Clinical differentiation of supravalvar, valvar or subvalvar obstruction is difficult, but the presence of an aortic click and a wide ascending aorta, without the murmur of aortic incompetence, suggests the presence of valvar obstruction. In most cases, left heart catheterization and selective angiography accurately reveal the nature of the obstruction. Severe disease, predisposing to sudden death, is indicated clinically by paradoxical splitting of the second sound, an electrocardiogram with left ventricular strain, and a vectorcardiogram with maximal posterior and leftward forces. A peak systolic gradient across the aortic valve of more than 50 mm. of mercury, or an aortic valve area of less than 0.5 sq. cm. per square meter of body surface, is the physiologic definition of critical stenosis. Surgical relief of aortic stenosis is indicated in all those with critical obstruction. The operative mortality rate in uncomplicated cases is less than 10 per cent, and satisfactory hemodynamic and electrocardiographic improvement may be expected in three fourths of the cases.

CRITICAL AORTIC STENOSIS WITH CONGESTIVE HEART FAILURE IN YOUNG INFANTS

A brief mention of this group of patients, of whom we have seen four in the past three years and who in many ways are similar to the infants with coarctation of the aorta and congestive heart failure, is indicated for a number of reasons.

To begin with, their clinical profile is totally different from that of patients with simple aortic stenosis; it resembles more that of infants with coarctation of the aorta and the hypoplastic left heart syndrome. These infants (less than two months of age) are critically ill, with left-sided and right-sided failure and cyanosis secondary to pulmonary venous unsaturation. On physical examination the classic loud stenotic murmur may not be obvious; the murmur may be only grade 2 in intensity, and, as a matter of fact, I know of one instance in which no murmur was heard. Digitalization, by increasing the cardiac output, may "bring out" the murmur of aortic stenosis. Also, the point of maximal intensity of the murmur may be at the lower left sternal border or even at the apex. A third sound and a mid-

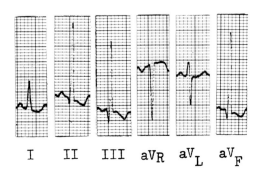

I   II   III   aVR   aVL   aVF

Figure 391. Tracing of infant with critical aortic stenosis and congestive heart failure.

V4R   V1   V2   V4   V5   V6

1/2 1/2

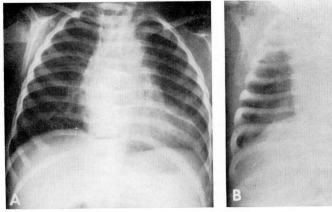

Figure 392. Preoperative (B) and postoperative (A) roentgenograms of infant in congestive heart failure with critical aortic stenosis.

diastolic rumble may be heard. The electrocardiogram commonly shows classic left ventricular hypertrophy (Fig. 391) with strain, and the roentgenogram reveals left ventricular and left atrial enlargement, with pulmonary venous congestion (Fig. 392). Cardiac catheterization reveals left ventricular hypertension with elevated end-diastolic pressure and a severe gradient across the aortic valve, left atrial and pulmonary arterial hypertension and pulmonary venous unsaturation.

The second reason for discussing these patients separately from those with simple aortic stenosis is that they represent real emergencies. Prompt surgical intervention, probably by a transaortic approach with inflow occlusion, or by means of a pump-oxygenator, may be lifesaving. Obviously, the risks of surgery are high, but for babies in this critical condition there really is no good alternative to operation unless prompt improvement in the congestive failure may be accomplished medically.

Differential Diagnosis

In the differential diagnosis, coarctation of the aorta should be considered first and foremost. If adequate blood pressure measurements are obtainable, there should be no problem. On the other hand, these infants may be in such profound shock that no accurate estimation of the blood pressure is possible. In many of these patients vigorous anticongestive measures may restore the circulation sufficiently within a few hours, so that the blood pressure can be measured.

One further point which distinguishes these infants from those with coarctation is that the patients in the latter group seldom, if ever, have electrocardiograms showing pure left ventricular hypertrophy and strain within the first few weeks. Therefore this type of tracing, with or without coarctation, should raise strong suspicions of aortic stenosis.

The second entity to be distinguished from aortic stenosis with congestive heart failure in infants is the hypoplastic left heart syndrome. On the whole, this is much more difficult than the differentiation from coarctation of the aorta, since the convenient tool of blood pressure measurement cannot be used as a differential diagnostic criterion. Furthermore, many of the patients with the hypoplastic left heart syndrome (see p. 578) have severe aortic stenosis or, more frequently, some aortic gradient. The maximal cardiac enlargement within the first day of life, and the total absence of left ventricular hypertrophy in the electrocardiogram of the patient with the hypoplastic left heart syndrome are the best clinical tools of differentiation.

Finally, the primary myocardial disease group (endocardial fibroelastosis and acute myocarditis, or the other members of this entity) should be considered in the differential diagnosis. The lack of a murmur, the poor cardiac beat and the fact that the onset occurs some weeks after birth are the only clinical signs suggesting primary myocardial disease.

Unless critical aortic stenosis may be excluded with certainty, left heart catheterization, probably through the inferior vena cava-foramen ovale approach, *is mandatory.* The technique is difficult, and the correct interpretation of the data is far from simple, particularly since all three of the conditions may coexist. We have seen babies with mild coarctation, severe aortic stenosis and considerable endocardial fibroelastosis. Where the hypoplastic left heart syndrome begins and critical, surgically correctible aortic stenosis ends may be extremely hard to determine in the individual case.

Summary

A critically ill newborn infant who has evidences of left-sided and right-sided failure, a murmur of aortic stenosis, a large heart with pulmonary venous congestion, and an electrocardiogram showing left ventricular hypertrophy with strain probably has critical aortic stenosis. Surgical intervention, after appropriate studies of the left side of the heart, should be considered seriously, but obviously carries very high risks.

AORTIC STENOSIS WITH COARCTATION OF THE AORTA

More than 10 per cent of our patients with proved aortic stenosis also had coarctation of the aorta. In most instances the stenosis was valvar, with a bicuspid valve, but two of the patients had subvalvar stenosis. The coarctation was at the usual location and was mild to moderate.

Clinical Picture

The clinical picture represents a composite of the two lesions. The patients have few, if any, symptoms. The auscultatory and radiologic findings can be predicted from a consideration of the two defects, but it may be worth while to stress the frequent occurrence of aortic regurgitation. The severe left ventricular hypertrophy shown in the electrocardiogram has already been stressed. Cardiac catheterization reveals a gradient across the aortic valve as well as across the coarcted segment. Which of the two lesions is the more significant may be deduced from the relative pressure drops across the two sites of obstruction. In most, but not all, of our patients the aortic valve obstruction seemed the more severe.

Course and Prognosis

The course in these patients is similar to that in patients having the separate lesions. Possibly the cumulative effects of the two may cause more trouble than either one alone, but I have no definite evidence in this regard.

Differential Diagnosis

In the differential diagnosis, simple aortic stenosis may be excluded easily by the relative hypertension of the arms. The problem of whether a patient with known coarctation of the aorta also has significant aortic stenosis is much more difficult. The presence of a loud stenotic murmur at the second right interspace certainly points in this direction. Further evidence may be furnished by the presence of the cardiographic abnormalities mentioned, particularly in a young person who does not have maximal systolic hypertension of the arms.

Treatment

The treatment depends on the severity of the respective lesions. In a patient with clear-cut severe aortic stenosis (proved by left heart catheterization) and trivial coarctation (indicated by blood pressure criteria), the aortic outflow tract should be opened at the appropriate time. In a patient who has severe coarctation of the aorta and a trivial murmur of aortic stenosis with no strain pattern in the electrocardiogram, the coarctation should be relieved first, without even performing left heart catheterization.

In patients in whom both defects are of approximately equal severity, it has been our custom to do an aortic valvotomy first, since it is believed that the strain of placing and then suddenly removing the aortic clamps in patients with significant aortic stenosis may prove to be too much for the myocardium. Resection of the coarctation can be carried out any time from two or three months to one or two years after the aortic valve surgery. *If any evidence of failure is on hand, appropriate anticongestive measures are indicated before operation.*

Summary

A patient with coarctation of the aorta who has a stenotic murmur at the second right interspace and whose electrocardiogram reveals severe left ventricular hypertrophy may also have aortic stenosis. Children with aortic stenosis and relative hypertension of the arms also have this combination. Surgery on the aortic valve is recommended first, unless there is clear-cut evidence that the coarctation is the more severe of the two obstructive lesions.

AORTIC STENOSIS AND MITRAL VALVE DISEASE

See Hypoplastic Left Heart Syndrome (p. 578).

MUSCULAR OR "FUNCTIONAL" SUBAORTIC STENOSIS

Brock[94] was the first to describe functional aortic obstruction in a patient with hypertensive cardiovascular disease. Since then, others[52, 88, 100, 506] have described examples of this entity, with or without associated valvar or vascular disease. Brent emphasized the familial occurrence of the entity.

Incidence

The incidence is hard to ascertain. Fourteen cases have been reported from the National Heart Institute.[100] We have had two proved (one at postmortem examination and one at operation) and two clinically suspected instances of this condition.

Anatomy

The most striking feature of this condition is that, although clinical and physiologic studies indicate maximal subvalvar obstruction, at operation

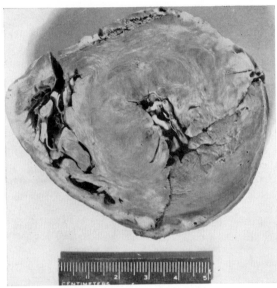

Figure 393.   Pathologic specimen from patient with muscular "functional" subaortic stenosis. Note the huge muscle mass practically obliterating the left ventricular cavity.

the aortic valve is normal and in diastole the subvalvar portion of the left ventricle is wide open. In systole, however, a strongly contracting outflow tract poses a formidable obstruction to left ventricular outflow. The surgical description—at cardiotomy, the musculature, during systole, strongly grabs the finger inserted from above into the left ventricular outflow tract—is the most graphic representation of the condition.

At postmortem examination the left ventricular cavity is almost completely obliterated by the greatly hypertrophied muscle mass (Fig. 393) involving, particularly, the interventricular septum. This huge septal mass protrudes into both ventricles, but obliterates principally the left ventricular outflow tract, up to a point 1 to 2 cm. below the valve. A small subvalvar chamber can be seen between the muscle mass and the aortic valve. The endocardium over this thick septal muscle is gray and opaque. Some encroachment of the mass on the orifice of the mitral valve may be noted also. Under the microscope the individual muscle fibers may be thickened, and patchy fibrosis, and even necrosis, may be seen.

Physiology

The severe subvalvar obstruction is a functional one in these patients, and as a consequence it does not exist throughout the whole of systole. A rapid ejection of blood occurs through the wide-open aortic orifice within the first quarter or half of the ejection period before the muscle clamps down on the outflow tract. After this the left ventricular pressure rapidly mounts to above the systemic level, but only a small trickle of blood is ejected. In our patients, and most of those described in the literature, there is a 100- to 150-mm. peak systolic gradient between the aorta and the left ventricle.

In the patients being discussed under this heading of functional, muscular subaortic stenosis, no known stimulus exists for the development of the maximal septal hypertrophy. It is clearly understood, however, that lesser degrees of this phenomenon may exist in a secondary fashion with stenosis of the aortic valve[294] or even with systemic hypertension.[94, 420]

Clinical Picture

Only the features distinguishing this entity from simple congenital aortic stenosis will be stressed. First, there is a strong familial tendency in some of these patients[88] toward sudden death. Second, usually the murmur is not discovered early in infancy, but syncope occurs at a relatively young age.

The findings at physical examination are interesting. The systolic murmur is likely to be maximal at the apex and the lower left sternal border, a protodiastolic blow is rare, and a mid-diastolic murmur is common. The vigorous carotid pulsations, with rapid upstroke, can be explained

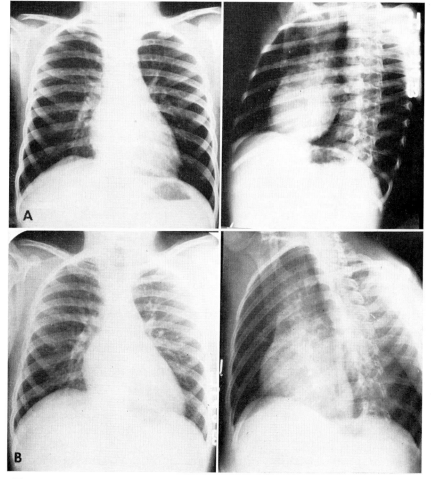

Figure 394. *A,* Posteroanterior and lateral roentgenograms of patient with muscular subaortic stenosis in 1953. *B,* Roentgenograms of same patient six years later. Note the progressive cardiac enlargement and increasing dominance of the left ventricle.

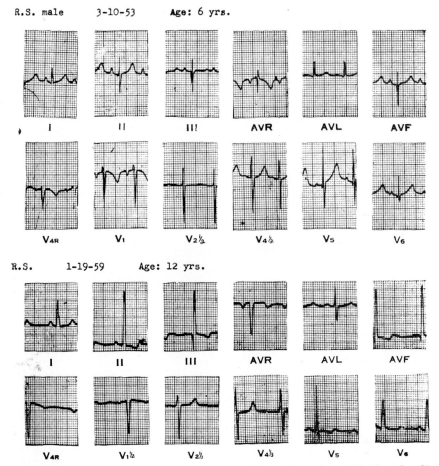

Figure 395. Progressive electrocardiographic changes in patient with "functional" or muscular subaortic stenosis. Note the development of left ventricular hypertrophy with strain over a six-year period. Note also the characteristic Q waves in aV_F, V₆ and lead III.

by the early rapid ejection period of the left ventricle. The roentgenograms show a small aorta, and there is no calcium in the aortic valve, even in older patients (Fig. 394). The electrocardiogram shows left ventricular strain, occasionally but not invariably, with deep left-sided Q waves (septal hypertrophy) (Fig. 395).

At catheterization a notch on the upstroke of the left ventricular pressure pulse (Fig. 388, *D*) at the level of the systemic systolic pressure may correspond to the "clamping down" of the outflow tract. Brockenbrough[100] drew attention to the fact that postextrasystolic beats in these patients are characterized by an increase in left ventricular pressure, with a corresponding decrease in systemic arterial pressure, because of the functional nature of the obstruction. Left ventricular angiograms are useful in demonstrating the variability of the obstruction throughout the heart cycle.

Course and Prognosis

This is a malignant disease, and sudden death is even more common in these patients, when they reach their twenties and thirties, than it is in those with severe aortic stenosis of the usual type.

Differential Diagnosis

The salient distinguishing features of this condition, as against simple congenital aortic stenosis, have already been enumerated. Critical rheumatic aortic stenosis, for all practical purposes, does not occur in children.

Treatment

Successful surgical treatment has been reported in two patients by Morrow and his co-workers from the National Heart Institute.[100] The operation consists in a longitudinal incision into the septal mass from below the aortic valve to the apex, similar to a Ramstedt procedure for pyloric stenosis. At The Children's Hospital Medical Center we have had only one successful experience with the operative treatment of this condition. The effectiveness of surgical treatment, on a long-term basis, is increasingly doubtful.

Summary

Functional subaortic stenosis is commonly a familial disease. It consists in functional obliteration of the left ventricular outflow by severe septal hypertrophy. On physical examination the murmur is maximal at the apex, the carotids are bounding, and the electrocardiogram shows evidences of maximal left ventricular hypertrophy. Cardiac catheterization and angiography are helpful in the diagnosis. Prognosis is poor; surgery is in the beginning stage.

CONGENITAL AORTIC RUNOFFS

As mentioned previously, a murmur characteristic of aortic regurgitation may be heard in patients with dominant aortic stenosis. In these children, however, the peripheral signs of free aortic regurgitation are usually missing; hence it may be assumed that the degree of insufficiency is minimal.

During the past years, however, we have encountered a number of children with the classic clinical picture of aortic regurgitation in whom, either because of their young age, the early discovery of the murmur or the absence of a rheumatic history, we have had to assume that the lesion was, indeed, congenital.

I would like to emphasize that the early discovery of the murmur (unless it falls within the first weeks or months of life) per se, is not enough to exclude rheumatic heart disease definitely. I can recall one patient, specifically, who had severe respiratory infections, and even a tonsillectomy, within the first two years of life, in whom an aortic diastolic murmur was heard by reliable observers when he was two and one-half years old. At operation, when he was fourteen years old, this boy had changes in the aortic valve characteristic of rheumatic heart disease.

Assuming, however, that rheumatic aortic regurgitation may be excluded, in one way or another, the following specific anatomic entities may be regarded as underlying the clinical profile of congenital aortic runoffs.

1. *Fenestration of aortic valve leaflets,* appearing like one or two discrete holes in the aortic valve cusps, may stimulate most closely the clinical and physiologic picture of rheumatic aortic regurgitation. This is a rare condition. We have seen only two such cases in our institution. There is no way this entity can be differentiated clinically or physiologically from rheumatic aortic regurgitation. I presume that more such cases will be discovered as surgery for aortic regurgitation gains momentum. Surgical closure of these isolated perforations is relatively simple.

2. *Ventricular septal defect with aortic regurgitation* (see p. 434).

3. *Bicuspid aortic valve probably with, but possibly even without, coarctation of the aorta* (see below).

4. *Coronary arteriovenous fistula* (see p. 515).

5. *Aneurysm of the aortic sinus* (see p. 511).

6. *Marfan's syndrome* with dilatation of the ascending aorta, the aortic valve ring and even all three aortic sinuses.

Other entities less likely to be considered pure aortic regurgitation, because of the sizable communication between the systemic and pulmonary circuits, but still to be discussed under the general heading of aortic runoffs, are (7) patent ductus arteriosus, (8) aortopulmonary window, and (9) persistent truncus arteriosus.

BICUSPID AORTIC VALVES

A note should be inserted here about congenital bicuspid aortic valves. I shall not discuss its differentiation from acquired bicuspidization, partly because the problem seldom arises in children, and partly because even the microscopic criteria for differentiation[214] are not uniformly accepted.

Congenital bicuspid aortic valve may be a solitary malformation, in which case a patient exhibits signs or symptoms of heart disease only if bacterial endocarditis develops. It has been taught that uncomplicated bicuspid aortic valve, without superimposed bacterial endocarditis, is compatible with completely normal cardiac findings.[683] Edwards,[215] in an interesting, speculative article, indicates that even the "perfect" bicuspid aortic valve may give rise to progressive aortic regurgitation which, later, may lead to calcification, endocarditis and even stenosis. Gelfman and Levine[272] found that in 80 per cent of their patients who had bicuspid valves there were no other associated anomalies.

Edwards[215] indicated that fully 75 per cent of all aortic coarctations have bicuspid valves. Abbott[1] estimated the frequency at only 25 per cent, Reifenstein[576] at 42 per cent. It may be assumed that the 20 per cent of the patients with coarctation of the aorta who have clinical aortic regurgitation probably also have bicuspid valves.[129, 147] That valvar congenital aortic stenosis may be associated frequently with bicuspid valves has already been mentioned[645] (see p. 547). Other less commonly associated lesions may be ventricular septal defect, transposition of the great arteries and aortic septal defect.

In summary, it may be stated that bicuspid aortic valve, as a solitary lesion, is probably rather common, but has no cardiac manifestation in childhood unless there is superimposed bacterial endocarditis. It may be stated also that if bacterial endocarditis develops in a patient without known pre-existing heart disease, a bicuspid aortic valve should be suspected. There is some evidence that in older patients even uncomplicated bicuspid aortic valves may become grossly incompetent or even stenotic. Bicuspid aortic valves are common concomitants of coarctation of the aorta, in which they may represent the anatomic basis of coexisting aortic stenosis and aortic regurgitation.

VASCULAR RINGS

Vascular rings are congenital anomalies of the aortic arch and its tributaries, causing varying degrees of compression of the trachea and the esophagus. Strictly speaking, since no cardiac dysfunction is connected with them, these lesions probably should not be discussed in a textbook on pediatric cardiology. A brief discussion is included, however, for the sake of completeness and because information about these anomalies is important to the pediatrician. Most of the data that follow have been compiled by Doctors Robert E. Gross[309] and Edward B. D. Neuhauser[312] of The Children's Hospital Medical Center of Boston.

Anatomy

Although, if one reviews the complicated development of the aortic arch and the branchial artery, one can easily recognize that there are innumerable possible variations and permutations on normal development, only those anomalies severe enough to cause symptoms of sufficient frequency to be of pratical significance will be discussed here. There are five such lesions: (1) double aortic arch (Fig. 396), (2) right aortic arch with a left ligamentum arteriosum (Fig. 397), (3) anomalous right subclavian artery (Fig. 398), (4) anomalous innominate artery (Fig. 399), and (5) anomalous left common carotid artery (Fig. 400). In all these anomalies the trachea and the esophagus, which normally lie behind the vascular structures, are surrounded by vessels.

Incidence

These lesions are comparatively common. Within ten years Gross[309] saw fifty-seven patients with vascular rings. Their relative frequency in his series is as follows: double aortic arch, twenty-one; right aortic arch with left ligamentum arteriosum, fifteen; anomalous subclavian arteries, twelve; anomalous innominate arteries, seven; anomalous left common carotid artery, two.

Physiology

The consequences of vascular rings can be measured in terms of encroachment on the trachea and the esophagus. If the esophagus is prin-

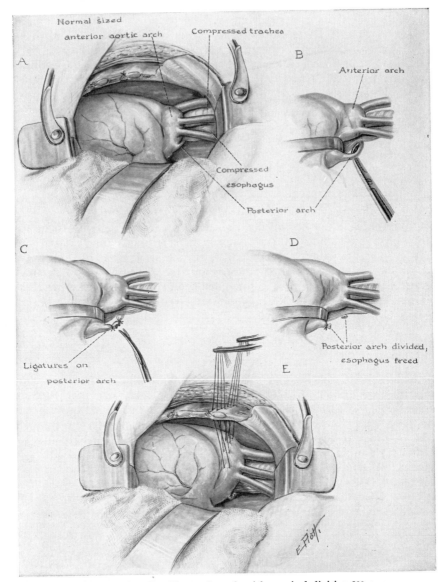

Figure 396. Double aortic arch with surgical division.[309]

cipally affected, swallowing difficulties and vomiting occur, whereas, if tracheal compression dominates, wheezing, cyanosis and frequent episodes of pneumonia may result.

Clinical Picture

The clinical picture varies considerably, depending on the nature of the malformation and the severity of the obstruction. Many of the malformations, particularly those of the anomalous right subclavian artery, cause no symptoms. Others may cause severe difficulties, even death in young infants.

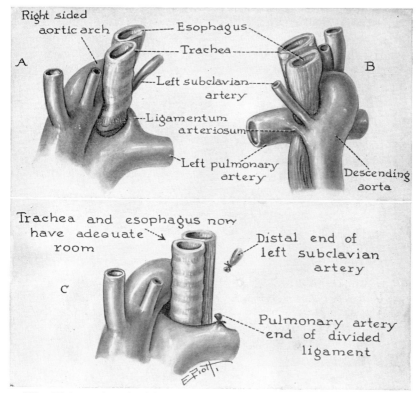

Figure 397. Right aortic arch with left ligamentum arteriosum and its surgical division.[309]

At physical examination the children with severe obstructions are extremely sick. The typical patient is a small, poorly developed baby with a great deal of wheezing and stridor. To reduce the tracheal compression to a minimum, the child tends to keep his head in hyperextension. Vomiting occurs frequently. Feeding exaggerates the stridor and the wheezing and may cause cyanosis. Many severe respiratory infections occur. During these infections the stridor and vomiting increase as well.

In some instances one is impressed by the fact that although these infants are hungry and start to eat eagerly, after a few mouthfuls they cannot swallow and may even regurgitate. In others small quantities may be taken easily, whereas large amounts cause discomfort and vomiting.

The heart, on physical examination, seems completely normal; the lungs may or may not show evidences of pneumonia. Mild abdominal distension is commonly present.

The electrocardiograms are well within normal limits.

Roentgenograms of the heart and cardiac fluoroscopy show no significant abnormalities. But by careful observation of the passage of barium along the esophagus, it is possible not only to establish the diagnosis of a vascular ring, but also often to identify the structures making up this constricting ring. Figures 401, 402 and 403 demonstrate the impression of the compressing vessels on the barium-filled esophagus. In order to ascertain the degree of compression on the trachea as well, a Lipiodol tracheogram should be obtained after the diagnosis of a vascular ring has been estab-

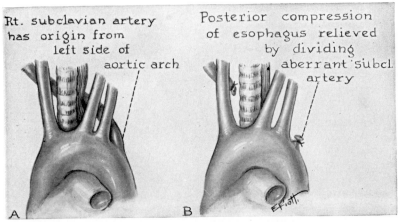

Figure 398.   Anomalous right subclavian artery and its surgical division.[309]

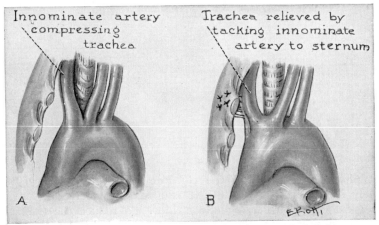

Figure 399.   Anomalous innominate artery with its surgical division.[309]

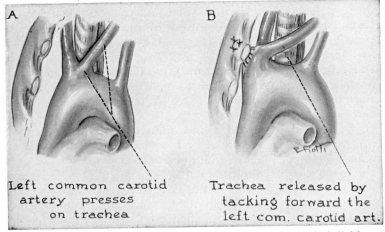

Figure 400.   Anomalous left common carotid artery and its surgical division.[309]

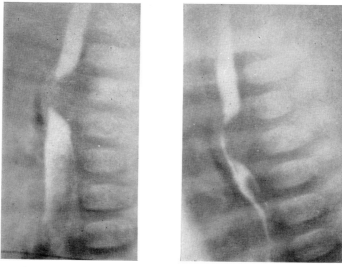

Figure 401. Esophagogram of patient with double aortic arch.

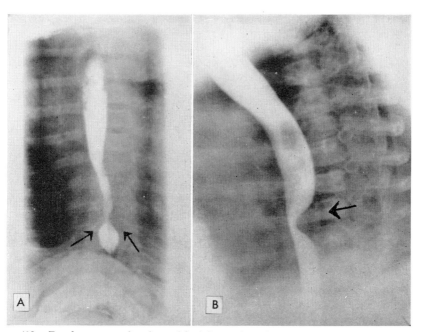

Figure 402. Esophagogram of patient with right aortic arch and left ligamentum arteriosum.

lished by the history, physical examination and roentgenogram of the barium-filled esophagus. A combined roentgenologic examination of this sort almost always reveals the full nature of the vascular anomaly. Figures 404, 405 and 406 are tracheograms of the three most common lesions.

Cardiac catheterization has not been been performed in any of our patients with this syndrome.

Angiocardiograms are seldom necessary; the diagnosis is usually clear

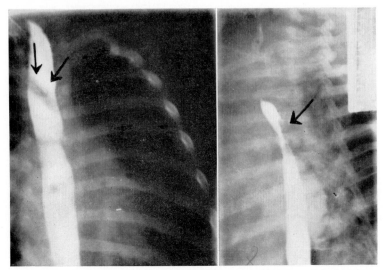

Figure 403.   Esophagogram of patient with anomalous right subclavian artery.

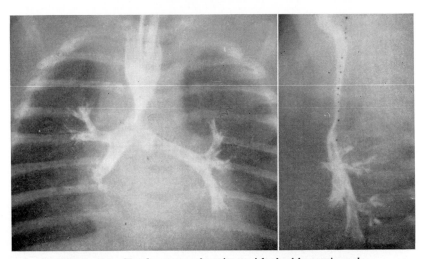

Figure 404.   Tracheogram of patient with double aortic arch.

from the roentgenologic studies of the barium-filled esophagus and the Lipiodol-filled trachea. In the few instances in which angiocardiography was performed the vascular structure was distinctly outlined.

Course and Prognosis

The symptoms of patients with vascular ring depend to a great extent on the nature of the anomaly and the severity of the compression. Children with double aortic arch usually have symptoms, consisting principally in respiratory embarrassment, early in infancy. A few infants are practically symptom-free, however. As a rule, patients with a right aortic arch and left ligamentum arteriosum do not have symptoms until later in childhood; the compression here also affects primarily the trachea, but it is not as severe as in patients with double aortic arch. In contrast to these two anomalies, the aberrant subclavian artery seldom cause any respiratory distress. The majority of the subclavian anomalies are completely asympto-

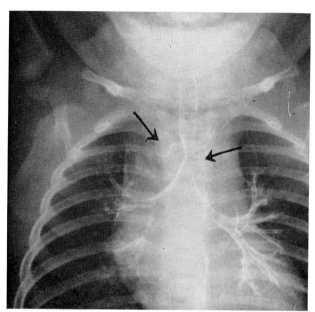

Figure 405.   Tracheogram of patient with right aortic arch and left ligamentum arteriosum.

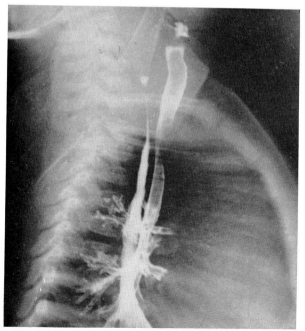

Figure 406.   Tracheogram of patient with anomalous innominate artery. Note the simultaneous filling of the esophagus and the trachea.

matic and are compatible with a normal life expectancy. In severe cases dysphagia may result.

The effects of anomalous innominate or left common carotid arteries are primarily respiratory and usually occur early in infancy.

Differential Diagnosis

Primarily the differential diagnosis of vascular rings concerns conditions causing repeated, chronic respiratory infections in infants and children. Among these, pancreatic fibrosis and tracheo-esophageal fistula, without esophageal atresia, should be considered and excluded by appropriate clinical, chemical and roentgenologic examinations.

Treatment

If the vascular rings cause symptoms and if there are radiologic evidences of compression, operation should be performed. The appropriate surgical techniques have been described in detail.[309] The aim of the surgical approach is to relieve the obstruction; in cases of double aortic arch, right aortic arch with left lingamentum arteriosum, and anomalous right subclavian artery, this is accomplished by severing the appropriate vessel. In cases of anomalous innominate or left common carotid arteries, obviously this cannot be accomplished without causing severe damage to the brain. Therefore, in these instances, the compression is relieved by simply pulling the vessels and fastening them anteriorly and to the side.

Summary

Anomalies of the aortic arch may cause compression of the esophagus and the trachea. Depending on the nature of the anomaly and the site of maximal compression, respiratory symptoms or dysphagia may dominate the picture. Particularly characteristic is the appearance of respiratory symptoms at feeding time. After preliminary barium studies of the esophagus and Lipiodol examination of the trachea, appropriate surgical repair is recommended if the symptoms are real and the compression is demonstrable.

THE HYPOPLASTIC LEFT HEART SYNDROME

The term "hypoplastic left heart syndrome," denoting obstructive valvar and vascular lesion on the left side of the heart resulting in more or less hypoplasia of the left ventricle, was coined by Lev.[418] Our own experiences have been summarized by Noonan.[536]

Incidence

This is not an uncommon anomaly. We have seen 100 patients with this syndrome in a 9-year period and consider it the most common cause of congestive heart failure in infants.[430] The experience at the Babies' Hospital in New York is similar to ours. Premature closure of the foramen ovale has been implicated in the etiology. There is a family history of other congenital anomalies, miscarriages or diabetes in more than a third of the patients.

Anatomy

A number of anatomic lesions, alone and in combination, may give rise to a hypoplastic left heart (Table 31, p. 797). Endocardial fibroelastosis of the secondary type is found in almost half of the patients. Usually the pulmonary artery is large, the arterioles are obstructed, and the right ventricle is hypertrophied and dilated. Noncardiac anomalies were associated with this syndrome in 37 per cent of our patients.

Physiology

The principal handicap is the elevated pressure in the left atrium, pulmonary vein and pulmonary artery, which places an undue burden on the right ventricle. A block at the aortic, aortic valvar or mitral valvar level is responsible for the left atrial hypertension. The left ventricular obstruction may be so maximal that the systemic output can be maintained only through the right ventricle via the pulmonary artery and the ductus arteriosus, in the manner of the fetal circulation. In contrast to the fetal circulation, however, the shunt through the atrial septum, if present, is from left to right.

AORTIC ATRESIA

Incidence

We have reported fifteen cases of pure aortic atresia.[536] Friedman and his associates[261] collected forty-four from the literature.

Clinical Picture

Most of these patients are critically ill within the first twenty-four to forty-eight hours of life, with cyanosis and combined right-sided and left-sided failure.

On physical examination, in addition to profound failure and cyanosis, one is impressed by the poor peripheral pulses, rapid respirations, and pallor. On auscultation systolic murmurs are not outstanding. As a matter of fact, in five out of ten of our patients none was heard; mid-diastolic murmurs were present in even fewer. Pulmonic closure is loud. The roentgenogram shows generalized cardiac enlargement early in life (Fig. 407). These are the patients who have the largest hearts within the first twenty-four to forty-eight hours. Pulmonary venous engorgment is evident in the films. Almost without exception, the electrocardiogram shows right ventricular hypertrophy and P pulmonale.

Cardiac catheterization is difficult in these critically ill, small babies. Meager observations indicate the following: (1) A left-to-right shunt is

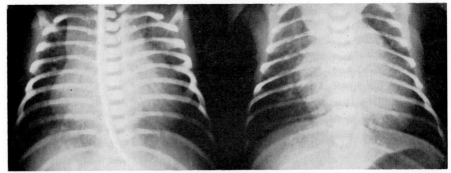

Figure 407. Posteroanterior films of the chests of two infants with aortic atresia. Note the cardiac enlargement, the dominant right atrium and right ventricle and the pulmonary vascular engorgement.

present at the atrial level. In most cases this is secondary to an atrial septal defect, but in at least one of our patients it was due to an anomalous pulmonary vein. There is systemic arterial unsaturation, due in part to pulmonary venous unsaturation and in part to a right-to-left ductal shunt. A ventricular shunt is rare. (2) Left atrial pressure is higher than right atrial pressure. Right ventricular and pulmonary arterial pressure is at systemic level or higher. Pulmonary venous wedge pressure is elevated. Systemic pressure is low-normal, but left ventricular pressure may be high. Usually there is a diastolic gradient across the mitral valve. (3) Pulmonary resistance is high. (4) The systemic flow is low-normal, but pulmonary flow may be slightly evelated (less than 50 per cent) because of the atrial left-to-right shunt. (5) The course of the catheter is not unusual. Passage through the mitral valve is difficult; passage across the aortic valve is impossible. The descending aorta may be entered through the ductus arteriosus. (6) Cine-angiography may demonstrate the prevailing shunt and, more importantly, the small left ventricular cavity.

Course and Prognosis

None of our patients lived beyond the fourth month of life, and most of them died within the first week.

Differential Diagnosis

The other entities making up the hypoplastic left heart syndrome group should be considered principally in the differential diagnosis. Although often no accurate distinction is possible without postmortem examination, the sudden onset of fatal congestive heart failure in an infant less than one week old with an extremely large heart strongly suggests this diagnosis. The only other important entity to be considered is critical aortic stenosis in infants who do not have a hypoplastic left heart. Often the distinction between these two situations is not possible without angiographic visualization of the cardiac chambers, but electrocardiographic evidence of severe left ventricular hypertrophy would certainly suggest severe aortic stenosis rather than atresia.

Treatment

Vigorous anticongestive measures represent the only medical approach to the problem. Surgically, the creation of a large atrial septal defect (if the ductus arteriosus remains open) may prove to be of some assistance.

MITRAL ATRESIA

Incidence

We have seen five patients with mitral atresia at The Children's Hospital Medical Center. Friedman reported eleven from the literature.[262]

Clinical Picture

Symptoms of cyanosis and congestive heart failure are noted somewhat later in these patients than in those of the previous group. On auscultation a harsh pansystolic murmur, due to ventricular septal defect or tricuspid regurgitation, is heard at the lower left sternal border. Associated coarctation of the aorta may be evidenced by relative hypertension of the arms. The roentgenograms and electrocardiograms are similar to those seen with aortic atresia, except that the cardiomegaly is not maximal and does not occur as early as it does in the previous group. Interestingly enough, an enlarged left atrium could be demonstrated on the roentgenogram in only one out of five patients (Figs. 408, 409).

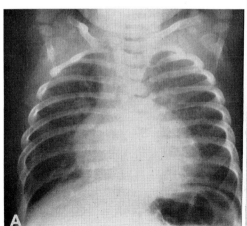
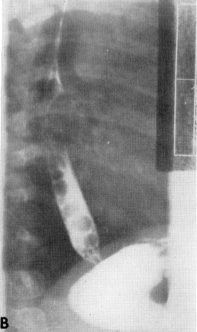

Figure 408. Posteroanterior and right anterior oblique films of patient with mitral atresia. Note the right-sided cardiac enlargement, the pulmonary vascular engorgement and the absence of left atrial enlargement.

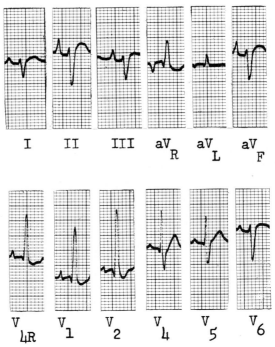

I   II   III   aV
R   aV
L   aV
F

V
4R   V
1   V
2   V
4   V
5   V
6

Figure 409. Electrocardiogram of patient with mitral atresia. Note the right axis deviation, minus 150 degrees, with a clockwise frontal plane loop, P pulmonale and right ventricular hypertrophy.

Results of *cardiac catheterization* are not significantly different from those described for patients with aortic atresia, except that *all* the blood entering the left atrium is shunted across the atrial septum into the right atrium, which then becomes a common mixing chamber. Naturally, in order to maintain a systemic flow, a right-to-left shunt across the ventricular septum is almost invariably present. Usually the ventricular septal defect is large and may actually result in an anatomic and physiologic single ventricle. Often the great arteries emerging from this single ventricle are transposed, or they may be in the corrected transposition relation to each other.

Course and Prognosis

It is possible for children with mitral atresia to live to the end of the first decade or even longer if both the atrial and the ventricular defects are large and if the pulmonic and systemic resistances are in a favorable relation to each other (just enough pulmonary stenosis to afford an adequate pulmonary flow, with systemic pressures in the ventricles, without flooding the lungs). Most patients, however, die within the first few months of life.

Differential Diagnosis

Mitral atresia is distinguished from other anomalies classified under the hypoplastic left heart syndrome by its common association with a single ventricle and by the abnormal takeoff of the great arteries. Furthermore, although these infants are critically ill, death usually does not occur within the first few days of life.

Treatment

As indicated, medical management may afford survival for a few months or even years. Creation of a large atrial septal defect has been helpful in two of our patients.

MITRAL STENOSIS

See page 586.

ATRESIA OF THE AORTIC ARCH

Incidence

We have six cases of this anomaly among our patients with the hypoplastic left heart syndrome. Kleinerman[399] reported 27 in 1958.

Clinical Picture

Since the interruption of the aortic arch usually occurs between the left common carotid and the insertion of the ductus arteriosus, cyanosis of the legs only would be expected. As a matter of fact, only one of our patients, and a small number in the literature, showed differential cyanosis. In most infants the cyanosis is generalized. Similarly, the expected relative hypertension of the arms is rarely noted. The reason for both these phenomena may be found in the presence of a large ventricular septal defect, anomalous origin of the brachiocephalic vessels, and congestive heart failure. At auscultation the systolic murmurs are nonspecific, as are the electrocardiograms and the roentgenograms.

We have made no *cardiac catheterization* studies of any of these infants, but in general the findings should not be too different from those described in the paragraphs on aortic atresia. A ventricular septal defect with a bi-directional shunt and a patent ductus arteriosus carrying pulmonary arterial blood into the descending aorta should be demonstrable by the course of the catheter, cine-angiography and oxygen saturation data.

Course and Prognosis

The longest survival reported among patients with this lesion was three years. Five of our six patients were dead before they were twenty days old.

Differential Diagnosis

Within the hypoplastic left heart group differentiation is possible only by means of most detailed cardiac catheterization and angiographic studies. In the rare instance in which differential cyanosis is present, the diagnosis may be made by clinical means. Obviously, it is almost impossible to differentiate between coarctation of the aorta with systemic right and left ventricles and aortic atresia with a hypoplastic left ventricle. I am sure that this distinction can be made only by the pathologist in most instances.

Treatment

Although, theoretically, a homograft or prosthesis may be inserted to correct the atresia of the aortic arch, we have never been able to accomplish this successfully. Even if it were possible, probably the presence of the other intracardiac and extracardiac anomalies would defeat the purpose of the operation. Anticongestive and antibiotic measures may prolong life for some weeks.

HYPOPLASIA OF THE AORTIC ARCH

Incidence

Hypoplasia of the aortic arch constitutes the largest group of patients within the hypoplastic left heart syndrome. More than two thirds of our patients had this anomaly. In most of them a patent ductus is present. Septal defects are demonstrable in half, mitral or aortic stenosis in a few.

Clinical Picture

Although, probably, of all the patients having the hypoplastic left heart syndrome, these are the least sick, still, 90 per cent of them have significant symptoms of respiratory distress, cyanosis and failure to thrive by the age of six weeks, and many considerably sooner.

There is relative hypertension of the arms. On auscultation, pulmonic

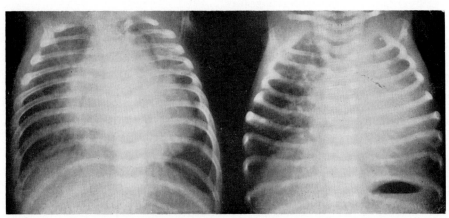

Figure 410. Posteroanterior films of patient with hypoplastic aortic arch. Note the essential similarity of the contour to those illustrated under aortic and mitral atresia.

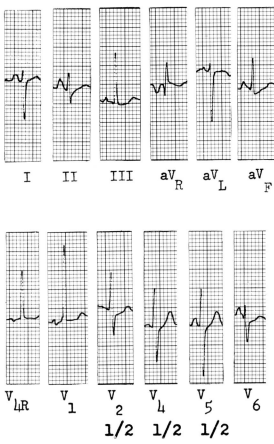

I   II   III   aV$_R$ aV$_L$ aV$_F$

V$_{4R}$ V$_1$ V$_2$ V$_4$ V$_5$ V$_6$

1/2   1/2   1/2

Figure 411. Electrocardiogram of patient with hypoplastic aortic arch. Note the right axis deviation, plus 135 degrees, with a clockwise frontal plane loop and right ventricular hypertrophy in the chest leads.

closure is uniformly loud, and in 80 per cent of the patients a harsh systolic murmur, grade 3 in intensity, or more, is present at the lower left sternal border. The electrocardiogram shows right ventricular hypertrophy, and roentgenologic examination reveals significant cardiac enlargement with pulmonary venous congestion (Figs. 410, 411).

Cardiac catheterization is somewhat more practical in these patients than in those having other varieties of this syndrome. The findings are, briefly, as follows: (1) There is a left-to-right, and occasionally a right-to-left, shunt at the ventricular level. A right-to-left shunt at the level of the ductus may also be present. (2) There is relative hypertension in the right brachial artery, and pulmonary venous pressure is elevated. (3) Pulmonary resistance is moderately high. (4) The systemic output is average, and the left-to-right shunt rarely equals systemic. (5) The catheter may pass across the ventricular septum or the ductus arteriosus from the right side and across the hypoplastic aortic arch in a retrograde fashion. (6) Cine-angiography may reveal the entire length of the hypoplastic segment of the aortic arch.

Course and Prognosis

Most of these infants, particularly those with severe associated anomalies, die within the first six weeks. Others with relatively uncomplicated lesions may live longer and may be operated on successfully as though they had simple preductal coarctation of the aorta. Still others may survive, like those with coarctation of the aorta with systemic right and left ventricle; the lesion remains inoperable, but the patients are not severely handicapped.

Differential Diagnosis

Often it is impossible to distinguish these infants from those with simple coarctation and congestive heart failure. On the whole, my view is that if they do not respond adequately to medical treatment, they are more likely to fall into the category of the hypoplastic left heart syndrome. Furthermore, the persistence of right ventricular hypertrophy in the electrocardiogram after the sixth month of age (in the few patients who survive that long) also points toward the hypoplastic left heart syndrome. Clearly, in many cases it is only a matter of semantics as to whether one classifies a patient as having coarctation with failure, or a hypoplastic aortic arch. Suggestions about the differential diagnosis of this entity are summarized in Table 32 (p. 798).

Treatment

The principles of management are the same as those outlined in the chapter on coarctation with congestive heart failure. Medical management should be tried first. If this fails, surgical intervention, at high risk, is completely justifiable.

Summary

As a group, patients with the hypoplastic left heart syndrome are critically ill young infants with left-sided and right-sided failure, pulmonary arterial hypertension and cyanosis. Among our patients this is the most common cause of congestive failure in the neonatal period. The differential diagnosis of the various entities is outlined in Table 32. The prognosis is almost uniformly poor. In selected cases palliative surgery, in terms of creation of an atrial septal defect or curative repair of the coarctation, may be indicated.

CONGENITAL MITRAL STENOSIS

In contrast to the patients with a hypoplastic left ventricle, a functioning left ventricle is present in the anomaly designated as "congenital mitral stenosis." The dividing line between the two malformations cannot be drawn sharply; in many instances the difference is quantitative rather than qualitative.

Incidence

This is a rare anomaly, indeed. Ferencz and her co-workers[242] were able to collect only thirty-four cases from the literature, to which they added nine of their own. We have seen five patients with congenital mitral stenosis within the past ten years. Starkey[664] reported the results of surgery on these patients.

Anatomy

Anatomically, the lesion is seldom an isolated one; associated endo-cardial fibroelastosis is usually found in those patients with severe stenosis who survive for more than a few days. Simultaneous involvement of the aortic valve and narrowing of the aorta are relatively common. A patent ductus arteriosus is present in almost half of the patients. Septal defects, except for an occasional patent foramen ovale, are rare. The consensus of almost all cardiologists is that whenever atrial septal defect with mitral stenosis is present (i.e. Lutembacher's syndrome), rheumatic etiology of the valvular lesion cannot be excluded with certainty. The involvement of the mitral valve is not too different from that in rheumatic heart disease; the leaflets are thickened, the commissures fused, and the chordae short-ened. All this may result in either a flat, diaphragm-like valve or a funnel-shaped one. In either case (and this may be the most outstanding characteristic) the texture of the valve is described as rubbery. Calcifications are rare.

Physiology

The hemodynamic consequences of congenital mitral stenosis are es-sentially the same as those outlined in the section on rheumatic mitral stenosis (p. 194). If a patent ductus arteriosus is associated with severe congenital mitral stenosis, the pulmonary vascular obstruction, secondary to the severe mitral block, may result in a right-to-left shunt through the ductus.

Clinical Picture

The clinical picture of congenital mitral stenosis varies considerably, depending on the severity of the lesion. Most infants with severe disease have symptoms within the first few months of life; occasionally a child may be free from symptoms for several years. Shortness of breath, exertional dyspnea and repeated, severe pulmonary infections are the most common symptoms. Cyanosis is mild. Interestingly enough, three of our five patients had bona fide syncopal attacks.

On physical examination underdevelopment is the most striking fea-ture; severe cyanosis is absent. Left chest prominence and a xiphoid type of impulse are usually present. Evidences of left-sided or right-sided con-gestive failure may be present, depending on the severity of the disease.

At auscultation, sinus rhythm is noted. Thus far we have not encoun-tered any patient with congenital mitral stenosis and atrial fibrillation. A loud first sound and an accentuated pulmonic closure are noted almost invariably. There is no opening snap, perhaps because of the rubbery nature of the valve. Keith[380] indicated that 15 per cent of these patients may have no murmur at all. We have noted a mid-diastolic rumble in all our patients, and four of the five even had a presystolic crescendo. An apical systolic murmur was present in three, and an equal number had a protodiastolic blow at the lower left sternal border.

The most characteristic roentgenologic finding is the presence of a prominent left atrium in the right anterior oblique view, with evidences of significant pulmonary venous congestion. Cardiac enlargement is only moderate and involves the right ventricle in addition to the left atrium (Fig. 412) and the pulmonary artery.

The electrocardiogram shows right ventricular hypertrophy, right axis deviation, P pulmonale and, occasionally, P mitrale (Fig. 413).

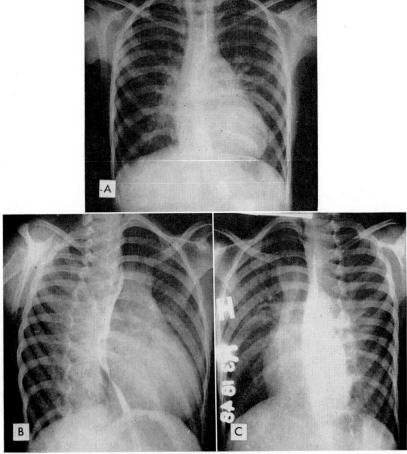

Figure 412. Posteroanterior and right anterior oblique views of patient with congenital mitral stenosis. Note the right ventricular enlargement, prominent main pulmonary artery segment and pulmonary vascular engorgement, particularly in the lower half of the lung field. Left atrial enlargement is demonstrated by the barium-filled esophagus in the posteroanterior and oblique views.

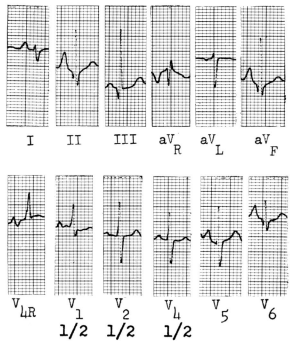

Figure 413. Electrocardiogram of patient with congenital mitral stenosis. Note the relatively mild right axis deviation, plus 105 degrees, with a clockwise frontal plane loop, right ventricular hypertrophy in the chest leads and combined atrial hypertrophy.

At *cardiac catheterization* (Fig. 414) the findings are identical with those described in the section on rheumatic mitral stenosis (p. 194), with increased pulmonary arterial pressure and pulmonary wedge pressure as high as 20 to 30 mm. of mercury.[458] In the cine-angiograms, delayed emptying of the left atrium is noted, together with the characteristic pattern of pulmonary venous drainage (p. 198) and a small but appreciable-sized left ventricular cavity.

Course and Prognosis

The prognosis for patients with congenital mitral stenosis varies considerably, depending on the severity of the stenosis and the associated defects. Infants with the most severe stenosis and left ventricular and aortic involvement resemble patients with a hypoplastic left ventricle and aortic atresia, in that they usually die within the first few weeks of life with pulmonary edema and congestive failure. Others, with relatively minor degrees of stenosis, may live for several years without severe disability. Eight of the ten patients described by Braudo and his associates[81] died at less than two years of age. Almost 50 per cent of Ferencz's[242] patients died at less than 6 months. At the time of operation our patients ranged from two and one-half to fifteen years of age, and one of the survivors is now twenty years old.

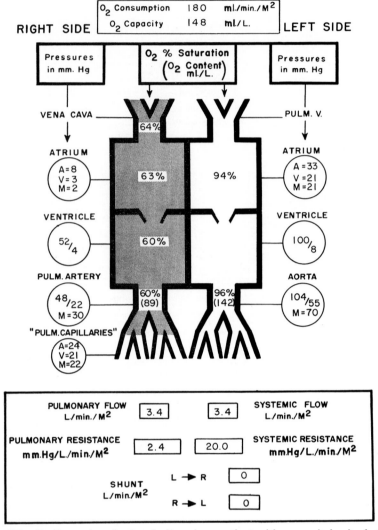

Figure 414. Cardiac catheterization findings in a patient with congenital mitral stenosis.

Differential Diagnosis

The differential diagnosis of congenital mitral stenosis is extremely difficult, often impossible.

Rheumatic Mitral Stenosis. The only way rheumatic mitral stenosis may be separated from congenital mitral stenosis, at present, is by considering the age at which heart disease was discovered. But since cases of rheumatic fever have been reported in young infants,[443] even this landmark may prove to be less reliable than was thought previously.

Hypoplastic Left Heart Syndrome. Although, as mentioned, no clear-cut dividing line exists, in all instances, between congenital mitral stenosis and the hypoplastic left heart syndrome with mitral and aortic valve involvement, still, the severe cyanosis, the cardiac enlargement and the early fatal termination usually identify a patient with an underdeveloped left ventricle. By outlining the size of the left ventricular cavity, cine-angiography may be helpful in the differential diagnosis.

Primary endocardial fibroelastosis and other members of the primary myocardial disease group without valve involvement may be identified by the absence of a murmur, by the left ventricular hypertrophy and the T-wave changes in the electrocardiogram and by the poor cardiac beat. At catheterization of the left side of the heart, no diastolic gradient can be found across the mitral valve, and the left atrial mean pressure equals the high left ventricular end-diastolic pressure.

Cor Triatriatum. It is difficult to distinguish cor triatriatum from congenital mitral stenosis without cardiac catheterization. At auscultation a diastolic rumble is rarely heard, and a murmur of mitral regurgitation is almost uniformly absent. Furthermore, left atrial enlargement is minimal. At cardiac catheterization the diagnostic clue is the finding of a pulmonary venous wedge pressure appreciably higher than left atrial pressure.

Pulmonary Vascular Obstruction. The diagnosis of the pulmonary vascular obstruction syndrome should never be made without identifying the associated septal defects or specifically excluding congenital mitral stenosis or cor triatriatum. Primary pulmonary vascular obstruction (essential pulmonary hypertension) is so rare in children that this diagnosis should be accepted with extreme reluctance and only if a septal defect is excluded by dye curves as well as angiograms and if a normal pulmonary venous wedge or left atrial pressure is clearly demonstrated.

Treatment

Congenital mitral stenosis may be treated surgically if the condition is uncomplicated and if coexisting endocardial fibroelastosis does not make all attempts at increasing left ventricular output futile. Bower and his associates[77] reported two cases in which surgical repair was attempted; one patient survived. Starkey[664] reported the results of surgery on five patients from our institution, with three survivors. One of these may be classified as having had a good result, the two others, only fair. It seems obvious from our experience, as well as that of others, that this is a difficult lesion to treat and that probably operation under direct vision, by means of the pump oxygenator, is the procedure of choice. The fear of creating mitral regurgitation in these grossly malformed valves is a justifiable one. Insertion of a prosthetic valve, some time in the future, may well be the only hope for ensuring adequate valve function in these patients.

At present, in my opinion, if the patient cannot be substantially improved by medical treatment, operation should be attempted in early infancy. If the child can survive, however, for a number of years, mitral valvuloplasty should be postponed until later, using the indications outlined in the section on rheumatic mitral stenosis (p. 201).

Summary

Congenital mitral stenosis should be suspected clinically in an infant who has evidences of pulmonary vascular obstruction, a large left atrium and a mitral diastolic murmur. At right heart catheterization pulmonary arterial hypertension and increased pulmonary venous wedge pressure are found; the diastolic gradient across the mitral valve may be demonstrated at left heart catheterization. The prognosis is poor in most instances. Operation, by means of the pump oxygenator, may be attempted with relatively high risks.

COR TRIATRIATUM

Incidence

Keith[380] collected 25 cases from the literature by 1958. We have had four patients at our institution.

Anatomy

The pulmonary veins enter a separate chamber at the superior dorsal aspect of the left atrium. If this chamber is completely separated from the left atrium, but communicates freely with the right atrium (Loeffler, type I), the anomaly should be considered under the heading of transposition of the pulmonary veins.

In the entity to be discussed here, the "third atrium," the receptacle of the pulmonary veins, is separated from the right atrium, but communicates through one or several small openings across a membrane with the "true" left atrium. This really amounts to "supravalvar mitral stenosis." The left atrium itself communicates with the atrial appendage and opens into the left ventricle through a normal, or relatively normal, mitral valve. Usually the foramen ovale is within the lower chamber (i.e. the left atrium proper), but occasionally it appears to open into the third atrium. The severity of the disease depends on the size of the orifice between the third chamber and the left atrium proper.

Physiology

The hemodynamic consequences are identical with those in mitral stenosis.

Clinical Picture

A few weeks after a normal birth these children with severe disease become dyspneic and show mild cyanosis and underdevelopment. Severe pneumonia and congestive heart failure ensue. The symptoms are indistinguishable from those seen with severe congenital mitral stenosis. Rarely, a patient with a relatively large communication between the third atrium and the left atrium may not show evidences of cardiac embarrassment until considerably later. In general, the findings at physical examination are similar to those presented by infants with congenital mitral stenosis and pulmonary vascular obstruction. Only in the auscultatory findings may there be some difference between the two conditions. None of our patients had the characteristic mid-diastolic rumble with presystolic accentuation. Keith referred to only one case in the literature with this finding.

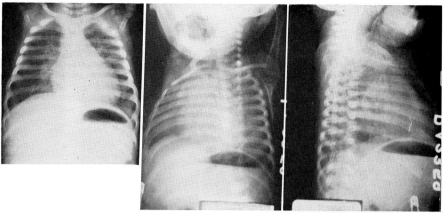

Figure 415. Three views of the heart of a patient with cor triatriatum. Note right atrial, right ventricular and possible left ventricular enlargement with prominent main pulmonary artery segment and pulmonary vascular engorgement.

The systolic murmur at the lower left sternal border, heard in half of the patients reported, is probably due to tricuspid regurgitation secondary to right-sided failure, rather than to mitral regurgitation. The absence of murmurs with evidences of pulmonary vascular obstruction does not exclude the diagnosis. Roentgenologic examination reveals right ventricular and pulmonary arterial enlargement with pulmonary venous congestion, but without a sizable left atrium (Fig. 415). The electrocardiographic findings are identical with those noted in congenital mitral stenosis.

At *cardiac catheterization* (Fig. 416) the findings in all but one respect are identical with those described in the section on mitral stenosis. The sole distinguishing feature is the appreciable gradient between the pulmonary capillary wedge and left atrial pressures, assuming that the latter was obtained by entering the lower chamber through the atrial septum. If the left atrium is approached through the back or if the foramen ovale opens into the third chamber, the pressure registered closely resembles that obtained from the pulmonary capillary wedge position. In other words, if an appreciable gradient is demonstrable between pulmonary capillary wedge and left atrial pressures, the diagnosis of cor triatriatum may be made with reasonable certainty. Absence of these findings does not exclude the diagnosis.

Course and Prognosis

Most infants with this anomaly succumb within the first few months of life, though exceptional patients with an adequate communication between the third chamber and the left atrium may survive until their teens and even to adulthood. Death occurs with pulmonary edema, pneumonia or chronic left-sided and right-sided failure.

Differential Diagnosis

Congenital Mitral Stenosis. See page 586.

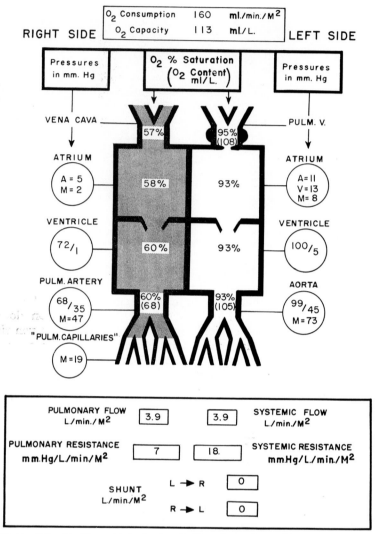

Figure 416.   Cardiac catheterization findings in patient with cor triatriatum.

Pulmonary Vascular Obstruction.   It should be emphasized here (see p. 607) that if the diagnosis of pulmonary vascular obstruction with congenital heart disease is to be made, the site of the septal defect must be identified. *The diagnosis of primary pulmonary vascular obstruction should never be made unless a low pulmonary capillary wedge pressure can be demonstrated. If this information is not available, I would recommend surgical exploration of the left atrium under direct vision to exclude cor triatriatum or mitral stenosis.*

The Hypoplastic Left Heart Syndrome.   See page 578.

Complete Transposition of the Pulmonary Veins with Pulmonary Arterial Hypertension.   This condition, which includes infants with subdiaphragmatic drainage, may pose a diagnostic problem. Within this group the patients with a large pulmonary flow may be identified relatively easily by the hyperkinetic impulse, the gallop rhythm and the large heart with active pulmonary vascular engorgement. Patients in whom the pulmonary flow is low and who have pulmonary vascular obstructive disease cannot be differentiated clinically from those with cor triatriatum; only cardiac catheterization, indicating identical saturations in the right atrium, the aorta and the pulmonary artery, reveals the correct diagnosis. It may be said here that functionally, and even anatomically, the two conditions are closely similar.

The Primary Myocardial Disease Group, Including Fibroelastosis. See Mitral Stenosis (p. 591).

Tumors of the Left Atrium. Only by angiography can a left atrial myxoma be differentiated from cor triatriatum with certainty. Of course, the episodic nature of the difficulties and the age of the patient may help in the differential diagnosis.

Treatment

The first successful repairs of cor triatriatum were reported by Vineberg[709] in 1956 and by Lewis[425] in the same year. In 1960 Therkelsen[689] reported one case in which surgery had been successful and indicated that a total of five had been operated on successfully up to that date.

As soon as the diagnosis is established, surgery under direct vision should be attempted. A blind procedure through the left atrial appendage may not allow adequate visualization. The operation consists in the creation of an adequate opening between the posterior chamber and the left atrium. In infants this is an exceedingly difficult procedure because of the very small structures and the posterior location of the third chamber. It is interesting to note that most of the successful case reports concerned older patients.

Summary

Patients with evidences of pulmonary vascular obstruction without a septal defect and with high pulmonary capillary wedge pressure should be suspected of having mitral stenosis or cor triatriatum. Although the correct diagnosis may not be established short of surgery, the latter anomaly may be suspected if the characteristic auscultatory and roentgenologic findings of mitral valve disease are absent and if a pressure gradient between the pulmonary capillaries and the left atrium can be demonstrated. Surgery carries high risks, but is recommended because of the poor prognosis of the disease.

CONGENTAL MITRAL REGURGITATION

Clinical evidences of mitral regurgitation in young children, or in patients with other congenital heart disease, should lead the cardiologist to the consideration of congenital mitral insufficiency. Within recent years a number of publications have focused attention on the medical and surgical aspects of this entity.[217, 568, 664, 679]

Anatomy

Congenital mitral incompetence may be associated with other congenital heart disease. In patients with endocardial cushion defect, a cleft mitral valve and anomalous insertion of the chordae are the anatomic explanations of functional incompetence (see p. 384). In patients with corrected transposition of the great arteries there may be either an Ebstein type of misplacement of the valve or short chordae tendineae (see p. 715). In children with severe coarctation of the aorta the valves themselves may be deformed, and it seems to me perfectly feasible that even a normal valve may become incompetent if the left ventricular pressure is so high that cardiac dilatation occurs. This may result in a vicious circle with progressively more mitral regurgitation, increased left ventricular volume and more dilatation of the valve ring. A dilated valve ring may also result from dilatation of the left ventricle such as is seen in patients with patent ductus arteriosus, ventricular septal defect or endorcardial fibroelastosis.

Solitary congenital mitral regurgitation may be seen in patients with Marfan's syndrome. Dilated valve rings, anomalously inserted short chordae or extra openings in one of the cusps have also been noted without any other congenital anomaly. Of ten patients described by Talver,[679] three had coarctation of the aorta, two had corrected transposition of the great arteries, and two had patent ductus arteriosus. In the remaining three patients the mitral incompetence was due to apparently primary dilatation of the valve ring, the anatomy also observed at surgery by Starkey[664] in our two patients.

Physiology

There is no difference between the physiologic effects of acquired and congenital mitral regurgitation except for the hemodynamic consequences of the associated lesions.

Clinical Picture

The clinical picture may be dominated by the associated lesions, and mitral regurgitation may manifest itself solely through the typical apical systolic murmur, the hyperdynamic left ventricular impulse and the left atrial enlargement on the roentgenogram.

In cases of solitary mitral regurgitation, the signs and symptoms are identical with those described in patients having rheumatic heart disease. In one of our patients the principal symptom was due to the compression of the left main bronchus and the left pulmonary artery by the giant left atrium (Fig. 417). Almost without exception the murmur is discovered within the first year of life.

Cardiac catheterization (Fig. 418) reveals findings similar to those encountered with rheumatic mitral incompetence. The only significant difference is that mild to moderate pulmonary arterial hypertension is

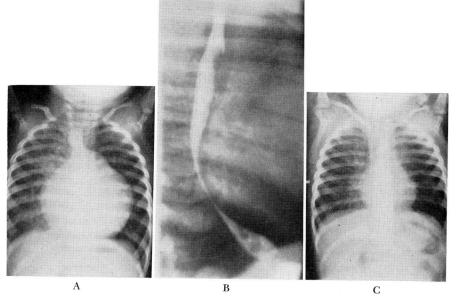

Figure 417. Preoperative and postoperative films of patient with congenital mitral regurgitation. *A,* Preoperative film showing the cardiac enlargement with a prominent main pulmonary artery segment. Note the obstructive emphysema of the left lung with deviation of the trachea to the right. *B,* The impression of the large left atrium on the barium-filled esophagus. It was this left atrium that, by compressing the left main bronchus, caused the emphysema. *C,* Postoperative film after repair of the mitral regurgitation and lobectomy.

a common concomitant of congenital mitral regurgitation (seven out of eight of Talver's patients). Paralleling the increased pulmonary arterial pressure is an increase in pulmonary capillary wedge pressure, with the typical pressure pulses (see p. 202). Left heart catheterization is useful principally in demonstrating, angiographically, the mitral regurgitation and the anatomy of the mitral valve. At present we have no truly reliable tools for quantitative estimation of the degree of insufficiency.

Course and Prognosis

The presence of mitral regurgitation aggravates the prognosis of coarctation of the aorta, ventricular septal defect or patent ductus arteriosus, and it may be the principal hemodynamic handicap in endocardial cushion defect, as well as in corrected transposition of the great arteries. As far as solitary mitral regurgitation is concerned, some of the small fenestrations of the valve may prove to be completely innocuous. On the other hand, in patients with wide mitral valve rings, chronic congestive heart failure may develop and may lead to early death. All the six patients with complete protocols in Talver's article had severe difficulties within the first decade. One of our patients, the boy with compression of the bronchus and pulmonary artery, was in severe difficulty in infancy, whereas the others failed to show significant symptoms until the second decade. Therefore it may be said that the prognosis of congenital mitral regur-

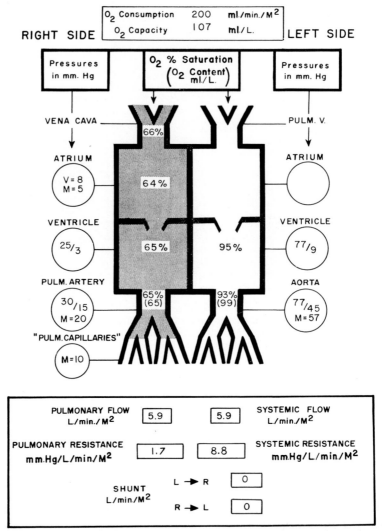

Figure 418. Cardiac catheterization findings in a boy with congenital mitral regurgitation.

gitation varies considerably and depends on the severity of the incompetence.

Differential Diagnosis

Within the framework of the congenital heart disease entities enumerated earlier (see p. 596), mitral regurgitation should be suspected clinically by the characteristic auscultatory and radiologic findings. The high pulmonary arterial or left atrial pressure, with its characteristic pressure pulse contour, and particularly cine-angiograms, with left ventricular injection, prove the diagnosis at catheterization.

The separation of rheumatic mitral incompetence from a congenital defect is extremely difficult, but may be made, on a presumptive basis, by age alone. Of course, the presence of associated congenital heart defects or Marfan's syndrome implies a congenital origin. Only direct visualization of the valve, with a left atrial biopsy, can substantiate the diagnosis. A small ventricular septal defect may be difficult, if not impossible, to differentiate clinically from rheumatic mitral regurgitation (see p. 410).

Treatment

In cases of mitral regurgitation with patent ductus arteriosus, ventricular septal defect or coarctation of the aorta, the latter defects should be treated surgically first. It may take a full year or two before optimal benefits from these procedures, in relation to the mitral incompetence, may be obtained. In patients with endocardial cushion defect, repair of the cleft mitral valve is part and parcel of the correction of the entire complex.

In patients with solitary congenital mitral regurgitation of appreciable severity and in patients whose associated lesions have been corrected without significantly influencing the incompetent mitral valve, repair (by means of the pump oxygenator) is indicated. In most instances this should consist in tightening the valve ring, reefing the enlarged left atrium and repairing the anomalous chordae. Both of our patients and six of Talver's improved appreciably postoperatively, but mortality statistics may not be taken too seriously in view of the small number of patients treated so far (Fig. 419). The optimal age for operation is probably between five and fifteen years.

Summary

Patients with congenital mitral regurgitation exhibit the signs and symptoms of rheumatic mitral regurgitation at a younger age, without a history of rheumatic fever, and often in association with other congenital

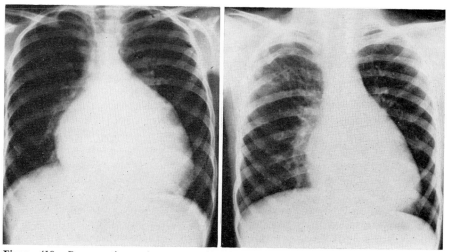

Figure 419. Preoperative and postoperative films of patient with congenital mitral regurgitation.

cardiac deformities. Surgical treatment is available for those with severe disease.

THE PULMONARY VASCULAR OBSTRUCTION SYNDROME

General Principles

The pulmonary arterial systolic pressure of normal persons is about one fourth or one fifth of the systemic arterial systolic pressure (Fig. 247). A significant elevation of pulmonary arterial pressure may be the result of either an increase in pulmonary blood flow (hyperkinetic) or a significant increase in pulmonary resistance, with normal or even diminished pulmonary blood flow (obstructive) (Fig. 247). In the pulmonary vascular obstruction syndrome the pulmonary arterial systolic pressure is elevated to levels identical with, or closely approximating, the systemic arterial pressure, because of an increase in pulmonary vascular resistance. Thus this syndrome becomes a physiologic entity with good correlations between the calculated resistance and the actual histologic picture of the pulmonary vasculature.[176] The increase in pulmonary vascular resistance may be restricted to the arteriolar level and, thus, associated with normal left atrial or pulmonary capillary wedge pressure (primary pulmonary arterial hypertension, "Eisenmenger's syndrome").[749] In another group of patients (those with left ventricular failure, mitral stenosis, cor triatriatum or transposition of the pulmonary veins with obstruction) obstructive pulmonary arterial hypertension is associated with, and may even be secondary to, increased left atrial and pulmonary capillary pressure. It is my view that these two entities, those with increased and those with normal left atrial pressure,[750] may not be as clearly separable as they seem at first glance. I have often wondered whether the increased pulmonary arteriolar resistance encountered in some patients with a large ventricular septal defect may not have been stimulated in the first place by high left atrial pressure, secondary to left ventricular failure. This unproved theory may explain why patients who have ventricular septal defects of the same size may or may not have pulmonary vascular obstructive disease; those without pulmonary arterial hypertension have a competent left ventricle operating at a low left atrial pressure even in the face of a large left-to-right shunt through a ventricular septal defect. In contrast, the patient with a similar-sized ventricular septal defect may have a relatively incompetent left ventricle, which needs a high filling pressure to accomplish the large output required because of the ventricular septal defect. This difference in left ventricular filling pressure would explain why pulmonary vascular obstructive disease develops in one patient and not in another.

Be that as it may, pulmonary arterial pressure which approximates systemic level, with relatively normal flow, is referred to in our institution as the pulmonary vascular obstruction syndrome. We exclude from this group patients with clear-cut cor pulmonale in whom clinically obvious parenchymatous or ventilatory factors are principally responsible for the pulmonary arterial hypertension. We include, however, patients with primary pulmonary hypertension,[207, 747] those with systemic and pulmonary communications in whom a dominant right-to-left shunt exists and, finally, those with pulmonary venous hypertension without shunts. Thus this syndrome encompasses all the conditions that Wood included in the definition of "Eisenmenger's syndrome," and more. It may be justifiable to ask why these varied pathologic entities should all be discussed under one heading. The answer is that *the clinician who first encounters these patients sees a relatively homogeneous clinical profile, irrespective of the underlying anatomy*.[176] Only after careful consideration of all the clinical and hemodynamic data will an accurate and therapeutically meaningful diagnosis emerge.

Incidence

The incidence of this condition cannot be estimated with any accuracy at this time. If only the patients with "essential" or "primary" pulmonary hypertension were considered, the incidence would be extremely low, particularly within the pediatric age group. If, however, patients with congenital heart disease and pulmonary vascular obstruction are included (which we consider reasonable), the incidence may easily be estimated at more than 10 per cent of all patients with congenital heart disease. Wood encountered "Eisenmenger's syndrome" in 8 per cent of his first 1000 cases of congenital heart disease.

Anatomy

The elastic fibers in the *large arteries* resemble the fetal pattern in the patients with common ejectile force (ventricular septal defect, patent ductus arteriosus, and so forth),[331] whereas in "acquired" pulmonary arterial hypertension these fibers have normal adult distribution (atrial septal defect). Atheromata, thrombosis or emboli are rare in children.

In the *medium-sized muscular arteries* the media seems thickened and resembles the fetal pattern. Intimal changes are almost never seen in infants and rarely in large numbers in patients less than eight to ten years of age.

As mentioned earlier (p. 420), the *small arterioles* may show "post-stenotic dilatation."

In primary pulmonary arterial hypertension the heart is normal except for right ventricular hypertrophy, though a patent foramen ovale may be present.

In pulmonary vascular obstruction associated with structural heart disease the following entities may be encountered:

(1) Diseases of the left side of the heart: (*a*) coarctation of the aorta, (*b*) aortic stenosis, (*c*) hypoplastic left heart syndrome, (*d*) primary myocardial disease, (*e*) mitral stenosis, and (*f*) cor triatriatum.

(2) Systemic to pulmonary communications: (*a*) truncus arteriosus, (*b*) aortopulmonary fenestration, (*c*) patent ductus arteriosus, (*d*) ventricular septal defect, (*e*) endocardial cushion defect, (*f*) secundum atrial septal defect, and (*g*) complete transposition of the pulmonary veins.

Physiology

Physiologically, as pointed out earlier, the greatly increased pulmonary resistance dominates the picture; figures calculated from the pressure gradients across the pulmonary bed and the pulmonary blood flow show that the pulmonary resistance is equal to or higher than the systemic resistance. This increase in resistance causes pulmonary and right ventricular hypertension and thus increases appreciably the work of the right ventricle, and occasionally even that of the right atrium. If the pressure in the right side of the heart is markedly elevated, a right-to-left shunt occurs either through a septal defect or through a forcibly opened foramen ovale.

Clinical Picture

Pulmonary vascular obstruction in young children may cause no symptoms at all. In older children, with more severe disease, exertional dyspnea, transient or permanent cyanosis, chest pain and syncope are noted. Wood[749] emphasized that hemoptysis is a frequent cause of death in adults with "Eisenmenger's syndrome." In contrast, primary pulmonary hypertension, according to him, is rarely accompanied by hemoptysis; the difference is thought to be due to the polycythemia which accompanies "Eisenmenger's syndrome." Squatting rarely occurs.

On physical examination the majority of these patients are fairly well developed. Cyanosis of mild degree, with slight clubbing, is frequently, though not invariably, present. The cardiac impulse is forceful and is localized at the xiphoid process. At auscultation the most outstanding finding is the greatly accentuated, even booming, rather narrow second sound at the pulmonary area.

It is worth emphasizing that in patients with ventricular septal defect and pulmonary vascular obstruction the second sound is often single, whereas in those with atrial septal defect and patent ductus arteriosus, splitting may be detected; in severe cases of primary pulmonary hypertension the second sound may even be widely split, with a late and loud pulmonary component. A pulmonic ejection click is common.

Of course, in patients with left-sided disease, the clinical manifesta-

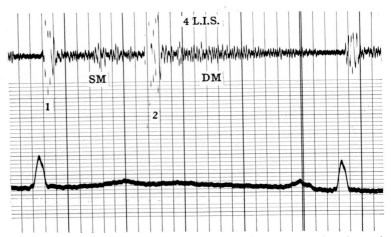

Figure 420. Phonocardiogram of patient with pulmonary vascular obstruction syndrome. Note the relatively unimpressive systolic murmur and the long loud diastolic murmur at the fourth left interspace.

tions of the underlying lesion may be more or less evident. It is important to emphasize, however, that the features of the pulmonary vascular obstruction syndrome may represent the dominant profile, irrespective of the underlying disease.

A grade 2 to 3 soft, blowing systolic murmur at the left sternal border is present in the majority, but not all, of the patients. Patients with maximal pulmonary vascular obstruction may have an early insufficiency blow at the left sternal border (Fig. 420). No mid-diastolic shunt rumble is audible at the apex in these children.

Roentgenologic examination reveals a moderate degree of right ventricular enlargement and a prominent main pulmonary arterial segment (Fig. 421). The pulmonary vasculature characteristically shows accentuated hilar markings with diminished peripheral vasculature. A "hilar dance" may be present at fluoroscopy. Only if the underlying disease is principally left-sided is there enlargement of the left atrium.

The electrocardiogram shows severe right ventricular hypertrophy

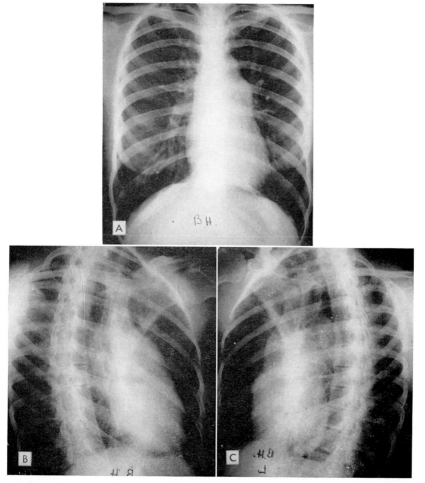

Figure 421. Posteroanterior and oblique roentgenograms of patient with pulmonary vascular obstruction.

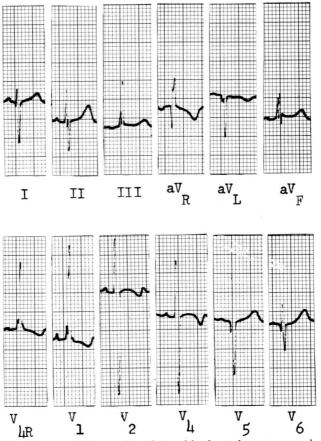

Figure 422. Electrocardiogram of patient with the pulmonary vascular obstructive syndrome. Note the moderate right axis deviation, plus 150 degrees, with a clockwise frontal plane loop and right ventricular hypertrophy.

with moderate P pulmonale (Fig. 422). Occasionally, P mitrale is encountered in the patients with left atrial enlargement.

Cardiac catheterization reveals the following (Fig. 423): (1) Oxygen determinations reveal no evidence of a significant left-to-right shunt at any level. More sensitive methods (hydrogen electrode) may reveal a minimal left-to-right shunt. Right-to-left shunts of varying severity may be demonstrated by means of arterial oxygen unsaturation in patients with pulmonary-systemic communications. (2) Right ventricular and pulmonary arterial systolic pressure at systemic level or higher, with elevated diastolic pressure, is uniformly present. Left atrial and pulmonary capillary pressures are elevated only in patients with left atrial or left ventricular disease. Measurement of the pulmonary wedge pressure may be difficult, if not impossible. (3) Total pulmonary resistance is markedly elevated (10 to 20 units per square meter). How much of this is due to increased resistance at the pulmonary venous level and how much at the pulmonary arteriolar level depends on the underlying disease. (4) Pulmonary flow is never significantly larger than systemic flow; often it is smaller because of a right-to-left shunt. (5) The course of the catheter depends on

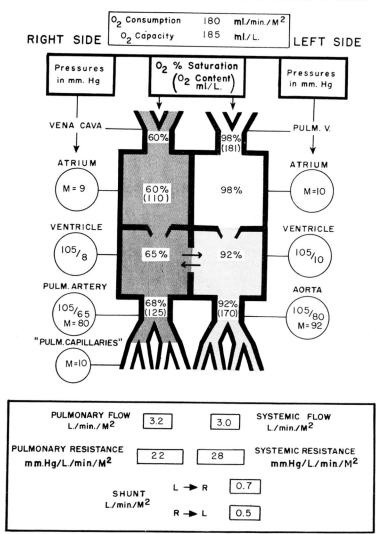

Figure 423. Catheterization findings of patient with the pulmonary vascular obstructive syndrome.

the underlying anomaly. (6) Cine-angiograms are helpful in demonstrating the constricted pulmonary arteries, and in patients with left-sided disease the dye lingers in the left atrium. (7) Dye-dilution curves and intracardiac phonocardiograms are not particularly helpful in the diagnosis except in identification of the accompanying defects.

In patients with pulmonary vascular obstruction syndrome cardiac catheterization and angiography entail a somewhat higher, but surely not prohibitive, risk.

Course and Prognosis

The course and prognosis of the pulmonary vascular obstruction syndrome clearly cannot be discussed without considering the associated anomalies, if they are present.

Primary pulmonary hypertension in infants and children is a rare and malignant disease, the downhill course of which must be measured in terms of months or a few years. The prognosis of pulmonary vascular obstruction secondary to left-sided failure is equally ominous, if not more so. Among the left atrial or pulmonary venous diseases, mitral stenosis is the only one that is likely to allow survival for some time without surgery. Pulmonary venous obstruction or cor triatriatum is likely to lead to death within the first year or even the first six months of life. The course in patients with pulmonary systemic communications and pulmonary vascular obstruction has already been described in some detail in the discussion of the respective lesion.

Suffice it to say here that the status of the pulmonary vascular resistance, as determined at cardiac catheterization, is comparatively stable throughout infancy and childhood in all but a minority of the patients with a ventricular or pulmonary arterial communication. Although it is fully possible that histologic changes are progressive, even in the early years, as far as the clinical picture is concerned there is very little change. Right ventricular and pulmonary arterial pressures and resistances, arterial saturation, heart size and the electrocardiographic findings are all unchanged or may even show improvement throughout the first and second decades. Toward the second half of the second decade, and surely in the third decade, the disease progresses rapidly downhill.[722] To a certain extent, secundum atrial defects are an exception to this rule in that, as mentioned earlier, pulmonary vascular obstruction may develop *in adult life,* and then may be rapidly progressive. Furthermore, patients with patent ductus arteriosus may also have a somewhat more rapid progression of the pulmonary vascular obstruction than occurs in patients with a ventricular septal defect.

In a discussion of "Eisenmenger's syndrome," Wood[749] stated that "recurrent hemoptysis begins in adult life and may prove fatal; if patients survive other risks, such as cerebral abscess, bacterial endocarditis, and ill-advised surgical intervention, they succumb finally to heart failure, usually in the fourth or fifth decade." Another way of putting it is by stating that the last time I discussed a patient with patent ductus arteriosus and pulmonary vascular obstruction in one of the neighboring institutions, it was pointed out that this man, at the age of thirty-five, was the first patient they had had for some years with this condition, at this age, who was *not* playing basketball. All this does not mean that one is unmindful of the definitely shortened life expectancy of these patients, as well as their debilitating symptomatology beginning at the second half of the second or third decade. What should be emphasized is that the day of doom may not be as imminent for many of these patients as it would appear at first glance. Furthermore, the risks of surgery should be considered with the thought in mind that the average age at death in Wood's series was thirty-three to thirty-six years, with maximum life expectancy between fifty-five and sixty-five years. Death in the pediatric age group, beyond early infancy and without extremely complex lesions, is rare. The onset of syncope and hemoptysis is an ominous prognostic sign.

One further point to be mentioned in the prognosis of these patients is the fact that sudden death is relatively common. It usually occurs in a syncopal attack, perhaps associated with convulsions and probably due to sudden decrease of the cardiac output as a result of increased pulmonary vascular obstruction. Also, I have seen death occur during cardiac catheterization, angiography, bone marrow biopsy and even while the circulation time was being determined by injection of Decholin.

Differential Diagnosis

The following entities are the principal ones to be considered:

Large Left-to-Right Shunt with or without Pulmonary Arterial Hypertension. The group as a whole may be identified on the basis of cardiac enlargement, uniformly plethoric lung fields, hyperdynamic cardiac impulse, left chest deformity and apical diastolic rumble. Individual members of the group (atrial defect, ventricular defect or patent ductus arteriosus) can usually be recognized clinically by the characteristic auscultatory phenomena, electrocardiograms and specific radiologic contours. Cardiac catheterization is frequently necessary to confirm the diagnosis.

Valvar Pulmonic Stenosis with Patent Foramen Ovale. Valvar pulmonic stenosis with patent foramen ovale may simulate the clinical picture of pulmonary vascular obstruction syndrome in many respects. Exertional dyspnea and mild cyanosis may constitute the presenting symptoms in both groups. It may be impossible to distinguish between the radiograms or the electrocardiograms in the two conditions. The physical examination, however, revealing the characteristic stenotic murmur at the left sternal border with an absent or decreased pulmonic second sound, usually establishes the diagnosis of pulmonic stenosis. Obviously, the surest diagnostic criterion of pulmonic stenosis is the demonstration of low pulmonary arterial pressure with a gradient across the right ventricular outflow tract.

Pulmonic Stenosis and Corrected Transposition of the Great Arteries with a Right-to-Left Shunt through a Ventricular Defect. Occasionally a patient with this group of anomalies may be confused with one having the pulmonary vascular obstruction syndrome, since the left-sided and anterior position of the aorta may cause a loud, single second sound at the second left interspace. The characteristic auscultatory findings, in addition to the roentgenologic contour and the abnormalities in the electrocardiogram, may be helpful in the clinical diagnosis, but cardiac catheterization studies are usually essential for complete analysis.

Cor Pulmonale. Cor pulmonale can be easily identified by the characteristic history, the physical examination and the pulmonary function studies.

Once the pulmonary vascular obstruction syndrome has been diagnosed on clinical grounds and pulmonary arterial hypertension, with markedly elevated pulmonary resistance, has been demonstrated at cardiac catheterization, it is extremely important that an accurate anatomic diagnosis be made also, since a number of conditions giving rise to the syndrome are surgically correctible, and in those which are not, the prognosis is variable, depending on the exact anatomic situation.

Physiologic studies should furnish answers to the following questions: (1) *Is there any left atrial hypertension?* This should be determined either by registering the pulmonary capillary pressure or by measuring left atrial pressure, using one of the methods discussed previously (see p. 139). *If this is not feasible and if no other anatomic diagnosis is established, surgical exploration of the left atrium and mitral valve is mandatory.* If there is no pulmonary venous or left atrial hypertension, all the conditions discussed under left-sided disease (see pp. 578-99) may be excluded. (2) *Is there any intracardiac or extracardiac shunt?* Selective cine-angiograms and dye-dilution curves, with injections into the right and left sides and sampling from both sides, may be necessary before the presence and location of a septal defect or patent ductus arteriosus may be detected. *Only if the answers to both questions are in the negative may the diagnosis of primary pulmonary hypertension be made.* The one exception to this statement is that a right-to-left shunt is possible with a patent foramen ovale, even in patients with primary pulmonary hypertension. Consequently, if only an atrial right-to-left shunt, without any previous evidence of a left-to-right shunt, is demonstrated in a patient with pulmonary vascular obstruction, probably the diagnosis of primary pulmonary hypertension may be made with assurance.

Treatment

Unfortunately no medical treatment is available for patients with the pulmonary vascular obstruction syndrome. A number of palliative measures will be mentioned briefly, with the understanding that nothing spectacular can be expected from them; at best the progression of the condition may be temporarily halted.

The avoidance of fatigue is important in the management of these children. Plenty of sleep at night and at least one or two hours of rest in the afternoon are mandatory. Prompt antibiotic treatment for, and even continuous chemoprophylaxis against, respiratory disease are recommended. The use of Gantrisin for chemoprophylaxis and one of the broad-spectrum antibiotics for treatment is advisable. Inhalation of oxygen for thirty minutes, two or three times a day, has been recommended without much proof of its efficacy. The intramuscular administration of Priscoline, an antispasmodic, has been recommended by Dresdale and his co-workers[207] to reduce the pulmonary vascular resistance. Grover and his associates[314] found the responses of the pulmonary resistance to Priscoline encouraging at cardiac catheterization. Our own experiments failed[604] to show any significant decrease in resistance at catheterization, under the influence of Priscoline, aminophylline or Reserpine. A long-term anticoagulant regimen has been recommended by Wood. I have had no experience with the efficacy of this treatment, but in view of the frequent occurrence of hemoptysis, I would not be too enthusiastic about it. Venesection, except in older patients with excessively high hematocrit levels (more than 85 per cent), also seems ineffective.

Surgical treatment of the various lesions accompanying pulmonary vascular obstruction has already been discussed in their respective chapters. *I would like to summarize the surgical treatment by saying that at present there is justification for surgical intervention only if a left-sided lesion is causing the vascular obstruction. In patients who have pulmonary-systemic communications without a net left-to-right shunt, there is no excuse for surgery today.* The problem of patients with borderline left-to-right shunts and atrial septal defect, ventricular septal defect or patent ductus arteriosus has already been discussed at length. A pulmonary banding procedure has been proposed for reversal of the pulmonary vascular obstructive changes in patients without a net left-to-right shunt. I have had no experience with this procedure, and results from elsewhere seem discouraging.

Summary

Pulmonary vascular obstruction is characterized by clinical and physiologic evidences of right ventricular and pulmonary arterial hypertension, secondary to severe increased pulmonary resistance, without a sizable left-to-right shunt. Exertional dyspnea, cyanosis, syncope and chest pain are the dominant symptoms. A booming pulmonary closure without a pronounced murmur, roentgenologic evidence of moderate right ventricular enlargement, and electrocardiographic evidence of severe right ventricular hypertrophy are the most important clinical features. The condition may or may not be associated with structural heart disease. Long-term prognosis is poor; surgical treatment is available only for patients with left-sided obstructive disease.

PRIMARY PULMONARY HYPERTENSION

This diagnosis may be arrived at only by exclusion. It represents obstructive pulmonary arterial hypertension of moderate or severe degree without intrinsic heart disease.

Incidence

It is difficult to arrive at the true incidence of this condition. Wood[747] cited it as 0.17 per cent of 10,000 patients surveyed by clinical means. Yu[757] stated that the total number of cases reported by 1958 was eighty-six. The female-to-male ratio is usually estimated to be between 3:1 and 4:1. Among the total number of cases reported, the number in children is small. By 1958 Keith was able to collect only 16 cases in patients less than 10 years of age. Yu estimated the percentage of those between the ages of 12 and 20 at 16 per cent. By 1958 the total number of patients less than 12 years old was eighteen. We have seen five such patients in our institution, three of whom were members of one family.

The etiology is not known. Husson,[354] Coleman[153] and Dresdale[206] are among the most recent authors to mention familial occurrence. Rawson[575] claimed a higher than usual incidence of collagen disease and Raynaud's disease in a family of patients with primary pulmonary hypertension. On the basis of microscopic findings in the pulmonary artery, Heath and Edwards[322] suggested that the condition is acquired.

Anatomy

Except for right ventricular and right atrial hypertrophy and an occasional patent foramen ovale, the heart is normal. The main pulmonary artery is dilated, but the elastic structure usually shows an adult pattern.[332] The principal changes are in the small muscular arteries and the arterioles, which show spotty, intimal proliferation and medial thickening. The larger vessels show changes of atherosclerosis and secondary thrombosis

Physiology

The pulmonary arterial hypertension imposes an appreciable amount of pressure-work on the right ventricle, which leads to an increase in ventricular filling pressure and right atrial hypertension.

Clinical Picture

The symptoms include fatigue, dyspnea and exercise intolerance. Syncope is common, and angina has been described in adults. Feeding troubles, vomiting and failure to thrive have been noted in the few infants described. Cyanosis is usually peripheral and is due to increased oxygen extraction, secondary to the low cardiac output. In some patients the high right atrial pressure forces the foramen ovale open, and central shunt cyanosis results. On physical examination one is impressed by the evidences of low output: small pulse, cold extremities and peripheral cyanosis. An A wave is seen at the jugular venous pulse. The pulmonary outflow tract is strongly pulsating. The cardiac impulse is heaving and is purely right ventricular. There is a pulmonic ejection click, and the second sound is closely split, with a booming pulmonic component at the second left interspace. A fourth sound may be heard at the lower left sternal border and the apex. Murmurs are absent in almost half of the patients.[757] The loudest systolic murmurs originate from tricuspid regurgitation; the pulmonary ejection murmur is not impressive. A Graham Steell murmur can be heard in about 25 per cent of the patients.

The most impressive feature in the roentgenogram is the prominent main pulmonary artery segment, which pulsates vigorously under the fluoroscope. The prominence of the hilar vessels contrasts sharply with the narrowness of the peripheral vasculature. There is enlargement of the right ventricle and the right atrium, and the aorta is small (Fig. 424).

The electrocardiogram reveals right ventricular and right atrial hypertrophy. In some small infants this may not be excessive, in spite of maximal pulmonary arterial hypertension (Fig. 425). Children have normal sinus

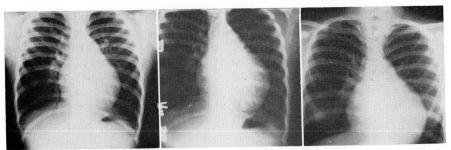

Figure 424. Progressive cardiac enlargement over a three-year period in patient with the pulmonary vascular obstructive syndrome.

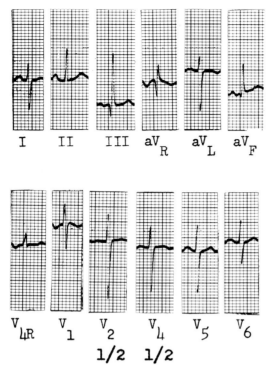

I   II   III   aV$_R$ aV$_L$ aV$_F$

V$_{4R}$ V$_1$ V$_2$ V$_4$ V$_5$ V$_6$

1/2 1/2

Figure 425. Relatively normal electrocardiogram in an infant with familial primary pulmonary vascular obstructive syndrome. Note the mean electrical axis of plus 120 degrees, the clockwise frontal plane loop and the right ventricular hypertrophy in the chest leads, which is not necessarily abnormal in an infant. A few weeks after this cardiogram had been taken the baby died in right-sided heart failure.

rhythm, but Wood[747] stated that atrial fibrillation is common in adults. The axis is to the right in the frontal plane, and the loop is clockwise.

At *cardiac catheterization* (Fig. 426) the following features are noted. (1) There is no evidence of a left-to-right shunt, but systemic arterial saturation may be lower than normal because of an atrial right-to-left shunt. Arterial oxygen saturation may vary from 70 to 95 per cent. Significantly, in contrast to patients with patent ductus arteriosus and pulmonary vascular obstructive disease, there is no difference between the oxygen saturation of the right brachial artery and that of the femoral artery. (2) Right ventricular and pulmonary arterial pressures are commonly at or even higher than systemic arterial pressure level. Right atrial mean pressure is high with giant A waves at 10 to 20 mm. of mercury. There is a significant pressure drop from right atrium to left atrium. Systemic arterial pressure is normal, as is pulmonary capillary wedge pressure. (3) Pulmonary resistance is markedly elevated (to as much as 10 to 25 units per square meter). (4) Cardiac output is low, between 1.5 and 2.5 liters per minute per square meter of body surface. (5) The course of the catheter is not unusual. (6) Cine-angiograms show the dye lingering in the right heart chambers and may show lack or arborization of the pulmonary vascular tree.

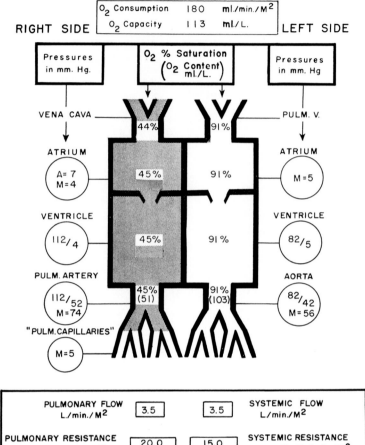

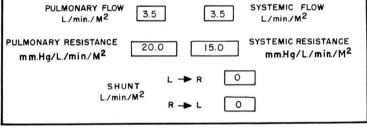

Figure 426.   Cardiac catheterization findings in patient with primary pulmonary vascular obstructive syndrome.

Course and Prognosis

In most cases the onset of symptoms is followed by death within a relatively short time. Three of our patients, who were members of one family, all died within the first six months, the other two within the first ten years of life. Keith placed the average time of death at eighteen months after the onset of symptoms. Yu indicated that death occurred eight to twelve months after the onset of congestive heart failure. Nevertheless patients have been known to be alive twelve years after the onset of symptoms. Death may occur suddenly, in syncope, or gradually, with evidences of chronic heart failure. In one adolescent girl death occurred after the onset of menses with profuse menorrhagia and syncope.

It should be re-emphasized that these patients are particularly prone to sudden death, which may occur at cardiac catheterization or even for no apparent reason at all.[124]

Differential Diagnosis

The differential diagnosis may be made only by exclusion. The principles have been outlined already (see Pulmonary Vascular Obstruction Syndrome, p. 600).

Treatment

No effective treatment is available today. One may attempt the use of anticoagulants, bed rest, oxygen inhalation or Priscoline, but there is no evidence that any of these measures alters the dismal prognosis to any appreciable degree.

Summary

Primary pulmonary arterial hypertension is a rare and relatively rapid fatal disease in infants and children. The etiology may be familial. The clinical picture is identical to that of the other types of pulmonary vascular obstruction. At cardiac catheterization neither evidences of left atrial hypertension nor those of a systemic-pulmonary communication may be found. Essentially, the diagnosis of idiopathic pulmonary hypertension is one of exclusion. No treatment, except supportive, is available.

PULMONIC STENOSIS

Until the introduction of cardiac catheterization into the clinical diagnostic laboratory, pulmonic stenosis was entirely an anatomic concept. According to this definition, patients whose right ventricular outflow tract was visibly obstructed had pulmonic stenosis. With the advent of cardiac catheterization the old anatomic definition was supplanted by a physiologic one—patients who have a systolic gradient between the right ventricle and the pulmonary artery (i.e. patients in whom the right ventricular systolic pressure is appreciably higher than the pulmonary arterial systolic pressure) are now considered to have pulmonic stenosis. This concept includes all patients with anatomic stenosis and, in addition, a large group of patients in whom the usual pathologico-anatomic methods fail to show an obstruction.

Incidence

Thus defined, pulmonary stenosis is present in 20 to 25 per cent of all patients with congenital heart disease. In about half of these the ventricular septum is closed; in the others a ventricular septal defect with more or less overriding of the aorta is present.

Anatomy

The anatomy of pulmonic stenosis has been beautifully summarized in a monograph by Sir Russell Brock.[93] He included eight varieties in his definition: (1) stenosis of the pulmonic valve with a normal aortic root, (2) infundibular stenosis with a normal aortic root, (3) pulmonary atresia, (4) tricuspid atresia, (5) tetralogy of Fallot, (6) the aorta and pulmonary artery both rising from the right ventricle, with pulmonic stenosis and septal defect, (7) transposition of the great vessels with pulmonic stenosis, and (8) common ventricle with pulmonic stenosis. The present chapter will include (1), (2), (3), (5) and (8) of Brock's subdivisions. There will be a separate discussion of (4). Numbers (6) and (7) will be taken up among the transpositions. In addition to these groups, we shall also discuss an embryologically different but physiologically similar group of patients—those with peripheral pulmonic stenosis. Supravalvar stenosis will be discussed within the framework of Brock's (1).

Physiology

The principal physiologic handicap in pulmonic stenosis is the difficulty in maintaining an adequate pulmonary blood flow across a reduced pulmonary orifice and accomplishing a pressure in the pulmonary artery which is significantly higher than left atrial pressure. The latter is predetermined by the pressure-volume characteristics of the left ventricle. In order to accomplish this, the right ventricle must work harder and produce more than the usual amount of pressure. If an opening exists between the two sides of the heart, and if the right ventricular outflow resistance equals or supersedes the total systemic resistance, a right-to-left shunt, with consequent cyanosis, results.

Because of the difference in symptoms, signs and prognosis, patients with pulmonary stenosis who have an intact ventricular septum will be discussed separately from those in whom pulmonic stenosis is associated with an open ventricular septum. A separate section will be devoted to patients who have pulmonic stenosis, a ventricular septal defect and right ventricular pressure greater than systemic level and to those children with unilateral pulmonary atresia. Furthermore, since its clinical features are so distinctive, peripheral pulmonic stenosis will be discussed separately. Also, pulmonary atresia with an underdeveloped right ventricle and an intact ventricular septum will be considered a separate entity. On the other hand, infundibular and valvar stenoses will be discussed within the groups associated with intact and open ventricular septums. Similarly, cases of pulmonary atresia and pulmonic stenosis will be regarded as parts of the tetralogy of Fallot syndrome.

PULMONIC STENOSIS WITH INTACT VENTRICULAR SEPTUM

This anomaly has been variously described as "pure pulmonic stenosis," "isolated pulmonic stenosis" and even "pulmonary stenosis with a normal aortic root."[22] Since the "purity" of the lesion is frequently contaminated and its "splendid isolation" is commonly invaded by an opening in the atrial septum, and because the position of the aortic root is difficult, if not impossible, to define in vivo, I prefer the simple anatomic description used in the heading.

Incidence

Pulmonic stenosis with intact ventricular septum is a common disease, although it was not recognized as such until the past decade. In 1947 Taussig,[682] in her excellent monograph, stated that she had not had the opportunity to study a proved case herself, and Currens and his associates[175] collected the first "large" series, consisting of 11 patients, in 1945. In contrast to this, at The Children's Hospital Medical Center in Boston we had studied 50 patients in detail, by cardiac catheterization, and had seen at least 3 times that many in whom the diagnosis was made on clinical grounds by 1954.[643] The number of cases diagnosed clinically or at cardiac catheterization in our institution is close to 500 (12 per cent) at present. Keith placed its incidence at 9.9 per cent of children with congenital heart disease. In Wood's series it was the third most common lesion, with a frequency of 12 per cent. The conservative estimate may be made that patients who have pulmonic stenosis and an intact ventricular septum constitute at least 10 to 15 per cent of all patients with congenital heart disease who live beyond infancy. The reason for this apparent change in incidence is hard to explain. In my opinion it is due to a clearer definition of the clinical profile revealed by cardiac catheterization; probably many of these patients were formerly classified as having Roger's disease or atrial septal defect.

Anatomy

Approximately four of five patients with this anomaly have valvar stenosis.[397, 643] Brock believed that the ratio is closer to 10:1. On the other hand, he emphasized the coexistence of secondary infundibular stenosis, particularly in severe cases of valvar obstruction in adults. Johnson[364] found this coexistence in 50 to 75 per cent of patients undergoing surgery. Supravalvar stenosis, consisting of a membrane-like structure about 1 cm. above the normal pulmonary valve, is rare. The cusps are usually fused into a membrane with a hole in the middle which varies in size. In patients with extreme stenosis the orifice is no more than 2 to 3 mm. in diameter, whereas with milder gradients the lumen may be 1 cm. The leaflets are thickened, sometimes even in young children. The subvalvar area may be underdeveloped, not posing an obstruction, and may show evidences of endocardial fibroelastosis. The valve ring may be small, but the main pulmonary artery, and particularly the left pulmonary artery, is dilated.

In the rare instances of organic primary infundibular stenosis with an intact ventricular septum there is a circumscribed muscular ring, about 1 cm. below the valve, separating the outflow portion of the right ventricle from a third, poststenotic, ventricle extending up to the normal valve. It is important to note that the papillary muscles of the tricuspid valve may originate from this muscular stenotic ring.

The excellent angiocardiographic studies of Kjellberg and his associates[397] clearly demonstrate the dome-shaped pulmonic valve protruding into the pulmonary artery during systole and collapsing back into the valve ring in diastole.

The right ventricular wall is thickened, and the main pulmonary artery is large and thin-walled. An explanation of the origin of this "poststenotic" dilatation of the pulmonary artery is contained in a classic paper by Emile Holman.[342] He demonstrated that the increased lateral pressure resulting from the deceleration of the high-velocity flow through a small orifice is probably responsible for this phenomenon. At the same time *the degree of poststenotic dilatation is surely not proportionate to the severity of the stenosis;* some of the patients with the mildest valvar stenosis may have the most pronounced poststenotic dilatation of the pulmonary artery. This well documented observation, supported by experimental evidence, led Van Buchem[701] to the assumption that the poststenotic dilation of the pulmonary artery is the result of a separate and distinct malformation of the artery itself.

Probe patency of the foramen ovale is fairly common; occasionally a secundum, or even a primum, atrial septal defect is present.

Physiology

The principal physiologic consequence of pulmonary stenosis with intact ventricular septum is an increase in right ventricular systolic pressure. But there are a few points worth discussing which clearly distinguish this variety of pulmonic stenosis, from the hemodynamic viewpoint, from other types of block (such as tetralogy of Fallot). The most important consideration is the fact that, for a comparable degree of pulmonic stenosis, patients with an intact septum may be able to establish a better pulmonary blood flow (and thus better exercise tolerance) than those who have pulmonic stenosis associated with a ventricular septal defect. This is accomplished at the price of a higher right ventricular pressure-work which the right ventricle is able to produce by virtue of its independence from the systemic circuit. As a consequence of this markedly increased pressure-work, severe right ventricular hypertrophy may be present, and eventually, if the stenosis is severe enough, cardiac dilatation, with congestive failure, may ensue. Cyanosis is a relatively late occurrence in these patients and may be the consequence of one of two mechanisms. It is either due to greatly diminished cardiac output and an increased oxygen extraction at the capillary level (peripheral cyanosis, p. 350) or is the result of a right-to-left shunt (central cyanosis, p. 351) through an atrial opening (atrial septal defect or patent foramen ovale) made possible by an appreciable increase in right atrial pressure and, thus, indicating high right ventricular end-diastolic pressure.

Clinical Picture

The clinical picture, as described in the paragraphs that follow, is based principally on data published in 1956 concerning 50 proved cases of pure pulmonic stenosis.[643] Subsequent observations have largely confirmed these data, with but a few significant modifications and additions. A considerable number—at least one fourth—of these patients are completely asymptomatic. Dyspnea and fatigue dominate the picture in the others, whereas cyanosis seems less severe and less frequent. Epistaxis, syncope and squatting occur, though not commonly (Fig. 427). Only rarely are symptoms present in infants; most patients do not have complaints until they reach the age of two to five years. Nevertheless we have seen more than a dozen small infants who have presented significant symptoms early in life. In one instance pulmonary valvotomy had to be performed, as an emergency procedure, on the third day of life.

On physical examination these youngsters are usually well developed and well nourished; the wide, pentagon-shaped face with high-colored cheeks and lips is almost recognizable at the bedside (Fig. 428). Definite cyanosis is present in no more than one third of the patients. Clubbing, if present, is mild. On careful inspection the veins in the neck may show a prominent A wave. A thrill is commonly present at the suprasternal notch, as well as at the upper left sternal border. The cardiac impulse is powerful and sustained and is maximal at the xiphoid process. Left chest prominence is rare.

The auscultatory phenomena are dominated by the stenotic systolic murmur (Figs. 120 to 130) at the second to fourth left interspace, with excellent transmission to the neck and back. It is interesting to note that this murmur is usually discovered early, often at birth and almost certainly

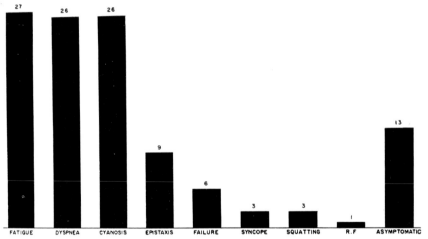

Figure 427.   Symptomatology of patients with pulmonary stenosis and intact ventricular septum.[643]

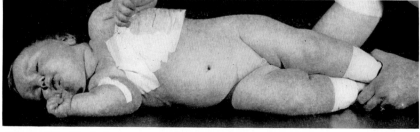

Figure 428.   Typical appearance of a patient with severe pulmonary stenosis and intact ventricular septum. This patient had been operated upon, as evidenced by the bandages across the chest. Note the chubby round face and good fat deposit over the legs.

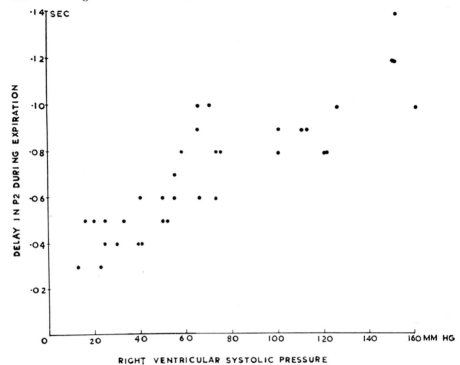

Figure 429.   The relation of right ventricular pressure to the delay in pulmonic closure during expiration.[412]

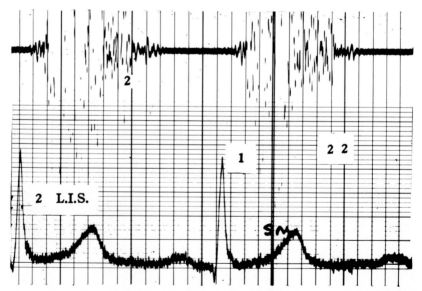

Figure 430.   Phonocardiogram of patient with moderately severe isolated pulmonic stenosis. Note the moderately well split second sound and pulmonic closure following aortic closure by about 0.06 second. The diamond-shaped murmur is composed of high frequency, high amplitude vibrations, with a midsystolic diamond beginning some time after the first sound.

within the first month of life. The first heart sound is usually unimpressive, although a systolic click, probably due to the jet of blood hitting the thin wall of the pulmonary artery, may be noted at the second to third left interspace. The click clearly varies with respirations and, on the whole, but surely not without exception, is the earmark of mild to moderate rather than maximal stenosis. The earlier the click, the more severe the stenosis.

Aortic closure is not remarkable, but pulmonic closure is late and of

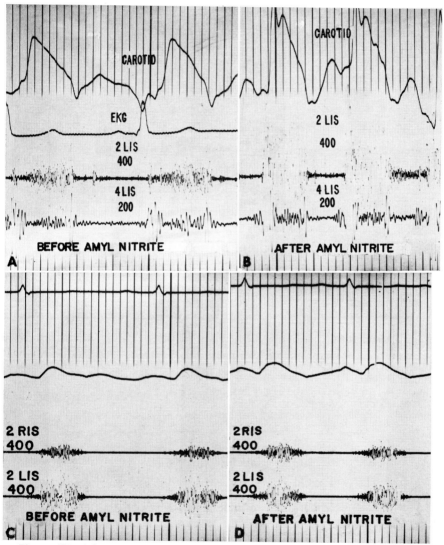

Figure 431. The effects of amyl nitrite on the intensity of the murmur of pulmonic stenosis. *A,* Note the murmur of severe pulmonic stenosis at the second left interspace, with a late crescendo of the murmur and a widely split second sound. *B,* Note the increase in the heart rate and in intensity of the murmur. *C,* At the second left interspace, note the diamond-shaped murmur with a midsystolic apex in another patient with severe pure pulmonic stenosis. *D,* Amyl nitrite has not appreciably increased the intensity of the murmur, though the heart rate has increased significantly.

low intensity. Leatham[412] (Fig. 429) was able to correlate the degree of splitting of the second sound with the severity of pulmonic stenosis. The wider the split, the more severe the obstruction. A pulmonic closure 0.08 to 0.10 second removed from aortic closure probably means a right ventricular pressure at or higher than systemic level. As a rule, the widely split second sound does not change with respiration, but moderate splitting does. A loud fourth sound is the earmark of severe stenosis with increased right atrial and right ventricular end-diastolic pressure.

The systolic murmur is diamond-shaped and consists of high-frequency vibrations (Fig. 430). The more severe the stenosis, the later the apex of the diamond and the longer the murmur (Fig. 120). In maximal pulmonic stenosis the systolic murmur clearly extends beyond aortic closure, giving the impression of a protodiastolic blow. It is interesting to contrast the behavior of the murmur in these patients with that in patients having tetralogy of Fallot. In the latter condition the apex of the murmur is

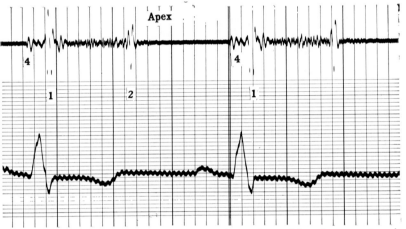

Figure 432. Phonocardiogram at the apex of a patient with pulmonary stenosis and intact ventricular septum. Note the loud fourth sound with rather unimpressive systolic murmur at this location.

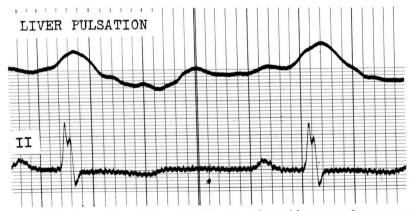

Figure 433. Presystolic pulsation of the liver in patient with severe pulmonary stenosis and intact ventricular septum. Liver tracing on top. Electrocardiogram as reference tracing on bottom.

early, and the more severe the stenosis, the shorter the systolic murmur becomes (Fig. 121). Vogelpoel and Schirer[710] stressed the influence of amyl nitrite on the nature of the murmur in pulmonic stenosis; they found that in patients with an intact ventricular septum the murmur becomes louder and longer, whereas in those with a ventricular septal defect and pulmonic stenosis both the duration and the intensity of the stenotic murmur lessen under the influence of amyl nitrite. Our own observations indicate that this differentiation is a useful one in most instances, but exceptions occur in patients with maximal pure pulmonic stenosis, in which neither the stroke volume of the right ventricle nor the speed of ejection increases after the administration of amyl nitrite, and only the right-to-left shunt becomes greater (Fig. 431). A right ventricular fourth sound is often heard in patients with severe pure pulmonic stenosis (Fig. 432). In fact, this may even extend into a presystolic murmur, due no doubt to some narrowing of the tricuspid valve.

Evidences of congestive failure are rare. Infants with the severest dis-

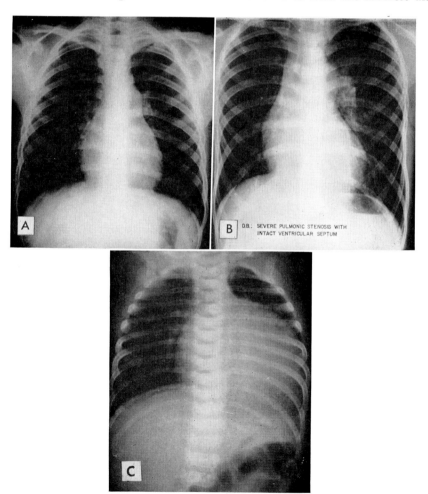

Figure 434. Posteroanterior views of three patients with pulmonary stenosis of varying severity. *A*, Mild; *B*, severe; *C*, very severe in congestive failure.

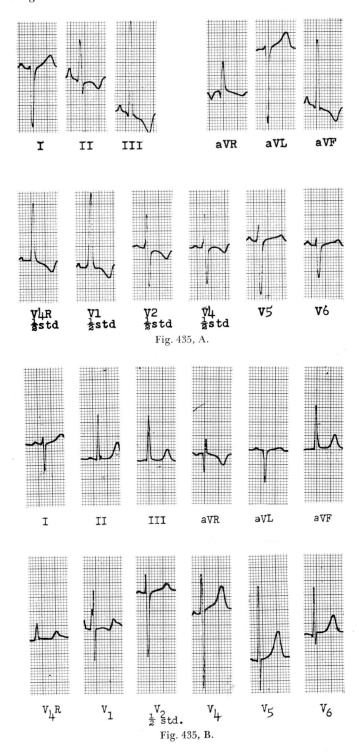

I   II   III   aVR   aVL   aVF

V4R   V1   V2   V4   V5   V6
½std   ½std   ½std   ½std

Fig. 435, A.

I   II   III   aVR   aVL   aVF

V4R   V1   V2   V4   V5   V6
               ½std.

Fig. 435, B.

ease and children around the age of puberty who have progressively severe
stenosis may show cardiac failure. In these children presystolic pulsation
of the liver may be noted (Fig. 433), and there may be little if any murmur
of pulmonic stenosis. A regurgitant murmur of tricuspid origin may be the
dominant auscultatory feature.

Roentgenologically, slight or moderate right ventricular enlargement
is seen in most of these children. Some patients with the mildest degrees
of obstruction have normal-sized hearts, whereas infants and children in
congestive failure may have unusually big hearts (Fig. 434). The enlargement involves principally the right ventricle and the right atrium; prominent main and left main pulmonary arteries indicate valvular obstruction.
Moderate or severe diminution of the pulmonary vasculature is seen in
about three fifths of the patients. At fluoroscopy the contractions of the
heart are powerful, except in patients with congesive failure. The prominent main pulmonary artery may show pulsations, but no expansile pulsation of the smaller pulmonary vessels is ever seen.

In all patients with moderate or severe stenosis the electrocardiogram
shows right ventricular hypertrophy; only ten of the fifty patients studied

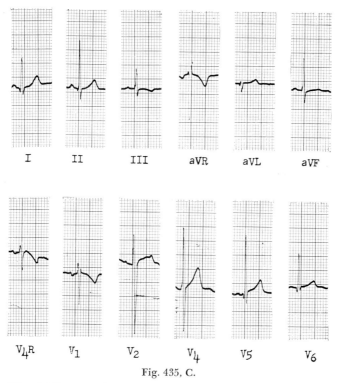

| I | II | III | aVR | aVL | aVF |

| V_4R | V_1 | V_2 | V_4 | V_5 | V_6 |

Fig. 435, C.

Figure 435. *A*, Electrocardiogram of patient with severe pulmonic stenosis. Note the
moderate right axis deviation, + 135 degrees, with a clockwise frontal plane loop, right
ventricular potentials extending through V_1, and prominent deep S waves in the left chest
leads. *B*, Electrocardiogram of moderate pulmonic stenosis. Note the mean electrical axis of
+ 105 degrees. The right ventricular voltages in the chest leads are not very tall; good left
ventricular voltages are present in the left chest leads. *C*, Electrocardiogram of patient with
trivial pulmonic stenosis. Note the mean electrical axis of + 75 degrees, with no evidence of
right ventricular hypertrophy in the chest leads.

in detail had normal tracings. Incomplete right bundle branch block is present in a considerable number of children; it dominates the picture in those with mild pulmonary obstruction. The tracings with the severest degrees of right ventricular hypertrophy are prone to show significant P pulmonale and changes in the S-T segment and the T wave from V_{1-4} or even V_5 (Fig. 435).

A semi-quantitative relation between the voltages in the right chest leads and the right ventricular systolic pressure has been demonstrated in our laboratory[143] (Fig. 436). It was found that although no *accurate* prediction of right ventricular pressure could be obtained from the voltages in the right chest leads of the electrocardiogram, there was good correlation for the regression equation of three times the voltage plus forty-seven. Furthermore, almost all patients with an R wave in V_1 of 20 mm. or more had at least systemic pressures in the right ventricle, and in those in whom, in addition, severe depression of the S-T segment and inversion of the T wave were noted, the systolic pressure in the right ventricle was likely to be more than 150 mm. of mercury. All these "quantitative" estimates are valid only in patients with intact ventricular septum and are more valid for children than adults.

Cardiac catheterization reveals the following (Fig. 437): (1) There is no evidence of a left-to-right shunt in the right heart chambers. Arterial unsaturation, usually slight, but occasionally as low as 50 per cent, is

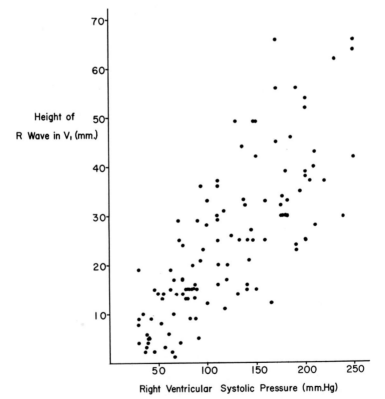

Figure 436. Scattergram of 119 observations of right ventricular systolic pressure and voltage of R wave in V_1. Note the good correlation with considerable scatter.[143]

present in patients with severe stenosis and is due to a right-to-left atrial shunt. (2) Right atrial A waves are tall (more than 5 mm. of mercury) in patients with severe pulmonic stenosis, particularly those with only a small foramen ovale. There is fair correlation between the right atrial A wave and right ventricular systolic pressure. There is a distinct systolic gradient between the right ventricle and the pulmonary artery, ranging from 30 to almost 200 mm. of mercury (Fig. 438). The shape of the withdrawal curve from the pulmonary capillary wedge position to the right ventricle should clearly indicate the nature of the obstruction (supravalvar, valvar or infundibular) (Fig. 439). The shape of the right ventricular pressure curve is triangular with a slow rise and descent and a peaked top. Characteristically, the left and right ventricular pressure tracings are different, both in terms of systolic pressure level and in the shape of the pressure pulse, in patients with severe as well as those with mild pulmonic stenosis with intact ventricular septum. There is, however, a sizable group of patients who have moderate pulmonic stenosis, in whom, perhaps fortuitously, the pressure pulses in the two ventricles are closely similar. Even in these patients, however, a clear difference (at least 10 mm. of mercury) between the pressures of the two ventricles may be demonstrated in the postextrasystolic beats.[340] Pulmonary arterial pressures look damped, and the mean ranges from 7 to 17 mm. of mercury. A Bernouilli effect (negative systolic pressure) is commonly noted in the pulmonary arterial pressure tracings of patients with severe valvar stenosis. (3) Pulmonary vascular resistance is obviously low, but resistance at the right ventricular outflow level may be maximal. Systemic resistance is normal. (4) The pulmonary and systemic blood flows are usually within normal limits, though in patients with a large atrial right-to-left shunt, pulmonary flow indices as low as 1 to 2 liters per minute per square meter may be observed. There is good correlation between pulmonary flow and arterial oxygen saturation.[340] Exercise increases right ventricular cardiac output by means of an increase in heart rate without much change in stroke volume in patients who do not have a significant right-to-left shunt. Right ventricular systolic pressure also increases on effort in these patients. In contrast, in patients who have a sizable atrial right-to-left shunt, no appreciable increase in right ventricular pressure occurs on effort, and the increased oxygen uptake is accounted for, almost entirely, by the increase in arteriovenous difference without much change in cardiac output, and there may even be a drop in stroke volume. (5) There is nothing unusual about the course of the catheter. The dangers of critically obstructing a markedly stenosed valve with the catheter in patients with low resting arterial saturation have already been mentioned.[552] (6) Cine-angiograms, with the patient in the left lateral position, are extremely useful in outlining the stenosis. The valve may be seen as a cone protruding into the lumen of the pulmonary artery in systole and falling back into the right ventricle in diastole. The size of the orifice may be measured in the beautiful selective angiograms of the Swedish group. The hypertrophied crista may clearly be seen encroaching on the infundibular area during systole. In the rare case of infundibular stenosis with intact ventricular septum, angiocardiograms reveal the unusual site of obstruction. (7) Dye-dilution curves, with injection into the right heart chambers and samples from the systemic artery, identify the site of the right-to-left shunt in patients with arterial unsaturation. Intracardiac

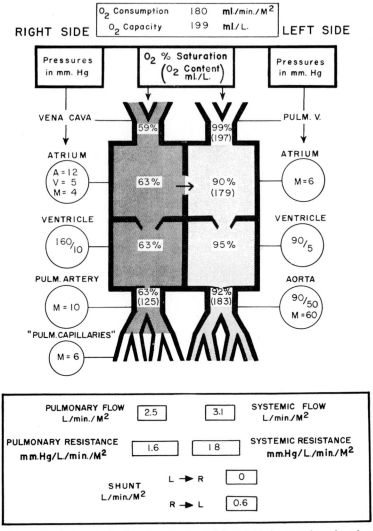

Figure 437. Catheterization findings in a patient with pulmonic stenosis and an intact ventricular septum

phonocardiograms demonstrate the late pulmonic closure and the stenotic murmur in the pulmonary artery.

Usually, cardiac catheterization is not needed to establish the diagnosis. The classic clinical profile of severe valvar pulmonic stenosis with intact ventricular septum may suffice, in experienced hands, to serve even as an indication for surgery. But physiologic studies are indicated if the clinical diagnosis is not clear or if the preoperative assessment of the severity of the lesion does not rest on firm grounds.

In correlating the clinical findings with catheterization data (Fig. 440), in respect to the severity of the malformation, it becomes evident that neither the intensity of the murmur nor the size of the heart may be used as reliable criteria. The presence of symptoms and the extreme degree

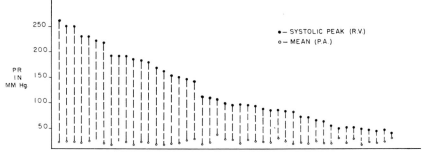

Figure 438. Pressure gradients in 45 patients with pulmonic stenosis with intact ventricular septum. Systolic peak pressure, top; mean pulmonary arterial pressure, bottom line. Note the relatively narrow fluctuation of the pulmonary arterial mean pressure and the wide variation of the right ventricular peak systolic pressure.[643]

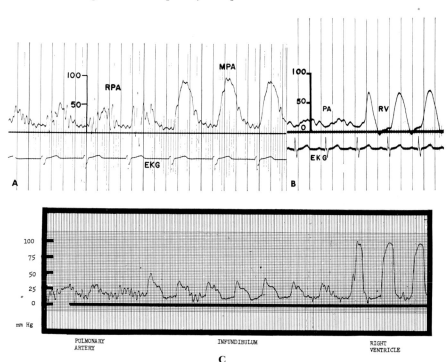

Figure 439.   Withdrawal tracings in patients with pulmonic stenosis. *A*, Stenosis of the right pulmonary artery. *B*, Valvar stenosis. *C*, Infundibular stenosis.

of pulmonary ischemia in correctly exposed films are fair indications of severe pulmonic stenosis. The presence of cyanosis, a tall A wave in the jugular venous pulse tracing, a loud fourth sound and P pulmonale all indicate significant right atrial hypertension and may be considered good indirect evidence of severe obstruction. Finally, a pulmonic closure which is delayed more than 0.08 second beyond aortic closure and electrocardiographic evidences of severe right ventricular hypertrophy, with or without strain (p. 76), may serve as conclusive proof that one is dealing with severe pulmonic stenosis with an intact ventricular septum.

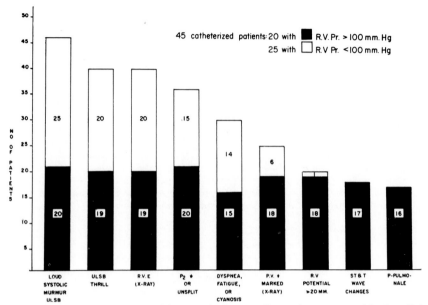

Figure 440. Correlation of right ventricular systolic peak pressure with the clinical picture in 45 patients with pulmonic stenosis and intact ventricular septum. For explanation, see text.[643]

Course and Prognosis

The prognosis in cases of pulmonary stenosis with intact ventricular septum is difficult to predict accurately at present because of the relatively short observation period available; as mentioned earlier, large numbers of these patients have not been observed clinically until the past ten years. On the basis of our own observations during these ten years, it seems that a number of fairly distinct categories may be outlined.

The first group of patients, those with the severest disease, exhibit evidences of congestive failure within the first year or even the first week of life. Anatomically, these patients have pinpoint stenosis of the pulmonary valve, but they probably constitute less than 10 per cent of the total number of patients with this disease. They are usually well developed babies who have a tinge of cyanosis, a large heart and electrocardiographic evidences of severe pulmonic stenosis. Unless they are operated on, these infants probably die within the first year or two of life.

The mild symptoms in the second group of children usually start within the first years of life. If the electrocardiographic criteria may be relied on, these youngsters have progressively higher right ventricular pressures through the years, with increasing fatigue and dyspnea and the late appearance of cyanosis. We know of at least one such child who died suddenly at the age of ten years, and others have been reported in the literature.[196, 480] This is a rare occurrence, however, particularly in contrast to aortic stenosis; the usual evolution is one of increasing symptoms, evidences of right-sided failure, and death in the late teens or twenties.

The patients in the third and final group do not have any symptoms throughout childhood; the right ventricular pressure, when measured, is less than 50 mm. of mercury, and the electrocardiogram fails to reveal evidences of progressively increasing right ventricular pressure through the years. It is this group of children—the asymptomatic, low-pressure group—about whom information is woefully lacking, particularly about their fate in adulthood. At present we do not even know whether the stenosis becomes relatively more or less severe as the years go by. Only careful observation through many decades will furnish a definite answer to this question. My clinical observations strongly suggest that these patients with the mildest degree of pulmonic stenosis almost never have progressive disease, at least during the first two decades.

Among the complications of pulmonic stenosis, the rare occurence of subacute bacterial endocarditis and the rather unlikely appearance of rheumatic fever may be mentioned. We have encountered one patient whose sudden catastrophic increase in symptoms was explained at postmortem examination on the basis of an infected vegetation obstructing an already small pulmonary orifice.

Differential Diagnosis

Tetralogy of Fallot. The most common problem in the differential diagnosis of pulmonary stenosis with intact ventricular septum is to distinguish it from tetralogy of Fallot.

The symptomatology of the two conditions shows slight but definite differences. In tetralogy of Fallot, usually, though not invariably, cyanosis and exertional dyspnea are present in almost equal degree at all times, while in pure pulmonary stenosis, fatigue and dyspnea are more prominent than cyanosis. Squatting and anoxic spells are more common in tetralogy of Fallot than in pulmonary stenosis with intact ventricular septum. Congestive failure—a real danger in patients with pure pulmonic stenosis—never occurs in children with tetralogy of Fallot.

On physical examination the finding of a giant A wave in the jugular venous pulse indicates pure pulmonic stenosis. If the stenotic murmur is heard best high at the left sternal border and has a late peak, lasting beyond aortic closure, and if pulmonic closure is delayed, the lesion is probably severe valvar pulmonic stenosis with an intact septum; the presence of a loud, single second sound (aortic closure) at the lower left sternal border strongly suggests tetralogy of Fallot, particularly if it is coupled with a stenotic murmur which has an early peak and is heard maximally at the lower left sternal border. Furthermore, whereas patients with maximal tetralogy of Fallot, particularly during anoxic spells, often have no murmur at all, patients with severe pure pulmonic stenosis almost always have a stenotic murmur. Exceptions to this rule have been described by others[684] and noted in our own series as well.

The electrocardiogram, as a rule, shows more severe degrees of right ventricular hypertrophy with strain and more P pulmonale in patients with severe isolated pulmonic stenosis than in those with tetralogy of Fallot. Also the transitional zone in the chest leads is further to the left in patients who have severe pulmonic stenosis and an intact ventricular septum.

The roentgenologic picture may be considerably different in the two conditions. In almost 25 per cent of the patients with tetralogy of Fallot there is a right aortic arch, whereas we have only seen this once in a patient who has pulmonic stenosis with an intact ventricular septum; only one additional case has been mentioned in the literature.[126] Other important radiologic differences between the two conditions are the frequent presence of a poststenotic dilatation and the occasional occurrence of much cardiac dilatation in severe pulmonic stenosis, whereas in tetralogy of Fallot the cardiac enlargement is always slight to moderate and the main pulmonary artery segment usually concave. At catheterization the triangular-shaped right ventricular pressure pulse, with postextrasystolic beats more than 10 mm. higher than normal beats, and clearly separated from the left ventricular pressure pulse contour, is the hallmark of an intact ventricular septum. The demonstration of valvar stenosis on the withdrawal tracing and the absence of a right-to-left shunt at the ventricular level point in the same direction.

The Left-to-Right Shunt Group.   Atrial septal defect, ventricular septal defect and patent ductus arteriosus—the left-to-right shunt group—are commonly mentioned in the differential diagnosis of "isolated" pulmonic stenosis. In my opinion the question need seldom, if ever, arise. The tumultuous cardiac impulse, the left chest deformity, the apical diastolic rumble and the pulmonary vascular engorgement with expansile pulsations all identify the left-to-right shunt group clearly. Individual lesions within the group can usually be identified on the basis of physical, electrocardiographic and roentgenologic examinations.

The Pulmonary Vascular Obstruction Syndrome.   The pulmonary vascular obstruction syndrome, and pulmonic stenosis with intact ventricular septum are discussed on page 607.

Pulmonary Atresia with Intact Ventricular Septum.   This condition should be considered in the differential diagnosis of newborns with evidences of cyanosis, right ventricular failure and pulmonary ischemia. The electrocardiogram is the most important tool in identifying this condition clinically, in that, in contrast to pulmonic stenosis associated with a functioning right ventricle, it shows left ventricular hypertrophy in the chest leads. The mean frontal plane axis is commonly between $+30$ and $+130$ degrees, distinguishing this entity from tricuspid atresia.

Carcinoid Disease.   Older children and adults with carcinoid of the bowel and metastases to the liver may, because of the increased serotonin excretion, show the hemodynamic consequences of pulmonic stenosis. The diagnosis may be suspected when patients with clinical evidences of pulmonic stenosis exhibit abdominal pain, diarrhea, flushing and generalized telangiectasia, and may be confirmed by the finding of a large amount of serotonin in the urine.

Ebstein's Anomaly.   Ebstein's anomaly should be considered in the differential diagnosis of only the severest degree of pulmonic stenosis, with congestive failure and cardiomegaly. The similarities are largely radiologic, both conditions being characterized by a large, poorly pulsating heart and diminished pulmonary vasculature. The differentiation rests on the following points: (1) The physical examination in Ebstein's disease fails to show the characteristic stenotic systolic murmur, but shows a triple or quadruple apical rhythm, with low-pitched systolic and diastolic murmurs. (2) The electrocardiogram in Ebstein's disease never shows much right ventricular hypertrophy, but rather the curious combination of a great deal of conduction disturbance with P pulmonale.

Aortic Stenosis.   See page 689.

Treatment

The treatment of pulmonic stenosis, if any, is surgical. Three main techniques are recommended; one is Brock's approach[90] to the pulmonary valve through the right ventricular musculature, the second is Swan's technique[67] of splitting the valve from the pulmonary arterial side during complete interruption of the circulation under hypothermia, and the most recent one is the open-heart technique, using the pump oxygenator. The excellent results of the two latter procedures and the fair results, at least in our hands, of the Brock technique have persuaded our surgical staff to approach the problem within recent years by means of open-heart surgery. Routinely, in our hospital, this is done through cardiopulmonary bypass and, only occasionally, in small infants, as an emergency procedure, do we use mild hypothermia and inflow occlusion. A shunt procedure is contraindicated; not only does it afford no significant relief, but it also may lead to progressive heart failure. The operative risks of pulmonary valvotomy (by means of the pump oxygenator) are less than 5 per cent. Virtually only small infants or those with a very poor myocardium and congestive heart failure represent significant risks. The results of the operation are gratifying. There is symptomatic improvement in all. In some cases the electrocardiogram may not show significant improvement for a year, but in most instances a dramatic drop in voltage occurs in the right chest leads, and an rsr' pattern appears within six to twelve months. The intensity of the stenotic murmur decreases, but only rarely does it disappear. The splitting of the second sound becomes normal. The murmur of pulmonary incompetence is common and may almost be considered a hallmark of successful valvotomy. Rarely, and only in patients with preoperative congestive heart failure, is there significant change in the roentgenologic contour (Fig. 442). We do not have postoperative catheterization studies in many of our patients; usually, the dramatic changes in the electrocardiogram are accepted as evidences of a satisfactory pressure drop.

The rare instance of infundibular pulmonic stenosis may also be successfully repaired by open-heart surgery, although the mortality risks (as well as the morbidity) are somewhat higher, since a ventriculotomy must be performed, whereas in valvar stenosis the obstruction may be approached from above. We have seen only a few patients with isolated infundibular stenosis; thus no significant mortality figures may be quoted.

Indications for pulmonary valvotomy can be summarized as follows:

1. *Young infants with the severest stenosis* and congestive failure should be subjected to operation as soon as the diagnosis is established.[277] Cardiac catheterization should be performed only if the cardiologist feels that the baby can tolerate the procedure and the delay of the operation. Actually, this is an emergency procedure. Anticongestive measures may be undertaken, but usually they are not successful and may waste precious time.

2. *Asymptomatic patients with the classic clinical profile of severe*

R.V. PRESSURE
(CATH.)

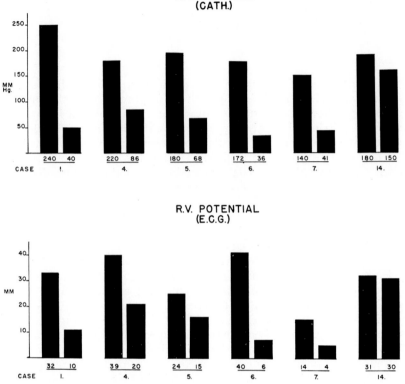

R.V. POTENTIAL
(E.C.G.)

Figure 441. Preoperative and postoperative right ventricular peak systolic pressures and preoperative and postoperative electrocardiograms in six patients with pulmonic stenosis and intact ventricular septum. Note the good parallelisms between pressure drops and drop in right ventricular voltages in the electrocardiogram. In Case 14 there has been a negligible drop both in electrocardiographic voltages and in right ventricular pressures. In all the others a significant drop in both occurred.[643]

valvar pulmonic stenosis and intact ventricular septum should be subjected to surgery, electively, between the ages of five and fifteen years. Earlier operation is indicated if the stenosis is deemed to be maximal or progressive by clinical and physiologic criteria. Preoperative catheterization is necessary if either the diagnosis or the assessment of the severity is in doubt. If the patient is subjected to surgery without benefit of preoperative catheterization studies, it is mandatory that the right ventricular pressure be measured on the operating table.

If catheterization criteria are demanded as operative indications, we regard a right ventricular pressure of more than 75 mm. of mercury at rest as the minimal requirement at the present time. Obviously, this figure is meaningless unless regarded in the general context of cardiac output, age, symptoms, personality, and many other variables.

3. *Asymptomatic patients with clinical or physiologic indications of mild pulmonic stenosis* should not be operated on at this time, but rather should be examined every six to twelve months to evaluate the progression of the condition. Cardiac catheterization is optional in this group of patients. As indicated previously, these children may have a mild form of the disease which may never need correction. The validity of this

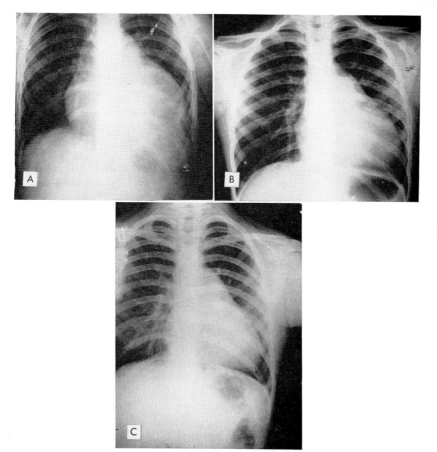

Figure 442. Changes in the heart size of patient with severe pulmonic stenosis and intact ventricular septum. *A,* The preoperative film; *B,* a year and a half after operation; *C,* three years after operation.

assumption can be tested only by careful follow-up examinations for many years.

4. *Asymptomatic patients with the clinical profile of trivial pulmonic stenosis* should not be catheterized or undergo operation. These are the children with the murmurs of valvar pulmonic stenosis and a loud click, but a normal second sound, normal electrocardiogram and, at roentgenologic examination, a prominent main pulmonary artery.

5. *Symptomatic patients with classic pulmonic stenosis* should be operated on without catheterization if the clinical evaluation indicates severe obstruction. If the clinical criteria of severity are equivocal, or even if they indicate trivial stenosis, these patients should be studied by cardiac catheterization; operation may be indicated if appropriate right ventricular pressures are obtained at rest or on exercise.

Among the postoperative complications, the development of the postpericardiotomy syndrome, congestive failure and arrhythmias should be mentioned. Medical treatment or surgical drainage of the effusion invariably clears up these complications. Careful postoperative supervision is essential for the discovery of these conditions.

One serious postoperative complication should be mentioned in this text for pediatric cardiologists, although it represents principally a surgical dilemma. This is the appearance of the so-called suicidal right ventricle. In effect, this consists in a postoperative clampdown of the infundibular area after successful valvotomy with resulting fatal right ventricular failure. In a recent article Brock[96] discussed this in detail and cogitated about a solution. The problem presents itself to the alert surgeon by the presence of a postoperative right ventricular pressure that is no lower and may even be higher than the preoperative value. The obvious question posed by this finding is whether, after valvotomy, the surgeon should also perform an infundibular resection. If so, how much residual right ventricular pressure serves as an indication for such a maneuver? Brock thought that it might be best not to try to relieve the residual, functional infundibular obstruction in patients with pure valvar stenosis. In his opinion, the dire consequences of ventriculotomy and infundibulectomy under these circumstances might outweigh the possible benefit. He believed that the functional infundibular stenosis would eventually resolve itself in the ensuing months, a phenomenon clearly described by Engle[228] and one which we have noted as well. This residual, functional, transient infundibular stenosis may be the anatomic basis for the persistent right ventricular hypertrophy shown in the electrocardiogram in the postoperative period of patients with successful valvotomy. Obviously, this "functional obstruction" should be sharply separated from organic, fibrous infundibular stenosis, which, of course, should be promptly treated surgically.

Fortunately, although extremely high right ventricular pressures have been encountered in our patients after valvotomy at the operating table, we have had no deaths from this cause, and within a year the electrocardiograms have shown significant improvement. The clinical picture of fatal "suicidal right ventricle" is one of a rapid downhill course with low cardiac output and right ventricular failure. Since most of our patients are children and adolescents, possibly our favorable experience with the syndrome may serve as an argument for operation at a younger age.

Summary

Pulmonic stenosis with an intact ventricular septum is characterized by a stenotic systolic murmur at the second left interspace, diminished and late pulmonary closure and evidences of right ventricular hypertrophy and enlargement. Patients with the milder form of the disease may be completely asymptomatic; others show dyspnea on exertion, fatigue and slight cyanosis. Clinical evidences of cyanosis, right atrial hypertension, right ventricular hypertrophy in the electrocardiogram and a widely split second sound indicate severe obstruction, the right ventricular pressures ranging from 75 to more than 200 mm. of mercury. Surgical relief of the obstruction, by means of open-heart surgery, is available at low risks.

PULMONIC ATRESIA WITH INTACT VENTRICULAR SEPTUM

This specific variant of pulmonic stenosis with intact ventricular septum should be mentioned briefly because of its characteristic clinical profile, its malignant course and the surgical challenge it presents.

Incidence

Only a dozen children with this anomaly have been recognized in our institution. Keith and his associates reported on 24 patients; they placed its occurrence at 1 per cent in their cases of congenital heart disease proved at postmortem examination. Recently Davignon[187] reviewed 20 cases taken from 800 proved instances of congenital heart disease at the Mayo Clinic.

Anatomy

In effect, pulmonic atresia with an intact ventricular septum corresponds to a hypoplastic right heart syndrome similar to that seen on the left side with aortic atresia. At the place where the three leaflets of the pulmonary valve ought to be, a diaphragm, consisting of the fused cusps, seals off the right ventricle from the pulmonary artery. The main pulmonary artery is small, but—and this is very important—patent in most patients. The cavity of the right ventricle is usually small. Of the twenty patients analyzed by the Mayo group, thirteen had truly hypoplastic right ventricles.[187] Greenwold and his associates[301] described a variation of this anatomic picture, in which the right ventricular cavity was normal in size, or even large, but the tricuspid valve was grossly deformed and incompetent and, in many ways, resembled Ebstein's malformation. This second type of abnormality was represented by seven of the twenty patients in the Mayo collection (type II). The presence of an opening in the atrial septum and a patent ductus arteriosus is mandatory for survival longer than a few hours. More often than not, there is endocardial fibroelastosis in the right heart chambers.

Physiology

The blood passing from the right atrium into the right ventricle is trapped. It can get back out through an incompetent tricuspid valve into the right atrium or, hypothetically, through the myocardial sinusoids. As a consequence of this "dead-end" right ventricle, all the blood representing the systemic, as well as the pulmonary, venous return enters the left atrium and the left ventricle. The pulmonary circulation can be maintained only through the patent ductus or an extensive bronchial network. This is different from tricuspid atresia, in which, in the majority of patients, the meager pulmonary circulation is maintained, at least in part, through a ventricular septal defect into the pulmonary artery. Furthermore, again in contrast to tricuspid atresia, by virtue of the intact ventricular septum, extremely high right ventricular pressures may be maintained.

Clinical Picture

In essence, the clinical profile is indistinguishable from that seen in infants with maximal pulmonic stenosis. There is cyanosis and severe right-sided failure within the first few days of life. Giant A waves at the jugular venous pulse may be discovered only by the careful observer, but the presystolic pulsation of the large liver is obvious. The heart size varies from relatively slight enlargement in the patients with a hypoplastic right ventricle to rather massive enlargement in those with the type II deformity. The cardiac impulse is maximal at the xiphoid process, and only a single second sound is heard at the lower left sternal border. If any murmur is present, usually it is the murmur of tricuspid regurgitation. If the ductus is open, cyanosis may be relatively mild, but a ductus murmur may possibly be heard. Except for the pulmonary ischemia, the roentgenologic image is rather inconstant. We have seen patients with relatively small hearts

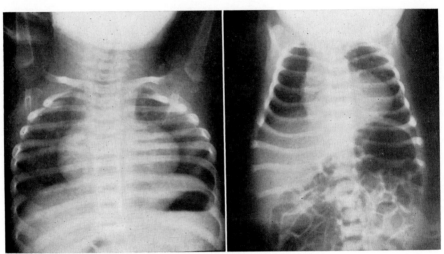

Figure 443.   Preoperative and postoperative films of patient with pulmonary atresia and intact ventricular septum.

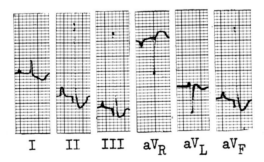

I   II   III   aV$_R$ aV$_L$ aV$_F$

Figure 444.   Electrocardiogram of patient with pulmonary atresia and intact ventricular septum. Note the mean electrical axis of plus 75 degrees, the left ventricular dominance of the chest leads and the digitalis effect.

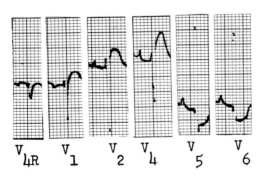

V$_{4R}$ V$_1$ V$_2$ V$_4$ V$_5$ V$_6$

and also those with cardiomegaly (Fig. 443). The electrocardiogram is the most characteristic part of the clinical picture. In contrast to tricuspid atresia, the main frontal plane axis is inferiorly directed (from $+30$ to $+130$ degrees). On the other hand, in contrast to tetralogy of Fallot, the chest leads show adult R/s progression (Fig. 444). These electrocardiographic features may not be fully developed until the end of the first week of life. Also, right ventricular hypertrophy may be present in some patients, making the picture indistinguishable from that of pure pulmonic stenosis.

Results of *cardiac catheterization* are indistinguishable from those for pure pulmonic stenosis except that at angiography no filling of the pulmonary artery from the right ventricle is visualized. The dye injected selectively into the right ventricle lingers in this chamber and then regurgitates through the tricuspid valve.

Course and Prognosis

Only patients with a sizable patent ductus arteriosus survive longer than the first week or two of life. All our patients died within the first month, most within the first ten days. Recently we had one patient nine months old (belonging in the type II category of the Mayo group) who died at operation. This is about the longest survival of a patient with this disease in the literature; the majority of the infants died at less than three months of age.

Differential Diagnosis

Tricuspid atresia and *severe tetralogy of Fallot* may be differentiated on the basis of the electrocardiogram. *Severe pulmonic stenosis with intact ventricular septum* is sometimes impossible to distinguish from the entity under discussion. In most instances the absence of a stenotic murmur and the frontal plane mean axis suggest pulmonary atresia. The markedly ischemic lung fields tend to separate this entity from anomalies involving the left side of the heart, such as *hypoplastic left heart syndrome, primary myocardial disease* and *cor triatriatum.*

Treatment

A small percentage of these patients may be salvaged by prompt surgical intervention. It is important to emphasize that, at least theoretically, inflow occlusion and approach to the pulmonary diaphragm from the pulmonary arterial side may be the quickest and least traumatic intervention. The other alternative is to perform a Brock procedure through the right ventricular wall, but the opening of the tense pericardium often results in sudden, irreversible cardiac arrest. Our surgical staff had dramatic success with this method in newborns, improving the arterial oxygen saturation occasionally from 20 to 80 per cent. *Although the diaphragmatic obstruction may be relieved, the small right ventricular cavity and the minute valve ring still may render survival impossible.* A Glenn procedure, consisting in anastomosis of the superior vena cava to the pulmonary artery, may be a more reasonable solution to the problem, but we have attempted it only twice for this type of anomaly, and we failed in both instances probably because of the small size of the vessels. Consideration may be given to a Potts or Blalock anastomosis, but the elevated left atrial pressure inherent in the postoperative period of these patients may aggravate the systemic congestion beyond the preoperative level unless a good-sized atrial defect is present. Taking everything into consideration, this approach may be the most practical one in the patient with truly hypoplastic right ventricle.

Summary

Pulmonic atresia with an intact ventricular septum presents the clinical and hemodynamic profile of maximal pulmonic stenosis in infants. The electrocardiogram reveals no right ventricular hypertrophy in the chest leads, however, if the patient is more than a few days old. The frontal plane axis may vary from normal to moderately right. Prompt surgical relief of the obstruction by means of pulmonary valvotomy or a shunt procedure may be lifesaving, but carries high risks. Without surgery, death ensues within the first few months of life.

PULMONIC STENOSIS WITH VENTRICULAR SEPTAL DEFECT AND RIGHT-TO-LEFT SHUNT (TETRALOGY OF FALLOT)

Pulmonic stenosis or atresia associated with a ventricular septal defect and dextroposed aorta, forming the anatomic basis of cyanotic congenital heart disease, was described about 180 years ago.[609] Almost 100 years later Fallot[239] defined this syndrome as consisting anatomically of four features—pulmonary stenosis or atresia, dextroposition of the aorta, ventricular septal defect and right ventricular hypertrophy. With the introduction of cardiac catheterization the physiology of this anatomico-clinical syndrome was revealed. The physiologic definition of tetralogy of Fallot is "the combination of a ventricular septal defect with pulmonic stenosis, right ventricular pressure in systemic range, and a shunt which is predominantly or exclusively right to left." Although the static term "tetralogy of Fallot" is being, and probably will be, used by everyone for many decades, my own objection to the term, based principally on an aversion to eponyms, finds a considerable amount of support in the many case reports of formes frustes of this disease, barely explainable on strict anatomic grounds.

Incidence

The tetralogy of Fallot is a common disease; it accounts for at least 15 per cent of all children more than 2 years of age who have congenital heart disease. It is the most common single lesion in patients with cyanotic disease who live beyond infancy. Wood[748] stated that Fallot's tetralogy accounts for two thirds of his patients with cyanotic congenital heart disease; Keith, quoting the Toronto Heart Registry, placed the figure at 50 per cent. If a person not well versed in the mysteries of pediatric cardiology simply made a diagnosis of tetralogy of Fallot in every cyanotic child more than 2 years old, he would probably be right close to 75 per cent of the time.

Anatomy

Embryologically, the combination of ventricular defect and pulmonary stenosis may be explained by a maldevelopment of the bulbus cordis from which the infundibulum and the proximal part of the pulmonary artery develop and which contributes significantly to the closure of the ventricular septum. Defects of the bulbus cordis occur between the fifth and seventh weeks of intrauterine life. The anatomy and embryology of Fallot's tetralogy have been masterfully described in a monograph by Brock.[93] I can scarcely do better than to refer the reader to this classic and to attempt here only a brief summary.

According to Brock (although not everyone agrees),[29, 111] pure infundibular stenosis is present in less than 50 per cent of the patients who have tetralogy of Fallot. The others have either pure valvar stenosis (35 per cent) or a combination of the two (22 per cent). The second point Brock stressed about the nature of the stenosis was that in all but the most severe cases, it is a localized obstruction, and the infundibular chamber (though hypoplastic) usually has an adequate lumen in children. In older patients, fibrosis, endocardial fibroelastosis and even calcification may contribute significantly to the organic obstruction. Angiographic studies show the contraction of the infundibulum during systole, thus contributing, in a functional sense, to the right ventricular obstruction.

The ventricular defect is usually in the anterior muscular septum just behind the crista and in close proximity to the medial leaflet of the tricuspid valve, if viewed from the right ventricle. The superior margin of the defect, as seen from the left ventricular side, is just below the right or posterior cusp of the aortic valve. The bundle of His runs dangerously close to the posterior margin of the defect.

The nature of the overriding of the aorta and its dependence on the ventricular septal defect has been discussed (see p. 403).

The degree of right ventricular hypertrophy depends principally on the severity of the pulmonary stenosis; usually the thickness of the right ventricle equals that of the left. The foramen ovale is patent in considerably more than the expected 20 to 25 per cent of these patients, and a right aortic arch is present in 25 per cent. Significant enlargement of the bronchial arteries occurs in patients with extreme tetralogy of Fallot. These collateral channels are sparse in infants, but gradually increase throughout childhood and adolescence. Occlusive changes[583] of pulmonary arterioles are common, particularly in patients beyond infancy and in those dying with anoxic spells. Keith estimated the presence of associated noncardiac anomalies at 20 per cent.

Physiology

In every patient with tetralogy of Fallot there exists a systolic pressure gradient between the right ventricle and the pulmonary artery. This results in a right ventricular outflow resistance that approximates or even supersedes the systemic resistance, thus causing a right-to-left shunt through a ventricular defect and essentially identical systolic pressure levels in the right ventricle and the systemic artery. The size of the right-to-left shunt may vary, depending on the ratio between the resistances in the two circuits, the size of the ventricular septal defect and on certain characteristics of the right ventricular contraction.

The handicaps resulting from this anomaly are twofold. First, because of the right-to-left shunt, central cyanosis of varying degree is present in most patients. Second, because of the pulmonary obstruction, which cannot be met with a right ventricular pressure appreciably higher than the systemic arterial pressure (owing to the presence of a ventricular defect), the pulmonary blood flow is limited, and exertional dyspnea is prominent. The presence of the ventricular septal defect thus places a ceiling (that of the systemic arterial pressure) on the pressure exerted by the right ventricle. This fact, although responsible for the limitation of exercise, also has the beneficial effect of protecting the right ventricle from doing too much pressure-work. This explains the observation that, although these patients may be extremely limited in their activities, cardiac failure is almost never seen during childhood.

Clinical Picture

Few children with tetralogy of Fallot are asymptomatic; most of them have the habit of squatting, they show evidences of cyanosis and dyspnea on exertion, and they are likely to have attacks of deep cyanosis, unconsciousness and convulsions.

The cyanosis is of the central type and is usually accompanied by clubbing. Exercise tolerance varies; some patients may be able to walk less than one block, while others may be able to walk a mile or more. When these children reach their limit, they usually squat for a few minutes and then get up and resume their previous activities. The nature of the anoxic spells has already been described (p. 353).

On physical examination these patients appear moderately underdeveloped; they rank between the tenth and the twenty-fifth percentiles on standard development charts. Cyanosis and clubbing of various degrees are evident. No giant A waves are visible in the jugular venous pulse. Left chest prominence is absent or minimal. The cardiac impulse is maximal at the xiphoid process, but there is some apical impulse as well. A thrill at the lower or mid-left sternal border is noted in more than half of the patients.

At auscultation the first heart sound is normal, and a constant aortic click may be heard at the apex in patients with severe disease. The aortic component of the second sound is loud and heard well at the lower left sternal border and the apex. Pulmonic closure, on the other hand, is of low intensity and almost always inaudible. Considerable argument centers around the question of whether this low-intensity, almost inaudible and most of the time unregisterable, pulmonic closure is widely separated from the aortic closure. In Leatham's[412] opinion, based on some external phonocardiographic evidence, pulmonic closure is markedly delayed. Feruglio[246] presented some intracardiac phonocardiograms proving the same point. Our own observations[340] indicate that with the two ventricles acting in unison the two sets of semilunar valves close nearly simultaneously, resulting in a narrow split. The widest separation between aortic closure and pulmonic closure we observed on external phonocardiograms was 0.07 second in a boy who had very little right-to-left shunt and acted, in essence, like a patient with an intact ventricular septum. Hopefully, this argument will be settled shortly by more extensive observations with intracardiac phonocardiograms. A few tracings we have obtained recently do, indeed, show sometimes, but not invariably, a low-intensity second sound in the pulmonary artery 0.08 to 0.10 second removed from aortic closure. Until this argument is settled definitely, for practical purposes it may be said that in patients with tetralogy of Fallot only a single loud second sound may be heard, corresponding to aortic closure, at the lower left sternal border and the apex. The second sound at the pulmonary area is diminished or absent. Third sounds or atrial sounds either are not heard or are insignificant. It is important to note that the second sound is never completely obliterated by the murmur; it always stops short of it.

The systolic murmur is usually stenotic, grade 3 to 5 in intensity, and is best heard at the mid or lower left sternal border. The apex of the diamond is early, within the first half of electrical systole. In contrast to

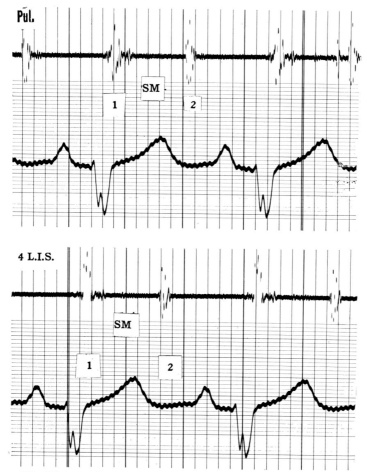

Figure 445. Phonocardiogram in a patient with severe tetralogy of Fallot. Note the relatively loud single second sound at the pulmonary area and the fourth left interspace and the slight systolic murmur.

pure pulmonic stenosis, the more severe the tetralogy of Fallot, the shorter the murmur. It is important to emphasize that the murmur never lasts beyond aortic closure (Fig. 121), and thus no illusion of a protodiastolic blow is created. In patients with absence of the pulmonary valve (see p. 441) a murmur of pulmonic incompetence may be heard. In the most severe cases of tetralogy of Fallot there may be only a slight murmur or none at all (Fig. 445). These are the ones in which practically no blood passes through the pulmonary obstruction. It is interesting to note the variability of the systolic murmur in these patients; although a child may have a grade 3 systolic stenotic murmur when feeling relatively well, at the height of an anoxic spell this same youngster may not have a murmur at all. With the improvement of the child's condition the murmur usually returns. These changes in auscultatory findings can be explained on the basis of variable volumes of blood, at variable velocities, traversing the stenotic right ventricular outflow tract at various times.

If an infundibular spasm really is the basis for the onset of anoxic spells, the disappearance of the murmur may be explained by the practically complete obliteration of the pulmonary flow. Some support for this theory of the origin of anoxic spells may be obtained from the efficacy of a thera-peutic trial with cyclopropane anesthesia, presumably relaxing a con-stricted infundibulum.[159] Furthermore, the effects of procaine (in a single case) on the spasm caused by the mechanical effects of the catheter point in the same direction.[80] In addition to infundibular spasm, an increase in the blood viscosity may also change the Reynold's number to an extent that no murmur is created. A continuous murmur is often heard in patients in whom there is no stenotic systolic murmur (Fig. 446). This is usually heard best at the second right and second left interspaces, as well as over the back, and can be explained on the basis of the wide network of bron-chial collaterals. In rare instances a continuous murmur localized to the second left intercostal space may be caused by a patent ductus arteriosus.

The roentgenologic picture (Fig. 447) is characterized by a relatively small heart of right ventricular contour and a poorly vascularized lung

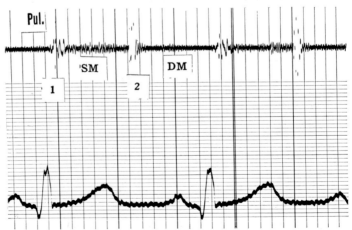

Figure 446. Phonocardiogram in patient with severe tetralogy of Fallot. Note the presence of a continuous murmur at the pulmonary area. Note the high-frequency, low-intensity vibration and the absence of the crescendic systolic element.

field (*coeur en sabot*). Any cardiac enlargement shown in the roentgenogram involves almost exclusively the right ventricle, and perhaps the right atrium. The main pulmonary arterial segment is small, even concave; the aorta, on the other hand, is large. A small, localized convexity corresponding to an infundibular chamber may be seen occasionally in a patient with low infundibular obstruction (Fig. 448). Aneurysmal dilation of the

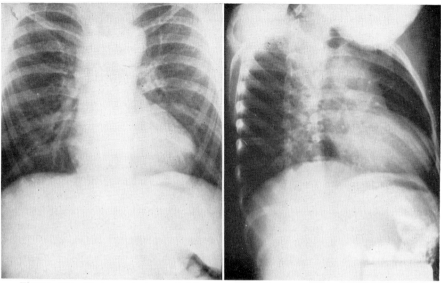

Figure 447. Posteroanterior and right anterior oblique roentgenograms of patient with severe tetralogy of Fallot. Note the large aorta, the right ventricular configuration with absence of the main pulmonary artery segment and the diminished pulmonary vasculature.

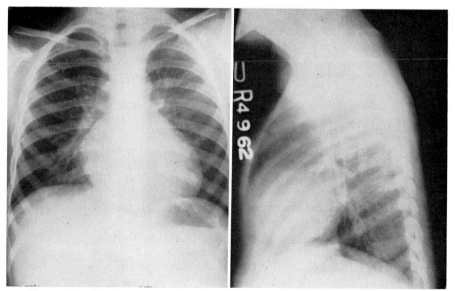

Figure 448. Roentgenogram of patient with severe tetralogy of Fallot and a sizable infundibular chamber. Note the convexity in the area of the main pulmonary artery segment, due to the sizable infundibular chamber.

left main pulmonary artery is seen in patients with tetralogy of Fallot and absence of the pulmonary valve.[496] The aortic arch is commonly on the right side. The peripheral pulmonary vasculature may be normal or diminished, and a pattern of collateral circulation may be noted in patients with the severest pulmonary stenosis.

The electrocardiogram is always abnormal. A moderate or severe degree of right ventricular hypertrophy is noted, with R waves of variable height in the right chest leads. Characteristically, there is an early transitional zone at V_2 or V_3. No good correlation exists between the QRS voltages and the right ventricular pressure in these patients. Evidence of additional left ventricular hypertrophy may sometimes be obtained from leads aV_F and V_{5-6} (Fig. 449).

The mean frontal plane axis is between $+90$ and $+150$ degrees. Left axis deviation between -90 and ±180 in patients with proved pulmonic stenosis and a ventricular septal defect may indicate that the right-to-left shunt is through an endocardial cushion defect. In newborns an upright T wave in V_1 may be the only indication of severe right ventricular hypertrophy.

Cardiac catheterization (Fig. 450) reveals the following: (1) In patients with mild tetralogy of Fallot a small increase in oxygen saturation may be noted at the right ventricular level, particularly if the catheter is placed in the vicinity of the defect in the outflow tract. The systemic arterial saturation is below normal in all patients, at least on effort, by definition. Resting saturations vary from 96 per cent in the patients with "pink tetralogies" to 50 per cent, or even 20 per cent, in those with pulmonary atresia. The difference between the oxygen saturation level at rest and that on exercise may sometimes be as great as 30 to 40 per cent. Left atrial saturation is normal in patients beyond infancy, and left ventricular saturation may be only slightly lower. In spite of the frequent occurrence of an opening in the atrial septum, a right-to-left shunt is rare, and its presence almost always indicates tricuspid valve disease or right ventricular failure. The full extent of unsaturation is noted only in the aorta or the peripheral arteries.

2. Right atrial pressure is nearly normal; A waves of 5 mm. of mercury or more are rare. The right ventricular pressure pulse is flat-topped and similar in height and configuration to the left ventricular pressure pulse tracing; rarely is there a difference of more than 5 mm. of mercury between simultaneously obtained right ventricular and left ventricular or aortic pressures (Fig. 451). Postextrasystolic beats seldom are more than 10 mm. higher than normal beats, and any change is reflected in left ventricular pressure as well. On the whole, pulmonary arterial mean pressures are somewhat lower (5 to 12 mm. of mercury) than those observed in patients with pulmonic stenosis and an intact ventricular septum, but a great deal of overlapping occurs. Systemic arterial pressures may be slightly elevated.

3. Pulmonic valve resistance is high, the vascular resistance low. Rarely a patient may show a high calculated vascular resistance (3 to 5 units), perhaps due to low flow and low left atrial pressure. Pulmonary vascular obstruction develops in a sizable proportion of the patients with long-standing, large shunts.

4. The systemic flow index is normal, the pulmonary index low (1 to 3 liters). There is good correlation between arterial oxygen saturation and pulmonary flow. On effort the oxygen consumption rises, pulmonary flow

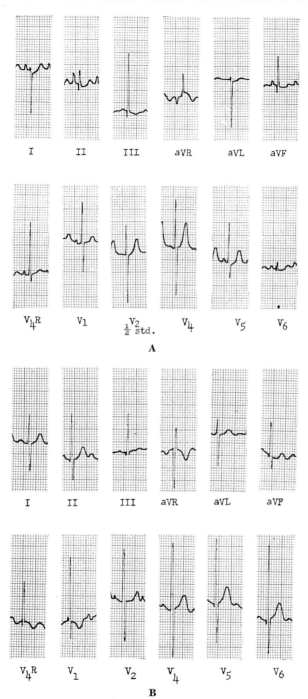

Figure 449. Two electrocardiograms of patients with tetralogy of Fallot syndrome. *A*, Pure right ventricular hypertrophy. *B*, Combined ventricular hypertrophy. Note the P pulmonale in *A*.

increases less than systemic flow, and the right-to-left shunt increases.

5. The passage of the catheter across the ventricular septum into the aorta is the only direct way of proving the presence of a ventricular septal defect. Blockage of the pulmonary orifice by the catheter may result in a severe drop in arterial oxygen saturation. On withdrawing the catheter from the pulmonary artery to the right ventricle, the nature of the obstruction is revealed (Fig. 438).

6. Cine-angiography and angiocardiography are vital tools in the preoperative evaluation of these patients. They shed light on the nature of the pulmonary obstruction and the size and position of the pulmonary arteries, both of which are of importance to the surgeon. I must draw the reader's attention to the magnificent discussion on this topic in the book on angiocardiography by Kjellberg and his associates.[397]

7. Dye-dilution curves may localize the site of the right-to-left shunt.

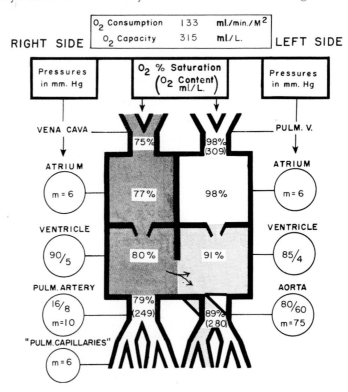

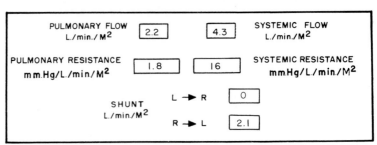

Figure 450.   Catheterization findings of patient with tetralogy of Fallot.

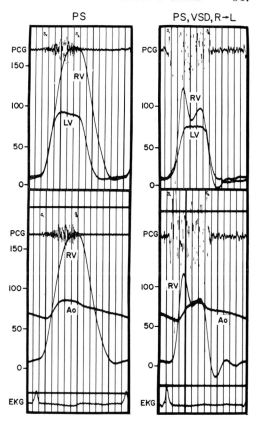

Figure 451. Simultaneous right ventricular and systemic pressure tracings in patient with pure pulmonic stenosis (PS) and tetralogy of Fallot (PS, VSD, R–7L). Note the close similarity between right ventricular and left ventricular or aortic pressure pulse in the latter, and also the wide difference in the former.

Cardiac catheterization is not necessary for the diagnosis of Fallot's tetralogy. In most instances the clinical profile is clear enough to allow accurate diagnosis and prognosis. The importance of physiologic studies, including angiography, lies in the light they shed on the detailed surgical anatomy, so indispensable for the operating surgeon.

Course and Prognosis

Approximately one third of the patients with the tetralogy of Fallot show cyanosis at birth. In another third blueness is first exhibited between the ages of one month and one year. The remainder of the patients do not have noticeable arterial unsaturation until they are well past the first year of life. A grouping of these patients according to the time of initial appearance of cyanosis is possible, and perhaps even useful if the reader realizes that most patients fall somewhere in between the three main groups.

Group 1 is made up of patients who are cyanotic at birth or shortly thereafter. They usually have the severest form of the disease, and they may be the ones in whom, because of the physiologic or anatomic obliteration of the pulmonary orifice, no stenotic systolic murmur is audible. The absence of any demonstrable flow through the pulmonary orifice and the presence of collaterals with a continuous murmur suggested the name "pseudotruncus," which has been applied to these patients. I prefer to designate these children as having pulmonary atresia with a ventricular septal defect or extreme tetralogy of Fallot, fully realizing that differentiation of this from a type IV truncus arterious may be impossible clinically, and even at postmortem examination. At four or five months of age these infants start to have anoxic spells (see p. 353) of increasing severity and frequency. Unless they are operated on, they rarely survive the first year of life. Death usually occurs in a major anoxic spell.

If they do survive the first twelve to eighteen months of life, living on their collateral network, they may live for several years, but are deeply cyanotic and polycythemic, with limitations of exercise. It is interesting to note that if pulmonary atresia is really present, they usually do not squat, since increasing the right ventricular output does not influence pulmonary flow. With all this they may be mentally alert, able to do school work and to occupy themselves in a sedentary fashion. They seldom survive the second decade, but their brief life span is often an inspiring example of the indomitable nature of the human spirit.

Group 2 is made up of patients whose cyanosis becomes obvious only after the first month of life, but before the end of the first year. This group is regarded as most typical of the tetralogy of Fallot syndrome. Anoxic spells also may appear in these patients at or about six months of age, but they are neither as numerous nor as severe as those noted in the first group of infants. Sometimes they take the form of irritable spells or prolonged crying episodes early in the morning. A loud systolic murmur is usually audible at the left sternal border; the murmur of collaterals is absent. When these children are able to walk (at one and a half to two and a half years of age), dyspnea, on exertion, and squatting become obvious. Symptoms are rather mild in favorable weather, but extremes in temperature are poorly tolerated. These children may run around and play satisfactorily in the house, but when they go out to the street or play area, they squat or ask to be picked up after they have walked a few hundred yards. A peculiar, irritating, hacking cough appears when they tire.

When school age is reached, the difficulties increase. Squatting is a socially unacceptable position, and dyspnea on exertion makes it impossible for them to play the games all children enjoy. The walk to school and the climbing of stairs become insurmountable obstacles. Without the help of an operation, life becomes less and less tolerable as the years go by. Perhaps the disease is harder for these youngsters to tolerate because, since they are not as sick as those in the first group, they may try to look and act like other children, and of course they fail. The patients in the first group are so completely different from the average youngster that they may be able to create a world of their own, a task sometimes simpler than attempting to become a member of a group that does not want you. Without operation the patients in the second group usually live through the second or even the third decade. Death occurs from anoxia, cerebral vascular accident, brain abscess, endocarditis or pulmonary hemorrhage. Congestive failure may be seen rarely in adults, or in patients with severe anemia, bacterial endocarditis, and/or aortic regurgitation. Obviously, heart failure also may be encountered in the postoperative state.

The third group of patients with tetralogy of Fallot do not show evidences of cyanosis until they are one year old or older. These are the children who sometimes are referred to as "acyanotic or pink tetralogies."[752] During infancy and early childhood they may show a characteristic picture of ventricular septal defect with pulmonary stenosis (p. 428). It is my belief that, early in life, these patients have a pulmonary outflow resistance considerably lower than the systemic resistance. As the child grows and as the right side of the heart hypertrophies, the pulmonary obstruction becomes more and more significant, and the predominantly left-to-right or balanced shunt through the ventricular defect becomes a dominantly right-to-left one. A loud systolic murmur is always present at the lower left sternal border; during infancy a diastolic rumble may be heard. These patients do not have anoxic spells, but dyspnea on exertion becomes more manifest through the years. Squatting may not appear until five or six years of age or even later. Cyanosis is minimal at rest, but becomes noticeable on exercise and in cold weather. Polycythemia is not present, but the levels for hemoglobin and erythrocytes are high normal. Sometimes with this minimal symptomatology, adaptation is extremely difficult for these children. For all practical purposes they look like everyone else, and still they cannot do nearly as much as can the majority of their contemporaries. Probably life expectancy should be placed between the second and fourth decades, or even higher in certain cases. Marquis[481] placed the number of patients reported surviving beyond forty years at twelve. The causes of death are the same as those mentioned in the discussion of the previous group.

Complications

Among the complications of tetralogy of Fallot, a number of rather important entities should be mentioned.

Brain Abscess. If signs and symptoms pointing to involvement of the central nervous system develop in a patient with tetralogy of Fallot, or other congenital heart disease with a right-to-left shunt, the diagnosis of a brain abscess should be thought of immediately. These patients are usually more than two years of age and are anoxic and polycythemic. A minor febrile illness, sore throat or upper respiratory tract infection occurs first. About seven to ten days later headaches may develop, vomiting occurs, and there are personality changes and, perhaps, focal neurologic lesions, with convulsions. Fever may or may not be present. The significance of papilledema may be hard to evaluate in a child with severe cyanotic disease. Changes in the motor and sensory spheres may be elicited, and pathologic reflexes may be present. A positive Kernig's sign may be noted. Laboratory examination may reveal leukocytosis, although brain abscess is one of the few instances in which a localized collection of pus may occur without an increase in the polymorphonuclear cell count. Lumbar puncture usually shows some increase in cerebrospinal fluid protein content; the cell count may or may not be increased, and the sugar content is usually normal. The electroencephalogram is not entirely dependable, but may indicate a localized process.

Under these circumstances, as stated before, the diagnosis of brain abscess should be suspected, and the advice and aid of a neurosurgical consultant should be sought. It may be preferable to adopt the conservative attitude of careful observation, or it may be better to proceed immediately by drilling burr holes over the right parieto-occipital region, the most common site of abscesses in this condition, or wherever the electroencephalogram shows localized abnormalities.[357] If the neurosurgical consultant prefers to watch the patient for a few hours or days, evidences of acute meningitis may manifest themselves as the abscess starts leaking. At this stage another lumbar puncture is indicated; this usually reveals a high cell count and a low sugar content. As soon as the diagnosis of brain abscess is made, surgical evacuation is indicated, with simultaneous antibiotic control of the infection. Matson,[491] surveying our experiences at The Children's Hospital Medical Center, reported on thirteen cases in a thirteen-year period, with six treated successfully by surgical means.

Why patients with tetralogy of Fallot are prone to the development of brain abscesses has not been satisfactorily explained. It is possible that infected emboli from the systemic venous reservoir are carried across the ventricular defect and propelled directly through the carotid arteries up to the central nervous system. It is also perfectly feasible that cerebral thrombi, inherent in the polycythemia of these patients, may become secondarily infected during a transient episode of bacteremia. Finally, infarction, due to anoxia rather than specific vascular occlusion, may be considered the precursor of brain abscess, in that this softened area may be especially susceptible to the transient bacteremia which occurs with even minor infections. It is interesting to note that positive blood cultures are rarely obtained in these patients and that bacterial endocarditis practically never accompanies brain abscess. The organism recovered from the abscess is usually the alpha streptococcus, although other etiologic agents such as *Hemophilus influenzae, Staphylococcus aureus,* gram-negative and gram-positive rods, and *Pseudomonas aeruginosa* have all been encountered. Under present-day antibiotic treatment the abscess is sterile in at least 25 per cent of the patients.

Hemiplegia.   Hemiplegia, without any evidence of a space-occupying lesion of the central nervous system, is probably due to cerebral thrombosis, embolism or profound anoxia. It usually occurs in infants less than two years of age with decided unsaturation. There is no clear-cut correlation between the hematocrit level and the occurrence of a cerebrovascular accident. As a matter of fact, Martelle and Linde[483] emphasized the role of relative anemia in the causation of cerebral vascular accidents. If one assumes that local anoxia may cause infarction, then the exaggeration of the effects of arterial unsaturation caused by the lower oxygen capacity may indeed predispose to damage of the central nervous system. Sometimes its appearance follows a severe anoxic spell; at other times it is noted immediately after a shunt operation. It may be more common in hot weather, with consequent dehydration, or during febrile illnesses, when the patient refuses to drink.

Obviously this condition, for which only palliative treatment and physiotherapy are available, should be carefully differentiated from a remediable brain abscess. If the clinical picture and the cerebrospinal fluid findings are equivocal, burr holes, or even exploration, may be indicated.

It may be possible to prevent this type of cerebrovascular accident by making certain that the patient has an adequate fluid intake under all circumstances and that any infections are promptly treated. I am not convinced of the value of venesection in these patients.

Relative Anemia and Polycythemia. One of the adaptative mechanisms of the organism to low arterial oxygen saturation is the increase in oxygen-carrying capacity (p. 352) of the blood by the development of polycythemia and increased hemoglobin content of the individual red cells. Indeed, it may be demonstrated that cyanotic infants with low erythrocyte counts and low hemoglobin levels perform less adequately and have considerably more symptoms than if their hemoglobin and red cell counts were raised to more adequate levels. The limiting factor of this mechanism is obviously the increasing viscosity of the blood. It may be seen from Figure 452 that when the hematocrit level reaches 65 to 70 per cent, further increase will entail a considerable rise in blood viscosity, resulting in impediment of blood flow, sludging and even decreased delivery of oxygen to the tissues.

On the basis of these observations a theory of optimal hematocrit

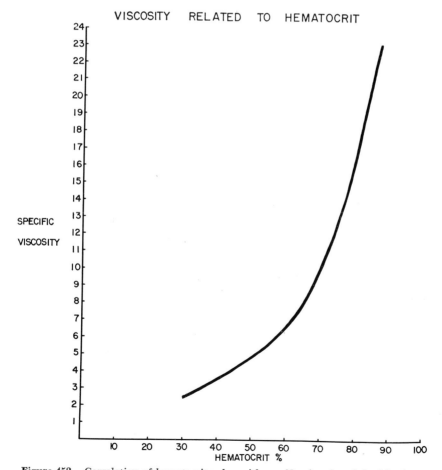

Figure 452.   Correlation of hematocrit value with specific viscosity of the blood.[600]

level for patients with cyanotic disease has been developed.[600] We have seen patients with severe arterial unsaturation and hemoglobin levels of 10 to 13 gm. per 100 ml. of blood, erythrocyte counts of 6 to 8 million and hematocrit levels of 40 per cent; these children have a relative hypochromic anemia easily correctable by iron administration. The resulting increase in hematocrit level is usually accompanied by symptomatic improvement until the level reaches 70 to 75 per cent, after which the symptoms observed at the low hemoglobin level recur.

At present it is our policy to treat with iron all patients with tetralogy of Fallot who are hypochromic, irrespective of the actual level of erythrocytes. We usually stop iron administration when the hematocrit level reaches 75 per cent. If, when the patient is first encountered, he has a hematocrit reading 85 per cent or more and is severely symptomatic, venesection may be cautiously attempted. If the removal of small increments of blood results in a decrease in symptoms, it may be repeated until the hematocrit level reaches 65 to 70 per cent. If, on the other hand, symptoms do not improve, or if they become aggravated by venesection, the procedure should be abandoned immediately. If the patient is relatively asymptomatic to begin with, venesection is not recommended at all, regardless of the level of the hematocrit.

In summary, I believe that patients with tetralogy of Fallot and appreciable arterial unsaturation probably function best with a hematocrit level of 55 to 75 per cent. If the values are lower than this, iron is indicated; if they are higher and the patient is severely symptomatic, venesection may be attempted cautiously.

Rheumatic Fever and Rheumatic Heart Disease. Rheumatic fever and rheumatic heart disease are rare in patients with tetralogy of Fallot.

Bacterial Endocarditis. Bacterial endocarditis represents a statistically significant danger for children with tetralogy of Fallot (see p. 214).

Hemorrhagic Disorders. These disorders, specifically hemoptysis due to rupture of the extensive collateral network into the alveoli or to infarction secondary to the pulmonary vascular obstruction, are comparatively common in older patients with tetralogy of Fallot, though unquestionably they occur less frequently than in patients with pulmonary arterial hypertension. Bleeding from the gastrointestinal tract is secondary to the low platelet counts and low fibrinogen levels. Paul[555] recently reported that the low platelet counts correlate well with anoxia in older patients. Younger patients, in whom anoxia does not cause the same degree of polycythemia that it does in older people, do not show the same degree of platelet deficiency.

Gout. Gout, as a complication of severe cyanotic heart disease, has been described recently by Somerville.[655] She described nine adults with this condition, the youngest being eighteen years old. Four of her patients had the tetralogy of Fallot; all of them were polycythemic, and the level of uric acid in the blood was elevated. We have seen this only once in a child with tetralogy of Fallot, but have observed it several times in patients with transposition of the great arteries.

Differential Diagnosis

Pulmonic Stenosis with Intact Ventricular Septum. See page 629.

Single Ventricle. See page 453.

Truncus Arteriosus. See page 505.

Tricuspid Atresia. Only on the basis of the electrocardiographic evidences of left ventricular hypertrophy can tricuspid atresia be differentiated from tetralogy of Fallot. In every other respect they may be indistinguishable from each other.

The Hypoplastic Left Heart Syndrome. This entity is rather difficult to confuse with Fallot's tetralogy because of the large heart, pulmonary venous congestion, very early cyanosis and congestive heart failure.

Complete Transposition of the Great Arteries. In the differential diagnosis of patients with severe cyanotic disease, the tetralogy of Fallot should be differentiated first from transposition of the great arteries.

Since only type IIA (transposition with pulmonic stenosis) has clear-cut pulmonary ischemia, this is the most difficult type to differentiate; even here, the absence of squatting, the somewhat larger heart, the stenotic murmur (often at the right side), the unusual mean electrical axis and the absence of severe right ventricular hypertrophy may furnish significant clinical clues. Often only cardiac catheterization and angiography, by demonstrating the anterior position of the aorta and a systemic arterial saturation lower than pulmonary arterial saturation, can definitely establish the diagnosis.

The other types of transposition, particularly in children and infants beyond the first few weeks of life, should present no particular problems, since the significant cardiac enlargement coupled with pulmonary vascular engorgement and physical underdevelopment should clearly identify transposition of the great arteries. Type I may be difficult to identify clinically within the first few days or weeks, but the absence of a murmur, the minor degrees of right ventricular hypertrophy and the pulmonary vasculature furnish helpful clues even in the very young.

Levocardia with Abdominal Situs Inversus and Absent Spleen. These patients, if the examination is restricted to the cardiovascular system, may look like typical patients with tetralogy of Fallot. If, however, an abdominal situs inversus is discovered on physical examination or at fluoroscopy, the suspicion of the absent spleen syndrome should be raised immediately. The comprehensive monograph of Ivemark[359] points out that this syndrome is almost never accompanied by a straightforward tetralogy of Fallot type of lesion, but includes, with a high statistical probability, lesions such as atrioventricularis communis, truncus arteriosus, pulmonary atresia or transposition of the great arteries.

Treatment

In 1945 Blalock and Taussig[62] reported the first results of their "shunt" operation, aimed at increasing the pulmonary blood flow by anastomosing a systemic artery (usually the subclavian) to the pulmonary artery. Potts and his associates[566] achieved the same purpose by establishing a direct connection between the aorta and the pulmonary artery. More recently Brock[91] advocated directly relieving the stenosis of the right ventricular outflow tract. Finally, Lillehei and his associates,[435] with the help of cross circulation, and the Mayo Clinic group,[210] with the aid of a pump oxygenator, were able to create a bloodless field in the heart and thus repair both the ventricular septum and the pulmonary stenosis in patients with tetralogy of Fallot. Since the publication of the first edition of this volume, open-heart repair with definitive correction of the tetralogy of Fallot by means of the pump oxygenator has been emphasized in the treatment of these children on a large scale all over the world. The use of cross circulation has been abandoned everywhere, to the best of my knowledge.

Thus a discussion of the surgical treatment of Fallot's tetralogy should be restricted to consideration of the three palliative procedures (Blalock, Potts, Brock) and complete correction by means of the pump oxygenator. Since everyone agrees that complete correction is surely the ultimate goal, it may be logical to take up the pros and cons of this procedure first and to consider the merits of the other three alternatives later.

In the first edition of this book I stated that "direct operation . . . will be the procedure of choice within a short time," and later on, "Since direct repair is just 'around the corner' . . ." Obviously, these views were far too optimistic. At the present writing, judged on the basis of the meager published data and innumerable informal conferences in dark bars at national meetings, complete repair in patients with cyanotic tetralogy of Fallot is still a difficult undertaking.[95, 374, 395, 630, 632] The risks quoted by various authors are between 15 and 25 per cent. It is difficult, however, to know exactly what the risk would be in an individual patient, since preoperative and postoperative oxygen saturation data are meager, the results for severely cyanotic patients and relatively acyanotic ones are lumped together, and the whole issue is rather confused. The mortality rate in infants is even higher than quoted; similarly, adult patients with scarred, and even calcified, outflow tracts and high hematocrit levels represent practically insurmountable problems.

Why do patients with tetralogy of Fallot tolerate complete repair so poorly? What are the immediate causes of death? Some of the complications which caused death in the past have been largely overcome: (1) complete heart block and (2) inadequate relief of the obstruction. Other factors are slowly being eliminated: (1) hemorrhage, (2) reopening of the ventricular septal defect, (3) insertion of too large a "patch" into the outflow tract of the right ventricle, and (4) technical errors resulting in severance of an anomalous right coronary artery or trauma to aortic valve cusps. The main cause of death in these children, irreversible arterial hypotension, is still left for the surgeon and the cardiologist to deal with and to explain.

Two theories have been proposed: (1) The arterial hypotension may be due to left ventricular failure caused by a small hypoplastic left heart which, postoperatively, is suddenly called on to accommodate a normal pulmonary venous return. In my opinion, this is not likely to be the cause of the catastrophe in most instances. Experience with the splendid results of shunt operations and a study of specimens obtained at postmortem examinations indicate that the left ventricle and left atrium, although smaller than the chambers on the right side, are certainly not abnormally small. (2) Pulmonary vascular obstruction at the arteriolar level, as demonstrated in the histologic specimens of Rich,[583] and more recently of Dammann and Ferencz,[182] may indeed be present in the patients with the smallest pulmonary flows and the most severe arterial unsaturation. It is possible that this represents the block between the right ventricle and the systemic artery which results in low cardiac output, irreversible postoperative hypotension and, later, low urinary output, acidosis and death. Furthermore, the effects of the large bronchial circulation on the pulmonary arteries during perfusion may also have to be taken into consideration.

In reviewing our data and those of others, one can barely escape the conclusion that the less cyanotic the child is, the more chance it has to survive operation. Consequently we do not hesitate to consider for operation patients belonging in group 3, i.e. patients with resting saturations in the upper eighties. Of course, the difficulties of perfusing children weighing less than 30 pounds would make us select the older children within this group. A mortality rate of 10 per cent may be predicted for these patients.[396] By the same token, under no circumstances should patients in group 1 (infants with maximal pulmonic stenosis and severe unsaturation) be considered for complete repair today. In regard to group 2 (patients beyond infancy, but with severe unsaturation), at this time we are somewhat reluctant to attempt complete repair; we would prefer one of the palliative approaches, if possible. I am sure that our positive approach to the patients in group 3 and our negative approach to those in group 1 will not change significantly within the next few years. I am almost certain that our cautious, hesitant approach toward patients in group 2 will change indeed. Either we will decide that all these patients need a first-stage palliative procedure to improve the state of the pulmonary vessels or we will improve our perfusion and operative techniques to a point at which direct operation may be offered as a one-stage procedure at an acceptable risk of ±10 per cent. Once these problems are worked out, I am certain that surgery at a younger age, when the infundibulum has not undergone irreversible scarring, will be preferred to operation in adults.

Probably, digitalis should be administered to all these patients in the postoperative period. Hemorrhage may be a real problem, particularly in the polycythemic older patients with low platelet counts and low fibrinogen levels. One hopes that heart block will not occur and that the pressor agents will not have to be used. If surgery is successful, these children show a truly miraculous change, with little murmur, pink lips and a normal exercise tolerance. The only adverse consequence is the presence of a larger heart than was noted preoperatively (Figs. 453, 454).

In the past, among the palliative operations, the Potts procedure (an aortopulmonary anastomosis) was preferred in our institution (Fig. 455). Although the postoperative cardiac enlargement is somewhat greater in these patients than in those with a Blalock shunt, the certainty of a persistent and adequate shunt was sufficiently tempting that most of our patients were operated on by this method until the advent of open-heart surgery. This is still a good operation, and Paul's review[553] indicated that the results are lasting and that in less than 20 per cent of the patients does pulmonary arterial hypertension develop within 10 years. At the same time, because the removal of a Potts shunt is considerably more difficult than the tying off of a Blalock anastomosis, the Potts operation is now our second choice among the shunt procedures.

If it is technically feasible, we now recommend a Blalock operation, a subclavian-pulmonary artery anastomosis, on the side opposite to the aortic arch, for shunt purposes. The indications for this operation are as follows: (1) Unquestionably, infants in group 1 who have anoxic spells should have a shunt. It may be advantageous from the viewpoint of the size of the

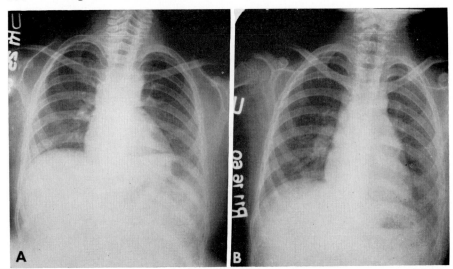

Figure 453. Preoperative and postoperative films of patient with tetralogy of Fallot. Note the disappearance of the concavity of the left heart border, filled in by the pericardial patch.

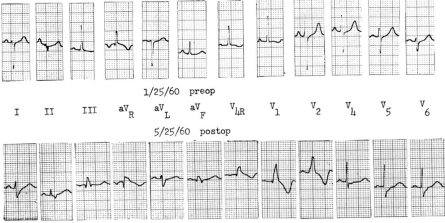

1/25/60 preop

I   II   III   aV$_R$ aV$_L$ aV$_F$ V$_{4R}$ V$_1$ V$_2$ V$_4$ V$_5$ V$_6$

5/25/60 postop

Figure 454. Preoperative and postoperative electrocardiograms of patient with tetralogy of Fallot. Note the right axis deviation, the right ventricular hypertrophy in the preoperative tracing and the development of complete right bundle branch block in the postoperative record.

subclavian artery to postpone this until the baby is a year or two old, but in critical situations one should not hesitate to operate even in the newborn period. Sometimes this may be an emergency lifesaving procedure. (2) Today we perform a shunt procedure on most children in group 2 if they have significant symptoms, preferably before they enter school. This gives us time to improve our technique of complete correction and may even make eventual repair easier. As indicated, this policy may become routine in the future or may give way to complete abandonment of the shunt technique and use of definitive repair in all group 2 patients. (3) Finally, extremely polycythemic adults with severe pulmonic stenosis

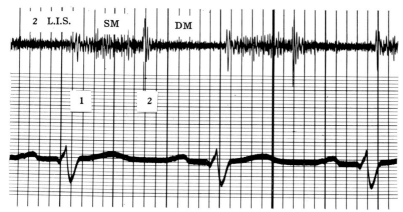

Figure 455. Continuous murmur after successful Potts procedure in patient who had tetralogy of Fallot.

may also benefit considerably from a shunt procedure, either as a permanent solution or as a first-stage operation before undertaking complete correction.

Sir Russell Brock[95] has been a long-time advocate and unsurpassed virtuoso of his procedure, consisting in infundibular resection without attacking the ventricular septal defect. This has been an excellent operation in his hands with mortality rates of ±15 per cent in children and adults.[128] We have not had much experience with it as a blind method, but have used it under direct vision in a few instances. Also, inadvertently, in some patients in whom complete repair was attempted, but whose ventricular septal defect reopened, this has been the end-result of an operation aimed at complete correction. The relief of the cyanosis and the improvement of exercise tolerance are good, but the price may have to be paid in terms of significant cardiac enlargement, pulmonary regurgitation (Fig. 456), pericardial effusion, and sometimes even severe, but fortunately transient, congestive heart failure. Brock believes that this may be a better "first-stage" operation than the shunt, since it at least alleviates one of the two principal malformations while preparing the pulmonary vascular bed and the left ventricle for the eventual complete repair. True as this may be, my own opinion is that the entrance into the pericardial cavity and the ventriculotomy may make complete repair more hazardous after a Brock than after a shunt operation. As far as I know, not enough patients have had complete repair after a Brock operation to settle this point. According to Wood,[744] their patients with a Brock procedure are doing so well that they cannot be persuaded to undergo a second procedure.

A few words about the results of the shunt operations. Paul,[553] reporting on his first 700 patients in whom a Potts anastomosis was made, found the over-all mortality to be 9 per cent, varying from 12 to 15 in infants to 4 per cent in children more than 3 years old. Approximately 70 per cent of the survivors had maintained an excellent or good status 10 years later. Among the complications should be mentioned significant cardiomegaly (15 per cent), dilatation of the pulmonary artery (40 per cent) and pulmonary arterial hypertension (in three out of eighteen). Paul thought that the size of the anastomosis, as reflected in the systemic arterial oxygen satu-

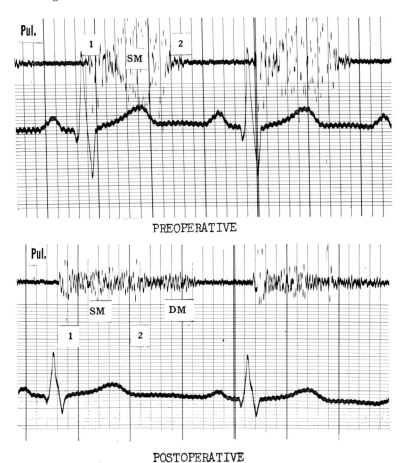

PREOPERATIVE

POSTOPERATIVE

Figure 456. Preoperative and postoperative phonocardiograms in a patient with tetralogy of Fallot who has undergone a Brock procedure. Note the appearance of long diastolic murmur in the postoperative record.

ration, might be the deciding factor responsible for the complications; an anastomosis no larger than 4 mm. and a postoperative arterial oxygen saturation of 90 per cent or less seem ideal.

Taussig,[683] reviewing the results of the Blalock-Taussig procedure, stated in the latest edition of her book that the mortality rate in the last 100 children was 2 per cent. She considered the ideal age for surgery between 8 and 12 years and stated that in this age group, 75 per cent maintain a satisfactory exercise tolerance, and only 5 per cent need a second operation within a 10-year period. Surgery in infants is more dangerous and the need for reoperation is greater (33 per cent). Our results, with 387 patients (223 Potts procedures and 164 Blalock operations), indicate a 6.5 per cent mortality rate in children and 10 per cent in infants.

The measure of the success of the operation can often be judged best by the development of a continuous, ductus-like murmur (Fig. 454) at the second interspace on the side of the operation. Usually, with the Potts procedure, the murmur is audible within the first day after operation, while with the Blalock operation the murmur may not be audible for a

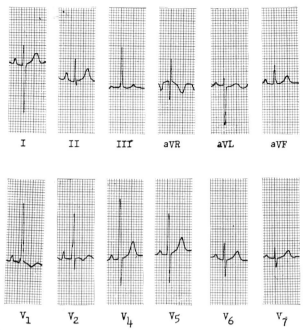

Figure 457. Electrocardiogram of patient with tetralogy of Fallot.

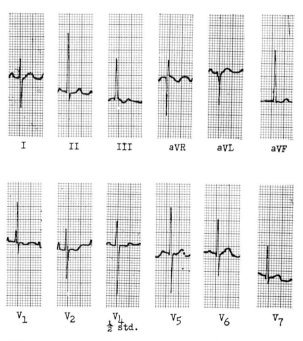

Figure 458. Electrocardiogram of the same patient as in Figure 457 after a Potts procedure. Note the increase in left ventricular potentials in leads aV_F and V_7. Also the increased voltages in leads II and III.

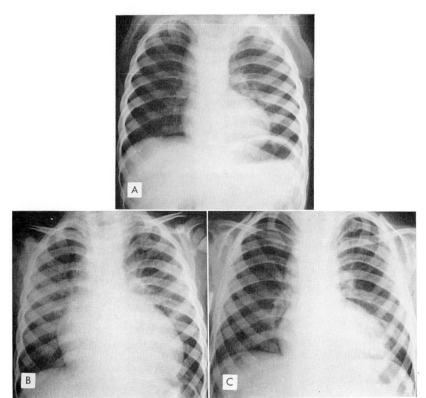

Figure 459. *A,* Posteroanterior view of typical tetralogy of Fallot. *B,* Posteroanterior view of the heart of the same patient after operation, showing cardiac enlargement and pulmonary vascular engorgement, three months later. *C,* Disappearance of pulmonary congestion and diminution of heart size after adequate anticongestive treatment.

week or more. Evidences of left ventricular hypertrophy become noticeable in the electrocardiogram (Figs. 457, 458); left ventricular and left atrial enlargement are commonly seen by x-ray. Pulmonary vascular engorgement of slight to moderate degree may be visible in the postoperative film.

If the operative shunt (usually the Potts type) is too large, the patient may go into congestive failure within the first week or two after operation. This is evidenced by a hyperdynamic cardiac impulse, pulmonary rales, systemic congestion, appearance of apical diastolic murmur, wide pulse pressure and cardiac enlargement. In most instances this can be remedied by vigorous anticongestive measures pursued for six to eighteen months. Eventually, perhaps through the development of some degree of pulmonary vascular obstruction, but more likely by means of ventricular hypertrophy, the circulation adjusts itself, and within one or two years the patient begins to show the full benefits of the operation (Fig. 459).

Of course, if evidences of congestive failure appear postoperatively in a patient thought to have tetralogy of Fallot, one must be certain that the preoperative diagnosis was not faulty and that the child is not suffering from pure pulmonic stenosis or a transposition of the great arteries, neither of which lends itself to symptomatic relief by means of this technique. If the diagnosis was wrong, obviously anticongestive measures will not satisfactorily solve the problem; the anastomosis may have to be closed and an appropriate operation, if technically possible, performed.

A word may be said here about the reasons why pure pulmonic stenosis and transposition of the great arteries do not respond well to a shunt procedure. In transposition of the great arteries the answer is simple. Diminished pulmonary blood flow is *not* the principal cause of cyanosis in these patients; furthermore, establishing an aortopulmonary anastomosis does not necessarily establish the type of shunt that is most useful under the given circumstances. Even if an aortopulmonary shunt is needed in transposition of the great arteries with pulmonic stenosis, without an appropriate-sized atrial septal defect such a shunt may have disastrous results.

Why patients with pulmonic stenosis of the isolated type respond poorly or even go into congestive failure after a shunt procedure has become clear only relatively recently. If the patient with this anomaly is not cyanotic, then obviously a shunt operation, recirculating fully oxygenated blood through the lungs, will not accomplish anything beneficial. If the patient's blood is unsaturated because of a right-to-left atrial shunt, then the cyanosis may be helped by the shunt operation, but it does not remedy the more serious underlying problem. As mentioned before, in patients with pure pulmonary stenosis a shunt from right to left will not occur until right atrial pressure is higher than left atrial pressure, i.e. until the right ventricular diastolic pressure is elevated. This, on the other hand, means right ventricular failure. In this situation, then, the basic difficulty is right ventricular failure, a condition not remediable at all by establishing an aortopulmonary shunt. (This is in contrast to tetralogy of Fallot, in which congestive failure does not occur in childhood.) Consequently patients with pure pulmonic stenosis and a right-to-left shunt go into congestive failure after a Potts procedure, principally because they would have done so anyhow. Another reason for the development of failure postoperatively is the fact that, as mentioned earlier, the increased left ventricular flow-work may easily lead to left ventricular failure in any patient after a shunt operation. Left ventricular failure, then, leads to left atrial and pulmonary capillary hypertension. This, on the other hand, leads to pulmonary arterial hypertension and increased right ventricular work.

The complications of tetralogy of Fallot enumerated on page 649 apparently do not occur any more frequently in patients after a shunt procedure than before, although recently more than the expected number of patients with bacterial endocarditis had had a previous shunt operation.

Medical management of these children is extremely important. Good dental hygiene and antibiotic prophylaxis, to avoid bacterial endocarditis, are mandatory. The maintenance of an adequate fluid intake, particularly in hot weather, is vital. The question of venesection and administration of iron, as well as the treatment of anoxic spells, has already been discussed. One of the most important aspects of the medical management is to decide when to intervene surgically. It is my view, at this time, that all patients with severe unsaturation should have a shunt operation at approximately two years of age, or sooner if anoxic spells occur. There seems to be little reason at this time to procrastinate. Complete correction is recommended for symptomatic patients with relatively good resting oxygen saturation (more than 80 per cent), with or without a previous shunt, at an age suitable to the surgeon. As surgical skill, perfusion technique and post-operative care improve, more and more patients will be subjected to surgery aiming at complete correction. In our hands, the Brock procedure is reserved as a first-stage operation for patients with pure valvar stenosis and those in whom, for technical reasons, a shunt cannot be performed.

Summary

Most patients more than two years of age with cyanotic congenital heart disease have pulmonary stenosis with a right-to-left shunt through a ventricular defect—i.e. the tetralogy of Fallot. The clinical profile is characterized by a small heart, a stenotic murmur at the left sternal border, a single second sound at the lower left sternal border, poorly vascularized lung fields and right ventricular hypertrophy. The principal handicaps resulting from this defect are anoxic spells during infancy and severe dyspnea on exertion throughout childhood and adult life. A shunt operation is a livesaving measure as far as the spells are concerned, and it affords symptomatic relief for the exercise intolerance. Eventually, complete repair of the ventricular defect and the pulmonary stenosis is desirable.

TETRALOGY OF FALLOT WITH UNILATERAL PULMONARY ATRESIA

A rather rare variant of Fallot's tetralogy in which only one main pulmonary artery is present will be discussed briefly because of the specific difficulties that this situation may present at the operating table.

Incidence

This apparently is a rare condition—we have found only nine such cases during the past fifteen years in our clinic.[528]

Anatomy

The anatomic situation is similar to that found in the classic tetralogy of Fallot. Pulmonary stenosis is associated with a ventricular defect, overriding aorta and right ventricular hypertrophy. The only distinguishing feature is that one pulmonary artery (usually the right) shows considerable poststenotic dilatation, while the other is hypoplastic or even completely absent (Fig. 460). The right ventricular obstruction may be valvar in some, whereas in others infundibular pulmonic stenosis is associated with an absent pulmonary valve.

Physiology

Hemodynamically, the situation is also practically identical with that found in tetralogy of Fallot, except that the circulation to the lung which is not supplied by a pulmonary artery, is exclusively through collateral channels. The lungs on the side where the pulmonary artery is absent are also hypoplastic, and differential spirometry shows poor respiratory function.

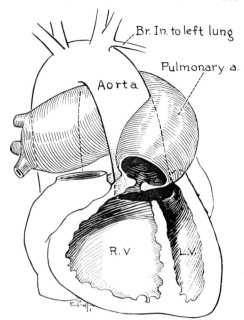

Figure 460. Diagrammatic presentation of tetralogy of Fallot with atresia of the left main pulmonary artery and dilatation of the right main pulmonary artery.[528]

Clinical Picture

In terms of symptomatology, the clinical picture cannot be distinguished from that of straightforward pulmonary stenosis with ventricular defect and a right-to-left shunt of rather severe degree. Interestingly enough, in older children hemoptysis may occur.

On physical examination the only distinguishing feature in these patients is that the stenotic murmur propagates almost exclusively to the side where the large main pulmonary artery is. This results in a murmur at the second right interspace (Fig. 461) in patients with levocardia and at the second left interspace in those with dextrocardia.

The electrocardiogram reveals the usual pattern of right ventricular hypertrophy.

The roentgenologic picture is the only truly diagnostic feature of this condition; these patients show diminution of the pulmonary vasculature and a small lung volume on one side, and a dilated main pulmonary artery with pulmonary vascular engorgement and even, occasionally, "hilar dance" on the other (Fig. 462).

At cardiac catheterization valvar pulmonic stenosis, with right ventricular hypertension in the systemic range, is encountered.

Angiocardiography is the most specific diagnostic tool, revealing the overriding aorta, a large right main pulmonary artery and no opacification of the left main pulmonary artery (Fig. 463).

Course and Prognosis

The expected course of this entity is difficult to outline with any accuracy because of the meager number of patients available. Some of our patients live restricted lives and are ten to fifteen years of age at present.

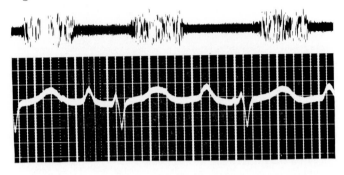

Second Right Interspace

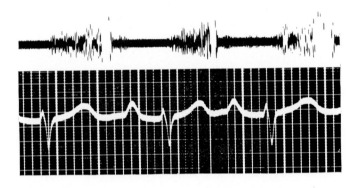

Second Left Interspace

Figure 461. Phonocardiogram of patient with atresia of the left main pulmonary artery. Note the loud murmur at the second right interspace with considerably fainter murmur at the second left interspace.[528]

One infant experienced severe pulmonary difficulties because of the compression of the right main bronchus by the aneurysmally dilated right main pulmonary artery; this infant died after an attempt at surgical correction. A fifth patient, with extremely severe symptoms, was successfully operated on.

Differential Diagnosis

Tetralogy of Fallot. Tetralogy of Fallot may be distinguished from this entity by the uniformly ischemic lung field and by the transmission of the systolic murmur to the left side of the chest if the heart is in the normal position.

Pulmonary Vascular Obstruction with Ventricular Defect and Right-to-Left Shunt. Pulmonary vascular obstruction with ventricular defect and right-to-left shunt may be confused with tetralogy of Fallot with unilateral pulmonary atresia because of the pulmonary plethora in one hemithorax.

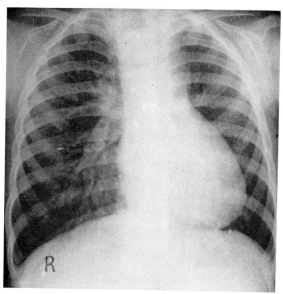

Figure 462. Posteroanterior roentgenogram of patient with atresia of the left main pulmonary artery. Note the ischemic left lung field with plethoric right lung field.

The presence of the stenotic murmur and the uneven distribution of the vasculature suggest the correct diagnosis rather easily.

Hemitruncus. Hemitruncus with a large pulmonary artery to one lung and no pulmonary artery to the other cannot be differentiated from this condition except by means of an angiocardiogram in the correct position.

Treatment

Because of technical difficulties, operation probably ought not to be recommended for the time being unless the symptoms are well nigh intolerable. In that case a right Blalock anastomosis to the large right main pulmonary artery is recommended. The operative risks are high. I do not know of any instance in which complete correction of this anomaly has been undertaken. It is hard to imagine how it could be performed successfully.

Summary

Patients who have a variant of tetralogy of Fallot, with unilateral atresia of one pulmonary artery and poststenotic dilatation of the other, may be recognized by the peculiar transmission of the murmur and the uneven distribution of the vascular pattern as shown on the roentgenogram. Since operation is fraught with more than average risk, it should not be recommended unless it is absolutely necessary. If a shunt procedure still seems desirable, the anastomosis should be effected to the large pulmonary artery rather than attempting to find a vessel in the completely undervascularized lung field.

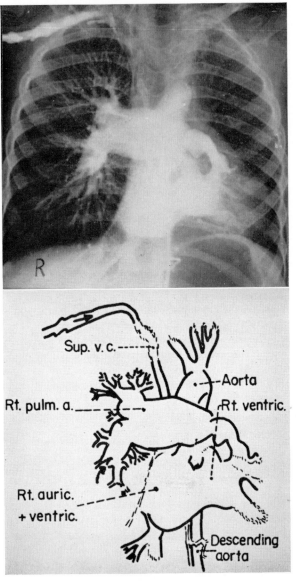

Figure 463.   Angiocardiogram with diagrammatic explanation in a patient with atresia of the left main pulmonary artery.[596]

PULMONIC STENOSIS WITH VENTRICULAR SEPTAL DEFECT AND RIGHT VENTRICULAR PRESSURE HIGHER THAN SYSTEMIC LEVEL

Another recently described variation of the tetralogy of Fallot syndrome should be mentioned briefly.[340] Patients with this combination of defects have all the anatomic features of Fallot's tetralogy, but the physiologic picture is different in one important respect; i.e. the right ventricular systolic pressure is appreciably higher than left ventricular pressure.

Incidence

We saw 10 patients with this syndrome between 1957 and 1959. In 1951 Soulie[658] reported 3 such cases. McGoon[466] described one in 1958. It is unquestionably a rare anomaly, but as often happens, once an entity is described, many more cases are recognized.

Anatomy

The most puzzling aspect of the syndrome is the location of the ventricular septal defect. What is the size and location of the septal opening that it does not allow for complete pressure equilibration? Perhaps, on the whole, the defect is somewhat smaller than the average seen in Fallot's tetralogy, but in only two out of ten patients was it considered truly small by the surgeon. The location of the defect may be more pertinent. In some patients the septal leaflet of the tricuspid valve covers it and may even adhere to it. In others the defect may be far posterior and inferior in the muscular septum and subject to closure during ventricular systole.

Physiology

The physiologic setup is closely similar to that described in the section on pulmonic stenosis with intact ventricular septum (p. 613), the only difference being that a right-to-left shunt through the ventricular septal defect is possible during the first part of the ejection period.

Clinical Picture

Clinically, for all practical purposes, these patients behave as though the ventricular septum was intact. The only difference is in the shape of

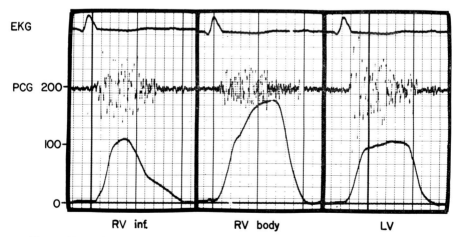

Figure 464. Phonocardiogram and pressure tracing in patient with pulmonic stenosis, ventricular septal defect, and right ventricular pressure higher than systemic level. Note the virtual identity of pressures in the right ventricular infundibulum and the notch on the upstroke of the right ventricular tracing corresponding to the level of the infundibulum. Note also in the phonocardiogram the early onset of the murmur.[340]

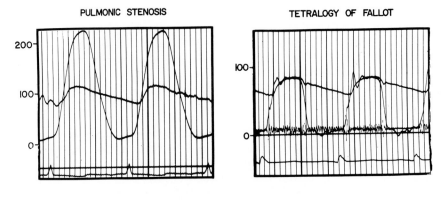

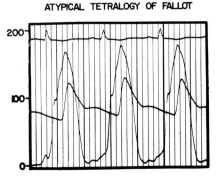

Figure 465. Right ventricular and systemic arterial pressures in pulmonic stenosis with intact ventricular septum, in the tetralogy of Fallot, and in a patient with pulmonic stenosis, ventricular septal defect and right ventricular pressure higher than systemic levels (atypical tetralogy of Fallot).[340]

the systolic murmur; the apex of the diamond occurs early, within the first half of electrical systole (Fig. 464). This is particularly unusual in view of the evidence of severe pulmonic stenosis obtainable through other parameters (the electrocardiogram, and so forth).

At *cardiac catheterization* the pressure relations are similar to those encountered in patients with pulmonic stenosis and intact ventricular septum, with a systolic gradient favoring the right ventricle over the systemic artery by 35 to 120 mm. of mercury in our patients. In spite of this, the presence of a ventricular septal defect could be demonstrated either by passage of the catheter, by dye-dilution curves or by angiography. Furthermore, the pulmonic stenosis was at the infundibular level, and the right ventricular pressure pulse tended to show a notch on the upstroke at the level of the systemic arterial systolic pressure (Fig. 465).

Course and Prognosis

No long-term follow-up of these patients is available, but I would think that their course should be similar to that encountered in patients with severe pulmonic stenosis and an intact ventricular septum.

Differential Diagnosis

It is extremely important from the therapeutic viewpoint to distinguish this entity from severe pulmonic stenosis with an intact ventricular septum. The following points may be useful in the differential diagnosis: (1) The presence of infundibular stenosis is suggested by auscultation, roentgenologic examination and cardiac catheterization. (2) The presence of a right-to-left shunt is implied by the presence of cyanosis and arterial unsaturation and proved by dye-dilution curves and angiography. (3) By demonstrating an early apex of the diamond-shaped murmur, the phonocardiogram also suggests the presence of a ventricular septal defect. (4) The shape of the right ventricular pressure pulse, with a notch on the ascending limb, implies a closing ventricular septal defect. In other words, this entity should be considered if a patient has the clinical profile of pure pulmonic stenosis, but has evidences of infundibular stenosis, an early systolic murmur and appreciable cyanosis. It is in these patients, particularly, that thorough physiologic studies are indicated preoperatively.

Treatment

At open-heart surgery not only must the right ventricular obstruction be relieved, but also the ventricular septal defect must be closed. Consequently, operation through the pulmonary artery is not sufficient; the ventricular septum also must be explored either through a ventriculotomy or from the atrium through the tricuspid valve.

Summary

Patients with the clinical profile of pure pulmonic stenosis should be suspected of having an associated ventricular septal defect if the obstruction seems infundibular, if the murmur is early and if there is cyanosis. The diagnosis may best be made at careful cardiac catheterization.

PERIPHERAL PULMONIC STENOSIS

Stenosis, or atresia, of one or more pulmonary arterial branches may be seen rarely as an isolated phenomenon or more commonly in association with other congenital cardiac malformations.

Peripheral Pulmonic Stenosis with Associated Anomalies

I shall only briefly refer to the fact that all patients with valvar pulmonic stenosis, tetralogy of Fallot, patent ductus arteriosus, ventricular septal defect, atrial septal defect, truncus arteriosus and tricuspid atresia may have constrictions in one or more pulmonary arterial branches. Stenosis of either pulmonary artery may be involved. As indicated, in patients with Fallot's tetralogy the left pulmonary artery is more commonly involved, whereas in the others the right one is more commonly affected. The stenosis may be demonstrated at angiography as a localized narrowing with post-

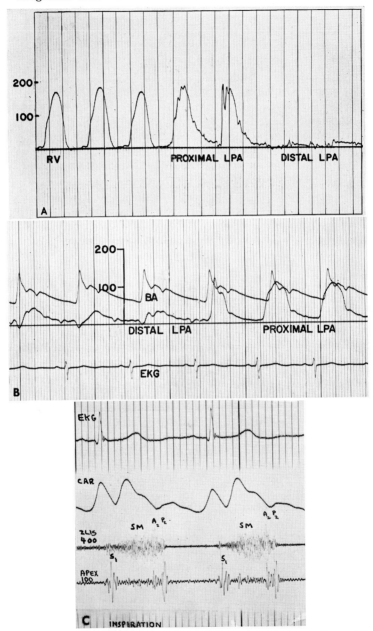

Figure 466. Pressure tracings and phonocardiogram in patient with peripheral pulmonic stenosis. *A,* Note the identity of systolic pressure, with minimal difference in diastolic pressure, in the right ventricle and the proximal portion of the left pulmonary artery. There is a sharp drop in systolic pressure on entering the distal portion of the left pulmonary artery. *B,* Note that the pressure in the proximal left pulmonary artery is closely similar to that in the brachial artery. Also note the damped tracing in the distal left pulmonary artery. *C,* Note the well split second sound at the apex and the second left interspace. Aortic closure is identified by the dicrotic notch in the carotid tracing. The diamond-shaped systolic murmur at the second left interspace has a late apex; it goes certainly beyond the aortic closure and may spread slightly beyond the pulmonic closure, as well.

stenotic dilatation or as a pressure gradient on withdrawal from the pulmonary capillary position (Fig. 466). Often, even at postmortem examination, these physiologic observations cannot be confirmed. The clinical recognition of peripheral pulmonic stenosis within the framework of the other anomalies mentioned is difficult, if not impossible. Occasionally a grade 2 to 3 midsystolic ejection murmur at the second left or right interspace, with good transmission over the lung fields, and rarely even assuming a continuous nature, is the only clue to the presence of this complicating anomaly. Gyllensward[318]stressed that an ordinary roentgenologic examination revealing dilated pulmonary vasculature in the periphery with the constricted vessels located centrally should also suggest this diagnosis. Unfortunately, in our hands neither the auscultatory nor the roengenologic findings have been characteristic enough to indicate the clinical diagnosis with any certainty. Among our cases diagnosed at cardiac catheterization there were twelve with various left-to-right shunts and nine with right-to-left shunts within the framework of the tetralogy of Fallot with unilateral pulmonary atresia (p. 662). More than thirty cases have been reported in the literature.[221, 238, 450]

Uncomplicated Peripheral Pulmonic Stenosis

Incidence

In this small group of patients peripheral pulmonic stenosis is the only significant cardiac defect. We have seen only three such patients, and fewer than twenty-five are mentioned in the literature.

Anatomy

The obstruction in these cases is multiple, by definition; supravalvar pulmonic stenosis consisting of a single obstructive site in the main pulmonary artery was discussed in the section on pulmonic stenosis with intact ventricular septum (p. 613). Beyond the obstruction there is poststenotic dilatation which may give rise to a picture resembling an arteriovenous aneurysm. It is possible that on one side there are obstructions in the main pulmonary arterial branch, while in the other lung the small vessels are involved and give rise to a hemangioma-like picture.

Physiology

Hypertension in the main pulmonary artery is the characteristic physiologic consequence of this lesion. It is interesting to note that the first such case described in Kjellberg's monograph was considered an example of essential pulmonary hypertension. This is understandable, since the hemodynamic consequences of the two entities are identical; the only difference is in the site of the obstruction.

Clinical Picture

A familial evidence of the anomaly has been noted by Van Epps[704] and by Gyllensward.[318]

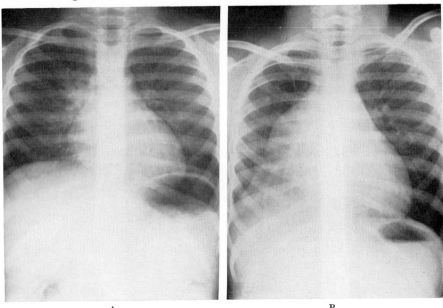

A   B

Figure 467. Preoperative and postoperative roentgenograms of patient with multiple peripheral pulmonic stenosis and proximal pulmonary arterial hypertension. *A,* Preoperative film. *B,* Film taken some months after the right upper and lower lobes were removed because of uncontrollable hemoptysis. Observe that the area of the right hilus in the preoperative film corresponds to the vascular malformation giving rise to the hemoptysis.

Among our patients, one was admitted with hemoptysis; the other two were asymptomatic. Dyspnea, fatigue and transient cyanosis may be the prevalent symptoms. On physical examination evidences of right ventricular enlargement are noted, and pulmonary closure is so loud that the pulmonary vascular obstruction syndrome is suspected. On the other hand, the second sound is well split, and a loud murmur of pulmonic stenosis is heard not only at the second left interspace, but also throughout the lung fields. In most instances the pulmonary arteries on both sides are involved, but occasionally unilateral lesions are found. In two thirds of our patients and in approximately one quarter of those in the literature, a continuous murmur was heard over the lung fields. I cannot state with any certainty whether this is the murmur of severe pulmonic stenosis alone or whether it originates from the arteriovenous aneurysm-like structures mentioned earlier.

Roentgenologic examination shows varying degrees of right ventricular and right atrial enlargement. In one of our patients the hemangioma-like pulmonary arteries were clearly seen in the roentgenogram (Fig. 467). Swedish workers have emphasized the poorly outlined, narrow hilar vessels in contrast to well marked, dilated peripheral pulmonary arteries. The electrocardiogram shows more or less right ventricular hypertrophy, depending on the severity of the obstruction (Fig. 468).

Cardiac catheterization reveals the following (Fig. 469): (1) A right-to-left shunt through a foramen ovale may result in more or less arterial unsaturation in patients with severe obstruction. (2) The pressures in the right atrium and right ventricle depend on the degree of obstruction.

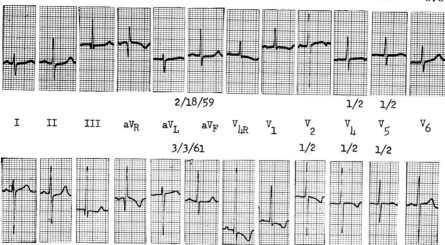

| I | II | III | aV_R | aV_L | aV_F | V_{4R} | V_1 | V_2 | V_4 | V_5 | V_6 |

2/18/59 ... 1/2 1/2

3/3/61 ... 1/2 1/2 1/2

Figure 468. Progressive right ventricular hypertrophy in patient with multiple peripheral pulmonic stenosis. Lobectomy was performed between the times the two electrocardiograms were made.

Two of our three patients had right ventricular pressures at or higher than systemic levels. The systolic pressure in the main pulmonary artery is identical to right ventricular pressure. If the peripheral branches can be penetrated by the catheter, a low, damped pressure is obtained with a gradient of 30 to 100 mm. of mercury. If only the left or the right pulmonary artery is involved, pressure in the right ventricle is normal at rest, but may increase on effort. (3) Resistance at these sites of obstruction may approximate systemic levels. (4) The pulmonary-systemic flow ratios depend on the extent and severity of the obstruction. Severe, bilateral involvement may be accompanied by low pulmonary flow and significant arterial unsaturation. (5) The only important feature of the course of the catheter is that, often, it may not be passed beyond the main pulmonary arterial branch. (6) Angiograms are the heart of the diagnosis. Beautiful pictures may be obtained, revealing the multiple, bilateral constrictions in the pulmonary arterial branches.

Course and Prognosis

The scarcity of the reported cases precludes an accurate appraisal of the course of these patients. All three of our patients are still alive and doing reasonably well, though their exercise tolerance is limited. One of Van Epp's patients died at six years of age.

Differential Diagnosis

Primary Pulmonary Hypertension. See page 609.

Valvar Pulmonic Stenosis with Intact Ventricular Septum. Only at catheterization may this differential diagnosis be made with certainty. The loud pulmonic closure, widely separated from aortic closure, and occasionally the continuous murmur may serve as clinical clues.

Pulmonary Vascular Obstruction Syndrome with a Septal Defect. The nature of the second sound, the lack of evidence of a left-to-right shunt

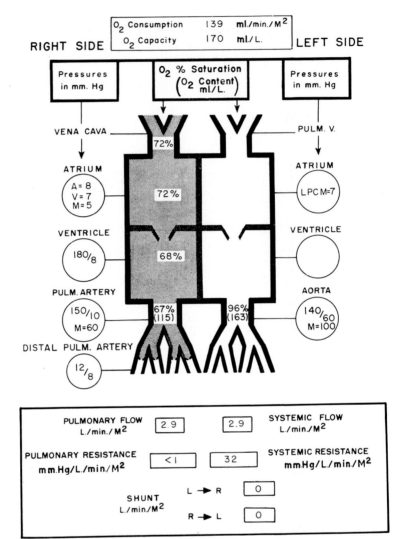

Figure 469. Catheterization findings in a patient with multiple, severe, peripheral pulmonic stenosis.

and the pulmonary vasculature (on the roentgenogram) tend to distinguish these two conditions.

Treatment

One look at the angiograms, revealing the multiplicity of constrictions, testifies to the unsurmountable obstacles to surgery. Only if, by some chance, the stenotic areas were restricted to the main branches could surgery conceivably be successful. We operated successfully on one of our patients. Surgery consisted in removal of two lobes of the right lung, the source of frequent and profuse hemoptysis.

Summary

Patients with evidences of pulmonary arterial hypertension, widely conducted stenotic, and even continuous, murmurs originating in the pulmonary artery and diminished pulmonary vasculature should be suspected of having multiple peripheral pulmonic stenosis. Cardiac catheterization reveals hypertension of the right ventricle and the main pulmonary artery. If the catheter can be passed beyond the main branches, a pressure gradient is obtained. Angiocardiography pictures the nature of the obstruction most graphically. Surgery is not available at present.

IDIOPATHIC PULMONARY REGURGITATION

Incidence

Whereas incompetence of the pulmonary valve in patients with pulmonary vascular obstruction (idiopathic, or associated with congenital heart disease or mitral stenosis) is a fairly common occurrence, pulmonary regurgitation as an isolated phenomenon is rare. Two such cases have been described by Kjellberg and his associates.[397] We have seen six such patients at the Children's Hospital Medical Center in Boston. This condition is also known as "idiopathic dilation of the pulmonary artery."

Anatomy

To the best of my knowledge, no anatomic studies are available in any patients with this syndrome. In all likelihood the condition is congenital.

Physiology

Patients with idiopathic pulmonary regurgitation are characterized by the presence of a loud, early, relatively low-frequency diastolic murmur in the pulmonary area and low diastolic pressure in the pulmonary artery, without any other hemodynamic abnormality. Physiologically, the results of even maximal pulmonary insufficiency are slight;[255] the normally low diastolic pressure in the pulmonary artery precludes the regurgitation of large volumes of blood during ventricular diastole. Acute experiments in dogs[40] indicate that surgically induced pulmonary regurgitation has no serious immediate consequences. That the situation from the long-term viewpoint may be different is suggested by the observation that cardiac enlargement and even congestive heart failure develop in an appreciable number of the dogs with pulmonary incompetence secondary to enucleation of the pulmonary valve.[573]

Clinical Picture

No symptoms attributable to heart disease are present. On physical examination the most striking finding is a loud, early diastolic murmur, even accompanied by a diastolic thrill at the second to fourth left interspace, with a decrescendo configuration (Fig. 470). A systolic murmur of lower intensity and frequency may also be heard in the same area; however, this lacks the typical characteristics of a stenotic murmur. The heart sounds are normal; interestingly enough, the pulmonary second sound is of only average intensity and splitting. The rest of the physical examination is entirely negative. Most important, the pulse pressure is well within normal limits.

Roentgenologically, no increase in the transverse diameter of the heart is noted. The main segment of the pulmonary artery is prominent and pulsates vigorously (Fig. 471). The pulmonary vasculature is well within normal limits.

The electrocardiogram is normal.

Cardiac catheterization shows normal hemodynamics, with the exception of a low pulmonary arterial diastolic pressure.

Angiocardiographic studies have not been performed on any of our patients.

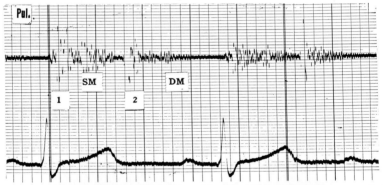

Figure 470. Phonocardiogram of patient with idiopathic pulmonary regurgitation.

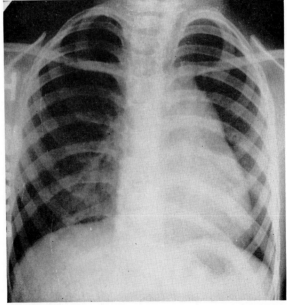

Figure 471. Posteroanterior roentgenogram of patient with idiopathic pulmonary regurgitation. Note the relatively normal-sized heart with prominent main pulmonary artery, but normal pulmonary vasculature.

Course and Prognosis

On the basis of limited personal experience, I believe that this condition is probably compatible with normal life expectancy and a fully active life. But recent reports of Engle[358] and Smith[647] described newborns in fatal congestive heart failure in whom congenital pulmonary insufficiency was the only cardiac lesion. Another report[220] described an adolescent with pulmonary regurgitation and cardiac enlargement. It is possible that the serious disease of these patients is due to a totally inadequate valve rather than to the slight functional incompetence commonly encountered clinically.

Differential Diagnosis

Aortic Regurgitation. Sometimes it is difficult to distinguish pulmonary from aortic regurgitation on the basis of the localization and the nature of the murmur alone. The most important points in differential diagnosis are the wide pulse pressure, the history of rheumatic fever and the high-frequency protodiastolic blow in patients with aortic regurgitation.

Patent Ductus Arteriosus or Ventricular Septal Defect with Aortic Regurgitation. Patent ductus arteriosus and ventricular septal defect with aortic regurgitation are relatively easily distinguished from idiopathic pulmonary regurgitation by the presence of pulmonary vascular engorgement in the roentgenogram. Occasionally cardiac catheterization is necessary to exclude the presence of a small left-to-right shunt.

Pulmonary Vascular Obstruction. Perhaps the most common cause of pulmonary insufficiency, pulmonary vascular obstruction, is distinguished from idiopathic pulmonary regurgitation on the basis of evidences of pulmonary arterial hypertension, such as a ringing pulmonary second sound, and evidences of right ventricular hypertrophy in the electrocardiogram.

Valvar Pulmonic Stenosis. Valvar pulmonic stenosis of maximal degree may be accompanied by a murmur suggestive of pulmonary regurgitation. As pointed out earlier, actually this is only a continuation of the systolic murmur beyond the aortic component of the second sound, a phenomenon relatively easily demonstrated phonocardiographically. Furthermore, the systolic murmur is always louder and stenotic in nature.

Ventricular Septal Defect with Absence of the Pulmonary Valve. As indicated before, this may be present either as a variant of the tetralogy of Fallot syndrome or superimposed on the clinical picture of a large ventricular septal defect. Both conditions should be easily distinguishable from the entity under discussion, in which, in essence, the only findings are the large main pulmonary artery and a protodiastolic blow in an otherwise healthy person.

Treatment

No treatment is necessary for idiopathic pulmonary regurgitation, beyond reassurance to the parents and the child.

Summary

An early diastolic murmur at the pulmonary area, accompanied by roentgenologic evidence of a large main pulmonary artery segment and perfectly normal hemodynamics, characterizes the syndrome of idiopathic pulmonary regurgitation. The condition is innocuous in the majority of patients.

TRICUSPID ATRESIA

In tricuspid atresia there is no direct communication between the right atrium and the right ventricle. The right atrial blood is shunted through a foramen ovale, or an atrial defect, into the left atrium, where complete mixture with the pulmonary venous blood occurs.

Incidence

Tricuspid atresia has been regarded as one of the rarest congenital cardiac diseases, but it must be considered in the differential diagnosis of every patient with cyanotic congenital heart disease. Brown,[102] in the last edition of his book, mentioned fifty cases collected from the literature; Abbott[1] reported sixteen in her series. Taussig, quoted by Keith, reported seventy-three patients operated on for this condition; Keith himself has collected forty-nine clinical cases. We have seen fifty proved cases at The Children's Hospital Medical Center in Boston within the past fifteen years. Thus, in my opinion, this anomaly may be more common than was hitherto suspected. Campbell[127] stated that patients with tricuspid atresia constitute about 5 per cent of the patients with cyanotic congenital heart disease. Wood placed the incidence at 1.5 per cent in his 900 cases of congenital heart disease, Keith at 3.2 per cent.

Anatomy

On the basis of the anatomic situation in the ventricles, Edwards and his co-workers[219] distinguished four types of tricuspid atresia, depending on whether or not the great arteries are transposed, whether a defect in the ventricular septum exists and whether there is stenosis of the pulmonary artery (Fig. 472).

Embryologically, the defect probably occurs by about the fourth or fifth intrauterine week and is due to an incomplete shift of the common atrioventricular canal, so that the ventricular septum, growing up from below, fails to divide it evenly. The lesions associated with tricuspid atresia, such as atrial defect, patent foramen ovale, patent ductus arteriosus or hypoplastic pulmonary artery, probably result from the altered hemodynamics caused by the tricuspid atresia. An atrial opening, in most instances a patent foramen ovale, is a sine qua non for survival. An associated large ventricular septal defect, amounting to a single ventricle, is usually accompanied by transposition of the great arteries.

Physiology

The physiologic consequences of tricuspid atresia are manifold.[69] The first and most important result is the presence of arterial unsaturation due

TRICUSPID ATRESIA — ANATOMICAL DIVISIONS
(EDWARDS)

I. NO TRANSPOSITION OF THE GREAT ARTERIES

a. WITHOUT VSD
   WITH PULMONARY ATRESIA AND
   A PATENT DUCTUS ARTERIOSUS

b. WITH SLIT-LIKE VSD,
   STENOTIC PULMONARY ARTERY

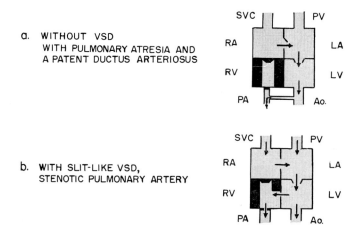

II. WITH TRANSPOSITION OF THE GREAT ARTERIES

a. WITH PULMONARY STENOSIS
   AND VSD

b. WITHOUT PULMONARY STENOSIS
   AND WITH VSD

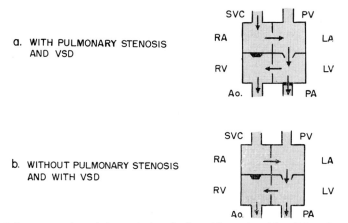

Figure 472.   Schematic presentation of the varieties of tricuspid atresia. (After Edwards.[219])

to a complete mixing of systemic venous and pulmonary venous blood in the left atrium. The degree of unsaturation depends on the ratio of pulmonary venous to systemic venous return within this common left atrial pool; this, in turn, is dependent entirely on the size of the pulmo nary blood flow. The larger the pulmonary blood flow, the less evident the cyanosis; thus patients of type Ia, Ib and IIb of Edwards's classifica tion have much cyanosis (Fig. 472). On the other hand, patients of type IIb, with large pulmonary blood flow, do not have to show definite cyanosis at all.

A second, and equally important, physiologic consequence of tricuspid atresia is the underdevelopment of the right ventricle in types Ia and Ib as a result of the inadequate blood flow through it. The third physiologic handicap, dependent on the size of the atrial septal opening, is the elevated right atrial pressure necessary to force the caval blood over to the left atrium; this, in turn, results in increased systemic venous pressure and, eventually, congestive failure. This, then, results in the paradoxical situation of right atrial hypertension without concomitant right ventricular hypertension.

Clinical Picture

The clinical picture to be described is based principally on the findings in our own proved cases of tricuspid atresia.

These children are all sick in early infancy. Severe cyanosis is the dominant symptom, except in those with single ventricle and transposition, with a large pulmonary blood flow. In addition, dyspnea, fatigue, anoxic spells and, of great importance, evidences of right-sided failure are observed. Squatting is rare in our experience, though Taussig mentioned that in her patients this was almost as frequent as it was in the children with tetralogy of Fallot.

At physical examination the majority of the infants are undernourished and poorly developed; cyanosis and clubbing are readily apparent. Left-sided chest prominence is absent; the thorax either is symmetrical or may show a slight bulge on the right side of the sternum. A thrill is palpable in only about a fourth of the patients. Considerable hepatomegaly, occasionally with presystolic pulsations, is present in more than half. The giant A waves in the jugular venous pulse, corresponding to the presystolic pulsations of the liver, are indicative of patients in whom the atrial septal opening is relatively small. Pulmonary rales and evidences of left-sided failure are uniformly absent. At auscultation the heart sounds are clear at the lower left sternal border. Only aortic closure can be heard well at the lower left sternal border in most instances. Pulmonic closure is usually absent, for obvious reasons, although in patients with an appreciably sized ventricular septal defect and, of course, in those with single ventricle and transposition both semilunar closures may be appreciated. A grade 3 to 4 harsh, blowing systolic murmur is audible at the lower left sternal border in more than half of the patients. In others, probably the sickest ones, only faint murmurs are audible. In almost 25 per cent of the infants, mostly those with the Ia type of defect, no murmurs are heard at all. The continuous murmurs of collaterals are rare. Interestingly enough, no atrial sound or diastolic murmur is present.

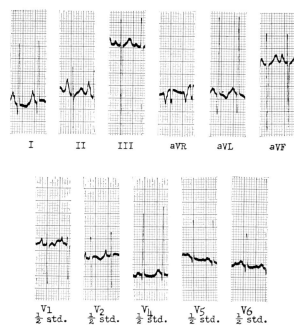

Figure 473. Electrocardiogram of patient with tricuspid atresia. Note left axis deviation (—45°), left ventricular hypertrophy and P pulmonale.

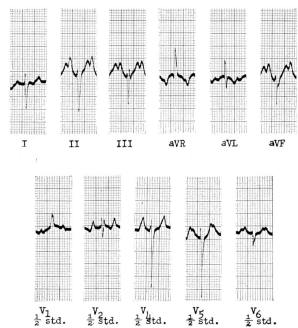

Figure 474. Electrocardiogram of patient with tricuspid atresia, showing extreme right axis deviation (—110°) with right ventricular hypertrophy in chest leads, but with a counterclockwise loop.

The electrocardiogram is always abnormal for the age of the patient. Left ventricular hypertrophy (or left ventricular dominance in young infants) or P pulmonale is noted in almost every instance; frequently both features are present in the same patient (Fig. 473). It is my impression that the patients with the most notable P pulmonale are those with the smallest atrial defects. Reviewing the electrocardiograms of twenty-three patients with proved uncomplicated tricuspid atresia, the frontal plane loop was inscribed counterclockwise in all, the mean electrical axis varying between +30 and —90 degrees in all but one. In the latter case the axis was at —110 degrees, also with counterclockwise inscription. Occasionally an infant may show right ventricular hypertrophy in the chest leads (Fig. 474) with the frontal plane as described, possibly because the exploring electrode in the V_1 position is directly over the small right ventricle.

The roentgenologic findings have been summarized by Wittenborg and his associates.[739] The classic picture (Fig. 475), characterized by the straight right border with a concave pulmonary artery segment in the anteroposterior view and the straight anterior border in the left anterior oblique projection, is certainly not the only radiologic configuration encountered in this disease. Depending on the size of the interatrial communication, and thus the size of the right atrium, either the classic picture or a *coeur en sabot* configuration (Fig. 476), or even the picture of dextrocardia (Fig. 477), may be encountered. Cardiac enlargement is always present and may vary from minimal to serious degree. The pulmonary vasculature is greatly diminished, except in the rare patient with complete transposition of the great arteries. [11 G] The main pulmonary artery segment is small or absent. The aortic arch is on the left in more than 90 per cent of the cases. No clear-cut differentiation between right and left ventricular enlargement is possible by radiologic means. Astley and his associates[25] described enlargement of the left atrium in the right anterior oblique and the posteroanterior view. In the latter projection this gives rise to a "square heart."

Cardiac catheterization reveals the following (Fig. 478): (1) There is a right-to-left shunt at the atrial level resulting in identical saturation in left atrium, left ventricle, right ventricle (if present) and both great arteries.

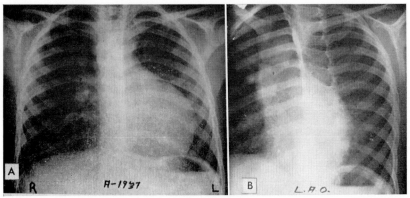

Figure 475. The classic radiologic picture of tricuspid atresia in the posteroanterior and the left anterior oblique views. Note the absent right border in the posteroanterior view and the cut-off anterior border in the left anterior oblique view.

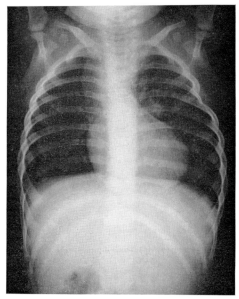

Figure 476.   *Coeur en sabot* configuration in a patient with tricuspid atresia.

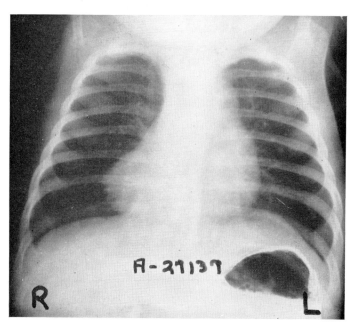

Figure 477.   Dextrocardia-like picture in patient with tricuspid atresia.

The systemic arterial saturation is directly proportionate to the pulmonary flow. (2) Right atrial pressure is elevated (mean, 5 to 10 mm. of mercury) with giant A waves. The height of the right atrial pressure and its relation to left atrial pressure depend on the size of the interatrial communication (Fig. 479). If the gradient between the right and left atrial mean pressures is 5 mm. or less, with closely similar phasic patterns, it may be assumed

that the interatrial communication is adequate. Left ventricular and systemic arterial pressures are normal. Right ventricular and pulmonary arterial pressures depend on the anatomic situation. In all but type IIb tricuspid
atresia, pulmonary arterial pressure is low, similar to that encountered
in Fallot's tetralogy. Right ventricular pressure is in systemic range. (3)
Pulmonary arterial resistance is low normal. (4) Pulmonary flow is low in
all but type IIb. Systemic flow is normal or increased. (5) The course of
the catheter is of considerable interest in that the right ventricle cannot
be entered from the right atrium. In inexperienced hands this, by itself,
does not prove the presence of tricuspid atresia. In our laboratory, however,
the assumption may be made that if our highly skilled people cannot cross
the tricuspid valve, it is almost certain to be atretic. The natural course
of the catheter is across the atrial septum into the left atrium and left

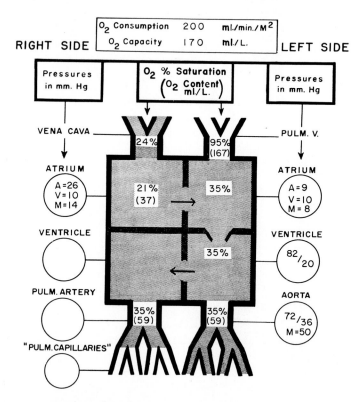

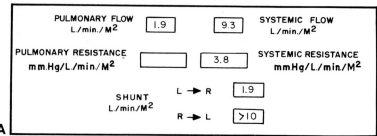

(See facing page for legend.)

ventricle. Usually only the aorta may be entered from the left ventricle, except in patients with transposition, where the natural bend is toward the pulmonary artery. (6) Cine-angiograms, with injection into the right atrium, prove conclusively the presence of an atretic tricuspid valve. The dye streams across the atrial septum, outlining (in the lateral position) the size of the atrial defect. Usually the relation of the great arteries is clearly evident. The right ventricle is hard to identify. As a matter of fact, one of the characteristic features of the examination is the appearance of a triangular filling defect at the place where the right ventricle is usually seen.

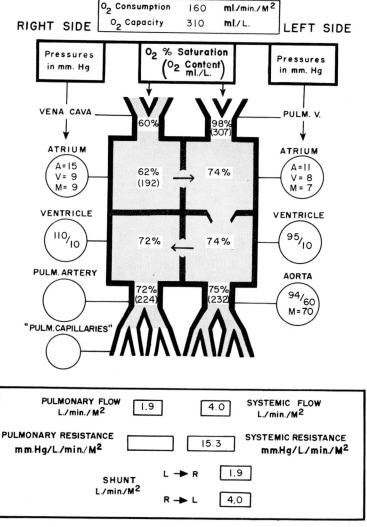

Figure 478. Catheterization findings in patients with tricuspid atresia. In neither diagram has the pulmonary artery been entered; thus the saturation figures are assumed. In *A* an appreciable gradient between right and left atrium exists, whereas in *B* the mean pressures are almost identical. Pulmonary flow is relatively larger in B, hence the higher arterial oxygen saturation.

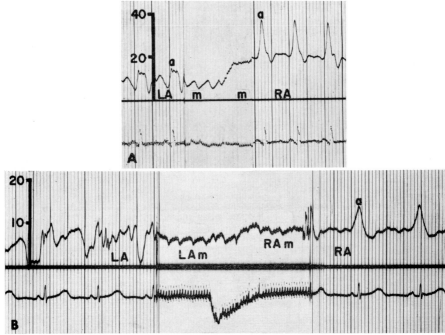

Figure 479. *A,* Large gradient between left and right atria, both in the phasic and the mean tracings, in patient with tricuspid atresia and a small foramen ovale. Notice particularly the huge A wave in the right atrium. *B,* Small mean gradient between right atrium and left atrium. Note, still, the sizable A wave in the right atrium. In this patient with tricuspid atresia a sizable atrial septal defect was present.

Course and Prognosis

Cyanosis, dyspnea and poor development are invariably noted in children less than six months old, and in most cases even at birth. Death usually occurs in congestive failure or in a severe anoxic spell within the first six to twelve months of life. A minority of the patients, usually those having a large atrial or ventricular defect, may survive without operation until their third or even sixth birthday. Among patients more than ten years of age who have not undergone operation, Keith placed survival at 10 per cent. Patients with tricuspid atresia may experience the usual complications of cyanotic congenital heart disease, i.e. hemiplegia, anemia, or polycythemia and subacute bacterial endocarditis. We have not yet encountered a patient with tricuspid atresia and brain abscess. Obviously, these patients do not live long enough to have rheumatic fever.

Differential Diagnosis

The differential diagnosis of tricuspid atresia involves the cyanotic group of congenital heart diseases in which there may be electrocardiographic evidences of left ventricular hypertrophy. Actually, only the following conditions need to be mentioned: single ventricle with or without transposition (p. 453), truncus arteriosus (p. 505), anomalous drainage of the entire caval system (p. 740), pulmonary atresia with intact ventricular septum (p. 634), complete atrioventricular canal (p. 384) and endocardial cushion defect with pulmonic stenosis.

Treatment

The treatment of patients with tricuspid atresia is surgical, but no truly corrective procedure is available at present even in institutions best equipped to perform open heart surgery. Only palliative procedures— Blalock's, Potts's or Glenn's—aimed at increasing the pulmonary blood flow, have been performed on these patients; these have been moderately successful. Our own experience with Potts's and Blalock's procedures indicates a 30 per cent mortality rate. Taussig quoted 35 per cent for Blalock operations. Within the last year half a dozen patients underwent the Glenn procedure at our institution (superior vena cava-pulmonary artery anastomosis) with success.

In contrast to other authors, I feel that preoperative cardiac catheterization is important in order to decide which surgical procedure would be optimal for the particular patient. The most important information to be obtained is the estimation of the gradient across the atrial septum. If there is no significant gradient, a Potts procedure on the left side is probably the procedure of choice. If there is a significant gradient between the right atrium and left atrium, I would recommend a Glenn procedure, if the patient is big enough. If this is technically impractical, a shunt procedure on the right side, coupled with enlargement of the atrial septal defect, is indicated.

Although the operative risks are relatively high and postoperative improvement is often not spectacular, I am more enthusiastic about recommending surgery today than I was in the past. This change in attitude has been brought about by the gradual improvement in surgical technique and the recognition that it is nearly inconceivable that complete repair will be feasible in the foreseeable future. Recognition of these facts and awareness of the high mortality rate of these patients during infancy lead us to a more aggressive policy. Of course, if possible, we like to postpone operation beyond infancy, but if the symptoms warrant it, we do not hesitate to proceed, even in the neonatal period. I am sure that this attitude has resulted in a much happier childhood for a number of these youngsters.

Of course, surgery along these lines, aiming at increasing the pulmonary flow, is indicated only in patients with greatly diminished pulmonary blood flow and severe cyanosis. The surgical treatment of patients in the IIb group will be discussed later (see Transposition of the Great Arteries, p. 699).

Summary

Patients with cyanotic congenital heart disease whose electrocardiograms indicate left axis deviation and left ventricular hypertrophy with P pulmonale are likely to have tricuspid atresia. This is a severe anomaly causing cyanosis at birth, and death usually within the first year of life. Palliative surgery is the only available treatment.

DOWNWARD DISPLACEMENT OF THE TRICUSPID VALVE
(EBSTEIN'S ANOMALY)

Incidence

Ebstein's malformation was first described about 100 years ago. Maude Abbott[1] did not mention any instance among her 1000 cases of congenital heart disease. We published reports of 10 cases from our institution in 1957,[492] and a review of the literature at that time revealed 80 cases. The total number reported by now is well over a hundred.

Anatomy

In Ebstein's disease the septal, and frequently the posterior, leaflet of the tricuspid valve is not attached in a normal fashion to the annulus fibrosus, but rather to the ventricular wall near the apex. The degree of malattachment and the structural deformities of the valve vary greatly, giving rise to the concept of a "spectrum" of Ebstein's malformations, ranging from extremely severe cases to "form fruste" varieties. The anterior leaflet is conventionally fixed to the annulus fibrosus. This anatomic constellation results in the upper part of the right ventricle being incorporated into the right atrium. Thus the portion of the heart above the apex of the tricuspid valve is huge and can be divided into a superior (atrial) and inferior (ventricular) portion; the border between the two is formed by the annulus fibrosus, to which only the anterior leaflet is attached. The ventricular cavity is small and consists only of the apical portion and the outflow tract of the right ventricle. The walls of both the right atrium and the right ventricle are thin and flabby. The infundibulum of the right ventricle is usually thick. The tricuspid valve is seldom stenotic, but may show a considerable amount of regurgitation. Either the foramen ovale is open, or an atrial septal defect is present. Pulmonic stenosis may be noted, and increasing attention is being paid to corrected transposition of the great arteries in association with left-sided Ebstein's deformity (see p. 713). In Gould's text, Edwards[214] mentioned that among ten cases of Ebstein's malformation five were full-blown instances, two were minor variations, and three were associated with corrected transposition of the great arteries.

The embryology of this malformation has not been clearly explained so far. It may be worth mentioning that Grant,[299] in a most stimulating article, suggested that the etiology lies in the abnormality of fusion between bulbar musculature and the invaginating ventricular septum.

Physiology

I have no clear-cut idea through what physiologic mechanisms the anatomic abnormality known as Ebstein's disease gives rise to the clinical picture to be described. It is difficult to imagine why hypoplasia of the right ventricle alone should result in the characteristic clinical profile, when complete experimental destruction[666] or bypassing[457] of the right ventricle may not cause any great circulatory alterations. Of course one may raise questions about the validity of comparing the acute experiment with the chronic situation existing in Ebstein's anomaly. Additional handicaps contributing to the physiologic picture are the varying degrees of tricuspid regurgitation, the right-to-left shunt through the atrial septum and, possibly, asynchronous or paradoxical contractions of the right heart chambers.

Clinical Picture

The symptomatology consists of mild cyanosis, dyspnea on exertion, fatigue and right-sided congestive failure. In approximately half of the reported cases the onset of symptoms occurred in infancy; the remaining patients were completely asymptomatic until the end of the first decade, or even into late adolescence. Anoxic spells and squatting are rare. Attacks of paroxysmal atrial tachycardia or atrial fibrillation may occur.

At physical examination these children are poorly developed, but reasonably well nourished. Slight cyanosis, at least partially suggestive of the peripheral type, is usually noted in at least half of the patients. As time goes on, cyanosis becomes increasingly noticeable and clearly central in type. Clubbing is slight. The neck veins are usually distended, and V waves may be prominent, but giant A waves are seldom, if ever, encountered. Mild left-sided chest deformity may be present. A thrill at the apex or lower left sternal border, noted in six of our ten children, was thought to be due to tricuspid regurgitation. The cardiac impulse is diffuse and feeble, extending from the xiphoid process to the apex. The liver is usually enlarged, but no presystolic pulsation is present. The extremities are cold and the pulses small, attesting to poor cardiac output.

At auscultation a characteristic triple or quadruple rhythm, at a slow rate and without clear-cut gallop quality, is the most striking feature; phonocardiographic analysis (Fig. 480) reveals the components to be the late first sound, the widely split second sound and the loud fourth sound. The pulmonary closure is diminished. A murmur of tricuspid regurgitation at the lower left sternal border or the apex is the most outstanding observation at auscultation. In addition, a "scratchy" diastolic murmur, consisting of low- to medium-frequency vibrations and extending through presystole, is heard in at least four out of five patients. These auscultatory phenomena are pathognomonic of the condition, and I have observed them in patients of varying ages from infancy to adulthood.

The electrocardiogram is also typical (Fig. 481). Large P pulmonale is clearly evident in most tracings. Conduction disturbances (prolonged P-R interval and incomplete or complete right bundle branch block) are the rule. The Wolff-Parkinson-White syndrome is a relatively frequent concomitant of the condition. No right ventricular hypertrophy is noted after early infancy. Left chest leads show average potentials. Figure 482 demonstrates the change in one patient, with characteristic right ventricular hypertrophy in early infancy and right bundle branch block, without clearcut right ventricular hypertrophy, four years later. Arrhythmias, such as premature beats, paroxysmal atrial tachycardia and atrial flutter, are common.

The roentgenologic picture is also characteristic. It consists of extreme cardiac enlargement, involving principally the right atrium, with diminished pulmonary vasculature (Fig. 483). The pulmonary artery segment

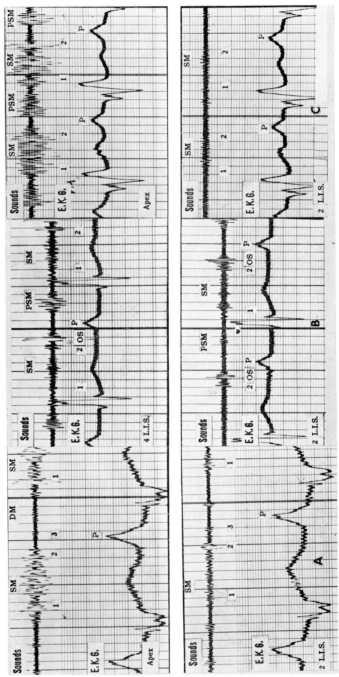

Figure 480. *A,* The murmur of tricuspid regurgitation at the apex with a low-frequency, low-intensity ejection murmur at the second left interspace. The well split second sound may be observed at the apex and the third sound demonstratd at the second left interspace. The first sound, well split second sound and the third sound add up to a quadruple rhythm. *B,* The loud presystolic murmur at the fourth left interspace, with a systolic murmur, a well split second sound and a loud opening sound. *C,* The almost continuous murmur consisting of the presystolic murmur and the regurgitant murmur at the apex.

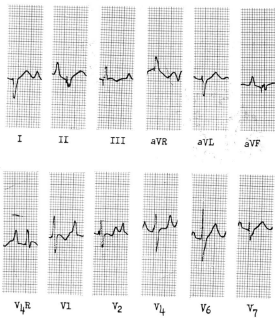

I   II   III   aVR   aVL   aVF

V_4R V1 V_2 V_4 V_6 V_7

Figure 481. Electrocardiogram of patient with Ebstein's disease. Note the P pulmonale with right axis deviation, incomplete right bundle branch block and questionable if any right ventricular hypertrophy.

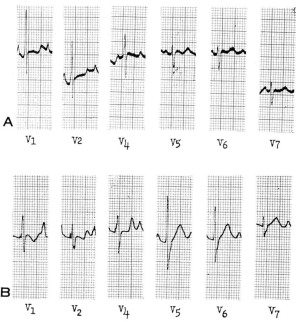

A

V_1 V_2 V_4 V_5 V_6 V_7

B

V_1 V_2 V_4 V_5 V_6 V_7

Figure 482. The development of the electrocardiogram in a patient with Ebstein's anomaly. *A,* Right ventricular hypertrophy in a child four months old, without significant P pulmonale. *B,* P pulmonale, disappearance of right ventricular hypertrophy and appearance of incomplete right bundle branch block, particularly in lead V_2.

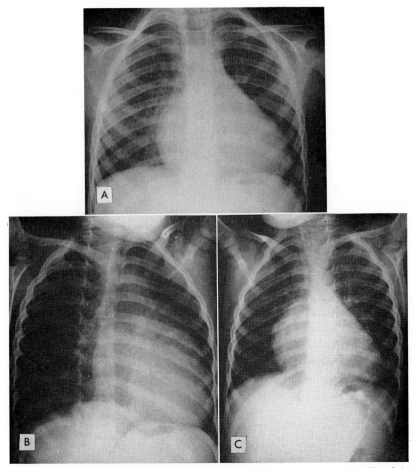

Figure 483.   Posteroanterior and oblique roentgenograms of patient with Ebstein's disease. Note the cardiac enlargement involving principally the right atrium and the diminished pulmonary vasculature.

is hypoplastic. At fluoroscopy the cardiac beat is feeble. The entire silhouette of the heart and its activity resembles that in cases of a large pericardial effusion or pure pulmonary stenosis in congestive failure.

The clinical picture, as described, is the profile of full-blown Ebstein's anomaly, corresponding to the pathologic picture of markedly deformed and misplaced septal and posterior tricuspid valve leaflets. In contrast to these are the instances of "forme fruste" of the disease, corresponding to relatively minor anatomic variations, represented by patients who may have only minor electrocardiographic abnormalities, minimal cardiac enlargement and faint murmurs. I think some of the patients belonging to this category may have been classified in the past as having "functional murmurs." Only skillfully performed catheterization studies or careful postmortem examination can distinguish this group of patients (Figs. 484, 485).

A further variation of this anomaly is seen in patients with severe pulmonic stenosis and an intact ventricular septum, in whom the tricuspid valve shows an Ebstein variation (Fig. 486, 487).

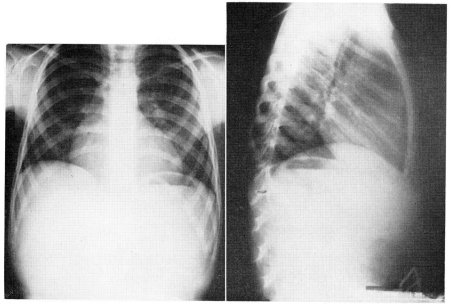

Figure 484. Posteranterior and right lateral views of the heart of a patient with mild Ebstein's disease.

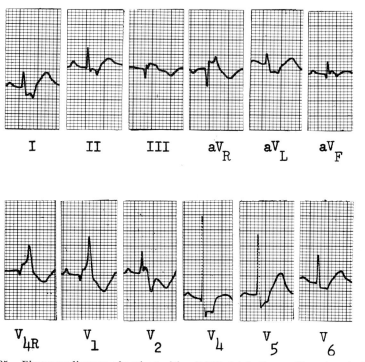

Figure 485. Electrocardiogram of patient with mild Ebstein's disease. Note that the P waves are not particularly tall and that there is intraventricular conduction disturbance.

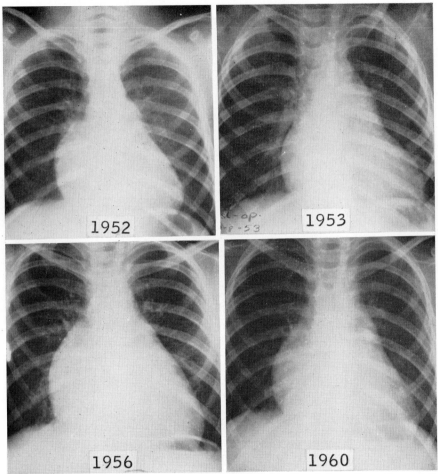

Figure 486. Serial roentgenograms of patient with Ebstein's malformation of the tricuspid valve and pulmonic stenosis. A Brock procedure was performed on this patient between 1952 and 1953, and another pulmonic valvotomy, with open-heart technique, between 1956 and 1960. Note the slight decrease in heart size after the first operation, with considerable progressive cardiac enlargement between 1953 and 1956, alleviated again by surgery.

Cardiac catheterization is fraught with more than average risk. We lost one patient during catheterization and another as a consequence of angiography. In our review in 1957 we found 5 five patients in the literature who died as a consequence of catheterization studies. This is a very high figure considering the rarity of the condition, and, in fact, Wood has stated that he will not wittingly proceed with catheterization again in a patient who has Ebstein's malformation.

Although at present I believe that catheterization studies should be made only with full recognition of the increased risks entailed in patients with suspected Ebstein's malformation, I suspect that the risks may not be quite as high today as they were in the past. Within the last few years we have catheterized patients with this disease without much trouble. I think that this change is probably due to the increased skill of catheteri-

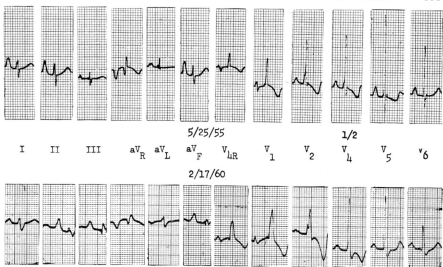

5/25/55   1/2

I   II   III   aV$_R$ aV$_L$ aV$_F$ V$_{4R}$ V$_1$ V$_2$ V$_4$ V$_5$ V$_6$

2/17/60

Figure 487. Electrocardiograms of patient with Ebstein's malformation and pulmonic stenosis. Note the P pulmonale with right ventricular hypertrophy in the tracing obtained in 1955 and the development of complete right bundle branch block after surgery.

zation teams and to the presence of continuous monitoring equipment and the availability of external defibrillators. In the past most of the deaths were due to arrythmias; today we are in a much better position (in a well equipped laboratory, with expert personnel and absence of amateurs) to cope with these than we were in the past. Our policy at present is not to catheterize patients in whom the diagnosis of Ebstein's malformation may be made with *certainty* on clinical grounds. On the other hand, if the diagnosis is in doubt and if an operable situation may not be definitely excluded, we proceed with studies, recognizing the somewhat increased risk.

Catheterization studies reveal[35, 706] the following (Fig. 488): (1) A left-to-right shunt at the atrial level occurs in about 25 per cent of the patients. In 50 per cent of the cases in the literature arterial unsaturation, due to an atrial right-to-left shunt and ranging from 66 to 91 per cent, was noted. (2) The right atrial mean pressure is only moderately elevated, and the pressure pulse may be normal or may show a dominant V wave (Fig. 489). Giant A waves are rare, but Blount and his associates[66] noted the transmission of a moderately high presystolic wave into the right ventricle and even to the pulmonary artery. The absence of striking abnormalities of the right atrial pressure pulse may be explained by the large right atrial cavity. The right ventricular pressure pulse is similar to that of the right atrium with increased end-diastolic pressure. Pulmonary arterial pressure is low and damped. We have seen two patients with a severe gradient across the pulmonary valve. (3) The calculated resistances are normal. (4) Systemic cardiac output is low; pulmonary flow is diminished to below systemic levels in patients with appreciable right-to-left shunts. (5) The course of the catheter is of interest in that it may easily coil in the huge right atrial cavity. Furthermore, because of the downward displacement of the tricuspid valve, right ventricular pressure pulses are first obtained when the catheter enters the usual position of the right ventricular outflow tract. (6) Cine-

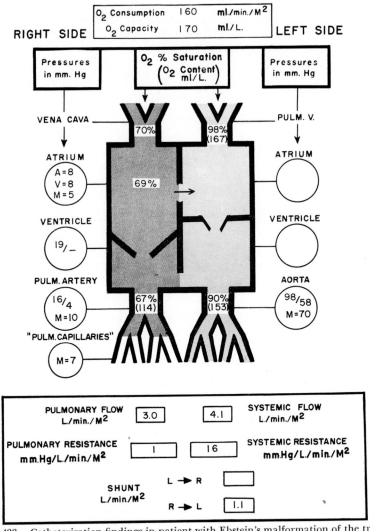

Figure 488. Catheterization findings in patient with Ebstein's malformation of the tricuspid valve.

angiography is not particularly useful in the diagnosis of Ebstein's malformation. (7) Intracardiac electrocardiograms[337] may be of diagnostic importance in that they reveal a right ventricular type of tracing in a catheter position where the pressure pulse still shows an atrial tracing. Dye curves reveal an atrial right-to-left shunt.

Course and Prognosis

Patients with the classic clinical picture of Ebstein's malformation usually die during the second decade. But we saw the malformation in a stillborn, and two patients are reported to have lived to the eighth decade and one died at sixty-one years of age.[229] Wood[748] emphasized that the early death usually associated with Ebstein's malformation is based on

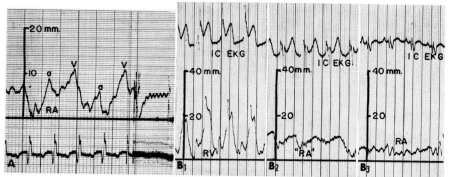

Figure 489. Pressure pulses and intracardiac electrocardiograms in patient with Ebstein's malformation. *A,* Right atrial pressure pulse with tall V wave and steep y descent. *B,* Intracardiac electrocardiogram on top and corresponding pressure pulse at bottom. B_1 indicates ventricular pressure pulse and electrocardiogram, B_2 atrial pressure pulse and ventricular electrocardiogram, and B_3 atrial pressure pulse and electrocardiogram.

observations made in severe cases; he thought, and I agree, that in many of the milder cases the prognosis may be much better. The cause of death may be congestive failure, arrythmia, disease of the central nervous system and even myocardial infarction. One of our patients in her teens was cyanotic, but well compensated, when living in Boston; she died in congestive heart failure a few months after she had moved to a high-altitude location.

Differential Diagnosis

Pure Pulmonic Stenosis.   See page 614.

Pericardial Effusion.   The principal similarity is a radiologic one. Nevertheless pericardial effusion may be identified on the basis of the absence of murmur, of triple or quadruple rhythm, of characteristic electrocardiographic findings and of cyanosis.

Total Anomalous Pulmonary Venous Drainage.   The similarity is principally an auscultatory one; both conditions are prone to exhibit triple or quadruple rhythms. Total transposition of the pulmonary veins is easily identifiable, however, by evidences of right ventricular hypertrophy in the electrocardiogram and pulmonary plethora in the roentgenogram.

Rheumatic Mitral Heart Disease.   Rheumatic mitral heart disease may have to be considered in the differential diagnosis because of the late appearance of symptoms and the presence of a diastolic murmur, coupled with what may be interpreted as an opening snap of the mitral valve. A careful review of the history and the auscultatory findings, together with the fact that roentgenologic examination reveals no enlargement of the left atrium, easily excludes the diagnosis of rheumatic mitral heart disease.

Treatment

Only symptomatic medical treatment is available for most of these patients. Surgical closure of an atrial septal defect was reported in one instance, without convincing beneficial effects.[754] Within recent years the Glenn operation (see Tricuspid Atresia, p. 687) has been recommended for treatment. Although it has proved to be a helpful palliative operation for patients with tricuspid atresia and maximal arterial unsaturation, and may hold some promise for patients with pulmonary atresia and an intact ventricular septum, we have not had the opportunity to treat any of our patients with Ebstein's malformation in this fashion. It would seem to me that in patients in whom anoxia is a severe handicap this would be indicated. Since the main cause of disability in patients with this syndrome is heart failure and arrythmia, it does not seem likely to me that anastomosis of the superior vena cava to the pulmonary artery would have much to offer to most of them. Furthermore, the tendency of these patients toward arrythmias, in general, would make me hesitant to suggest surgical intervention unless anoxia is indeed severe.

Summary

Patients with slight cyanosis, definite dyspnea on exertion and congestive heart failure may be suspected of having Ebstein's anomaly of the tricuspid valve. The clinical diagnosis is based on the presence of a triple rhythm, with systolic and diastolic murmurs, a large heart with ischemic lung fields, electrocardiographic evidences of P pulmonale without right ventricular hypertrophy, serious conduction disturbances and the Wolff-Parkinson-White syndrome. These patients are prone to sudden death in arrhythmias and heart failure. Only symptomatic medical treatment is available for the majority. A Glenn procedure may be helpful for those with severe anoxia.

17

THE TRANSPOSITIONS

COMPLETE TRANSPOSITION OF THE GREAT ARTERIES

Incidence

Complete transposition is rarely seen in patients beyond infancy, but it is almost the most significant lesion encountered in the newborn period. Keith considered this anomaly to be the most common cause of congestive heart failure within the first two months of life and the second in frequency from three to six months. Abbott found forty-nine cases in her series. Campbell estimated[127] that 8 per cent of his patients with cyanotic congenital heart disease had transposition of the great arteries. Wood placed the frequency at less than 5 per cent of his cyanotic patients. Keith, reviewing 4 publications, placed the incidence at 7.8 per cent in cyanotic patients. A recent publication from our department[537] reviewed our experiences with fifty patients who had transposition and were studied at cardiac catheterization. These represent but one third of our total cases, but the discussion to follow will be based principally on this article.

Anatomy

Complete transposition of the great arteries is an embryologic defect caused by a straight-line division of the bulbar trunk instead of the usual spiralling division at the fifth to seventh intrauterine week. There are three principal anatomic characteristics of complete transposition of great arteries (Fig. 490). (1) There is a change in the anteroposterior relation between the aorta and pulmonary artery; the aorta is anterior and the pulmonary artery is posterior. (2) The change in the frontal plane, in the left-to-right

I. NORMAL

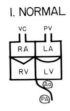

2. COMPLETE TRANSPOSITION

Without inversion (common)   With inversion (rare)

3. INCOMPLETE TRANSPOSITION (Partial inversion)

Taussig-Bing   Double outlet RV

Without transposition (common)   With transposition (rare)

4. CORRECTED TRANSPOSITION (Transposition + inversion + functional correction)

Transposition = Change in A-P relation
Inversion = Change in L→R relation

Figure 490. Schematic presentation of transposition of the great arteries in patients with situs solitus. Note in the normal patient that the tricuspid valve is over the right side, the mitral valve over the left side, the aorta is posterior and the pulmonary artery anterior. The aorta is also to the right and the pulmonary artery to the left. In complete transposition the position of the atrioventricular valve is the same as in the normal. In the common forms, without inversion, only the anteroposterior relation of the great arteries is changed, whereas in the rare form associated with inversion, left-to-right relations are reversed. In incomplete transposition (partial inversion) the left-to-right relation of the great arteries are disturbed. In the common form of the Taussig-Bing syndrome the anteroposterior relations are not disturbed, whereas in the exceptional variety they are. In both instances the pulmonary artery overrides both ventricles and the aorta is completely inverted. In the double-outlet right ventricle only the aorta is inverted, without transposition. Finally, in corrected transposition, not only are the anteroposterior relations and the left-to-right relations reversed, but also functional correction is accomplished by alignment of the aorta to the left atrium and pulmonary veins via the tricuspid valve.

direction, is not nearly as great; the aorta may be to the right, directly in front of or slightly to the left of the pulmonary artery. The latter structure ascends straight, however, and parallel to the aorta, not crossing it. (3) Finally, and most interestingly, the pulmonary artery originates exclusively from the left ventricle, and the aorta from the right ventricle.

Usually the atria are in their proper relation to the veins, and they open, through appropriate atrioventricular valves, into appropriate ventricles. The right coronary artery usually originates from the posterior and the left coronary from the left anterior aortic cusp.

Associated anomalies must include communications between the systemic and pulmonary circuits at the atrial, ventricular or pulmonary arterial level in order to allow survival for even a few days. The ventricular septum is open in 60 to 80 per cent of the patients, depending on the source of the patient material. Frequently the ventricular septal defect is so large that, in effect, one is dealing with a single ventricle. In all those in whom the ventricular defect is closed and in many of those in whom it is open, an atrial septal defect or patent foramen ovale is present. The ductus arteriosus is anatomically patent in at least half of the patients. Pulmonic stenosis is relatively rare; 5 per cent in anatomic series[419] and 20 per cent in our clinically studied material. Additional malformations may include tricuspid atresia, mitral stenosis or mitral atresia, atrioventricularis communis and dextrocardia or levocardia with abdominal situs inversus.

Pulmonary vascular obstructive changes are described with increasing frequency after early infancy.[145, 243]

Physiology

The physiologic handicaps resulting from complete transposition of the great arteries are extremely serious.[125, 537] First and foremost is the deficient oxygen supply to the tissues resulting from the inability to transfer adequate quantities of well oxygenated pulmonary venous blood to the systemic circuit. A second and equally far-reaching consequence is that cardiac dilatation and myocardial failure ensue within a few weeks or months. The cause of this is most likely the high cardiac output of both circuits and the poor coronary oxygen supply to this maximally overloaded myocardium. Of course, not only is the output of both ventricles increased in most instances, but, as an added handicap, both ventricles operate at systemic pressure levels as well. The underdevelopment of these children is probably related more to the presence of congestive heart failure than to anoxia.

Clinical Picture

The division of patients with transposition of the great arteries into four physiologic groups may serve as a useful classification for the understanding of the various clinical profiles encountered (Table 33, p. 799).

The predominance of males (4 to 1) has been commented on by many observers. It is interesting to note that diabetes occurs rather frequently in the family history. The average birth weight of our patients was 7 pounds 5 ounces, but many of them were rather large babies. One may speculate on the association of these weights with the history of diabetes in the family.

Cyanosis and congestive heart failure are the most common symptoms. Rarely is transposition discovered accidentally because of the presence of a heart murmur. In almost four out of five patients, cyanosis is discovered at birth; there were only three patients out of our fifty in whom cyanosis was not commented on until they were one year old. The patients in group IIC are the ones with the least cyanosis. Four out of five children with transposition show evidences of congestive heart failure; for all practical purposes only those with pulmonic stenosis (group IIA) escape this complication. Anoxic spells are noted in some small infants. Chest pain is not too uncommon in older children. Squatting almost never occurs.

At physical examination the gross physical underdevelopment is immediately apparent. As a matter of fact, the wasted body, with the large square head (Fig. 491), maximal cyanosis and clubbing, with varices over the

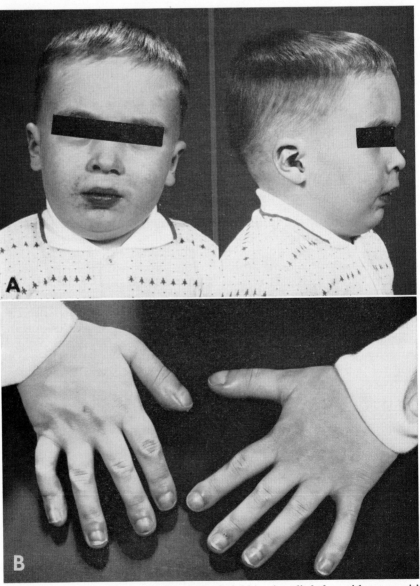

Figure 491. *A,* "Square head" and (*B*) maximal clubbing in a little boy with transposition of the great arteries and pulmonic stenosis.

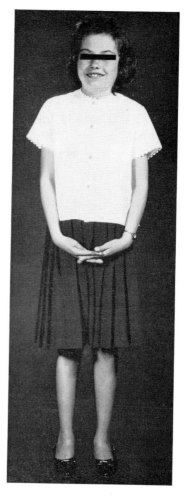

Figure 492. Teenager with transposition of the great arteries and pulmonary vascular obstructive disease. This young lady goes to school and lives an almost normal existence.

fingers, presents a characteristic appearance, easily recognizable at the bedside. It is interesting to note that with the good birth weight, growth retardation may not become evident until the patient is two or three months of age. It is also worth noting that, on the whole, the patients in group IIA show the best developmental pattern. Motor development is severely retarded, but intellectual development, even in the patients with the most severe cyanosis, may not be affected.

The posteroanterior diameter of the chest seemed to be increased in the majority of our patients, and the left side of the chest was also prominent. Usually the first sound is not remarkable, but a constant systolic click is common. The second sound is usually not split; it is loud over the midsternum and even at the second left interspace and probably represents aortic closure. A third heart sound is commonly heard. A systolic murmur is almost invariably present, but in at least 25 per cent of our patients, particularly those in groups I and IIB, it was grade 2 or less in intensity. Systolic murmurs of grade 4 intensity are rare. In more than half of our patients, particularly those in groups IIB and C, a diastolic murmur (mid-diastolic-protodiastolic) was heard.

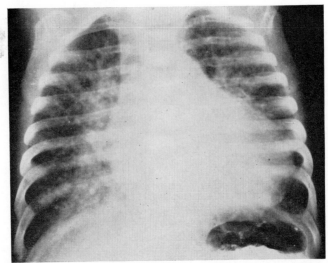

Figure 493. Typical roentgenogram of patient with transposition of the great arteries with a "long bulge" on the left border and pulmonary vascular engorgement. This silhouette in a cyanotic patient is practically diagnostic.

The roentgenologic examination is helpful in the sense that it reveals cardiac enlargement with pulmonary vascular engorgement in a patient with cyanosis. Over and beyond this, in regard to specific clues, chamber enlargement or characteristic patterns (egg-shaped with narrow waist, Fig. 17, or a long bulge in the left midsegment,[24] Fig. 493), it is somewhat less dependable. On the whole, the egg-shaped silhouette is seen more in group I, a normal or prominent main pulmonary artery suggests IIB or C, and IIA looks like the picture of tetralogy of Fallot, with a small heart and diminished pulmonary vasculature (Fig. 494). There is a great deal of overlapping among the various types. The rapid increase in heart size within a relatively short time, early in infancy, has been emphasized by Keith and his associates[382] (Fig. 495). The electrocardiogram is of considerable interest. Mild to severe right axis deviation ($+100$ to -150 degrees) (Fig. 496) can be seen in all patients except those belonging in group IIC; the mean electrical axis in this group ranges from $+100$ to -90 degrees. Moderate degrees of right ventricular hypertrophy are seen in patients in groups I and IIA, whereas combined or even left ventricle hypertrophy of mild degree was noted in those in groups IIB and C. P mitrale is rare and is seen almost exclusively in patients in groups IIC, whereas P pulmonale is seen in the majority of the others.

Cardiac catheterization reveals the following (Fig. 497): (1) An increase in oxygen saturation at the right atrial or ventricular level occurs in all patients. In most instances the principal increase seems to occur at the ventricular level, though in some, particularly those in group I, it actually occurs at the atrial level. A left-to-right shunt at the ductal level is not likely to occur and is almost impossible to prove. There is a right-to-left shunt (aortopulmonary) through the patent ductus arteriosus in some patients in group IIA. In the others the right-to-left shunt occurs at either the ventricular or the atrial level, or both. Arterial oxygen saturation varies from 12 to 85 per cent and is always lower than pulmonary arterial saturation. The

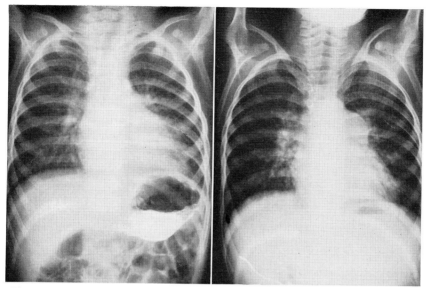

Figure 494.   Roentgenograms of a patient with transposition of the great arteries and pulmonary vascular obstruction, taken four years apart. Note the appearance of the dilated pulmonary artery in the later film.

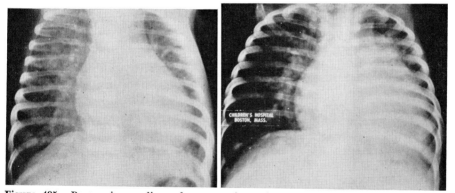

Figure 495.   Progressive cardiac enlargement in patient with transposition of the great arteries, ventricular septal defect and a large flow.

highest arterial oxygen saturations occur in patients in group IIC (60 to 85 per cent), the lowest in patients in group I. (2) There is moderate elevation of the left and right atrial pressures. Right ventricular and left ventricular pressure pulses are closely similar, even in the majority of patients in group I. Systemic arterial pressure pulses show a rapid upstroke and relatively wide pulse pressure. The pulmonary arterial pressure pulse in patients in group IIA looks damped, with a low mean pressure; in the others it is similar in contour to the systemic arterial tracing. (3) Systemic resistance is within normal limits. Pulmonary resistance is elevated in about 30 per cent of all patients, regardless of age. As has been indicated (p. 701), there seems to be definite histologic evidence of the progression of the pulmonary vascular obstruction in these patients. (4) The patients with severe arterial

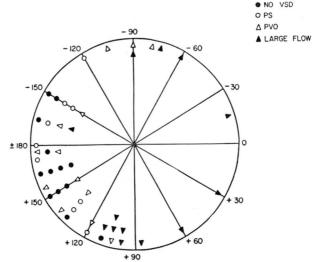

Figure 496. Distribution of the mean electrical axis in a group of fifty patients with transposition of the great arteries.[537]

unsaturation have large systemic flows. As a matter of fact, a good correlation may be established between arterial oxygen content and systemic flow (Fig. 498). Of course, the pulmonary flows are largest in the patients with the highest oxygen saturations, i.e. group IIC, and lowest in groups IIA and B (Fig. 499). It is important to stress that the size of the pulmonary flow depends on the resistance to left ventricular outflow (pulmonic stenosis or pulmonary vascular obstruction) and on the size of the communication between the two systems. The higher the resistance and the larger the communication, the smaller the pulmonary flow. (5) We were able to enter all four chambers of the heart in thirty-nine of our fifty patients. The pulmonary artery cannot be entered in patients in group I; it is easiest to approach in those in group IIC. When the pulmonary artery is entered, it is always found to be posterior to the aorta, but it may be on either side of the crista supraventricularis. (6) Cine-angiography is important in the diagnosis of transposition of the great arteries in that it may be the only means of demonstrating the relations between the great arteries, as well as the location and direction of the shunts. The aorta is anterior and fills exclusively from the right ventricle.

Course and Prognosis

Transposition of the great arteries is an extremely severe disease. Hanlon and Blalock[323] could find only 6 children mentioned in the literature before 1948 who lived to be more than 10 years old. Keith indicated that the average age of 70 patients was 8.4 weeks and that 90 per cent died at less than 7 months of age. He spoke of a "benign group" of patients, having a ventricular septal defect and pulmonary vascular obstruction or pulmonic stenosis, who could survive for many years.

Seventeen of our 50 patients were more than 3 years old at the completion of our survey in 1959; half of these are now 10 years old or older;

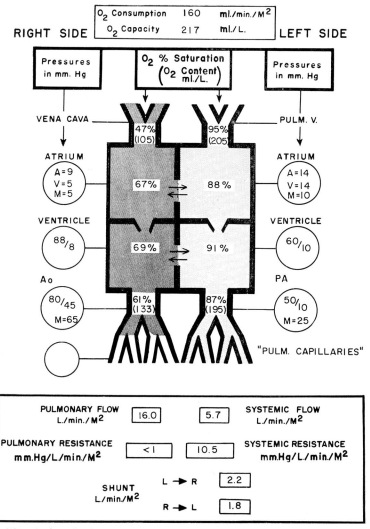

Figure 497. Catheterization findings in patient with transposition of the great arteries.

most belong in groups IIA and B. I believe that patients in groups I and IIC have the poorest prognosis. At least half of these patients die within the first four months of life.

In most instances the cause of death is congestive heart failure and anoxia. Myocardial infarction, thromboembolic phenomena or aspiration may be contributing causes. It is important to stress that most of the patients in whom congestive heart failure fails to develop within the first year of life survive for some years, and may even improve with time. Contrariwise, evidences of heart failure within the first month of life almost invariably indicate early fatal termination. The presence of heart failure at any time indicates a poor prognosis.

Because of the vigorous anticongestive and anti-infectious measures pediatricians have seen fit to take in the hopes of eventual corrective sur-

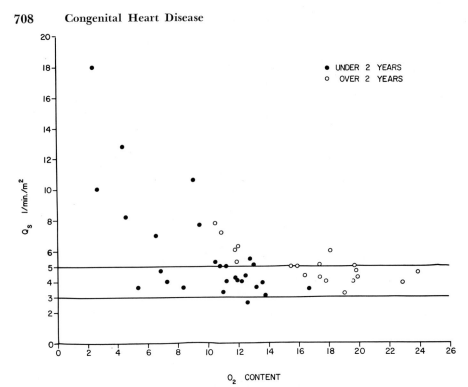

Figure 498. Relation of oxygen content to systemic flow in patients with transposition of the great arteries. Note that the patients with relatively normal oxygen content have relatively normal systemic output. Those with the most severe unsaturation have the highest output.[537]

gery, I am sure that transposition of the great arteries does not have the dismal outlook today that it had some years ago.

Differential Diagnosis

Tetralogy of Fallot.   See page 653.
Hypoplastic Left Heart Syndrome.   See page 578.
Truncus Arteriosus.   See page 505.
Complete Transposition of the Pulmonary Veins with Pulmonary Arterial Hypertension.   These critically ill small babies, like those with transposition of the great arteries, may be deeply cyanotic and have pulmonary plethora. The differential diagnosis may rest on the following characteristics of pulmonary venous transposition: (1) The over-all cardiac enlargement is only mild to moderate. (2) The pulmonary vascular engorgement is almost exclusively passive. (3) The electrocardiogram shows right ventricular hypertrophy with complete R/s reversal. (4) At auscultation a quadruple rhythm is often heard.
Coarctation of the Aorta with Systemic Right and Left Ventricles. See page 542.

Treatment

Medical treatment should aim at the control of congestive heart failure

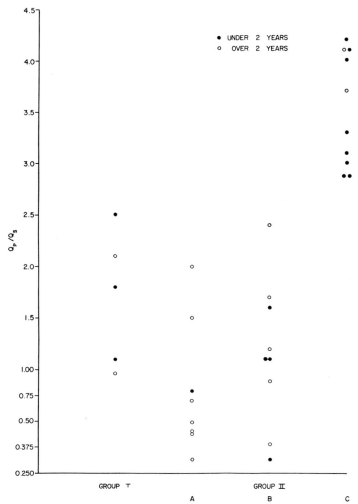

Figure 499.   Systemic flow ratios in the four physiologic groups. Note that patients in group II C have the highest pulmonary blood flows.[537]

and infection. Careful attention should be paid to the hematologic status, particularly in relation to arterial oxygen saturation (see p. 651).

Surgical treatment is still far from ideal.[434, 518] Complete correction, by means of the Senning procedure[631] (redirecting the venous inflow through an atrial transplant) was successful in one of Senning's patients, and in four of Kirklin's eleven patients.[394] Unfortunately, further experience with this method has not been particularly successful, and some of Kirklin's patients have died since the original report. Ingenious methods for a transplant on the arterial side have been devised in the laboratory,[355] but to my knowledge, not a single patient has survived any such operation.

This dismal review of the procedures aimed at complete correction leaves the field wide open for conservative medical management and palliative surgery. At present our policy is *not* to operate on patients with ventricular septal defect and pulmonic stenosis, because of the relatively good prognosis, unless they are severely anoxic. In this event, a Blalock procedure is the operation of choice. *Patients in group I need surgery early.* In our institution the creation of a large atrial septal defect[61] seems to help these infants as well as others who have inadequate mixing at the atrial or ventricular level. Surgery can and should be performed within the first few weeks of life. I believe that the group at the Children's Memorial Hospital prefers Baffes's procedure[27] (anastomosis of the inferior vena cava to the left atrium and the right pulmonary vein to the right atrium) for these babies. Patients in group IIC should have the pulmonary artery banded if they are in severe heart failure. Patients in group IIB, like those in IIA, may be treated conservatively unless anoxia is severe, in which case Baffes's procedure is recommended.

A physiologic classification of these patients is imperative for an intelligent therapeutic approach. Therefore cardiac catheterization with angiography is recommended for all symptomatic patients suspected of having complete transposition of the great arteries. The risk of the various palliative procedures is hard to assess because of the small number of cases reported and because of the variations in patients. Still, it can be said that the Blalock procedure may carry a 15 to 25 per cent risk in these patients. An equal risk should be assigned to the creation of an atrial septal defect. The risks of Baffes's procedure or of banding of the pulmonary artery may be estimated at 25 per cent. Cooley,[539] using the Blalock-Hanlon technique, recently reported a mortality rate of 18 per cent in his last 23 patients; Baffes's[28] mortalities in 1958 revealed a 34.6 per cent immediate and an 8 per cent late mortality.

Summary

Infants with early cyanosis, progressive cardiac enlargement and pulmonary plethora should be suspected of having complete transposition of the great arteries. Four physiologic groups may be distinguished, each characterized by a clinical profile. Infants with an intact ventricular septum and those with a large ventricular septal defect and large pulmonary flow are the sickest, whereas those with a ventricular septal defect and pulmonic stenosis or pulmonary vascular obstruction have a somewhat better prognosis. No complete surgical correction is available at present, but various palliative operations may prove helpful.

INCOMPLETE TRANSPOSITION OF THE GREAT ARTERIES (PARTIAL INVERSION)

INVERSION OF THE AORTA WITH AN OVERRIDING PULMONARY ARTERY (THE TAUSSIG-BING SYNDROME)

A variation of complete transposition of the great arteries of some clinical significance was described in 1949 by Taussig and Bing.[685] These authors defined the syndrome as consisting of (1) an overriding large pulmonary artery, (2) a transposed aorta, and (3) a ventricular septal defect.

Incidence

This condition is rare. We have recognized two such cases at post-mortem examination during the past ten years. Kjellberg and his associates reported three instances[397] Beuren[56] found a total of fourteen cases in the files of the Johns Hopkins Hospital. Three of these were proved at post-mortem examination; the others were diagnosed by catheterization and angiography. This author quoted another nine case reports from the literature.

Anatomy

There seems to be some confusion as to what belongs anatomically in the Taussig-Bing group. The fact that the aorta originates from the right ventricle seems clear enough; equally indispensable is the "overriding" of the pulmonary artery, i.e. its communication with both the right and the left ventricles (a "levoposition" of this vessel). What does not seem altogether clear is whether the aorta is anterior, as in "complete" transposition, or posterior, as in the normal situation. In Taussig and Bing's original description the aorta was posterior, but in some of Beuren's patients the aorta was anterior. In a critical review of the literature Beuren found both types of hearts, those with an anterior and those with a posterior aorta, included in the definition of the Taussig-Bing syndrome. Interestingly enough, no patient with pulmonic stenosis is included in the syndrome, but I am sure that these may be forthcoming.

It seems to me that perhaps both variations should be included in this syndrome, recognizing, in effect, the incompleteness of the transposition (Fig. 490).

Physiology

The situation cannot be distinguished from complete transposition of the great arteries with a ventricular septal defect and pulmonary vascular obstruction (group IIB).

Clinical Picture

The clinical picture has not been sufficiently well outlined to be presented in any authoritative fashion. Taussig and Bing, in their original article,[685] mentioned that, clinically, these patients resemble those with the "Eisenmenger complex" except that their cyanosis dates back to birth. The patient on whom Taussig based her statement was a 5½-year-old girl; one of three patients presented by Kjellberg and his associates[397] was nine years old. Thus it is obvious that the prognosis for these youngsters is not quite as poor as that for some of the patients with complete transposition of the great arteries. It may correspond, roughly, to the outlook for children with type IIB transposition.

At physical examination the findings apparently present a combination of transposition of the great arteries and large ventricular septal defect. Cyanosis and clubbing are severe, left chest deformity may be present, and sometimes a thrill is palpable. The pulmonary second sound is loud. A systolic murmur and thrill may be noted at the left sternal border. The electrocardiogram shows right ventricular hypertrophy. Roentgenologically, cardiac enlargement with pulmonary plethora is noted, with fullness of the main pulmonary artery segment.

At cardiac catheterization the following findings are mentioned in the literature: (1) The pulmonary arterial oxygen content is significantly higher than the systemic arterial oxygen content. (2) There is right ventricular and pulmonary arterial hypertension at systemic level. (3) The aorta and the pulmonary artery communicate directly with the right ventricle. (4) Pulmonary resistance is elevated.

Angiocardiography is the only definite method, short of postmortem examination, of making this diagnosis.

Course and Prognosis

The course of this anomaly is not known beyond the fact that cyanosis begins early and that survival for a few years is possible.

Differential Diagnosis

The distinction between the Taussig-Bing syndrome and complete transposition of the great arteries with ventricular septal defect and pulmonary vascular obstruction is almost impossible on clinical grounds and extremely difficult short of a postmortem examination. *It is well worth while to remember, however, that ventricular defect, pulmonary vascular obstruction and normal takeoff of the great arteries (Eisenmenger's syndrome) rarely produce clinical cyanosis in children.* If such is noted within this physiologic framework, some abnormality of the origin of the great arteries should be suspected.

Treatment

Conservative medical management of the physiologic consequences of severe cyanotic disease and pulmonary vascular obstruction may give these unhappy children as good a life as anything at present. If surgery is contemplated, Baffes's procedure or enlargement of the atrial septal defect may be of some benefit.

Summary

The Taussig-Bing syndrome, an incomplete form of transposition of the great arteries in which the aorta originates from the right ventricle and there is "overriding" of the pulmonary artery, cannot be distinguished by clinical means from complete transposition with a ventricular defect and pulmonary vascular obstruction. Physiologic studies may reveal the relation of the great arteries. No satisfactory treatment is available.

INVERSION OF THE AORTA WITH NORMAL ORIGIN OF THE PULMONARY ARTERY (DOUBLE-OUTLET RIGHT VENTRICLE)

These rare malformations were summarized by Neufeld[532] in 2 separate publications in 1961. He reported fourteen new cases. In 1957 Witham[738] described 4 patients. In essence, these are incomplete transpositions, in that, as in the Taussig-Bing syndrome, the anterior-posterior relations of the great arteries may be normal, but the aorta originates from the right ventricle (Fig. 490). This results in a situation in which the great arteries, looked at externally or at surgery, seem normal; actually, however, they lie in the same sagittal plane, both originating from the right ventricle. The only outlet to the left ventricle is through the ventricular septal defect. Depending on whether there is obstruction to the outflow into the pulmonary artery, these patients may present the clinical picture of Fallot's tetralogy or of a ventricular septal defect with pulmonary vascular obstruction. The only clinical clue leading to suspicion of this anomaly is an electrocardiogram characteristic of endocardial cushion defect (see p. 387). This type of tracing is not a sine qua non of the malformation, nor does its presence establish the diagnosis of a double-outlet right ventricle. If such a tracing is found within the framework of Fallot's tetralogy or a ventricular septal defect, however, the origins of the great arteries should be outlined with more than usual care before operation is contemplated. Consideration of this presently inoperable situation should serve as a further warning against indiscriminate attempts at open-heart surgery in patients with ventricular septal defect or Fallot's tetralogy.

Summary

A double-outlet right ventricle is another form of incomplete transposition of the great arteries; the aorta and pulmonary artery both originate from the right ventricle. Depending on the status of the pulmonary outflow tract, the clinical picture may resemble that of Fallot's tetralogy or of a large ventricular septal defect. The endocardial cushion type of electrocardiogram may suggest the clinical diagnosis, but even the most careful physiologic studies may fail to confirm it. The condition is presently inoperable.

CORRECTED TRANSPOSITION OF THE GREAT ARTERIES (TRANSPOSITION PLUS INVERSION PLUS FUNCTIONAL CORRECTION)

Although corrected transposition of the great arteries has been known to pathologists for almost a hundred years,[590] it was not until Anderson[18] presented his fourteen cases with good clinical descriptions that the condition became well known to cardiologists. An excellent classification, on anatomic grounds, was presented by Cardell in 1956.[139] Recently the Mayo group[616] summarized their experiences with 33 cases and estimated the number reported in the literature as 100. Abbott found 6 cases among her 1000 postmortem examinations. The data presented in the following paragraphs are based on a hitherto unpublished review of 35 cases collected from our files between 1952 and 1959 by Dr. James L. Reynolds. I shall discuss here only the patients with corrected transposition of the great arteries and situs solitus. The situs inversus group will be discussed among the dextrocardias.

Incidence

The incidence of corrected transposition of the great arteries among our catheterized patients is approximately 3 per cent.

Anatomy

The definition of corrected transposition consists of three components (Fig. 490): (1) *transposition,* i.e. a reversal of the anteroposterior relations between the aorta and pulmonary artery; (2) *inversion,* indicating a complete reversal of the great arteries in the left-to-right direction. As a consequence of these changes the *aorta is always anterior and occupies the left border of the heart* (Fig. 500). For the purposes of this discussion, *in an anatomic sense, this particular position of the great arteries, combining transposition with inversion, is what is meant by corrected transposition.* (3) *Functional correction (the location of the aorta on the left side)* allows the aorta to communicate with the left chambers, and furnishes it with pulmonary venous blood *if the atria and their venous drainage stay in their normal position.*

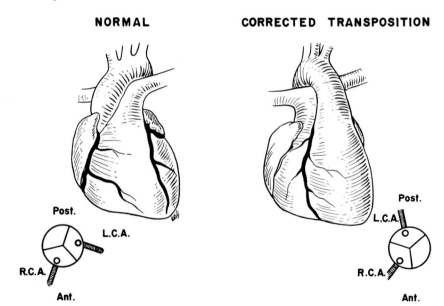

NORMAL   CORRECTED TRANSPOSITION

Figure 500.   External view of the heart and the great arteries in a normal person and in one with corrected transposition of the great arteries. Note that the left border of the heart in the patient with corrected transposition is occupied by the aorta, not the pulmonary artery. Note also the anterior position of the aorta. In the inset, origin of the coronary arteries from the aortic sinuses is illustrated. Note the left coronary originating from the posterior sinus and the right from the right anterior.

The ventricles and their respective atrioventricular valves usually do not stay in their normal position; they undergo inversion as well. Consequently, in the typical case of corrected transposition of the great arteries, the aorta is on the left side and anterior, communicating with an anatomic right ventricle which receives pulmonary venous blood from an anatomic left atrium through an anatomic tricuspid valve.

A variation of this situation is present when the heart is in the right side of the chest, in the situs inversus position, in which case the aorta is on the right side and anterior, but still communicates with an anatomic right ventricle and a functional and anatomic left atrium. This is a relatively rare condition. In the recent Mayo series the ratio between situs solitus and situs inversus corrected transposition of the great arteries was 10:1. Finally, I would like to mention that inversion of the great arteries (aorta to the left) may be seen in rare instances in patients with complete, functionally uncorrected, transposition, in which case the left-sided and anterior aorta communicates with an anatomic left ventricle, but always with a functional and anatomic right atrium. As emphasized before, in the usual case of complete transposition, the aorta is to the right or directly in front of the pulmonary artery, and only rarely in the position of complete inversion, to the left of it (Fig. 490).

Inherent in the anatomic situation outlined above are two important facts. (1) The coronary arteries are inverted (Fig. 500), the right coronary originating from the right and the left coronary artery from the posterior sinus; the noncoronary cusp is anterior. (2) The atrioventricular valves are in an abnormal position, in that the mitral valve opens into the pulmonary and the tricuspid into the aortic ventricle. Postmortem examination revealed more or less severe anomalies of the left atrioventricular valve in seven of our eight patients. These varied from simple regurgitation to full-blown Ebstein's malformation, and even atresia. Associated lesions included ventricular septal defect (three fourths of the patients), pulmonic stenosis (half of the patients) and, in rare instances, aortic stenosis, patent ductus arteriosus and atrial septal defect. As a rule, the ventricular defect is large. The right-sided ventricle, giving rise to the pulmonary artery, is usually much larger than the left-sided cavity. Frequently the left-sided ventricle is only a rudimentary chamber coalescing with the outflow portion of the large ventricle and contributing to the formation of a subaortic chamber. A "false septum," consisting, in fact, of the crista supraventricularis, forms a "septal defect" separating the large inflow portion of the right-sided ventricle from the small outflow portion (Fig. 501).

Pulmonic stenosis may be subvalvar or valvar. Aortic stenosis is rare and almost always subvalvar. In patients with pulmonic stenosis a ventricular septal defect in usually present, though we had one patient with an intact ventricular septum proved at postmortem examination, and Anderson mentioned three others with this condition. We had one patient with combined aortic and pulmonic stenosis and a single ventricle.

Only rarely does corrected transposition occur without associated anomalies. I had the opportunity to discuss one of these infants who died in paroxysmal atrial tachycardia at a clinicopathologic conference recently; there was one in the series presented by the Mayo Clinic group, Cardell mentioned two and Schaefer and Rudolph,[614] one.

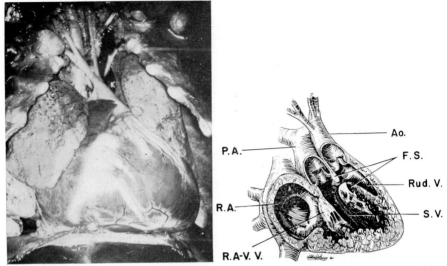

Figure 501. Photograph and schematic drawing of patient with corrected transposition of the great arteries and single ventricle. Note that the aorta originates from a rudimentary ventricle separated by a false septum (*F. S.*), corresponding to the right ventricular infundibulum, from the single ventricle (*S.V.*) created by the fusion of the left ventricle and the inflow portion of the right ventricle.

Physiology

It has been stated that corrected transposition of the great arteries, per se, does not entail any derangement of the normal cardiodynamics. One of the patients of the Mayo Clinic series, who died at the age of sixty, may be cited in support of this contention.

My own opinion is that the associated functional anomalies of the conduction system and the atrioventricular valves, and the impulse formations, are so integrally associated with the anomaly that the patient surely faces severe functional hazard, even in the rare instance of anatomically "pure" corrected transposition of the great arteries.

The physiologic consequences are those associated with atrioventricular block, paroxysmal tachycardia, mitral regurgitation, ventricular septal defect, pulmonic stenosis, pulmonary arterial hypertension, and so forth.

Clinical Picture

The history of these patients depends almost exclusively on the associated anomalies. The frequency of fatigue, dyspnea, cyanosis, congestive heart failure or underdevelopment is about the same in these children as in the group with identical cardiac defects without corrected transposition. Only the presence of atrioventricular block and paroxysmal atrial tachycardia modifies the course of the underlying malformation. The murmur is usually heard at birth; in only 15 per cent of our patients was it discovered after they were 6 months of age.

At physical examination many of them are underdeveloped, but this is surely a rule with many exceptions. A male-to-female ratio of 2:1 or 3:1

is noted. The findings at physical examination, roentgenologic examination and electrocardiography are those expected from the underlying malformation with the following exceptions:

1. At physical examination, evidences of mitral regurgitation, in terms of both a hyperkinetic left ventricle and an apical systolic murmur, are present in approximately 50 per cent of the patients. Since the pulmonary artery emerges from the heart on the right side, the murmur of pulmonic stenosis, if present, is best heard at the second right interspace. Aortic closure, by the same token, is heard on the left side. This may give rise to the paradoxical situation of a patient with evidences of pulmonic stenosis, having a systolic murmur at the second right interspace and a loud aortic closure at the pulmonic area (Fig. 502). Similarly, in patients with aortic stenosis and corrected transposition the systolic murmur is heard best at the second left interspace.

2. The roentgenologic profile of corrected transposition is distinguished by the unusual cardiac waist. The emergence of the aorta on the left results in a narrowing of the right upper border and in a shoulder-like, gentle, sloping prominence on the midleft cardiac border, corresponding to the ascending aorta. Below this is the medially shifted left main pulmonary artery (Fig. 503). The left atrium is enlarged in two thirds of the patients. None of these features is present in all patients, and the roentgenograms may give no clue at all to the presence of corrected transposition. If a good aortic knob can be visualized at the usual place, this may be used as evidence against corrected transposition of the great arteries.

3. The electrocardiogram contributes more than any other clinical tool to the diagnosis of corrected transposition of the great arteries. The following features may be noted: (*a*) In at least a third of the patients there is an atrioventricular conduction disturbance ranging from first- to third-degree block. This may be present with or without a ventricular septal defect. As a matter of fact, I think that among patients with ventricular septal defects, probably those with corrected transposition are most likely to have heart block (Fig. 504). (*b*) Atrial arrhythmias, ranging from supra-

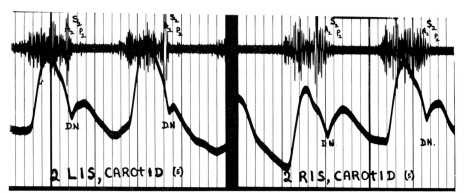

Figure 502. Phonocardiogram of patient with corrected transposition, ventricular septal defect and pulmonic stenosis. Note the well split second sound and the loud aortic component at the second left interspace. Note also that the murmur of pulmonic stenosis is loudest at the second right interspace. The second sound is split 0.06 second. First (aortic) component is loud and maximal at 2LIS. The murmur of pulmonic stenosis is maximal at 2RIS. DN refers to the dicrotic notch of the carotid pulse tracing.

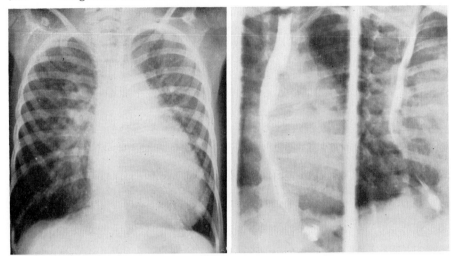

Figure 503. Posteroanterior and right oblique roentgenograms of a patient with corrected transposition of the great arteries and ventricular septal defect. Note the evidence of left-to-right shunt with pulmonary plethora. The convex left border is caused by the ascending aorta. Left atrial enlargement is indicated on the barium-filled esophagus and is secondary to mitral regurgitation.

ventricular premature beats through paroxysmal atrial tachycardia, and even atrial fibrillation, are seen in another third of the patients. The Wolff-Parkinson-White syndrome is common. The presence of atrial fibrillation or flutter in a youngster who does not have acute rheumatic fever should raise the suspicion of corrected transposition of the great arteries (Fig. 505). (c) In more than three fourths of the patients there is absence of the q waves in the left chest leads associated with right axis deviation and right ventricular hypertrophy, with a qR pattern in V_1 (Fig. 506). (d) Atrial hypertrophy, left or combined, is the rule, with few exceptions.

At *cardiac catheterization* the findings are obviously dominated by the associated defects. The following features are common, however, to patients with corrected transposition, irrespective of the underlying lesions. (1) A complete study with exploration of all chambers is hard to accomplish. Paroxysmal atrial tachycardia is common, as is the creation of heart block. The position of the tricuspid valve is shifted medially, and the pulmonary artery may not be entered from the usual position. The catheter almost preferentially crosses the ventricular septum and enters the aorta before it enters the pulmonary artery. A catheter study replete with arrythmias and failure to enter the pulmonary artery suggests the presence of corrected transposition of the great arteries. (2) Often the position of the great arteries can best be outlined by means of angiography. This clearly shows the aorta occupying the left border in the posteroanterior view and the pulmonary artery being posterior in the left lateral view. Sometimes the retrograde passage of the catheter outlines the characteristic location of the aorta (Fig. 507). (3) The systemic arterial saturation is higher than, or at least equal to, pulmonary arterial saturation. This differentiates the condition from complete transposition of the great arteries with inversion. The oxygen data often suggest the presence of a single ventricle (Fig. 508).

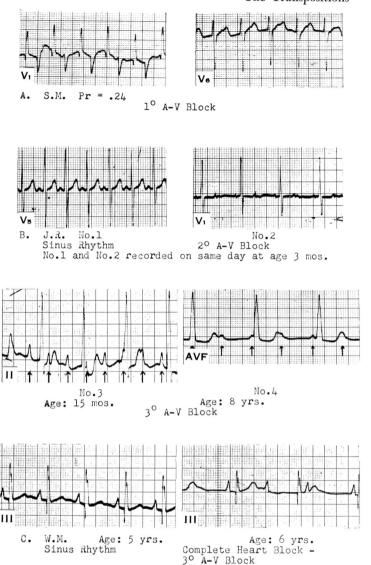

Figure 504. Varying degrees of atrioventricular block in corrected transposition of the great arteries. Patient A had first-degree atrioventricular block with a P-R interval of 0.24 second. Patient B had sinus rhythm and 2:1 atrioventricular block on the same day and third-degree atrioventricular block (complete heart block) at fifteen months and at eight years. Complete heart block developed in patient C between five and six years of age.

Course and Prognosis

Because of the complex and often irremediable associated cardiac defects, corrected transposition bears a serious prognosis. Most patients die in congestive heart failure, secondary to ventricular septal defect with pulmonary arterial hypertension and mitral regurgitation, or in anoxia due to severe pulmonic stenosis and a right-to-left shunt. A sizable number die in arrhythmias, some early in infancy. In many of the cases published

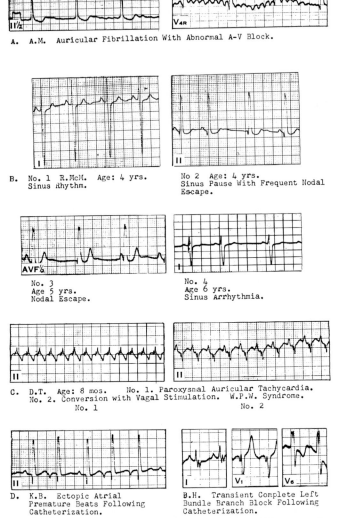

A. A.M. Auricular Fibrillation With Abnormal A-V Block.

B. No. 1 R.McM. Age: 4 yrs.
    Sinus Rhythm.

No 2 Age: 4 yrs.
Sinus Pause With Frequent Nodal
Escape.

No. 3
Age 5 yrs.
Nodal Escape.

No. 4
Age 6 yrs.
Sinus Arrhythmia.

C. D.T. Age: 8 mos.   No. 1. Paroxysmal Auricular Tachycardia.
    No. 2. Conversion with Vagal Stimulation. W.P.W. Syndrome.
              No. 1   No. 2

D. K.B. Ectopic Atrial
    Premature Beats Following
    Catheterization.

B.H.   Transient Complete Left
Bundle Branch Block Following
Catheterization.

Figure 505. The spectrum of arrhythmias seen in patients with corrected transposition of the great arteries. Patient A.M. had atrial fibrillation with atrioventricular block. Patient R.McM. had sinus rhythm, sinus pauses and frequent nodal escape at four years of age. The same patient had some nodal escape at five years and sinus arrhythmia at six years. Patient D.T. had paroxysmal atrial tachycardia converted to sinus rhythm with a Wolff-Parkinson-White syndrome. In patient K.B. ectopic atrial premature beats developed after cardiac catheterization. In patient B.H. complete left bundle branch block developed after cardiac catheterization.

recently, death occurred during or after attempted surgical correction; five of the ten patients in our series and seven of the fifteen from the Mayo Clinic group died as a result of operation. Schiebler[616] stated that the patients either die within the first year of life or survive beyond the age of fifteen years, a prognosis equally valid for uncomplicated ventricular septal defect.

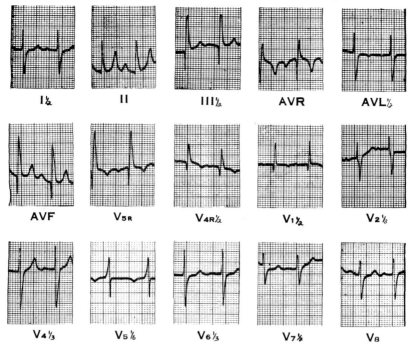

Figure 506. Typical electrocardiogram of patient with corrected transposition of the great arteries. Note the prolonged P-R interval and the deep Q waves in the right chest leads, without any Q as far left as V_8. Note also the right axis deviation and right ventricular hypertrophy.

Differential Diagnosis

Since the few patients with uncomplicated corrected transposition of the great arteries are not likely to seek medical advice, the problem of differential diagnosis arises only in the evaluation of the associated anomalies. If the question is raised, the position of the great arteries should be outlined by catheterization or angiography. Furthermore, simultaneous determinations of the oxygen saturation in the pulmonary artery and a systemic artery should be obtained to exclude complete transposition.

The following clues may be important in the recognition of corrected transposition with various associated anomalies: (1) arrythmias, atrioventricular conduction disturbances and the Wolff-Parkinson-White syndrome, (2) roentgenologic silhouette with left atrial enlargement and a "shoulder" at the left upper border, corresponding to the ascending aorta, (3) absence of the q waves in the left chest leads with right ventricular hypertrophy, (4) a murmur of pulmonic stenosis on the right side, with a loud second sound at the second left interspace, or a murmur of aortic stenosis at the second left interspace, (5) catheterization plagued by arrythmias, with inability to enter the pulmonary artery.

Treatment

Medical treatment of the consequences of the associated anomalies and

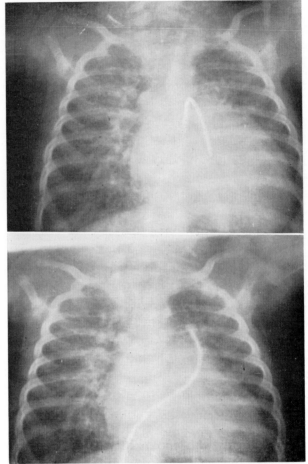

Figure 507. Typical course of the catheter in patient with transposition of the great arteries. Note the medially placed pulmonary artery in the upper film and the laterally placed aorta in the lower film.

of the arrythmias should be handled in routine fashion. Surgical treatment is difficult because of (1) the tendency toward heart block and arrythmias, (2) the frequent occurrence of a single ventricle with a rudimentary outflow chamber, which is inoperable, (3) the frequently anomalous course of the coronary artery which interferes with conventional ventriculotomy technique, and (4) irremediable left atrioventricular valve anomaly.

In spite of the increased risks of surgery, some patients with severe disease should still be submitted to operation, but, at present, if at all possible, I would postpone operation. The rare patient with pulmonic stenosis and intact ventricular septum may be operated upon without appreciably higher than average risks.

Summary

Patients in whom the aorta, carrying pulmonary venous blood, emerges to the left of and anterior to the pulmonary artery have corrected transposition of the great arteries. More than 90 per cent of these patients have

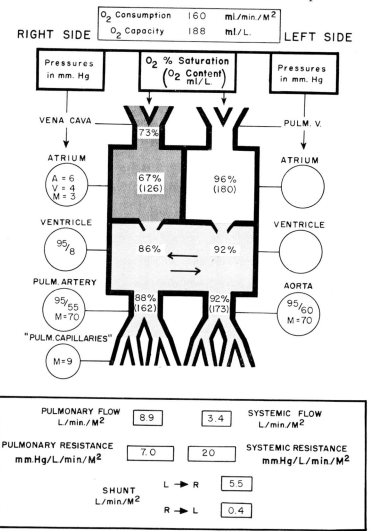

Figure 508. Cardiac catheterization findings in patient with corrected transposition of the great arteries.

associated anomalies, among which ventricular septal defect, pulmonic stenosis and mitral regurgitation should be mentioned first. Heart block and paroxysmal atrial tachycardia are common. Auscultation, roentgenologic examination and, especially, electrocardiography should suggest the diagnosis, but only exact delineation of the position of the great arteries at catheterization or angiography can confirm it. Because of the high risks, on the whole, operation should be postponed if possible.

COMPLETE TRANSPOSITION OF THE PULMONARY VEINS

In complete transposition of the pulmonary veins—total anomalous pulmonary venous connection—all the pulmonary and systemic veins enter the right atrium. The systemic circuit is supplied with blood from this common pool by means of a right-to-left shunt through an interatrial communication (patent foramen ovale or atrial septal defect).

Incidence

Abbott reported only four cases in her series of 1000 congenital malformations. Smith[646] collected 75 cases from the literature in 1951. Burroughs and Edwards,[116] surveying the literature up to 1956, collected 188 cases; 119 of these were not associated with any other major cardiac anomaly. Guntheroth[316] summarized our experiences with 20 patients studied between 1950 and 1956. Since then we have seen over thirty patients with this condition. Keith estimated the incidence at 2 per cent of all cardiac malformations.

Anatomy

Embryologically, this anomaly can probably be explained by the failure of a connection to develop between the atrial portion of the heart and the pulmonary portion of the splanchnic plexus and by a persistence of the more primitive connection between the latter and the systemic venous system.

Darling, Rothney and Craig[184] proposed an anatomic classification of

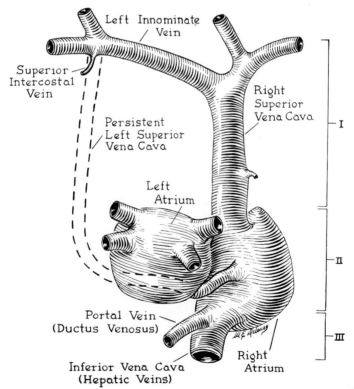

Figure 509. Diagrammatic representation of the various types of total transpositions of the pulmonary veins.[184]

complete transposition of the pulmonary veins on the basis of the entry of these structures into the right side of the heart (Fig. 509). In type I the connection is through one common channel to the left or right superior vena cava. In type II it is to the right atrium or the coronary sinus. In type III the connection is to the portal system. In type IV it is through multiple channels to two or more of the previously mentioned sites.

Type I seems to be the most common variety of the syndrome, representing about 55 per cent of the total number of cases reported in the literature. Type II is noted in 30 per cent, type III in 12 per cent and type IV in 3 per cent.[380] It is worth emphasizing that, with the exception of type IV (a total of 15 cases among the 188 collected by Edwards[116]), all veins enter a single site It should be stressed further that in most instances the pulmonary veins form a single trunk *before* entering the systemic venous channel. This is the rule *without exception* if the point of entry is distal to the superior vena cava; rare exceptions may be found if the point of entry is the superior vena cava, the right atrium or the coronary sinus.

Associated intracardiac anomalies may be encountered, but will not be discussed here. The probability of associated anomalies is particularly great if the point of entry is a persistent left superior vena cava; associated anomalies almost never occur if the point of entry is the coronary sinus.

Physiology

Total anomalous pulmonary venous drainage represents a profound derangement of the normal circulatory pattern. The right side of the heart and the pulmonary arterial system is called on to handle a much greater than average volume of blood, while the left-sided output is low normal. This situation, roughly analogous to the physiology of atrial septal defect of the secundum type (except for a slight degree of arterial unsaturation), is tolerated relatively well for many years. Difficulties arise when, in addition to the increased volume work, the right ventricle is also confronted by pulmonary arterial hypertension. This group of critically ill infants have pulmonary arterial hypertension secondary to pulmonary venous hypertension. Most of the patients with subdiaphragmatic drainage (type III) belong in this category, but a sizable number of patients with types I and II belong here as well. The fact that pulmonary venous obstruction is present is the important determining factor in the etiology of this syndrome, rather than the point of entry in the right side of the heart.

The obstruction to pulmonary venous flow may be localized at the point of entry into the systemic venous structure, or may be represented by a long narrow channel without any single point of obstruction. Furthermore, pulmonary venous hypertension may be associated with a large pulmonary flow and slight obstruction (hyperkinetic), in which case cyanosis is slight, or with maximal obstruction (localized or diffuse) with low pulmonary flow and severe cyanosis (Table 34, p. 799). *The point of obstruction to the pulmonary venous flow may be anywhere from the atrial septum backward to the cavae, sinus venosus,* and so forth.

Clinical Picture

Patients without Significant Pulmonary Arterial Hypertension. As mentioned earlier, all these children (less than 25 per cent of the total) have type I or II transposition, according to Darling's classification. I would like to emphasize, however, that most of the patients in these two anatomic groups *do* have critical pulmonary arterial hypertension. The symptoms in the children with near normal pulmonary arterial pressures are similar to those of patients with secundum atrial septal defect. There may be early, transient cyanosis within the first few weeks of life, but afterward these patients do relatively well, with only minor degrees of fatigue, dyspnea and cyanosis. One boy with this type of lesion, who lived in Maine, used to go hunting with his father when he was eighteen years old.

On physical examination these patients are fairly well developed and well nourished. Cyanosis and clubbing are slight. There is left chest prominence, and the hyperdynamic cardiac impulse is maximal at the xiphoid process. The jugular venous pulse shows a prominent V wave with deep x and y troughs. The liver may or may not be enlarged, depending on the state of compensation. At auscultation one is impressed by the quadruple or quintuple rhythm, consisting of a first sound, a well split second sound and a third and/or fourth sound (Fig. 510). Pulmonic closure is normal in intensity, and the splitting is fixed. A soft ejection murmur, grade 2 to 3 in intensity, is heard at the pulmonary area; occasionally this may assume a stenotic nature in patients who have some pulmonary gradient. A mid-diastolic or presystolic rumble is heard almost without exception (Fig. 511). Keith described a continuous murmur corresponding to a "pulmonary venous hum" at the second left interspace (Fig. 512).

In essence, the roentgenologic picture shows pulmonary vascular engorgement with right ventricular, pulmonary arterial and right atrial enlargement. In addition (Fig. 15), certain specific contours may be recognized, such as the figure-of-eight (snowman) configuration of the left superior vena cava-left innominate vein drainage.[649] Another, less typical configuration consists in a prominence of the coronary sinus itself, projecting either posteriorly at the left atrial level or at the right heart border, adjoining the right atrium (Fig. 513).

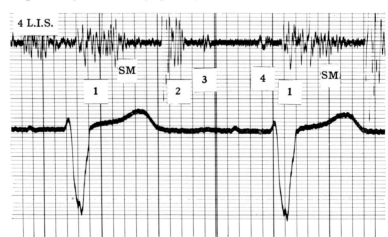

Figure 510. Phonocardiogram of patient with total transposition of the pulmonary veins. Note the systolic murmur and the four heart sounds.

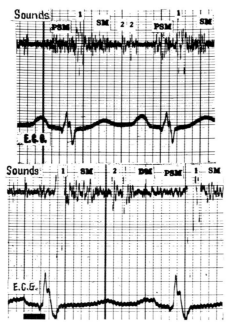

Figure 511.   Systolic and diastolic murmurs in two cases of total transposition of the pulmonary veins.

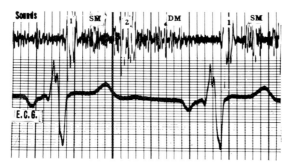

Figure 512.   Continuous murmur in a patient with total transposition of the pulmonary veins.

Electrocardiographically, right ventricular and right atrial hypertrophy is the rule without exception (Fig. 514). In the patients with the most severe disease a complete reversal of the R/s progression is noted. I do not believe that the qR pattern is particularly specific for these patients.

In summary, the clinical picture of these patients closely resembles that of a secundum atrial septal defect except for the presence of minimal cyanosis, somewhat more pronounced symptomatology, electrocardiographic evidence of more severe right ventricular hypertrophy and, occasionally, a specific rentgenographic contour.

Patients with Pulmonary Arterial Hypertension.   These patients comprise close to 80 per cent of the children with total anomalous pulmonary venous connections. These infants are sick; half of them die within the

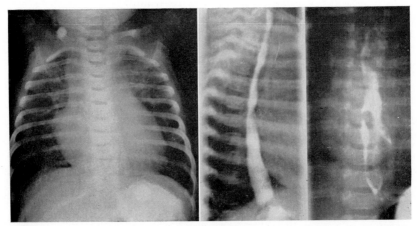

Figure 513. Posteroanterior roentgenogram of a patient in whom all the pulmonary veins drained into the coronary sinus. Note the typical bulge in the right cardiac border forming a double contour. That this double contour is not caused by an enlarged left atrium is shown by the posteroanterior and right anterior oblique esophagograms adjoining the posteroanterior film.

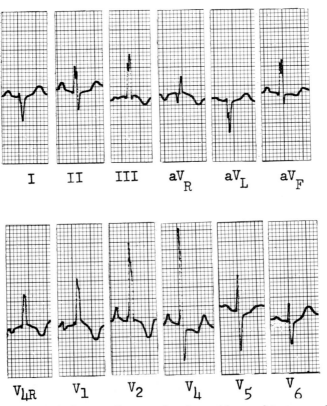

Figure 514. Typical electrocardiogram of patient with complete transposition of the pulmonary veins. Note the right axis deviation, plus 165 degrees and right ventricular hypertrophy in the chest leads, with complete R-S reversal.

first three months of life; two thirds, by six months; and most, by a year. The onset of symptoms rarely occurs within the first week, but commonly begins within the first four to six weeks of life. The degree of cyanosis and its time of onset correlate well with the severity of the disease. In addition to cyanosis, tachypnea, congestive heart failure, vomiting and underdevelopment feature prominently in the symptomatology. The common physiologic denominator is pulmonary hypertension; anatomically, all patients with subdiaphragmatic and close to 75 per cent with supradiaphragmatic drainage have pulmonary hypertension.

At physical examination the cyanosis is moderate to severe. The respirations are rapid, and evidences of right-sided failure are obvious. The liver is large and pulsatile, and the peripheral pulses are poor. At auscultation one is impressed by the gallop rhythm and the loud pulmonic closure. The murmurs are similar to those mentioned earlier in patients without pulmonary arterial hypertension except that, perhaps, they are less prominent in the patients with pulmonary hypertension. Keith indicated that a third of the patients may have no murmur at all.

Roentgenologically, two types of pictures may be recognized. In the patients with maximal cyanosis, small pulmonary flow and severe pulmonary venous obstruction, the heart is small and the lung fields reveal severe pulmonary venous congestion, almost resembling critical mitral stenosis or even miliary tuberculosis (Fig. 515). This picture was formerly thought to be characteristic only of patients with subdiaphragmatic drainage. In the patients with hyperkinetic pulmonary hypertension, large pulmonary flow and moderate cyanosis, there is rapidly progressive right

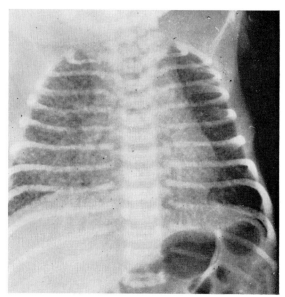

Figure 515. Typical posteroanterior roentgenogram of patient with complete transposition of the pulmonary veins and pulmonary vascular obstruction. Note the small heart and the granular lung fields. Formerly, this picture was thought to be characteristic only of subdiaphragmatic drainage. Actually, this film was obtained from a patient whose pulmonary veins entered the superior vena cava, but pulmonary vascular obstruction was present.

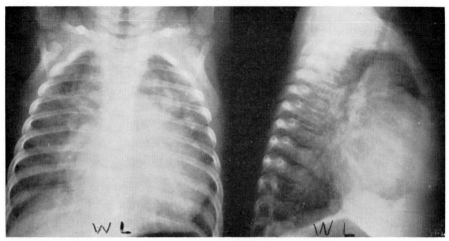

Figure 516. Posteroanterior and right lateral views of patient with complete transposition of the pulmonary veins and hyperkinetic pulmonary arterial hypertension.

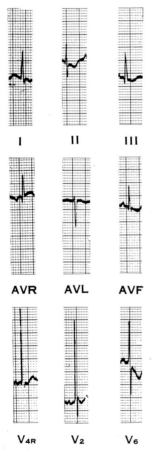

I   II   III

AVR   AVL   AVF

V₄ᵣ   V₂   V₆

Figure 517. Typical electrocardiogram of a six-day-old baby with total anomalous pulmonary venous drainage into the superior vena cava, with obstruction and low pulmonary flow. This tracing was from the same patient whose roentgenogram is shown in Figure 515.

ventricular and right atrial enlargement. The lung field show active, as well as passive, engorgement (Fig. 516). The specific contours described earlier are seldom seen in young infants. The electrocardiograms always show severe right ventricular hypertrophy, with complete R/s reversal, and right atrial hypertrophy with a clockwise frontal plane loop (Fig. 517).

Cardiac catheterization (Figs. 518, 519) reveals the following: (1) The most characteristic feature of the anomaly is the practical identity of oxygen saturation from right atrium to pulmonary artery and systemic artery. In the patients having anatomic types I and II, a minimal, but persistent, difference in oxygen saturation is noted, saturation in the pulmonary artery being higher than that in the systemic artery. This is due to the fact that the unsaturated blood from the inferior vena cava drains

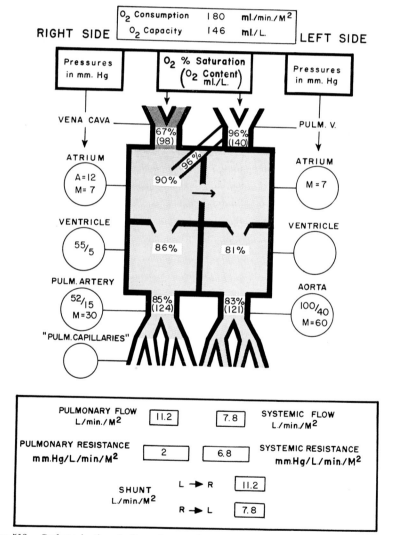

Figure 518. Catheterization findings in a patient with complete transposition of the pulmonary veins and mild pulmonary arterial hypertension.

directly through the foramen ovale into the left atrium. A high oxygen saturation is noted in the superior vena cava in patients with the type I anomaly. In those with a type III anomaly the high saturation is noted in the inferior vena cava and may not even extend into the right atrium. In these patients the systemic arterial oxygen saturation is higher than that in the pulmonary artery. In patients belonging to the type II group the rise is first observed in the right atrium or the coronary sinus. Systemic arterial saturation varies from 93 per cent in those with large pulmonary flow and low pulmonary resistance to 20 per cent in patients with small pulmonary flow and maximal pulmonary vascular obstruction. (2) Right atrial pressure is more or less elevated, the mean values in our patients varying from 3 to 15 mm. of mercury. There is always a gradient between right atrial and left atrial pressure, favoring the right; its magnitude depends on the

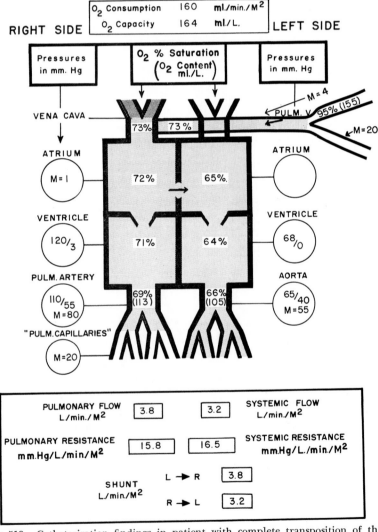

Figure 519. Catheterization findings in patient with complete transposition of the pulmonary veins with severe pulmonary hypertension.

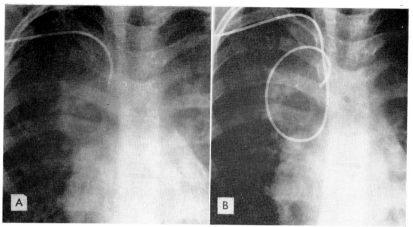

Figure 520.   Course of the catheter into the dilated superior vena cava. *A*, Catheter just entering the superior vena cava. *B*, Catheter coiling up in this huge structure.

size of the atrial defect. Right ventricular and pulmonary arterial pressures
are at systemic levels in these critically ill infants and children with much
elevation of the pulmonary capillary pressure, but are normal or only
slightly elevated in the relatively asymptomatic older patients. On the
whole, systemic arterial pressures are within normal limits. (3) Systemic
resistance is always normal; pulmonary resistance is greatly elevated in the
critically ill children. (4) Systemic flow is within normal limits; pulmonary
flow varies tremendously. In patients with maximal pulmonary vascular
obstruction, pulmonary blood flow equals systemic flow, whereas in the
relatively asymptomatic older patient the pulmonary-systemic flow ratio
may be as high as 5. The ratio in patients with hyperkinetic pulmonary
arterial hypertension is midway between the two extremes. (5) The catheter
often coils in the dilated superior vena cava (Fig. 520). The anomalously
connected pulmonary vein may be entered from the right side of the heart.
(6) Angiocardiograms or cine-angiograms are indispensable tools for outlining the exact anatomy.

Course and Prognosis

As described earlier, the prognosis for patients with pulmonary arterial
hypertension is poor; death usually occurs within the first few weeks or
months of life. The more severe the obstruction, the smaller the pulmonary
flow and the deeper the cyanosis, the poorer is the prognosis. Some of the
children with appreciable pulmonary hypertension of the hyperkinetic
variety may live four or five years (Fig. 521), but most of those with maximal
obstruction die before they are three months old.

The prognosis for patients without pulmonary arterial hypertension
resembles that for those with large atrial septal defect of the secundum
type. Survival through the second decade, without significant symptoms,
is not unusual.[633]

Differential Diagnosis

Secundum Atrial Septal Defect.   This should be differentiated from

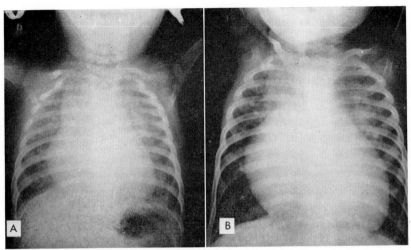

Figure 521. Rapid progressive cardiac enlargement in a patient with total transposition of the pulmonary veins. *A,* Posteroanterior roentgenogram in a child two years of age. *B,* Posteroanterior roentgenogram in the same patient three months later.

complete transposition of the pulmonary veins without pulmonary arterial hypertension. The virtual identity of saturations between systemic and pulmonary arteries is rare in simple atrial defect. In other words, arterial unsaturation almost never occurs in patients with atrial septal defect who do not have pulmonary arterial hypertension, except in certain specific anatomic situations (see p. 370). Furthermore, dye-dilution curves, with injection into left and right pulmonary arteries, are identical in patients with complete transposition of the pulmonary veins.

Single Atrium. This anomaly is almost always associated with a cushion defect type of electrocardiogram, with a counterclockwise frontal plane loop, in contrast to the secundum type of loop displayed by total anomalous pulmonary venous connection. In addition, the pulmonary arterial saturation is never higher than systemic arterial saturation in patients with a single atrium unless it is associated with transposition of the great arteries.

Complete Transposition of the Great Arteries. In small infants this anomaly should be thought of in the clinical differentiation of complete transposition of the pulmonary veins and pulmonary arterial hypertension, since in both there is early cyanosis, congestive heart failure and pulmonary plethora. The severe degree of right ventricular hypertrophy in the electrocardiogram, the quadruple rhythm and the onset of symptoms later than the first two weeks of life favor the diagnosis of transposition of the pulmonary veins. Of course, at catheterization, the patients with transposition of the great arteries do not show an increase in oxygen content at the right atrial level.

Mitral Stenosis and Cor Triatriatum. On clinical grounds these may be indistinguishable from complete transposition of the pulmonary veins and maximal pulmonary vascular obstruction. Left atrial enlargement and the late onset of symptoms are clinical clues to left atrial disease. Often only cardiac catheterization, revealing the high oxygen content in the right atrium, superior vena cava or inferior vena cava (type III), can clinch the diagnosis.

The Hypoplastic Left Heart Syndrome. This syndrome may have to be differentiated from the entity under discussion. Clinically, congestive heart failure within the first days of life, the absence of active pulmonary vascular engorgement, the large left atrium and evidences of aortic disease favor the hypoplastic left heart syndrome. Oxygen saturations at catheterization clearly indicate the correct diagnosis.

Ebstein's Anomaly. Only gallop rhythm in a child with a large heart and slight cyanosis should suggest Ebstein's anomaly in the differential diagnosis. Even without cardiac catheterization the ischemic appearance of the lung fields would exclude anomalous pulmonary venous connection.

Treatment

Surgical attempts at correction have been reported since 1947.[79] There were no spectacular successes[117, 381, 511] until the introduction of the pump oxygenator into the treatment of this anomaly. In a recent publication Cooley and Collins[162] reported on ten patients. The first three were treated without cardiopulmonary bypass and died; the last seven, for whom the pump oxygenator was used, survived. In 1959 Senning[531] reported 2 cases with one survivor. Bahnson and his collaborators,[31] in a study of patients with complete and incomplete transposition of the pulmonary veins, reported thirty-six patients treated surgically, with twenty-three survivors.

In our institution six patients with complete transposition of the pulmonary veins, without pulmonary arterial hypertension (types I and II), were treated successfully by means of cardiopulmonary bypass. The operation consists in creation of a large anastomosis between the common pulmonary venous trunk and the left atrium, with simultaneous shifting of the atrial septum to allow for a larger left atrial cavity. The anomalous communication between the pulmonary vein and the right atrium is closed, and the atrial septal defect is repaired. If the pulmonary veins enter the coronary sinus, then, by means of a simple shift of the atrial septum, the entire coronary sinus drainage is directed into the left atrium. This results in complete hemodynamic correction with slight residual arterial unsaturation.

These methods of operation are highly satisfactory in children who have a normal or only moderately elevated pulmonary arterial pressure and an adequate mitral valve and left ventricle. If the left heart cavities or the atrioventricular valve is so small that it cannot handle the entire pulmonary venous return, this kind of approach may result in fatal pulmonary edema. Thus it is mandatory that left atrial pressure be measured after the anastomosis between the pulmonary venous trunk and the left atrium has been established, and *before* all communications between the left atrium and right atrium are permanently severed. If a significant increase in pressure is observed, an "escape valve" from the pulmonary vein-left atrial system to the right atrium should be preserved, either by creation of an atrial defect or by only partial obliteration of the anomalous connection to the right atrium. This, then, may be attended to some time later, during a second operation.

This type of surgery is not adequate for the young, critically ill infant with pulmonary venous obstruction. Here the problem is much like that encountered in patients with cor triatriatum. The principal objective of surgery is relief of the obstruction. Whether this may be accomplished successfully depends on the nature and location of the block. If the common trunk lies directly behind the left atrium, the problem may be solved rather easily by connecting these two structures. But even if the anatomic setup lends itself to correction, the small size of the infant, the hazards of perfusion and the difficulty in correctly identifying the minute structures make this a formidable surgical undertaking. Nevertheless, in view of the hopeless prognosis for these babies, surgery should be attempted.

Summary

As a rule, patients with complete transposition of the pulmonary veins are critically ill infants with cyanosis, congestive heart failure and pulmonary plethora. Catheterization reveals systemic arterial saturation at the right atrial level and pulmonary arterial hypertension. A minority of the patients with total anomalous pulmonary venous connection are older children with a clinical profile similar to that of secundum atrial septal defect. They have only minimal arterial unsaturation, and the right atrial saturation is practically at systemic level. Pulmonary arterial pressure is only slightly elevated. In the former group, surgery is mandatory, but extremely difficult; safe and effective surgery is available for the latter group, as an elective procedure.

INCOMPLETE (UNILATERAL) TRANSPOSITION
OF THE PULMONARY VEINS

Incidence

Incomplete transposition of the pulmonary veins is a fairly common condition; at least 100 cases have been reported in the literature, and it has been estimated that the anomaly is discovered in close to 0.7 per cent of routine postmortem examinations.[349] We encountered 11 patients with this syndrome from 1950 to 1956. Among 92 patients with an atrial left-to-right shunt observed at Johns Hopkins Hospital, 38 per cent were found to be due to anomalous pulmonary venous drainage.[31]

Anatomy

If one or more, but not all, of the pulmonary veins enter the right atrium instead of the left, incomplete transposition of the pulmonary veins exists. Almost without exception, this incomplete anomalous drainage involves only one lung. In other words, if the anomalous pulmonary venous drainage involves both lungs, all the veins drain into the right atrium; conversely, if only some of them drain into the right atrium, only one lung is involved. The drainage from the right lung is involved almost twice as often as that from the left lung. An atrial septal defect of the ostium secundum type is associated with this condition almost exclusively in patients with anomalous drainage from the right lung. The point of entry to the right side of the heart from the right lung, in order of preference, is superior vena cava, inferior vena cava and right atrium proper. In most instances of anomalous drainage of the left lung the left superior vena cava receives the pulmonary venous blood.

The embryologic explanation underlying this anomaly is probably similar to that discussed in the section on complete transposition of the pulmonary veins (p. 724).

Physiology

The physiologic consequences of partial anomalous pulmonary venous drainage are essentially the same as those of atrial septal defect. It results in a left-to-right shunt at the atrial level, and in an appreciable number of instances it is associated with an atrial defect.

Clinical Picture

For practical purposes the clinical profile in this condition cannot be distinguished from that of atrial septal defect. Leatham[412] maintained that the splitting of the second sound is not fixed if partial anomalous venous connection is not associated with an atrial septal defect. Furthermore, occasionally, alert radiologists may identify the anomalous course of the pulmonary veins in the posteroanterior roentgenogram. The crescent-shaped course of the lower right pulmonary vein draining into the inferior vena cava (Fig. 522), the straight upper right pulmonary vein, draining into and distending the right superior vena cava, and the upper left pulmonary vein crossing over and distending the innominate vein may all furnish

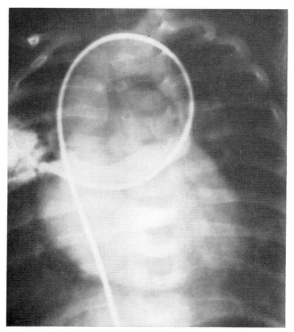

Figure 522.   Crescent-shaped pulmonary vein entering the right atrium.

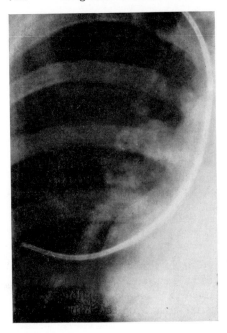

Figure 523. Passage of the catheter into pulmonary vein from right atrium.

clues to the correct diagnosis. Occasionally isolated distention of the right atrium may raise a suspicion of incomplete transposition of the pulmonary veins.

Cardiac catheterization may furnish the only more or less definite clue, suggesting the diagnosis of partial anomalous pulmonary venous drainage by passage of the catheter into a pulmonary vein from the right side of the heart (Fig. 523). This, by itself, does not unequivocally establish the diagnosis unless the pulmonary vein is entered from the superior vena cava and the increase in oxygen content is also at the superior vena cava level. Even though the pulmonary vein is catheterized from what seems to be the right atrium, one may, in fact, have already traversed an atrial defect or foramen ovale, and may have approached the lung from the left atrium. The only way to prove with certainty that some of the pulmonary veins drain into the right atrium is to demonstrate, by means of dye-dilution techniques, a difference in circulation times between the left pulmonary artery and the systemic artery, and the right pulmonary artery and the systemic artery.[676] Obviously the lung which has the anomalous drainage will have a significantly longer circulation time than the one which drains directly into the systemic circuit.

Results of angiocardiography, even with the selective technique, have been disappointing as far as accurately outlining the point of entry of the pulmonary vein is concerned.

Course and Prognosis

The statement is repeatedly encountered in the literature that if less than 50 per cent of the pulmonary veins drain into the right atrium and unless the condition is associated with another major intracardiac anomaly, normal life expectancy may be predicted. Since, as was stated previously, incomplete transposition of the pulmonary veins does not usually involve more than 50 per cent of the lungs, it would follow that most patients with partial anomalous pulmonary venous drainage have a normal life expectancy. This is not true, however. I have analyzed the available data in the literature in this respect (Table 35, p. 799), and it is clear that although some patients do indeed live normal life spans, others do not, and in some the age at death is not known. Consequently, in my opinion, a prediction as to how long a patient with incomplete transposition of the pulmonary veins will live should be based on the individual merits of the case, much as it is in patients with atrial septal defect. It is impossible to determine from the size of an atrial defect how large a left-to-right shunt exists. In the same fashion the number of abnormally draining veins is only one of the deciding factors in the prognosis of incomplete transposition of the pulmonary veins. The status of the vascular resistance and the functional condition of the myocardium are equally important in determining the ultimate effects of this anomaly.

Therefore, depending on the number of veins involved, the presence or absence of an associated atrial septal defect, and a number of other factors, incomplete transposition of the pulmonary veins may cause more or less embarrassment of the circulation. If difficulties arise, they consist in right-sided failure and the other consequences of atrial septal defect. No worth-while figures on the average life expectancy of these patients exist.

Differential Diagnosis

The problems in differential diagnosis outlined in the section on atrial septal defect are applicable to partial anomalous pulmonary venous drainage. The differentiation from atrial septal defect by means of cardiac catheterization and dye-dilution curves, as well as a few clinical clues, has been outlined earlier in this section.

Treatment

Surgical treatment of this anomaly can be accomplished on the basis of the indications and by means of the techniques outlined in the section on atrial defect (see p. 381). Fortunately, in the hands of our surgical team at The Children's Hospital Medical Center, the technical difficulty in coping with partial pulmonary venous anomaly has not been difficult, even if the preoperative diagnosis was atrial septal defect.[715] In case only one lobe of one lung is involved, lobectomy may be the preferred operative approach.

Summary

Partial transposition of the pulmonary veins usually involves one lung only. The signs, symptoms and laboratory data are practically identical with those of atrial septal defect. Cardiac catheterization, with special techniques, may distinguish between these two conditions. Indications and techniques for operation are identical with those discussed in the section on atrial septal defect.

TRANSPOSITION OF THE VENAE CAVAE

A few words may be said about anomalies of the vena cava. A persistent left superior vena cava may occur as an isolated anomaly; more commonly, however, it is associated with other types of congenital heart disease. At The Children's Hospital Medical Center we have seen it associated with transposition of the great arteries, partial or complete transposition of the pulmonary veins, septal defects, patent ductus arteriosus and tetralogy of Fallot. In all these cases the left superior vena cava entered the coronary sinus and drained, through it, into the right atrium. The course of the vessel may be seen in the ordinary roentgenogram, but is clearer in a venous angiogram (Fig. 524). From all outward appearances this anomaly had no functional significance, but it can be extremely annoying at cardiac catheterization if an approach is made through the left arm.

Of considerable functional significance, however, is the rare instance in which both venae cavae empty into the left atrium, together with the pulmonary veins. This is analogous to complete transposition of the pulmonary veins. We have never encountered a case of this type in our clinic. Taussig[682] described the clinical picture of complete transposition of the cavae, and Friedlich and his associates[260] analyzed the physiologic data. According to these authors, if both venae cavae drain into the left atrium, a situation exists which is similar to that of tricuspid atresia with underdeveloped right ventricle.

Tuchman and his associates[699] reported the first case, and Davis and his co-workers,[188] the second case, of isolated drainage of the left superior vena cava into the left atrium. The diagnosis may be made with certainty only at cardiac catheterization, but it may be suspected on the basis of

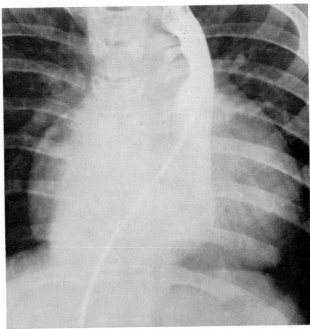

Figure 524. Angiogram indicating drainage of left superior vena cava into coronary sinus.

mild cyanosis without exercise intolerance, evidence of left ventricular hypertrophy in the electrocardiogram and roentgenograms suggesting the presence of a left superior vena cava.

We have seen two patients, in the second and third decades, respectively, who had the inferior vena cava draining into the left atrium. The signs and symptoms were the same as those described for the anomalously draining left superior vena cava, except that in the roentgenogram the inferior vena cava was absent from its usual place.[265, 683] Surgery is possible for these conditions.

DEXTROCARDIA

The literature on dextrocardia is full of conflicting and confusing statements, starting with the definition of the term. For the purposes of this discussion, dextrocardia denotes a heart in the right side of the thorax, the apex pointing to the right (Fig. 525).

Anatomy

Accepting this definition of dextrocardia, one must exclude from this discussion *extrinsic dextrocardia,* in which the heart is in the right side of the chest because something pushes or pulls it over (diaphragmatic hernia, pulmonary fibrosis, cystic disease of the lungs).

One is left with mirror-image dextrocardia with abdominal heterotaxia and *dextroversion with or without abdominal heterotaxia.*

In mirror-image dextrocardia the mirror is in the sagittal plane, the

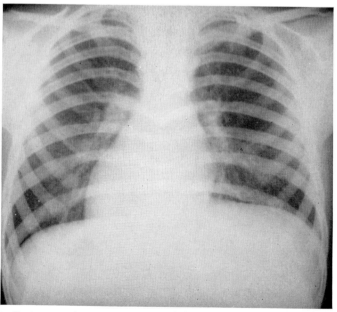

Figure 525. Posteroanterior roentgenogram of the heart in a patient with dextrocardia.

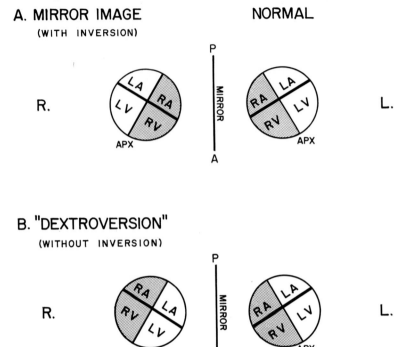

Figure 526. Diagrammatic presentation of dextrocardia: *A*, mirror image; *B*, dextroversion.

apex points to the right, and the anteroposterior relations are preserved, but there is inversion, i.e. a reversal of the left-to-right relation of the atria and the ventricles (Fig. 526).

Clinical recognition of mirror-image dextrocardia rests on the following observations: (1) There is *complete inversion* of the thoracoabdominal organs *without structural deformity*. The stomach bubble is on the right, the liver is on the left, the ascending colon is to the left, the descending colon to the right, the left lung has three lobes and the right, two. The spleen is always under the right side of the diaphragm. (2) *There is no significant congenital heart disease*. According to Grant,[297] among more than 1000 patients with mirror-image dextrocardia, only 5 were noted to have congenital heart disease. Keith placed the incidence of congenital heart disease in patients with dextrocardia and abdominal situs inversus at 3 per cent. This contrasts with Arcilla and Gasul's[20] figures of 55 per cent; however, the number in the latter series is small (eleven) and is derived from a very active cardiac service, representing highly selected material. (3) *The electrocardiogram, reflecting the inversion* of the cardiac chambers, shows an inverted P_1, QRS_1 and T_1. (4) *Bronchiectasis* with paranasal sinusitis is frequently associated with mirror-image dextrocardia (Kartagener's syndrome).[54]

In dextroversion with or without abdominal heterotaxia, the heart is again, of course, in the right side of the chest. It does not represent a mirror image, however, since there is no inversion or exchange in the left-to-right relation, but merely a reversal in the interoposterior direction.

The left ventricle and left atrium are anterior, the right ventricle is posterior and superior (Fig. 526).

Clinical recognition of dextroversion is based on the following observations: (1) There may or may not be thoracoabdominal heterotaxia. *If there is abdominal situs inversus, it is usually incomplete* and may be accompanied by *structural deformity.* The spleen may be absent in 20 per cent of these patients. (2) *There is a more than 90 per cent probability of associated congenital heart disease,*[428] particularly transposition of the great arteries or truncus arteriosus. Other deformities which may be present are single ventricle, tricuspid atresia, pulmonic stenosis, complete transposition of the pulmonary veins, single atrium and corrected transposition. Keith stressed the great rarity of Fallot's tetralogy, saying that "the three cases listed are by no means clear-cut." Arcilla[20] cited one case proved at postmortem examination. (3) In the electrocardiogram *the P axis is normal,* but, because of the associated anomalies, the QRS and T axes are highly variable. Often there is inversion of T_1 and a deep Q_1.

Clinical Picture

As indicated, mirror-image dextrocardia with complete situs inversus should not give any symptoms except those referable to Kartagener's triad. The unusual location of the heart may be easily missed even by competent observers unless the apex of the heart is always carefully palpated. Auscultation is not a reliable tool for the discovery of dextrocardia. Fluoroscopy is, of course, the best tool; the roentgenograms alone may be misleading, the view of the common tendency to look at films in the conventional position and to disregard the sometimes not too clearly visible markings of left and right. The cardiogram is pathognomonic, with inverted P_1, QRS_1 and T_1, upright P_{aVR} and inverted P_{aVL} (Fig. 48). Congenital heart disease is rare.

In contrast, children with dextroversion are usually referred to the physician because of congenital heart disease. Eighty per cent of them are cyanotic, and most have diminished pulmonary blood flow. Simple tetralogy of Fallot with dextroversion is exceedingly are; usually surgically incorrectible defects are found. The cardiogram is variable, depending on the intrinsic heart disease, but, unless arrythmia is present, the P axis is normal.

The physiologic data obtained at *cardiac catheterization* are useful in that they outline the nature of the pulmonary outflow tract and delineate the relation of the individual chambers to each other. In our hands, however, the complete anatomic and physiologic diagnosis is not much closer to reality after these time-consuming studies than it was before.

Course and Prognosis

The prognosis in dextrocardia depends entirely on the accompanying abnormalities. The "mirror-image" type, as mentioned, is often accompanied by bronchiectasis.[110] Many of the patients with dextroversion die in infancy because of incorrectable congenital heart disease. Others follow a course similar to that of patients with the tetralogy of Fallot or transposition of the great arteries with pulmonic stenosis.

Differential Diagnosis

Dextrocardia itself should be differentiated only from conditions in which the heart is pushed or pulled over into the right side of the thorax because of extracardiac conditions. Usually this is possible without much difficulty on the basis of the radiologic picture and a history indicating that the displacement of the heart was not present at birth. The accompanying intracardiac lesions are hard to evaluate with or without elaborate laboratory studies.

Treatment

Patients with Kartagener's syndrome (bronchiectasis, sinusitis and situs inversus) should be cared for according to the usual medical and surgical principles underlying the treatment of bronchiectasis.

After careful clinical and physiologic evaluation, patients with cyanotic congenital heart disease and diminished pulmonary arterial pressure should probably be operated on, using either Potts's or Blalock's technique. Multiple anomalies and the unusual anatomy of the great vessels are common enough to make the operative risk high. Only patients with severe disease should be considered candidates for operation.

Summary

In dextrocardia the heart is in the right side of the chest, the apex pointing to the right. Mirror-image dextrocardia is always accompanied by complete thoracoabdominal heterotaxia and seldom by intrinsic congenital heart disease. Conversely, patients with dextroversion have only partial or no situs inversus, but the incidence of congenital heart disease is 90 per cent or more. In most of these patients the congenital heart disease consists of complex cyanotic lesions, with transposition or one of its variants. Only palliative surgery is available, and at high risks.

LEVOCARDIA WITH ABDOMINAL SITUS INVERSUS

Levocardia, for the purposes of this discussion, denotes a heart in the left hemithorax, the apex pointing to the left; this of course is the normal position of the heart. In the patients under discussion the heart in this normal position is associated with transposed abdominal viscera, structural congenital cardiac anomaly and, commonly, absence of the spleen. The pathogenesis of this condition is not known; Forgacs[254] thought that the change in relations between the liver and the heart is responsible for the venous drainage into the left rather than the right side of the heart, and the consequent abnormalities in septation and the development of the cono-truncus structures. The insult producing this developmental anomaly probably occurs between the third and fourth embryonic weeks.

Incidence

The rarity of this condition has been pointed out by Campbell and

Forgacs,[130] who were able to report only 14 cases of their own and 19 from the literature between 1947 and 1955. Keith collected sixty-two cases from the literature in which the diagnosis was proved at postmortem examination and added four of his own.

Anatomy

Campbell and Forgacs[130, 132] divided their patients into two groups: one group, in which the venous (right) atrium and the superior vena cava are transposed to the left side, is clinically recognizable by an inverted P wave in lead I and by the fact that the aortic arch is on the right. In the second group, the more common one, the venous atrium and the superior vena cava remain on the right, and P_1, in the electrocardiogram, is upright; the aortic arch in these patients may be left-sided or right-sided. Keith's designation of the first group as being characterized by inversion (27 per cent) and the second by not having inversion (67 per cent) seems most logical to me (Fig. 527). Patients in both these groups have partial or complete transposition of the great vessels, septal defects and pulmonary stenosis.

Our own experience indicates that endocardial cushion defects associated with common truncus arteriosus, pulmonary stenosis, transposition of the great arteries and anomalous systemic or pulmonary venous connections are the most common lesions encountered. Fallot's tetralogy or simple septal defects are rare in patients with levocardia, and these diagnoses should be made only with extreme reluctance, on the basis of incontrovertible evidence. Probably in less than 10 per cent of the patients with levocardia and abdominal situs inversus is the heart structurally normal.

The degree of heterotaxia varies; seldom is it complete. Splenic abnormalities ranging from absence of the organ to multiple spleens are found in more than half of the patients. Howell-Jolly bodies are common in the blood smear.

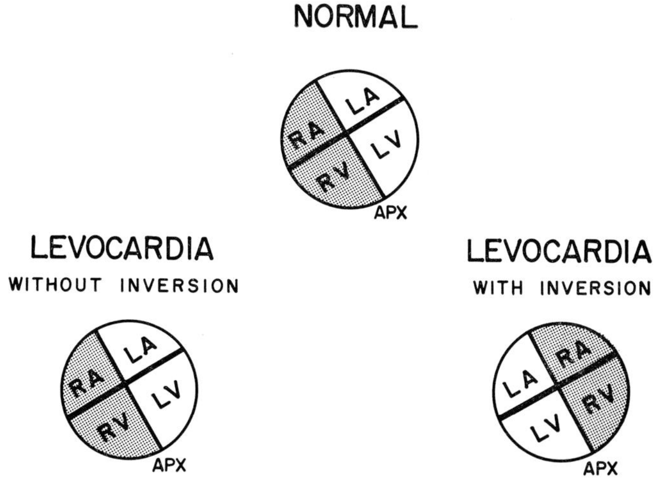

Figure 527. Diagrammatic presentation of levocardia with or without inversion.

Clinical Picture

The clinical, catheterization and angiographic pictures, as well as the natural history of the disease, are determined by the particular type of congenital heart disease which accompanies this syndrome. The oldest patient mentioned by Campbell and Forgacs was nineteen years old. Keith stated that only 6 per cent survive beyond the age of 5 years. Most of those described in the literature have died in infancy or early childhood. None of the children we examined post mortem had lived to be one year old. Inadequate pulmonary blood flow is almost invariably encountered; cyanosis is usually severe.

Differential Diagnosis

The most important point to remember about these patients is that they often resemble those with a simple, uncomplicated tetralogy of Fallot, which in fact they almost never prove to be. The presumptive diagnosis in every one of Young and Griswold's[756] eight cases was tetralogy of Fallot; we have made the same error ourselves. The only way this pitfall may be avoided is to follow the course of the ingested barium until it has gone below the diaphragm at fluoroscopy and to take careful note of the position of the stomach.

Treatment

Because of the presence of cyanosis in a patient with ischemic lung fields, the shunt operation seems a logical approach to the problem. But the complicated anatomic situation does not lend itself easily to this type of correction. Potts's or Blalock's procedure may be the only salvation for these patients, but operation should not be proposed lightly, since the surgical mortality rate is certainly higher than average. Campbell and Forgacs[130] described their operative experience as "less fortunate" than Young and Griswold's,[756] who themselves lost three of eight patients (all those less than two years of age). Considering the fact that most of these patients die before they reach one year of age, these figures demonstrate the seriousness of this situation, with or without surgical intervention.

Summary

Levocardia with abdominal situs inversus is usually accompanied by severe cyanotic congenital heart disease. The clinical profile may resemble that of a patient with a severe degree of tetralogy of Fallot, but, anatomically, truncus arteriosus, transposition of the great vessels, pulmonic stenosis, endocardial cushion defects and systemic or pulmonary vascular anomalies are the most common abnormalities found. Most patients die in infancy; a shunt procedure may be attempted in patients with definite pulmonary ischemia, but the mortality rate is high.

REFERENCES

1. Abbott, M.: *Atlas of Congenital Cardiac Diseases.* New York, American Heart Association, 1936.
2. Abrahams, D. G., and Wood, P. H.: Pulmonary Stenosis with Normal Aortic Root. *Brit. Heart J.,* 13:519, 1951.
3. Adams, C. W.: Postviral Myopericarditis Associated with the Influenza Virus. *Am. J. Cardiol.,* 4:56, 1959.
4. Adams, F. H., and Katz, B.: Endocardial Fibroelastosis; Case Report with Special Emphasis on the Clinical Findings. *J. Ped.,* 41:141, 1952.
5. Adams, F. H., and Lind, J.: Physiologic Studies on the Cardiovascular Status of Normal Newborn Infants (with Special Reference to the Ductus Arteriosus). *Pediatrics,* 19:431, 1957.
6. Adams, P., Jr., Anderson, R. C., Lillehei, C. W., and Meyne, N.: Reversibility of of Pulmonary Hypertension Following Closure of Ventricular Septal Defects. *Am. J. Dis. Child.,* 98:558, 1959.
7. Agorogianiss, S.: Personal communication to the author.
8. Alimurung, M. M., Eley, R. C., and Massell, B. F.: Paroxysmal Auricular Tachycardia; Report of Case with Persistent Ectopic Auricular Pacemaker, without Sinoauricular Node Activity. *Am. Heart J.,* 40:468, 1950.
9. Alimurung, M. M., Rappaport, M. B., and Sprague, H. B.: Variations in First Apical Sound Simulating So-Called "Presystolic Murmur of Mitral Stenosis," Phonocardiographic Study. *New England J. Med.,* 241:631, 1949.
10. Alimurung, M. M., Herrera, F., Guytingco, A., and Cruz, P. M.: Heart Disease in the Philippines. A Seven Year (1947–1953) Postwar Survey of Four Manila General Hospitals. *Am. Heart J.,* 50:293, 1955.
11. Alimurung, M. M., Joseph, L. G., Craige, E., and Massell, B. F.: Q-T Interval in Normal Infants and Children. *Circulation,* 1:1329, 1950.
12. Alimurung, M. M., Joseph, L. G., Nadas, A. S., and Massell, B. F.: Unipolar Precordial and Extremity Electrocardiogram in Normal Infants and Children. *Circulation,* 4:420, 1951.
13. Allison, P. R., and Linden, R. J.: The Bronchoscopic Measurement of Left Auricular Pressure. *Circulation,* 7:669, 1953.
14. Altschule, M. D.: *Physiology in Diseases of the Heart and Lungs.* Cambridge, Harvard University Press, 1949.
15. Alzamora, V., and others: On the Possible Influence of Great Altitudes on the Determination of Certain Cardiovascular Anomalies. *Pediatrics,* 12:259, 1953.
16. American Heart Association: Recommendations for Human Blood Pressure Determinations by Sphygmomanometers. New York, 1951.
17. Andersen, D. H., and Kelly, J.: Endocardial Fibro-elastosis. I. Endocardial Fibro-elastosis Associated with Congenital Malformations of the Heart. II. A Clinical and Pathologic Investigation of Those Cases without Associated Cardiac Malformations, Including Report of Two Familial Instances. *Pediatrics,* 18: 513, 539, 1956.
18. Anderson, R. C., Lillehei, C. W., and Lester, R. G.: Corrected Transposition of the Great Vessels of the Heart. A Review of 17 Cases. *Pediatrics,* 20:626, 1957.
19. Andrews, G. W. S., Pickering, G. W., and Sellors, T. H.: Aetiology of Constrictive Pericarditis, with Special Reference to Tuberculous Pericarditis, Together with Note on Polyserositis. *Quart J. Med.,* 17:291, 1948.
20. Arcilla, R. A., and Gasul, B. M.: Congenital Dextrocardia. Clinical Angiocardiographic and Autopsy Studies on Fifty Patients. *J. Pediat.,* 58:39, 1961.
21. Ash, R.: First Ten Years of Rheumatic Infection in Childhood. *Am. Heart J.,* 36:89, 1948.

747

22. Ash, R., Rubin, M. I., and Rappaport, M.: Electrocardiographic Variations in Acute Glomerulonephritis. *Am. J. Dis. Child.*, 67:106, 1944.

23. Ashman, R., and Hull, E.: *Essentials of Electrocardiography for the Student and Practitioner of Medicine.* 2nd ed. New York, Macmillan Company, 1941.

24. Astley, R., and Parsons, C.: Complete Transposition of the Great Vessels. *Brit. Heart J.*, 14:13, 1952.

25. Astley, R., Oldham, J. S., and Parsons, C.: Congenital Tricuspid Atresia. *Brit. Heart J.*, 15:287, 1953.

26. Auld, W. H. R., and Watson, H.: Fibroelastosis of the Heart in Adolescence. *Brit. Heart J.*, 19:186, 1957.

27. Baffes, T. G.: A New Method for Surgical Correction of Transposition of the Aorta and Pulmonary Artery. *Surg., Gynec. & Obst.*, 102:227, 1956.

28. Baffes, T. G., and Potts, W. J.: Surgical Correction of Transposition of the Aorta and the Pulmonary Artery. *Progr. in Cardiovasc. Dis.*, 1:102, 1958.

29. Baffes, T. G., Johnson, F. R., Potts, W. J., and Gibson, S.: Anatomic Variations in the Tetralogy of Fallot, *Am. Heart J.*, 46:657, 1953.

30. Bahn, R. C., Edwards, J. E., and DuShane, J. W.: Coarctation of the Aorta as a Cause of Death in Early Infancy. *Pediatrics*, 8:192, 1951.

31. Bahnson, H. T., Spencer, F. C., and Neill, C. A.: Surgical Treatment of 35 Cases of Drainage of the Pulmonary Veins to the Right Side of the Heart. *J. Thoracic Surg.*, 36:777, 1958.

32. Bailey, C. P.: The Surgical Treatment of Mitral Stenosis (Mitral Commissurotomy). *Dis. of Chest*, 15:377, 1949.

33. Bailey, C. P., and others: Congenital Interatrial Communications: Clinical and Surgical Considerations with a Description of a New Surgical Technique: Atriosepto-pexy. *Ann. Int. Med.*, 37:888, 1952.

34. Bain, H. W., McLean, D. M., and Walker, S. J.: Epidemic Pleurodynia (Bornholm Disease) Due to Coxsackie B-5 Virus. *Pediatrics*, 27:889, 1961.

35. Baker, C., Brinton, W. D., and Channell, G. D.: Ebstein's Disease. *Guy's Hosp. Rep.*, 99:247, 1950.

36. Baker, L. A., and Musgrave, D.: Study of Mitral Stenosis in Patients Who Survived Age of 50. *An. Int. Med.*, 26:901, 1947.

37. Barber, J. M., Magidson, O., and Wood, P.: Atrial Septal Defect, with Special Reference to the Electrocardiogram, the Pulmonary Artery Pressure, and the Second Heart Sound. *Brit. Heart J.*, 12:277, 1950.

38. Barcroft, J.: *Researches of Pre-natal Life.* Oxford, Basil, Blackwell & Mott, Ltd., 1944.

39. Barber, A. C.: The Pathogenesis of Sodium Retention in Congestive Heart Failure. *Metabolism*, 5:480, 1946.

40. Barger, A. C., Roe, B. B., and Richardson, G. S.: Relation of Valvular Lesions and of Exercise to Auricular Pressure, Work Tolerance, and to Development of Chronic Congestive Failure in Dogs. *Am. J. Physiol.*, 169:384, 1952.

41. Barger, A. C., Ross, R. S., and Price, H. L.: Reduced Sodium Excretion in Dogs with Mild Valvular Lesions of the Heart, and in Dogs with Congestive Failure. *Am. J. Physiol.*, 180:249, 1955.

42. Barger, A. C., Rudolph, A. M., and Yates, F. E.: Sodium Excretion and Renal Hemodynamics in Normal Dogs, Dogs with Mild Valvular Lesions of the Heart and Dogs in Frank Congestive Heart Failure. (Abstr.) *Am. J. Physiol.*, 183:595, 1955.

43. Barnes, A. R., and Burchell, H. B.: Acute Pericarditis Simulating Acute Coronary Occlusion; Report of 14 Cases. *Am. Heart J.*, 23:247, 1942.

44. Baronofsky, I. D., Gordon, A. J., Grishman, A., Steinfeld, L., and Kreel, I.: Aorticopulmonary Septal Defect: Diagnosis and Report of Case Successfully Treated. *Am. J. Cardiol.*, 5:273, 1960.

45. Bayer, O., Loogen, F., and Wolter, H. H.: The Mitral Opening Snap in the Quantitative Diagnosis of Mitral Stenosis. *Am. Heart J.*, 51:234, 1956.

46. Bayley, R. H.: On Certain Applications of Modern Electrocardiographic Theory to the Interpretation of Electrocardiograms Which Indicate Myocardial Disease. *Am. Heart J.*, 26:769, 1943.

47. Bazett, H. C.: An Analysis of the Time Relationship of the Electrocardiogram. *Heart*, 7:353, 1920.

48. Beattie, E. J., Jr., Cooke, F. N., Paul, J. S., and Orbison, J. A.: Coarctation of the Aorta at the Level of the Diaphragm Treated Successfully with a Preserved Human Blood Vessel Graft. *J. Thoracic Surg.*, 21:506, 1951.

49. Beck, W., Swan, H. J. C., Burchell, H. B., and Kirklin, J. W.: Pulmonary Vascular Resistance after Repair of Atrial Septal Defects in Patients with Pulmonary Hypertension. *Circulation*, 22:938, 1960.

50. Becu, L. M., and others: Anatomic and Pathologic Studies in Ventricular Septal Defect. *Circulation*, 14:349, 1956.

51. Bellet, S.: *Clinical Disorders of the Heart Beat.* Philadelphia, Lea & Febiger, 1953.

52. Bercu, B. A., and others: Pseudoaortic Stenosis Produced by Ventricular Hypertrophy. *Am. J. Med.*, 25:814, 1958.

53. Berg, J. M., Crome, L., and France, N. E.: Congenital Cardiac Malformations in Mongolism. *Brit. Heart J.*, 22:331, 1960.

54. Bergstrom, W. H., Cook, C. D., Scannell, J., and Berenberg, W.: Situs Inversus, Bronchiectasis, and Sinusitis: Report of a Family with Two Cases of Kartagener's Triad and Two Additional Cases of Bronchiectasis among Six Siblings. *Pediatrics*, 6:573, 1950.

55. Besterman, E.: Atrial Septal Defect with

Pulmonary Hypertension. *Brit. Heart J.,* 23:587, 1961.

56. Beuren, A.: Differential Diagnosis of the Taussig-Bing Heart from Complete Transposition of the Great Vessels with a Posteriorly Overriding Pulmonary Artery. *Circulation,* 21:1071, 1960.

57. Bing, R. J., Vandam, L. D., and Gray, F. D., Jr.: Physiological Studies in Congenital Heart Disease. I. Procedures. *Bull. Johns Hopkins Hosp.,* 80:107, 1947; II. Results of Preoperative Studies in Patients with Tetralogy of Fallot. *Ibid.,* 80:121, 1947.

58. Bing, R. J., Handelsman, J. C., Campbell, J. A., Griswold, H. E., and Blalock, A.: The Surgical Treatment and Physiopathology of Coarctation of the Aorta. *Ann. Surg.,* 128:803, 1948.

59. Björk, V. O., Malmström, G., and Uggla, L. G.: Left Auricular Pressure Measurements in Man. *Ann. Surg.,* 138:718, 1953.

60. Björk, V. O., Crafoord, C., Jonsson, B., Kjellberg, S. R., and Rudhe, V.: Atrial Septal Defects; A New Surgical Approach and Diagnostical Aspects. *Acta chir. Scandinav.,* 107:466, 1954.

61. Blalock, A., and Hanlon, C. R.: Surgical Treatment of Complete Transposition of Aorta and Pulmonary Artery. *Surg., Gynec. & Obst.,* 90:1, 1950.

62. Blalock, A., and Taussig, H. B.: The Surgical Treatment of Malformations of the Heart, *J.A.M.A.,* 128:189, 1945.

63. Bland, E. F., and Jones, T. D.: Rheumatic Fever and Rheumatic Heart Disease; A Twenty-Year Report on 1000 Patients Followed Since Childhood. *Circulation,* 4:836, 1951.

64. Bland, E. F., White, P. D., and Garland, J.: Congenital Anomalies of Coronary Arteries: Report of Unusual Case Associated with Cardiac Hypertrophy. *Am. Heart J.,* 8:787, 1933.

65. Bland, E. F., White, P. D., and Jones, T. D.: Development of Mitral Stenosis in Young People, with Discussion of Frequent Misinterpretation of Middiastolic Murmur at Cardiac Apex. *Am. Heart J.,* 10:995, 1935.

66. Blount, S. G., Jr., McCord, M. C., and Gelb, I. J.: Ebstein's Anomaly. *Circulation,* 15:210, 1957.

67. Blount, S. G., Jr., McCord, M. C., Mueller, H., and Swan, H.: Isolated Valvular Pulmonic Stenosis. Clinical and Physiologic Response to Open Valvuloplasty. *Circulation,* 10:161, 1954.

68. Blount, S. G., Jr., Swan, H., Gensini, G., and McCord, M. C.: Atrial Septal Defect: Clinical and Physiologic Response to Complete Closure in Five Patients. *Circulation,* 9:801, 1954.

69. Blount, S. G., and others: Physiological Studies in Congenital Heart Disease. XII. The Circulatory Dynamics in Patients with Tricuspid Atresia. *Bull. Johns Hopkins Hosp.,* 89:235, 1951.

70. Blumberg, R. W., and Lyon, R. A.: Endocardial Sclerosis. *Am. J. Dis. Child.,* 84:291, 1952.

71. Blumenthal, S., Griffiths, S. P., and Morgan, B. C.: Bacterial Endocarditis in Children with Heart Disease. A Review Based on the Literature and Experience with 58 Cases. *Pediatrics,* 26:993, 1960.

72. Blumgart, H. L., Gargill, S. L., and Gilligan, D. R.: Studies on the Velocity of Blood Flow. XV. The Velocity of Blood Flow and Other Aspects of the Circulation in Patients with "Primary" and Secondary Anemia and in Two Patients with Polycythemia Vera. *J. Clin. Invest.,* 9:679, 1931.

73. Bonham-Carter, R. E., Walker, C. H. M., Daley, R., Matthews, M. B., and Medd, W. E.: Patent Ductus Arteriosus with an Abnormal Aortic Valve. *Brit. Heart J.,* 17:255, 1955.

74. Boone, J. A., and Levine, S. A.: The Prognosis in "Potential Rheumatic Heart Disease" and "Rheumatic Mitral Insufficiency." *Am. J. M. Sc.,* 195:764, 1938.

75. Borst, H. G., McGregor, M., Whittenberger, J. L., and Berglund, E.: Influence of Pulmonary Artery and Left Atrial Pressures on Pulmonary Vascular Resistance. *Circulation Research,* 4:393, 1956.

76. Bower, B. D., Gerrard, J., and MacGregor, M. E.: Acute Benign Pericarditis, a Report of 4 Cases in Childhood. *Brit. M.J.,* 1:244, 1953.

77. Bower, B. D., Gerrard, J. W., D'Abreu, A. L., and Parsons, C. G.: Two Cases of Congenital Mitral Stenosis Treated by Valvotomy. *Arch. Dis. Childhood,* 28:91, 1953.

78. Brannon, E. W., Merrill, A. J., Warren, J. V., and Stead, E. A., Jr.: The Cardiac Output in Patients with Chronic Anemia as Measured by the Technique of Right Atrial Catheterization. *J. Clin. Invest.,* 24:332, 1945.

79. Brantigan, O. C.: Anomalies of the Pulmonary Veins. *Surg., Gynec. & Obst.,* 84:653, 1947.

80. Braudo, J. L., and Zion, M. M.: The Cyanotic (Syncopal) Attack in Fallot's Tetralogy. *Brit. M.J.,* 1:323, 1959.

81. Braudo, J. L., Javett, S. M., Adler, D. I., and Kessel, I.: Isolated Congenital Mitral Stenosis. Report of Two Cases with Mitral Valvotomy in One. *Circulation,* 15:358, 1957.

82. Braudo, J. L., Nadas, A. S., Rudolph, A. M., and Neuhauser, E. B. D.: Atrial Septal Defects in Children. A Clinical Study with Special Emphasis on Indications for Operative Repair. *Pediatrics,* 14:618, 1954.

83. Braunwald, E., and Morrow, A. G.: A Method for the Detection and Estimation of Aortic Regurgitant Flow in Man. *Circulation,* 17:505, 1958.

84. Idem: Left Ventriculo-Right Atrial Com-

munication: Diagnosis by Clinical, Hemodynamic and Angiographic Methods. *Am. J. Med.,* 28:913, 1960.

85. Braunwald, E., Lombardo, C. R., and Morrow, A. G.: Drainage Pathways of Pulmonary Veins in Atrial Septal Defect. *Brit. Heart J.,* 22:385, 1960.

86. Braverman, I. B., and Gibson, S.: The Outlook for Children with Congenital Aortic Stenosis. *Am. Heart J.,* 53:487, 1957.

87. Brent, L. B., Fisher, D. L., and Taylor, W. J.: Familial Muscular Subaortic Stenosis. (Abstr.) *Circulation,* 20:676, 1959.

88. Brent, L. B., and others: Familial Muscular Subaortic Stenosis; An Unrecognized Form of "Idiopathic Heart Disease," with Clinical and Autopsy Observations. *Circulation,* 21:167, 1960.

89. Broadbent, J. C., Wood, E. H. and Burchell, H. B.: Left-to-Right Intracardiac Shunts in the Presence of Pulmonary Stenosis. *Proc. Staff Meet., Mayo Clin.,* 28:101, 1953.

90. Brock, R. C.: Pulmonary Valvulotomy for the Relief of Congenital Pulmonary Stenosis. *Brit. M. J.,* 1:1121, 1948.

91. Idem: Congenital Pulmonary Stenosis. *Am. J. Med.,* 12:706, 1952.

92. Idem: Discussion; in C. R. Lam, Ed.: *Henry Ford Hospital International Symposium on Cardiovascular Surgery.* Philadelphia, W. B. Saunders Company, 1955, p. 409.

93. Brock, R.: *The Anatomy of Congenital Pulmonic Stenosis.* New York, Paul B. Hoeber, Inc., 1957.

94. Idem: Functional Obstruction of the Left Ventricle; Acquired Aortic Subvalvar Stenosis. *Guy's Hosp. Rep.,* 106:221, 1957.

95. Idem: The Surgical Treatment of Fallot's Tetralogy. *Guy's Hosp. Rep.,* 108:314, 1959.

96. Idem: The Surgical Treatment of Pulmonary Stenosis. *Brit. Heart J.,* 23:337, 1961.

97. Brock, R., and Ross, D. N.: The Sinus Venosus Type of Atrial Septal Defect. *Guy's Hosp. Rep.,* 108:291, 1959.

98. Brock, L. L., and Siegel, A. C.: Studies on the Prevention of Rheumatic Fever: The Effect of Time of Initiation of Treatment of Streptococcal Infections on the Immune Response of the Host. *J. Clin. Invest.,* 32:630, 1953.

99. Brock, R., Milstein, B. B., and Ross, D. N.: Percutaneous Left Ventricular Puncture in Assessment of Aortic Stenosis. *Thorax,* 11:163, 1956.

100. Brockenbrough, E. C., Braunwald, E., and Morrow, A. G.: A Hemodynamic Technic for the Detection of Hypertrophic Subaortic Stenosis. *Circulation,* 23:189, 1961.

101. Brotmacher, L., and Campbell, M.: The Natural History of Ventricular Septal Defect. *Brit. Heart J.,* 20:97, 1958.

102. Brown, J. W.: *Congenital Heart Disease.* 2nd ed. New York, Staples Press, Ltd., 1950.

103. Burack, W. R., Pryce, J., and Goodwin, J. F.: A Reversible Nephrotic Syndrome Associated with Congestive Heart Failure. *Circulation,* 18:562, 1958.

104. Burch, G. E.: *A Primer of Venous Pressure.* Philadelphia, Lea & Febiger, 1950.

105. Idem: *A Primer of Congestive Heart Failure.* Springfield, Ill., Charles C Thomas, 1954.

106. Burch, G. E., and Walsh, J. J.: Cardiac Enlargement Due to Myocardial Degeneration of Unknown Cause. *J.A.M.A.,* 172:207, 1960.

107. Burch, G. E., and Winsor, T.: Physiological Studies on 5 Patients Following Ligation of Inferior Vena Cava. *Proc. Soc. Exper. Biol. & Med.,* 53:135, 1943.

108. Idem: *A Primer of Electrocardiography.* Philadelphia, Lea & Febiger, 1945.

109. Burchell, H. B., and Edwards, J. E.: Aortic Sinus Aneurysm with Communications into Right Ventricle and Associated Ventricular Septal Defect. *Proc. Staff Meet., Mayo Clin.,* 26:336, 1951.

110. Burchell, H. B., and Pugh, D. G.: Uncomplicated Isolated Dextrocardia ("Dextroversio Cordis" Type). *Am. Heart J.,* 44:196, 1952.

111. Burke, E. C., Kirklin, J. W., and Edwards, J. E.: Sites of Obstruction to Pulmonary Blood Flow in the Tetralogy of Fallot: An Anatomic Study. *Proc. Staff Meet., Mayo Clin.,* 26:498, 1951.

112. Burnard, E. D.: A Murmur from the Patent Ductus Arteriosus in the Newborn Baby. *Brit. M.J.,* 1:806, 1958.

113. Idem: The Cardiac Murmur in Relation to Symptoms in the Newborn. *Brit. M.J.,* 1:134, 1959.

114. Burnard, E. D., and James, L. S.: The Cardiac Silhouette in Newborn Infants: A Cinematographic Study of the Normal Range. *Pediatrics,* 27:713, 1961.

115. Idem: Radiographic Heart Size in Apparently Healthy Newborn Infants: Clinical and Biochemical Correlations. *Pediatrics,* 27:726, 1961.

116. Burroughs, J. T., and Edwards, J. E.: Total Anomalous Pulmonary Venous Connection. *Am. Heart J.,* 59:913, 1960.

117. Burroughs, J. T., and Kirklin, J. W.: Complete Surgical Correction of Total Anomalous Pulmonary Venous Connection: Report of Three Cases. *Proc. Staff Meet., Mayo Clin.,* 31:182, 1956.

118. Burwell, C. S., and Blalock, A.: Chronic Constrictive Pericarditis; Physiologic and Pathologic Considerations. *J.A.M.A.,* 110:265, 1938.

119. Burwell, C. S., and Robin, E. D.: Some Points in the Diagnosis of Myocardial Fibrosis. *Tr. A. Am. Physicians,* 67:67, 1954.

120. Idem: Diagnosis of Diffuse Myocardial Fibrosis. *Circulation,* 20:606, 1959.

121. Butler, S., and Levine, S. A.: Diphtheria as Cause of Late Heart Block. *Am. Heart J.,* 5:592, 1930.

122. Bywaters, E. G. L., and Thomas, G. T.: Prevention of Rheumatic Fever Recurrences. *Brit. M.J.*, 2:350, 1958.

123. Cabrera, E., and Monroy, J. R.: Systolic and Diastolic Loading of the Heart. I. Physiologic and Clinical Data. *Am. Heart J.*, 43:661, 1952.

124. Caldini, P., Gensini, G. G., and Hoffman, M. S., Primary Pulmonary Hypertension with Death during Right Heart Catheterization. A Case Report and a Survey of Reported Fatalities. *Am. J. Cardiol.*, 4:519, 1959.

125. Campbell, J. A., Bing, R. J., Hendelsman, J. C., Griswold, H. E., and Hammond, M.: Physiological Studies in Congenital Heart Disease. VIII. The Physiological Findings in 2 Patients with Complete Transposition of the Great Vessels. *Bull. Johns Hopkins Hosp.*, 84:269, 1949.

126. Campbell, M.: Simple Pulmonary Stenosis; Pulmonary Valvular Stenosis with a Closed Ventricular Septum. *Brit. Heart J.*, 16:273, 1954.

127. Idem: Selection of Patients for Surgery in Congenital Heart Disease. *Brit. M. Bull.*, 11:178, 1955.

128. Idem: Late Results of Operations for Fallot's Tetralogy. *Brit. M. J.*, 2:1175, 1958.

129. Campbell, M., and Baylis, J. H.: The Course and Prognosis of Coarctation of the Aorta. *Brit. Heart J.*, 18:475, 1956.

130. Campbell, M., and Forgacs, P.: Laevocardia with Transposition of the Abdominal Viscera. *Brit. Heart J.*, 15:401, 153.

131. Campbell, M., and Kauntze, R.: Congenital Aortic Valvular Stenosis. *Brit. Heart J.*, 15:179, 1953.

132. Campbell, M., and Reynolds, G.: The Significance of the Direction of the P Wave in Dextrocardia and Isolated Laevocardia. *Brit. Heart J.*, 14:481, 1952.

133. Campbell, M., and Suzman, S.: Coarctation of the Aorta. *Brit. Heart J.*, 9:185, 1947.

134. Campbell, M., and Thorne, M. G.: Congenital Heart Block. *Brit. Heart J.*, 18:90, 1956.

135. Campbell, M., and Turner-Warwick, M.: Two more Families with Cardiomegaly. *Brit. Heart J.*, 18:393, 1956.

136. Campbell, M., Reynolds, G., and Trounce, J. R.: Six Cases of Single Ventricle with Pulmonary Stenosis. *Guy's Hosp. Rep.*, 102:99, 1953.

137. Campeau, L. A., Ruble, P. E., and Cooksey, W. B.: Congenital Absence of the Pulmonary Valve. *Circulation*, 15:397, 1957.

138. Capps, J. A., and Coleman, G. H.: *An Experimental and Clinical Study of Pain in the Pleura, Pericardium, and Peritoneum.* New York, Macmillan Company, 1932.

139. Cardell, B. S.: Corrected Transposition of the Great Vessels. *Brit. Heart J.*, 18:186, 1956.

140. Carmichael, D. B., Sprague, H. B., Wyman, S. M., and Bland, E. F.: Acute Nonspecific Pericarditis. Clinical, Laboratory, and Follow-up Considerations. *Circulation*, 3:321, 1951.

141. Castellanos, A., Pereiras, R., and García, A.: "La angio-cardiografia radioopaca." *Arch. Soc. estud. clin. Habana*, 1937, 31, nos. 9–10.

142. Cayler, G. G., Mays, J., and Riley, H. D., Jr.: Cardiorespiratory Syndrome of Obesity (Pickwickian Syndrome) in Children. *Pediatrics*, 27:237, 1961.

143. Cayler, G. G., Ongley, P., and Nadas, A. S.: Relation of Systolic Pressure in the Right Ventricle to the Electrocardiogram. *New England J. Med.*, 258:979, 1958.

144. Cayler, G. G., Rudolph, A. M., and Nadas, A. S.: Systemic Blood Flow in Infants and Children. *Pediatrics*, to be published.

145. Char, F., Adams, P., Jr., and Anderson, R. C.: Electrocardiographic Findings in One Hundred Verified Cases of Ventricular Septal Defect. *Am. J. Dis. Child.*, 97:48, 1959.

146. Chin, E. F., and Ross, D. N.: Myxoma of the Left Atrium; Successful Surgical Removal under Hypothermia. *Brit. M.J.*, 1:1447, 1957.

147. Christensen, N. A., and Hines, E. A., Jr.: Clinical Features in Coarctation of the Aorta: A Review of 96 Cases. *Proc. Staff Meet., Mayo Clin.*, 23:339, 1948.

148. Christie, A.: Normal Closing Time of the Foramen Ovale and the Ductus Arteriosus. *Am. J. Dis. Child.*, 40:323, 1930.

149. Civin, W. H., and Edwards, J. E.: Pathology of Pulmonary Vascular Tree; Comparison of Intrapulmonary Arteries in Eisenmenger's Complex and in Stenosis of Ostium Infundibuli Associated with Biventricular Origin of the Aorta. *Circulation*, 2:545, 1950.

150. Clark, L. C., Jr., and Bargeron, L. M., Jr.: Detection and Direct Recording of Left-to-Right Shunts with the Hydrogen Electrode Catheter. *Surgery*, 46:797, 1959.

151. Coburn, A. F.: *The Factor of Infection in the Rheumatic State.* Baltimore, Williams & Wilkins Company, 1931.

152. Idem: Salicylate Therapy in Rheumatic Fever; Rational Technic. *Bull. Johns Hopkins Hosp.*, 73:435, 1943.

153. Coleman, P. N., Edmunds, A. W. B., and Tregillus, J.: Primary Pulmonary Hypertension in Three Sibs. *Brit. Heart J.*, 21:81, 1959.

154. Collett, R. W., and Edwards, J. E.: Persistent Truncus Arteriosus: Classification According to Anatomic Types. *S. Clin. N. Amer.*, 29:1245, 1949.

155. Collins, D. M., East, T., Godfrey, M. P., Harris, and Oram, S.: Ventricular Septal Defect with Pulmonary Stenosis and Aortic Regurgitation. *Brit. Heart J.*, 20:363, 1958.

156. Combined Rheumatic Fever Study Group:

A Comparison of the Effect of Prednisone and Acetylsalicylic Acid on the Incidence of Residual Rheumatic Heart Disease. *New England J. Med.*, 262:895, 1960.

157. Committee of the American Rheumatism Association: Primer on the Rheumatic Diseases. Part 1. *J.A.M.A.*, 171:1205, 1959.

158. Committee on Standards and Criteria for Programs of Care of the Council of Rheumatic Fever and Congenital Heart Disease of the American Heart Association: Jones Criteria (Modified) for Guidance in the Diagnosis of Rheumatic Fever. *Circulation*, 13:617, 1956.

159. Condon, H. A., and Lee, P. F.: Functional Infundibular Stenosis Treated by Cyclopropane Anaesthesia. *Anaesthesia*, 15:45, 1960.

160. Cone, T. E., Jr., Allen, M. S., and Pearson, H. A.: Pheochromocytoma in Children. Report of Three Familial Cases in Two Unrelated Families. *Pediatrics*, 19:44, 1957.

161. Cooley, D. A.: Personal communication to the author.

162. Cooley, D. A., and Collins, H. A.: Anomalous Drainage of Entire Pulmonary Venous System into the Left Innominate Vein. *Circulation*, 19:486, 1959.

163. Cooley, D. A., McNamara, D. G., and Latson, Jr.: Aorticopulmonary Septal Defect: Diagnosis and Surgical Treatment. *Surgery*, 42:101, 1957.

164. Cooley, D. A., Morris, G. C., Jr., and Cora, A. S.: Cardiac Myxoma. Surgical Treatment in Four Cases. A.M.A. *Arch. Surg.*, 78:410, 1959.

165. Cooley, J. C., and others: Coarctation of the Aorta Associated with Patent Ductus Arteriosus. *Circulation*, 13:843, 1956.

166. Coombs, C. F.: *Rheumatic Heart Disease.* New York, William Wood & Company, 1924.

167. Cooper, A. S.: Idiopathic Pulmonary Hemosiderosis. Report of a Case in an Adult Treated with Triamcinolone. *New England J. Med.*, 263:1100, 1960.

168. Corday, E., Gold, H., and Jaffe, H. L.: Radioiodine Treatment of Paroxysmal Supraventricular Tachycardia in the Euthyroid Patient. *Circulation*, 17:900, 1958.

169. Cori, G. T.: Glycogen Structure and Enzyme Deficiencies in Glycogen Storage Disease. *Harvey Lect.* (1952–3), 48:145, 1954.

170. Cossio, P., Dambrosi, R. G., and Warmford-Thomson, H. F.: The First Heart Sound in Auricular and Ventricular Extrasystoles. *Brit. Heart J.*, 9:275, 1947.

171. Cournand, A., Baldwin, J. S., and Himmelstein, A.: *Cardiac Catheterization in Congenital Heart Disease: A Clinical and Physiological Study in Infants and Children.* New York, Commonwealth Fund, 1949.

172. Crafoord, C., and Nylin, G.: Congenital Coarctation of the Aorta and Its Surgical Treatment. *J. Thoracic Surg.*, 14:347, 1945.

173. Craige, E., Alimurung, M. M., Bland, E. F., and Massell, B. F.: The Q-T Interval in Rheumatic Fever. *Circulation*, 1:1338, 1950.

174. Crandell, F.: The Heart in Progressive Muscular Dystrophy. *Am. J.M. Sc.*, 231:659, 1956.

175. Currens, J. H., Kinney, T. D., and White, P. D.: Pulmonary Stenosis with Intact Interventricular Septum. Report of 11 Cases. *Am. Heart J.*, 30:491, 1945.

176. Cutler, J. G., Nadas, A. S., Goodale, W. T., Hickler, R. B., and Rudolph, A. M.: Pulmonary Arterial Hypertension with Markedly Increased Pulmonary Resistance; The Pulmonary Vascular Obstruction Syndrome. *Am. J. Med.*, 17:485, 1954.

177. Cutler, J. G., Ongley, P. A., Shwachman, H., Massell, B. F., and Nadas, A. S.: Bacterial Endocarditis in Children with Heart Disease. *Pediatrics*, 22:706, 1958.

178. D'Heer, H. A. H., and Van Nieuwenhuizen, C. L. C.: Diagnosis of Congenital Aortic Septal Defect. Description of Two Cases and Special Emphasis on a New Method Which Allows an Accurate Diagnosis by Means of Cardiac Catheterization. *Circulation*, 13:58, 1956.

179. Daeschner, C. W., Moyer, J. H., and Able, L. W.: Pheochromocytoma in a Four-Year Old Child; Renal Hemodynamic, Pharmacologic, and Radiographic Studies. *J. Pediat.*, 45:141, 1954.

180. Dalton, J. C., Pearson, R. J., and White, P. D.: Constrictive Pericarditis: A Review and Long-Term Follow-up of 78 Cases. *Ann. Int. Med.*, 45:445, 1956.

181. Dammann, J. F., Jr., and Ferencz, C.: Clinico-anatomic Correlations; in C. R. Lam, Ed.: *Henry Ford Hospital International Symposium on Cardiovascular Surgery.* Philadelphia, W. B. Saunders Company, 1955.

182. Idem: The Significance of the Pulmonary Vascular Bed in Congenital Heart Disease. I. Normal Lungs. II. Malformations of the Heart in Which There Is Pulmonary Stenosis. III. Defects between the Ventricles or Great Vessels in Which Both Increased Pressure and Blood Flow May Act upon the Lungs and in Which There Is a Common Ejectile Force. *Am. Heart J.*, 52:7, 210, 1956.

183. Danforth, W. H., Ballard, F. B., Kako, K., Choudhury, J. D., and Bing, R. J.: Metabolism of the Heart in Failure; in Symposium on Congestive Heart Failure. New York, The American Heart Association, Inc., 1960, p. 31.

184. Darling, R. C., Rothney, W. B., and Craig, J. M.: Total Pulmonary Venous Drainage into the Right Side of the Heart; Report of 17 Autopsied Cases Not Associated with Other Major Cardio-

vascular Anomalies. *J. Lab. Investigation,* 6:44, 1957.

185. Davidsen, H. G., Fabricus, J., and Husfeldt, E.: Five Cases of Congenital Aneurysm of the Aortic Sinuses (of Valsalva) and Notes on the Prognosis. *Acta med. scandinav.,* 160:455, 1958.

186. Davidson, J. D., Waldmann, T. A., Goodman, D. S., and Gordon, R. S., Jr.: Protein-Losing Gastroenteropathy in Congestive Heart Failure. *Lancet,* 1:899, 1961.

187. Davignon, A. L., Greenwold, W. E., DuShane, J. W., and Edwards, J. E.: Congenital Pulmonary Atresia with Intact Ventricular Septum; Clinicopathologic Correlation of Two Anatomic Types. *Am. Heart J.,* 62:591, 1961.

188. Davis, W. H., Jordaan, F. R., and Synman, H. W.: Persistent Left Superior Vena Cava Draining into the Left Atrium, as an Isolated Anomaly. *Am. Heart J.,* 57:616, 1959.

189. Dawes, G. S.: Changes in the Circulation at Birth. *Brit. M. Bull.,* 17:148, 1961.

190. Dawes, G. S., Mott, J. C., Widdicombe, J. G., and Wyatt, D. G.: Changes in the Lungs of the Newborn Lamb. *J. Physiol.,* 121:141, 1953.

191. Dennis, J. L., Hansen, A. E., and Corpening, T. M.: Endocardial Fibroelastosis. *Pediatrics,* 12:130, 1953.

192. Dexter, L., and others: Studies of Congenital Heart Disease. I. Techniques of Venous Catheterization as a Diagnostic Procedure. *J. Clin. Invest.,* 26:547, 1947; II. Pressure and Oxygen Content of Blood in Right Auricle, Right Ventricle, and Pulmonary Artery in Control Patients, with Observations on Oxygen Saturation and Source of Pulmonary "Capillary" Blood. *Ibid.,* 26:554, 1947. III. Venous Catheterization as a Diagnostic Aid in Patent Ductus Arteriosus, Tetralogy of Fallot, Ventricular Septal Defect and Auricular Septal Defect. *Ibid.,* 26:561, 1947.

193. Idem: Aortic Stenosis. *Arch. Int. Med.,* 101:254, 1958.

194. Diamond, I.: The Hamman Rich Syndrome in Childhood: Report of a Case with Unilateral Pulmonary Arterial and Venous Stenosis and Arteriovenous Occlusion *Pediatrics,* 22:279, 1958.

195. Dieuaide, F. R.: Observations on Respiratory Cases in Ventricular Paroxysmal Tachycardia. *Bull. Johns Hopkins Hosp.,* 35:229, 1924.

196. Dimond, E. G., and Lin, T. K.: The Clinical Picture of Pulmonary Stenosis (without Ventricular Septal Defect). *Ann. Int. Med.,* 40:1109, 1954.

197. Dines, D. E., Edwards, J. E., and Burchell, H. B.: Myocardial Atrophy in Constrictive Pericarditis. *Proc. Staff Meet., Mayo Clin.,* 33:93, 1958.

198. Dingle, J. H., and others: Study of Illness in Group of Cleveland Families; Plan of Study and Certain General Observations. *Am. J. Hyg.,* 58:16, 1953.

199. Dock, W.: Mode of Production of the First Heart Sound. *Arch. Int. Med.,* 51:737, 1933.

200. Donovan, M. S., Neuhauser, E. B. D., and Sossman, M. C.: The Roentgen Signs of Patent Ductus Arteriosus. *Am. J. Roentgenol.,* 50:293, 1943.

201. Dorfman, A., Gross, J. I., and Lorincz, A. E.: The Treatment of Acute Rheumatic Fever. *Pediatrics,* 27:692, 1961.

202. Dow, J. D.: The Radiological Diagnosis of the Sinus Venosus Type of Atrial Septal Defect. *Guy's Hosp. Rep.,* 108:305, 1959.

203. Dow, J. W.: Unpublished data.

204. Dow, J. W., and Dexter, L.: Circulatory Dynamics in Atrial Septal Defect. (Abstr.) *J. Clin. Invest.,* 29:809, 1950.

205. Downing, D. F.: Recatheterization of the Right Heart in Ventricular Septal Defect. *Am. Heart J.,* 57:669, 1959.

206. Dresdale, D. T., Michtom, R. J., and Schultz, M.: Recent Studies in Primary Pulmonary Hypertension, Including Pharmacodynamic Observations on Pulmonary Vascular Resistance. *Bull. New York, Acad. Med.,* 30:195, 1954.

207. Dresdale, D. T., Schultz, M., and Michtom, R. J.: Primary Pulmonary Hypertension. I. Clinical and Hemodynamic Study. *Am. J. Med.,* 11:686, 1951.

208. Dressler, W.: Pulsations of the Wall of the Chest. *Arch. Int. Med.,* 60:225, 437, 441, 654, 663, 1937.

209. DuShane, J. W., Weidman, W. H., Brandenburg, R. O., and Kirklin, J. W.: The Electrocardiogram in Children with Ventricular Septal Defect and Severe Pulmonary Hypertension. *Circulation,* 22:49, 1960.

210. DuShane, J. W., and others: Ventricular Septal Defects with Pulmonary Hypertension. *J.A.M.A.,* 160:950, 1956.

211. Edmonds, H. W., and Seelye, W. B.: Endocardial Sclerosis; A Review of Changing Concepts with Report of 6 Cases. *Pediatrics,* 7:651, 1951.

212. Edwards, J. E.: Functional Pathology of the Pulmonary Vascular Tree in Congenital Cardiac Disease. *Circulation,* 15:164, 1957.

213. Idem: Editorial. *Circulation,* 17:1001, 1958.

214. Idem: Congenital Malformations of the Heart and Great Vessels; in S. E. Gould: *Pathology of the Heart.* Springfield, Ill., Charles C Thomas, 1960, p. 266.

215. Idem: The Congenital Bicuspid Aortic Valve. *Circulation,* 23:485, 1961.

216. Edwards, J. E., and Burchell, H. B.: Specimen Exhibiting the Essential Lesion in Aneurysm of the Aortic Sinus. *Proc. Staff Meet., Mayo Clin.,* 31:407, 1956.

217. Idem: Pathologic Anatomy of Mitral Insufficiency. *Proc. Staff Meet., Mayo Clin.,* 33:497, 1958.

218. Edwards, J. E., Douglas, J. M., Burchell, H. B., and Christensen, N. A.: Pathol-

ogy of the Intrapulmonary Arteries and Arterioles in Coarctation of the Aorta Associated with Patent Ductus Arteriosus. *Am. Heart J.*, 38:205, 1949.

219. Edwards, J. E., and others: *An Atlas of Congenital Anomalies of the Heart and Great Vessels.* Springfield, Ill., Charles C Thomas, 1953.

220. Ehrenhaft, J. L.: Discussion of Physiologic Observations in Experimental Pulmonary Insufficiency. *J. Thoracic Surg.*, 30: 641, 1955.

221. Eldridge, F., Selzer, A., and Hultgren, H.: Stenosis of a Branch of the Pulmonary Artery. An Additional Cause of Murmurs over the Chest. *Circulation*, 15: 865, 1957.

222. Ellis, F. H., Jr., Brandenburg, R. O., Callahan, J. A., and Marshall, H. W.: Open Heart Surgery for Acquired Mitral Insufficiency. A.M.A. *Arch. Surg.*, 79:222, 1959.

223. Ellis, F. H., Jr., Brandenburg, R. O., and Swan, H. J. C.: Defect of the Atrial Septum in the Elderly. *New England J. Med.*, 262:219, 1960.

224. Ellis, F. H., Kirklin, J. W., Swan, H. J. C., DuShane, J. W., and Edwards, J. E.: Diagnosis and Surgical Treatment of Common Atrium (Cor Triloculare-Biventriculare). *Surgery*, 45:160, 1959.

225. Engle, M. A.: Ventricular Septal Defect in Infancy. *Pediatrics*, 14:16, 1954.

226. Engle, M. A., and Glenn, F.: Primary Malignant Tumor of the Heart in Infancy; Case Report and Review of the Subject. *Pediatrics*, 15:562, 1955.

227. Engle, M. A., and Ito, T.: The Postpericardiotomy Syndrome. *Am. J. Cardiol.*, 7:73, 1961.

228. Engle, M. A., Holswade, G. R., Goldberg, H. P., Lukas, D. S., and Glenn, F.: Regression, After Open Valvotomy, of Infundibular Stenosis Accompanying Severe Valvular Pulmonic Stenosis. *Circulation*, 17:862, 1958.

229. Engle, M. A., Payne, T. P. B., Bruins, C., and Taussig, H. B.: Ebstein's Anomaly of the Tricuspid Valve. Report of 3 Cases and Analysis of Clinical Syndrome. *Circulation*, 1:1246, 1950.

230. Ernstene, A. C.: Differentiation of Changes in Q-T Interval in Hypocalcemia and Hypopotassemia. *Am. Heart J.*, 38:260, 1949.

231. Evans, J. R., Rowe, R. D., and Keith, J. D.: Spontaneous Closure of Ventricular Septal Defects. *Circulation*, 22: 1044, 1960.

232. Idem: The Clinical Diagnosis of Atrial Septal Defect in Children. *Am. J. Med.*, 30:345, 1961.

233. Evans, J. W., Harris, T. R., and Brody, D. A.: Ruptured Aortic Sinus Aneurysm; Case Report, with Review of Clinical Features. *Am. Heart J.*, 61:408, 1961.

234. Evans, W.: Familial Cardiomegaly. *Brit. Heart J.*, 11:68, 1949.

235. Idem: Polythelia in Cardio-atrial Disease. *Brit. Heart J.*, 21:130, 1959.

236. Evans, W., and Wright, G.: Electrocardiogram in Friedreich Disease. *Brit. Heart J.*, 4:91, 1942.

237. Facquet, J., Lemoine, J. M., Alhomme, P., and Lefebvre, J.: La mesure de la pression auriculaire gauche par voie transbronchique. *Arch. mal. coeur*, 45:741, 1952.

238. Falkenbach, K. H., Zheutlin, N., Dowdy, A. H., and O'Loughlin, B. J.: Pulmonary Hypertension Due to Pulmonary Arterial Coarctation. *Radiology*, 73:575, 1959.

239. Fallot, A.: *Contribution à l'anatomie pathologique dela maladie bleue (cyanose cardiaque).* Marseille, Barlatier-Feissat, 1888.

240. Farber, S., and Hubbard, J.: Fetal Endomyocarditis: Intra-uterine Infection as Cause of Congenital Cardiac Anomalies. *Am. J. M. Sc.*, 186:705, 1933.

241. Feinstein, A. R., and DiMassa, R.: Prognostic Significance of Valvular Involvement in Acute Rheumatic Fever. *New England J. Med.*, 260:1001, 1959.

242. Ferencz, C., Johnson, A. L., and Wiglesworth, F. W.: Congenital Mitral Stenosis. *Circulation*, 9:161, 1954.

243. Ferguson, D. J., Adams, P., and Watson, D.: Pulmonary Arteriosclerosis in Transposition of the Great Vessels. *Am. J. Dis. Child.*, 99:653, 1960.

244. Ferrer, M. I., Harvey, R. J., Cournand, A., and Dickinson, W. R.: Cardiocirculatory Studies in Pulsus Alternans of the Systemic and Pulmonary Circulations. (Abstr.) Second World Congress of Cardiology and the 27th Annual Scientific Sessions of the American Heart Association, Washington, D.C., Sept. 12–17, 1954. American Heart Association, Inc., 1954, p. 51.

245. Ferrer, M. I., and others: Circulatory Effects of Mitral Commissurotomy, with Particular Reference to Selection of Patients for Surgery. *Circulation*, 12:7, 1955.

246. Feruglio, G. A., and Gunton, R. W.: Intracardiac Phonocardiography in Ventricular Septal Defect. *Circulation*, 21: 49, 1960.

247. Fey, L. D., and Mills, M. A.: Fulminating Trichinosis with Myocarditis. *Northwest Med.*, 53:701, 1954.

248. Fiedler, A.: Ueber akute interstitielle Myokarditis. *Zentralbl. f. inn. Med.*, 21: 212, 1900.

249. Finkel, S., and Baldwin, J. S.: Q-T Interval during Active and Inactive Rheumatic Fever. *Pediatrics*, 9:410, 1952.

250. Finland, M.: Treatment of Bacterial Endocarditis. *New England J. Med.*, 250: 372, 419, 1954.

251. Fisher, D. L.: The Use of Pressure Recordings Obtained at Transthoracic Left Heart Catheterization in the Diagnosis of Valvular Heart Disease. *J. Thoracic Surg.*, 30:379, 1958.

252. Idem: Catheterization of the Left Heart: in H. A. Zimmerman.[763]

253. Ford, R. V., Rochelle, J. B., Handley,

C. A., Moyer, J. H., and Spurr, G. L.: Choice of a Diuretic Agent Based on Pharmacological Principles. *J.A.M.A.,* 166:129, 1958.

254. Forgacs, P.: Congenital Heart Disease with Isolated Inversion of the Abdominal Viscera. *Brit. Heart J.,* 9:27, 1947.

255. Fowler, N. O., Mannix, E. P., and Noble, W.: Some Effects of Partial Pulmonary Valvectomy. *Circulation Research,* 4:8, 1956.

256. Freundlich, E., Engle, M. A., and Goldberg, H. P.: Coarctation of Aorta in Infancy. Analysis of a 10-Year Experience with Medical Management. *Pediatrics,* 27:427, 1961.

257. Friedberg, C. K.: Subacute Bacterial Endocarditis; Revision of Diagnostic Criteria and Therapy. *J.A.M.A.,* 144:527, 1950.

258. Friedberg, C. K.: *Diseases of the Heart.* 2nd ed. Philadelphia, W. B. Saunders Company, 1956.

259. *Ibid.,* p. 861.

260. Friedlich, A. L., Bing, R. J., and Blount, S. G., Jr.: Physiological Studies in Congenital Heart Disease; Circulatory Dynamics in Anomalies of Venous Return to Heart, Including Pulmonary Arteriovenous Fistula. *Bull. Johns Hopkins Hosp.,* 86:20, 1950.

261. Friedman, S., Murphy, L., and Ash, R.: Aortic Atresia with Hypoplasia of the Left Heart and Aortic Arch. *J. Pediat.,* 38:354, 1951.

262. Idem: Congenital Mitral Atresia with Hypoplastic Nonfunctioning Left Heart. *Am. J. Dis. Child.,* 90:176, 1955.

263. Friedman, S., Ash, R., Harris, T. N., and Lee, H. F.: Acute Benign Pericarditis in Childhood; Comparisons with Rheumatic Pericarditis, and Therapeutic Effects of ACTH and Cortisone. *Pediatrics,* 9:551, 1952.

264. Fyler, D. C., Rudolph, A. M., Wittenborg, M. H., and Nadas, A. S.: Ventricular Septal Defect in Infants and Children. *Circulation,* 18:833, 1958.

265. Gardner, D. L., and Cole, L.: Long Survival with Inferior Vena Cava Draining into Left Atrium. *Brit. Heart J.,* 17:93, 1955.

266. Gasul, B. M., and Loeffler, E.: Anomalous Origin of the Left Coronary Artery from the Pulmonary Artery (Bland-White-Garland Syndrome): Report of 4 Cases. *Pediatrics,* 4:498, 1949.

267. Gasul, B. M., Egbert, H. F., and Raul, C.: The Diagnosis of Aortic Septal Defect by Retrograde Aortography. Report of 6 Cases. *Circulation,* 4:251, 1951.

268. Gasul, B. M., Dillon, R. F., Vrla, V., and Hait, G.: Ventricular Septal Defects, Their Natural Transformation into Those with Infundibular Stenosis or into the Cyanotic or Noncyanotic Type of Tetralogy of Fallot. *J.A.M.A.,* 164:847, 1957.

269. Gasul, B. M., and others: Congenital Coronary Arteriovenous Fistula. Clin-ical, Phonocardiographc, Angiocardiographic and Hemodynamic studies in Five Patients. *Pediatrics,* 25:531, 1960.

270. Idem: Angiocardiography in Congenital Heart Disease Correlated with Clinical and Autopsy Findings; A Five-Year Clinical and Pathological Study of Thirty-Four Cases in Infants and Young Children out of a Series of Eleven Hundred Patients and Four Hundred Twenty-Five Angiocardiograms. *Am. J. Dis. Child.,* 85:404, 1953.

271. Geiger, A. J.: Letter to the Editor. Manipulative Augmentation of Pericardial Rubs. *J.A.M.A.,* 176:1053, 1961.

272. Gelfman, R., and Levine, S. A.: The Incidence of Acute and Subacute Bacterial Endocarditis in Congenital Heart Disease. *Am. J. M. Sc.,* 204:324, 1942.

273. Gerbode, F., Hultgren, H., Melrose, D., and Osborn, J. J.: Syndrome of Left Ventricular-Right Atrial Shunt. Successful Surgical Repair of Defect in Five Cases, with Observations of Bradycardia on Closure. *Ann. Surg.,* 148:433, 1958.

274. Gerbode, F., Johnston, J. B., Robinson, S., Harkins, G. A., and Osborn, J. J.: Endocardial Cushion Defects: Diagnosis and Technique of Surgical Repair. *Surgery,* 49:69, 1961.

275. Gibson, S.: Unpublished data.

276. Idem: Auricular Fibrillation in Childhood and Adolescence. *J.A.M.A.,* 117:96, 1941.

277. Gibson, S., White, H., Johnson, F., and Potts, W. J.: Congenital Pulmonary Stenosis with Intact Ventricular Septum. *Am. J. Dis. Child.,* 87:26, 1954.

278. Gifford, R. W., Jr., Roth, G. M., and Kvale, W. F.: Evaluation of New Adrenolytic Drug (Regitine) as Test for Pheochromocytoma. *J.A.M.A.,* 149:1628, 1952.

279. Gilbert, J. W., Jr., Morrow, A. G., and Braunwald, E.: The Results of Open Commissurotomy in Acquired Calcific Aortic Stenosis: Clinical and Hemodynamic Studies in Patients Operated upon with General Hypothermia. *Ann. Surg.,* 151:1, 1960.

280. Glass, I. H., Mustard, W. T., and Keith, J. D.: Coarctation of the Aorta in Infants. A Review of Twelve Years' Experience. *Pediatrics,* 26:109, 1960.

281. Glover, J. A.: Quoted by Wood.[746]

282. Gold, H., and others: Comparison of Chlorothiazide and Meralluride. New Rapid Method for Quantitative Evaluation of Diuretics in Bed Patients in Congestive Heart Failure. *J.A.M.A.,* 173:745, 1960.

283. Goldberg, H., Bakst, A. A., and Bailey, C. P.: The Dynamics of Aortic Valvular Disease. *Am. Heart J.,* 47:527, 1954.

284. Goldberg, H. P., Glenn, F., Dotter, C. T., and Steinberg, I.: Myxoma of the Left Atrium: Diagnosis Made during Life with Operative and Postmortem Findings. *Circulation,* 6:762, 1952.

285. Goldberger, E.: *Unipolar Lead Electro-*

cardiography and Vectocardiography, Including the Standard Leads, the aV and V Leads, the Cardiac Arrhythmias and the Principles of Vectocardiography. 3rd ed. Philadelphia, Lea & Febiger, 1953.

286. Goldenberg, M., and Aranow, H., Jr.: Diagnosis of Pheochromocytoma by the Adrenergic Blocking Action of Benzodioxan. *J.A.M.A.*, 143:1139, 1950.

287. Golinko, R. J., and Rudolph, A. M.: A Valve for Respiratory Studies in Infants. *Pediatrics,* 27:645, 1961.

288. Goodman, L. S., and Gilman, A.: *The Pharmacological Basis of Therapeutics; A Textbook of Pharmacology, Toxicology, and Therapeutics for Physicians and Medical Students.* 2nd ed. New York, Macmillan Company, 1955.

289. Goodwin, J. F., Hollman, A., Cleland, W. P., and Teare, D.: Obstructive Cardiomyopathy Simulating Aortic Stenosis. *Brit. Heart J.,* 22:403, 1960.

290. Gore, I., and Saphir, O.: Myocarditis; Classification of 1402 Cases. *Am. Heart J.,* 34:827, 1947.

291. Idem: Myocarditis Associated with Acute and Subacute Glomerulonephritis. *Am. Heart J.,* 36:390, 1948.

292. Gorlin, R., and Gorlin, S. G.: Hydraulic Formula for Calculation of Area of Stenotic Mitral Valve, Other Cardiac Valves and Ventral Circulatory Shunts. *Am. Heart J.,* 41:1, 1951.

293. Gorlin, R., Lewis, B. M., Haynes, F. W., Spiegl, R. J., and Dexter, L.: Factors Regulating Pulmonary Capillary Pressure in Mitral Stenosis. IV. *Am. Heart J.,* 41:834, 1951.

294. Gorlin, R., McMillan, I. K., Medd, W. E., Matthews, M. B., and Dalby, R.: Dynamics of the Circulation in Aortic Valvular Disease. *Am. J. Med.,* 18:855, 1955.

295. Gorlin, R., Sawyer, C. G., Haynes, F. W., Goodale, W. T., and Dexter, L.: Effects of Exercise on Circulatory Dynamics in Mitral Stenosis. III. *Am. Heart J.,* 41: 192, 1951.

296. Gorlin, R., and others: Studies on the Circulatory Dynamics in Mitral Stenosis. II. Altered Dynamics at Rest. *Am. Heart J.,* 41:30, 1951.

297. Grant, R. P.: The Syndrome of Dextroversion of the Heart. *Circulation,* 18:25, 1958.

298. Grant, R. P., and Estes, E. H., Jr.: *Spatial Vector Electrocardiography.* Clinical Electrocardiographic Interpretation. Philadelphia, The Blakiston Company, 1952.

299. Grant, R. P., Downey, F. M., and MacMahon, H.: The Architecture of the Right Ventricular Outflow Tract in the Normal Human Heart and in the Presence of Ventricular Septal Defects. *Circulation,* 24:223, 1961.

300. Grant, R. T.: Development of the Cardiac Coronary Vessels in the Rabbit. *Heart,* 13:261, 1926.

301. Greenwold, W. D., DuShane, J. W., Burchell, H. B., Bruwer, A., and Edwards, J. E.: Congenital Pulmonary Atresia with Interventricular Septum: Two Anatomic Types. *Circulation,* 14: 945, 1956.

302. Griffiths, A. L.: Hypertension of Renal Origin in Childhood. *Arch. Dis. Childhood,* 25:81, 1950.

303. Griffiths, S. P.: Bacterial Endocarditis Associated with Atrial Septal Defect of the Ostium Secundum Type. *Am. Heart J.,* 61:543, 1961.

304. Grishman, A., and Scherlis, L.: *Spatial Vectorcardiography.* Philadelphia, W. B. Saunders Company, 1952.

305. Groom, D.: A High Sensitivity Pickup for Cardiovascular Sounds. *Am. Heart J.,* 54:592, 1957.

306. Gross, P.: Concept of Fetal Endocarditis; General Review with Report of Illustrative Case. *Arch. Path.,* 31:163, 1941.

307. Gross, R. E.: Coarctation of the Aorta. Surgical Treatment of One Hundred Cases. *Circulation,* 1:41, 1950.

308. Idem: Surgical Closure of an Aortic Septal Defect. *Circulation,* 5:858, 1952.

309. Idem: *The Surgery of Infancy and Childhood;* Its Principles and Techniques. Philadelphia, W. B. Saunders Company, 1953.

310. Gross, R. E., and Hubbard, J. P.: Surgical Ligation of a Patent Ductus Arteriosus. Report of First Successful Case. *J.A.M.A.,* 112:729, 1939.

311. Gross, R. E., and Longino, L. A.: The Patent Ductus Arteriosus; Observations from 412 Surgically Treated Cases. *Circulation,* 3:125, 1951.

312. Gross, R. E., and Neuhauser, E. B. D.: Compression of the Trachea or Esophagus by Vascular Anomalies: Surgical Therapy in 40 Cases. *Pediatrics,* 7:69, 1951.

313. Gross, R. E., Watkins, E., Pomeranz, A., and Goldsmith, E. I.: A Method for Surgical Closure of Interauricular Septal Defects. *Surg., Gynec. & Obst.,* 96:1, 1953.

314. Grover, R. F., Reeves, J. T., and Blount, S. G., Jr.: Tolazoline Hydrochloride (Priscoline), an Effective Pulmonary Vasodilator. *Am. Heart J.,* 61:5, 1961.

315. Guntheroth, W. G., and Nadas, A. S.: Blood Pressure Measurements in Infants and Children. *Pediat. Clin. N. Amer.,* 2: 257, 1955.

316. Guntheroth, W. G., Nadas, A. S., and Gross, R. E.: Transposition of the Pulmonary Veins. *Circulation,* 18:117, 1958.

317. Gurewich, V., Sasahara, A. A., Quinn, J. S., Peffer, C. J., and Littmann, D.: Aortic Pressures during Closed-Chest Cardiac Massage. *Circulation,* 23:593, 1961.

318. Gyllensward, A., Lodin, H., Lundberg, A., and Möller, T.: Congenital, Multiple Peripheral Stenoses of the Pulmonary Artery. *Pediatrics,* 19:399, 1957.

319. Haggerty, R. J., and Eley, R. C.: Letter to the Editor: Varicella and Cortisone. *Pediatrics,* 18:160, 1956.

320. Haggerty, R. J., Maroney, M. W., and Nadas, A. S.: Essential Hypertension in Infancy and Childhood. *Am. J. Dis. Child.,* 92:535, 1956.

321. Hakkila, J., Frick, H. M., and Halonen, P. I.: Pericarditis and Myocarditis Caused by Toxoplasma: Report of a Case and Review of the Literature. *Am. Heart J.,* 55:758, 1958.

322. Halliday-Smith, K. A.: Some Auscultatory and Phonocardiographic Findings Observed in Early Infancy. *Brit. M.J.,* 1:756, 1960.

323. Hanlon, C. R., and Blalock, A.: Complete Transposition of the Aorta and the Pulmonary Artery. *Ann. Surg.,* 127:385, 1948.

324. Hansen, W. R., McClendon, R. L., and Kinsman, J. M.: Auricular Fibrillation; Hemodynamic Studies before and after Conversion with Quinidine. *Am. Heart J.,* 44:499, 1952.

325. Harken, D. E., Ellis, L. B., and Norman, L. B.: The Surgical Treatment of Mitral Stenosis. *J. Thoracic Surg.,* 19:1, 1950.

326. Harken, D. E., Black, H., Ellis, L. B., and Dexter, L.: The Surgical Correction of Mitral Insufficiency. *J. Thoracic Surg.,* 28:604, 1954.

327. Harley, H. R. S.: The Sinus Venosus Type of Interatrial Septal Defect. *Thorax,* 13:12, 1958.

328. Harrison, T. R.: *Failure of the Circulation.* 2nd ed. Baltimore, Williams & Wilkins Company, 1939.

329. Harvey, R. M., and Ferrer, M. I.: A Clinical Consideration of Cor Pulmonale; in *Symposium on Congestive Heart Failure.* New York, The American Heart Association, Inc., 1960, p. 776.

330. Hay, J. D., and Keidan, S. E.: Persistent Ectopic Auricular Tachycardia in Children. *Brit. Heart J.,* 14:345, 1952.

331. Heath, D., and Best, P. V.: The Tunica Media of the Arteries of the Lung in Pulmonary Hypertension. *J. Path. & Bact.,* 76:165, 1958.

332. Heath, D., and Edwards, J. E.: Configuration of Elastic Tissue of Pulmonary Hypertension. *Circulation,* 21:59, 1960.

333. Heiner, D. C., and Nadas, A. S.: Patent Ductus Arteriosus in Association with Pulmonic Stenosis. A Report of Six Cases with Additional Noncardiac Congenital Anomalies. *Circulation,* 17:232, 1958.

334. Hektoen, L.: Congenital Aortico-pulmonary Communication: Communication between Aorta and Left Ventricle under Semilunar Valve. *Tr. Chicago Path. Soc.,* 4:97, 1900.

335. Hellerstein, H. K., Levine, B., and Feil, H.: Electrocardiographic Changes Following Carotid Sinus Stimulation in Paroxysmal Supraventricular Tachycardia. *J. Lab. & Clin. Med.,* 38:820, 1951.

336. Hench, P. S., Kendall, E. C., Slocumb, C. H., and Polley, H. F.: The Effect of a Hormone of the Adrenal Cortex (17 Hydroxy-11-Dehydrocorticosterone: Compound E) and of Pituitary Adrenocorticotropic Hormone on Rheumatoid Arthritis; Preliminary Report. *Proc. Staff Meet., Mayo Clin.,* 24:181, 1949.

337. Hernandez, F. A., Rochkind, R., and Cooper, H. R.: The Intracathetary Electrocardiogram in the Diagnosis of Ebstein's Anomaly. *Am. J. Cardiol.,* 1:181, 1958.

338. Hill, L. F., Hubbard, J. P., Harris, T. N., Jackson, R. L., and Wheatley, G. M.: Rheumatic Fever: Summary of Present Concepts. *Pediatrics,* 3:680, 1949.

339. Hirsch, J. G., and Flett, D. M.: Sinus Bradycardia in Acute Rheumatic Fever. *Ann. Int. Med.,* 36:146, 1952.

340. Hoffman, J. I. E., Rudolph, A. M., Nadas, A. S., and Gross, R. E.: Pulmonic Stenosis, Ventricular Septal Defect and Right Ventricular Pressure above Systemic Level. *Circulation,* 22:405, 1960.

341. Hollman, A., Goodwin, J. F., Teare, D., and Renwick, J. W.: A Family with Obstructive Cardiomyopathy (Asymmetrical Hypertrophy). *Brit. Heart J.,* 22:449, 1960.

342. Holman, E.: "On Circumscribed Dilatation of an Artery Immediately Distal to a Partially Occluding Band": Poststenotic Dilatation. *Surgery,* 36:3, 1954.

343. Holman, E., and Willett, F.: Results of Pericardiectomy for Constrictive Pericarditis. *J.A.M.A.,* 157:789, 1955.

344. Horlick, L., and Merriman, J. E.: Myxoma of the Left Atrium Simulating Mitral Stenosis with Cerebral Emboli. *Canad. M.A. J.,* 77:582, 1957.

345. Hotchkiss, W. S.: Patent Ductus Arteriosus and the Occasional Cardiac Surgeon. *J.A.M.A.,* 173:244, 1960.

346. Hufnagel, C. A.: Surgical Treatment of Aortic Insufficiency, in C. R. Lam, Ed.: *Henry Ford Hospital International Symposium on Cardiovascular Surgery.* Philadelphia, W. B. Saunders Company, 1955.

347. Idem: Direct Approaches for the Treatment of Aortic Insufficiency. *Am. Surg.,* 25:321, 1959.

348. Hufnagel, C. A., and Conrad, P. W.: Direct Treatment of Aortic Regurgitation. (Abstr.). *Circulation,* 24:961, 1961.

349. Hughes, C. W., and Rumore, P. C.: Anomalous Pulmonary Veins. *Arch. Path.,* 37:364, 1944.

350. Hull, E.: Cause and Effects of Flow through Defects of Atrial Septum. *Am. Heart J.,* 38:350, 1949.

351. Hultgren, H. N.: Discussion; in Congenital Heart Disease. Report of the Fourteenth M. & R. Pediatric Research Conference. Columbus, Ohio, M. & R. Laboratories, 1955, p. 33.

352. Hultgren, H., Selzer, A., Purdy, A., Holman, E., and Gerbode, F.: The Syn-

drome of Patent Ductus Arteriosus with Pulmonary Hypertension. *Circulation,* 8:15, 1953.

353. Hurtado, A.: *Aspectos fisiológicos y patológicos de la altura.* Lima, Ed. Rímac, 1943.

354. Husson, G. S., and Wyatt, T. C.: Primary Pulmonary Obliterative Vascular Disease in Infants and Young Children. *Pediatrics,* 23:493, 1959.

355. Idriss, F. S., Goldstein, I. R., Grana, L., Grench, D., and Potts, W. J.: A New Technic for Complete Correction of Transposition of the Great Vessels; An Experimental Study with a Preliminary Clinical Report. *Circulation,* 24:5, 1961.

356. Illingworth, R. S., and others: Acute Rheumatic Fever in Children. A Comparison of 6 Forms of Treatment in 200 Cases. *Lancet,* 2:653, 1957.

357. Ingraham, F. D., and Matson, D. D.: *Neurosurgery of Infancy and Childhood.* Springfield, Ill., Charles C Thomas, 1954.

358. Ito, T., Engle, M. A., and Holswade, G. R.: Congenital Insufficiency of the Pulmonic Valve. A Rare Cause of Neonatal Heart Failure. *Pediatrics,* 28:712, 1961.

359. Ivemark, B. I.: Implication of Agenesis of the Spleen on the Pathogenesis of Cono-truncus Anomalies in Childhood: An Analysis of the Heart Malformations in the Splenic Agenesis Syndrome, with Fourteen New Cases. *Acta paediat.,* 44: Suppl. 104, 1955.

360. James, L. S.: Discussion; in Report of the thirty-seventh Ross Conference on Pediatrics. Columbus, Ohio, Ross Laboratories, 1961, p. 67.

361. Jannach, J. R.: Myocarditis in Infancy with Inclusions Characteristic of Psittacosis. A.M.A. *J. Dis. Child.,* 96:734, 1958.

362. Javett, S. N., and others: Myocarditis in the Newborn Infant. A Study of an Outbreak Associated with Coxsackie Group B Virus Infection in a Maternity Home in Johannesburg. *J. Pediat.,* 48:1, 1956.

363. Jhaveri, S., Czoniczer, G., Reider, R. B., and Massell, B. F.: Relatively Benign 'Pure' Mitral Regurgitation of Rheumatic Origin: A Study of Seventy-Four Adult Patients. *Circulation,* 22:39, 1960.

364. Johnson, A. M.: Hypertrophic Infundibular Stenosis Complicating Simple Pulmonary Valve Stenosis. *Brit. Heart J.,* 21:429, 1959.

365. Idem: Norepinephrine and Cyanotic Attacks in Fallot's Tetralogy. *Brit. Heart J.,* 23:197, 1961.

366. Johnson, J., and Kirby, C. K.: Surgical Treatment of Ventricular Fibrillation. *Ann. Surg.,* 134:672, 1951.

367. Jones, A. M., and Langley, F. A.: Aortic Sinus Aneurysms. *Brit. Heart J.,* 11:325, 1949.

368. Jones, T. D.: Diagnosis of Rheumatic Fever. *J.A.M.A.,* 126:481, 1944.

369. Jones, T. D., and Bland, E. F.: Rheumatic Fever and Heart Disease. Completed Ten-Year Observations on 1000 Patients. *Tr. A. Am. Physicians,* 57:267, 1942.

370. Joseph, M. C., and Tenckhoff, L.: Sinus Arrhythmia in Rheumatic Fever. *Am. Heart J.,* 61:634, 1961.

371. Katz, L. N.: The Lewis A. Conner Memorial Lecture: The Performance of the Heart. *Circulation,* 21:483, 1960.

372. Kay, E. B., and Zimmerman, H. A.: Surgical Treatment of Mitral Stenosis by Open Technique. *J.A.M.A.,* 173:1644, 1960.

373. Kay, E. B., Mendelsohn, D., Jr., and Zimmerman, H. A.: Surgical Treatment of Aortic Valvular Disease with Artificial Valves. (Abstr.) *Circulation,* 24:969, 1961.

374. Kay, E. B., Nogueira, C., Mendelsohn, D., Jr., and Zimmerman, H. A.: Corrective Surgery for Tetralogy of Fallot. *Circulation,* 24:1342, 1961.

375. Kay, J. H., and Thomas, V.: Experimental Production of Pulmonary Insufficiency. *Arch. Surg.,* 69:646, 1954.

376. Keith, J. D.: Personal communication to the author.

377. Idem: Congenital Heart Disease; in L. Parsons: *Modern Trends in Paediatrics.* London, Butterworth & Co., 1951.

378. Idem: The Diagnosis of Ventricular Septal Defect. Second World Congress on Cardiology, Washington, D.C., September, 1954.

379. Keith, J. D., and Manning, J.: Personal communication to the author.

380. Keith, J. D., Rowe, R. D., and Vlad, P.: *Heart Disease in Infancy and Childhood.* New York, Macmillan Company, 1958.

381. Keith, J. D., Rowe, R. D., Vlad, P., and O'Hanley, J. H.: Complete Anomalous Pulmonary Venous Drainage. *Am. J. Med.,* 16:23, 1954.

382. Keith, J. D., Neill, C. A., Vlad, P., Rowe, R. D., and Chute, A. L.: Transposition of the Great Vessels. *Circulation,* 7:830, 1953.

383. Kellaway, G.: Acute Anoxic Cardiac Failure in Pulmonary Heart Disease. *Lancet,* 2:768, 1959.

384. Kelly, J. J., Jr., and Lyons, H. A.: Atrial Septal Defect in the Aged. *Ann. Int. Med.,* 48:267, 1958.

385. Kelson, S. R., and White, P. D.: Notes on 250 Cases of Subacute Bacterial (Streptococcal) Endocarditis Studied and Treated between 1927 and 1939. *Ann. Int. Med.,* 22:40, 1945.

386. Kennedy, J. A.: A New Concept of the Cause of Patency of the Ductus Arteriosus. *Am. J. M. Sc.,* 204:570, 1942.

387. Kibrick, S., and Benirschke, K.: Severe Generalized Disease (Encephalohepatomyocarditis) Occurring in the Newborn Period and Due to Infection with Coxsackie Virus, Group B; Evidence of Intrauterine Infection with This Agent. *Pediatrics,* 22:857, 1958.

388. Kilburn, K. H., Eagan, J. T., Sieker, H. O., and Heyman, A.: Cardiopulmonary Insufficiency in Myotonic and Progressive Muscular Dystrophy. *New England J. Med.*, 261:1089, 1959.

389. Kiloh, G. A.: Pure Aortic Stenosis. *Brit. Heart J.*, 12:33, 1950.

390. Kirkendall, W. M., Culbertson, J. W., and Eckstein, J. W.: Renal Hemodynamics in Patients with Coarctation of the Aorta. *J. Lab. & Clin. Med.*, 53:6, 1959.

391. Kirklin, J. W.: Discussion; in C. R. Lam, Ed.: *Henry Ford Hospital International Symposium on Cardiovascular Surgery*. Philadelphia, W. B. Saunders Company, 1955, p. 364.

392. Kirklin, J. W., and DuShane, J. W.: Repair of Ventricular Septal Defect in Infancy. *Pediatrics*, 27:961, 1961.

393. Kirklin, J. W., and Mankin, H. T.: Open Operation in the Treatment of Calcific Aortic Stenosis. *Circulation*, 21:578, 1960.

394. Kirklin, J. W., Devloo, R. A., and Weidman, W. H.: Open Intracardiac Repair for Transposition of the Great Vessels: 11 Cases. *Surgery*, 50:58, 1961.

395. Kirklin, J. W., Ellis, F. H., Jr., McGoon, D. C., DuShane, J. W., and Swan, H. J. C.: Surgical Treatment for the Tetralogy of Fallot by Open Intracardiac Repair. *J. Thoracic Surg.*, 37: 22, 1959.

396. Kirklin, J. W., Payne, W. S., Theye, R. A., and DuShane, J. W.: Factors Affecting Survival after Open Operation for Tetralogy of Fallot. *Ann. Surg.*, 152: 485, 1960.

397. Kjellberg, S. R., Mannheimer, E., Rudhe, U., and Jonsson, B.: *Diagnosis of Congenital Heart Disease*. Chicago, Year Book Publishers, Inc., 1955.

398. Idem: *Diagnosis of Congenital Heart Disease*. 2nd ed. Chicago, Year Book Publishers, Inc., 1959.

399. Kleinerman, J., Yang, W. M., Hackel, D. B., and Kaufman, N.: Absence of Transverse Aortic Arch. *Arch. Path.*, 65:490, 1958.

400. Korner, P. I., and Shillingford, J. P.: The Quantitative Estimation of Valvular Incompetence by Dye Dilution Curves. *Clin. Sc.*, 14:553, 1955.

401. Kouwenhoven, W. B., Jude, J. R., and Knickerbocker, G. G.: Closed-Chest Cardiac Massage. *J.A.M.A.*, 173:1064, 1960.

402. Kurtz, C. M.: *Orthodiascopy:* An Analysis of over Seventeen Hundred Orthodiascopic Examinations. New York, Macmillan Company, 1937.

403. Kuttner, A. G.: Prevention of Rheumatic Fever and Rheumatic Heart Disease. *Postgrad. Med.*, 14:429, 1953.

404. Kuttner, A. G., and Markowitz, M.: The Diagnosis of Mitral Insufficiency in Rheumatic Children. *Am. Heart J.*, 35:718, 1948.

405. Kuttner, A. G., and Reyersbach, G.: Prevention of Streptococcal Upper Respiratory Infections and Rheumatic Recurrences in Rheumatic Children by Prophylactic Use of Sulfanilamide. *J. Clin. Invest.*, 22:77, 1943.

406. Lagerlöf, H., and Werko, L.: Studies on Circulation of Blood in Man; Pulmonary Capillary Venous Pressure Pulse in Man. *Scandinav. J. Clin. & Lab. Invest.*, 7:147, 1949.

407. Landtman, B.: Heart Arrhythmias in Children. *Acta paediat.*, 34: Suppl. 1, 1947.

408. Lang, H. T., Jr., and Nadas, A. S.: Coarctation of the Aorta with Congestive Failure in Infancy—Medical Treatment. *Pediatrics*, 17:45, 1956.

409. Lange, R. L., and Hecht, H. H.: Quantitation of Valvular Regurgitation From Multiple Indicator- Dilution Curves. *Circulation*, 18:623, 1958.

410. Laubry, C., and Pezzi, C.: Quoted by Wood, Magidson, and Wilson.[752]

411. Lavenne, F., Tyberghein, J., Brasseur, L., and Meersseman, F.: Complexe d'Eisenmenger avec insuffisance pulmonaire par absence de valvules. *Acta cardiologica*, 9:249, 1954.

412. Leatham, A.: Auscultation of the Heart. *Lancet*, 2:703, 757, 1958.

413. Leatham, A., and Vogelpool, L.: The Early Systolic Sound in Dilatation of the Pulmonary Artery. *Brit. Heart J.*, 16:21, 1954.

414. Lees, M. H., Hauck, A. J., Starkey, G. W. B., Nadas, A. S., and Gross, R. E.: Congenital Aortic Stenosis: Operative Indications and Surgical Results. *Brit. Heart J.*, 24:31, 1962.

415. Leight, L., Snider, T. H., Clifford, G. O., and Hellems, H. K.: Hemodynamic Studies in Sickle Cell Anemia. *Circulation*, 10:653, 1954.

416. Lepeschkin, E., and Surawicz, B.: The Measurement of the Q-T Interval of the the Electrocardiogram. *Circulation*, 6: 378, 1952.

417. Lepeschkin, E.: *Modern Electrocardiography*. Baltimore, Williams & Wilkins Company, 1951, Vol. 1.

418. Lev, M.: Pathologic Anatomy and Interrelationship of Hypoplasia of the Aortic Tract Complexes. *Lab. Invest.*, 1:61, 1952.

419. Lev, M., Alcalde, V. M., and Baffes, T. G.: Pathologic Anatomy of Complete Transposition of the Arterial Trunks. *Pediatrics*, 28:293, 1961.

420. Levine, H. J., Wagman, R. J., Neill, W. A., Krasnow, N., and Gorlin, R.: The New Concept of Subaortic Stenosis. Proceedings of the New England Cardiovasc. Soc., 1960-61, p. 27.

421. Levine, S. A.: *Clinical Heart Disease*. 4th ed. Philadelphia, W. B. Saunders Company, 1951.

422. Idem: *Clinical Heart Disease*. 5th ed. Philadelphia, W. B. Saunders Company, 1958.

423. Levine, S. A., and Harvey, W. P.: *Clinical Auscultation of the Heart*. 2nd ed.

760   References

Philadelphia, W. B. Saunders Company, 1959.

424. Lewis, D. H., Deitz, G. W., Wallace, J. D., and Brown, J. R., Jr.: Present Status of Intracardiac Phonocardiography. *Circulation,* 18:991, 1958.

425. Lewis, F. J., Varco, R. L., Taufic, M., and Niazi, S. A.: Direct Vision Repair of Triatrial Heart and Total Anomalous Pulmonary Venous Drainage. *Surg., Gynec. & Obst.,* 102:713, 1956.

426. Lewis, T.: Observations upon Flutter and Fibrillation. I. Regularity of Clinical Auricular Flutter. *Heart,* 7:127, 1920.

427. Idem: *Diseases of the Heart Described for Practitioners and Students.* 2nd ed. New York, Macmillan Company, 1937.

428. Lichtman, S. S.: Isolated Congenital Dextrocardia; Report of Two Cases with Unusual Electrocardiographic Findings; Anatomic, Clinical, Roentgenologic and Electrocardiographic Studies of Cases Reported in the Literature. *Arch. Int. Med.,* 48:683, 1931.

429. Idem: Treatment of Subacute Bacterial Endocarditis; Current Results. *Ann. Int. Med.,* 19:787, 1943.

430. Liebman, J., and Nadas, A. S.: Heart Disease in the Newborn. *Pediat. Clin. N. Amer.,* 5:1087, 1958.

431. Idem: The Vectorcardiogram in the Differential Diagnosis of Atrial Septal Defect in Children. *Circulation,* 22:956, 1960.

432. Likoff, W., and Uricchio, J. F.: Results of Mitral Commissurotomy. Clinical Status of 200 Patients 5 to 8 Years after Operation. *J.A.M.A.,* 166:737, 1958.

433. Liljestrand, G., and Steinström, N.: Clinical Studies on the Work of the Heart during Rest. II. The Influence of Variations in the Haemoglobin Content in the Blood Flow. *Acta med. Scandinav.,* 63:130, 1925.

434. Lillehei, C. W., and Varco, R. L.: Certain Physiologic, Pathologic, and Surgical Features of Complete Transposition of the Great Vessels. *Surgery,* 34:376, 1953.

435. Lillehei, C. W., and others: Direct Vision Intracardiac Surgery by Means of Controlled Cross Circulation or Continued Arterial Reservoir Perfusion for Correction of Ventricular Septal Defects, Atrioventricularis Communis, Isolated Infundibular Pulmonic Stenosis and Tetralogy of Fallot; in C. R. Lam, Ed.: *Henry Ford Hospital International Symposium on Cardiovascular Surgery.* Philadelphia, W. B. Saunders Company, 1955, p. 371.

436. Lind, J.: Quoted by Wilson, J. G.: Fetal Circulation and Early Postnatal Changes, in Congenital Heart Disease. Report of the Fourteenth M. & R. Pediatric Research Conference. Columbus, Ohio, M. & R. Laboratories, 1955, p. 27.

437. Lind, J., and Wegelius, C.: Angiocardiographic Studies in Children. *Advances in Pediatrics,* 5:154, 1952.

438. Linde, L. M., Adams, F. H., and O'Loughlin, B. J.: Endocardial Fibroelastosis. Angiocardiographic Studies. *Circulation,* 17:40, 1958.

439. Little, R. C.: Volume Elastic Properties of the Right and Left Atrium. *Am. J. Physiol.,* 158:237, 1949.

440. Littmann, D., and Schaaf, R. S.: Therapeutic Experiences with Subacute Bacterial Endocarditis, with Special Reference to the Failures. *New England J. Med.,* 243:248, 1950.

441. Logan, A., and Turner, R.: Surgical Treatment of Mitral Stenosis, with Particular Reference to the Transventricular Approach with a Mechanical Dilator. *Lancet,* 2:874, 1959.

442. Logue, R. B., and Hanson, J. F.: Heart Block; Study of 100 Cases with Prolonged P-R Interval. *Am. J. M. Sc.,* 207:765, 1944.

443. Logue, R. B., and Hurst, J. W.: Rheumatic Fever during the First Few Years of Life and Its Differentiation from Endocardial Fibrosis. *Am. J. M. Sc.,* 223:648, 1952.

444. Long, R. T. L., Braunwald, E., and Morrow, A. G.: Intracardiac Injection of Radioactive Krypton: Clinical Applications of New Methods for Characterization of Circulatory Shunts. *Circulation,* 21:1126, 1960.

445. Lord, J. W., Jr., Imparato, A. M., Hackel, A., and Doyle, E. F.: Endocarditis Complicating Open-Heart Surgery. *Circulation,* 23:489, 1961.

446. Lown, B., and Levine, S. A.: *Current Concepts in Digitalis Therapy.* Boston, Little, Brown & Co., 1954.

447. Idem: *Atrial Arrhythmias.* New York, Landsberger Medical Books, Inc., 1958.

448. Lown, B., Ganong, W. F., and Levine, S. A.: The Syndrome of Short P-R Interval, Normal QRS Complex and Paroxysmal Rapid Heart Action. *Circulation,* 5:693, 1952.

449. Lown, B., Wyatt, N. F., Crocker, A. T., Goodale, W. T., and Levine, S. A.: Interrelationship of Digitalis and Potassium in Auricular Tachycardia with Block. *Am. Heart J.,* 45:589, 1953.

450. Luan, L. L., D'Silva, J. L., Gasul, B. M., and Dillon, R. F.: Stenosis of the Right Main Pulmonary Artery. Clinical, Angiocardiographic and Catheterization Findings in Ten Patients. *Circulation,* 21:1116, 1960.

451. Lucas, R. V., Jr., St. Geme, J. W., Jr., Anderson, R. C., Adams, P., Jr., and Ferguson, D. J.: Maturation of the Pulmonary Vascular Bed. A Physiologic and Anatomic Correlation in Infants and Children. *Am. J. Dis. Child.,* 101:467, 1961.

452. Luckey, E. H., and Rubin, A. L.: The Correction of Hyponatremia in Congestive Heart Failure; in *Symposium on Congestive Heart Failure.* New York, The American Heart Association, Inc., 1960, p. 69.

453. Luisada, A. A.: *The Heart Beat:* Graphic Methods in the Study of the Cardiac Patient. New York, Paul B. Hoeber, Inc., 1953.

454. Idem: Notation of Phonocardiographic Waves. *Am. J. Cardiol.,* 4:40, 1959.

455. Lundsgaard, C., and Van Slyke, D. D.: Cyanosis. *Medicine,* 2:1, 1923.

456. Lurie, P. R.: Postural Effects in Tetralogy of Fallot. *Am. J. Med.,* 15:297, 1953.

457. Idem: Personal communication to the author.

458. Lurie, P. R., and Shumacker, H. B., Jr.: Mitral Commissurotomy in Childhood. *Pediatrics,* 13:454, 1954.

459. Lynfield, J., Gasul, B. M., and Luan, L. L.: Serial Physiologic Studies of the Natural Course of 33 Infants and Children with Ventricular Septal Defects. (Abstr.) *Circulation,* 20:733, 1959.

460. Lynfield, J., Gasul, B. M., Arcilla, R., and Luan, L. L.: The Natural History of Ventricular Septal Defects in Infancy and Childhood. Based on Serial Cardiac Catheterization Studies. *Am. J. Med.,* 30:357, 1961.

461. Lyon, E.: Probleme der cardiovasculären Komplikationen nach Pockenschutzimpfung. *Med. Klin.,* 52:1947, 1957.

462. Lyon, R. A., and Rauh, L. W.: Extrasystoles in Children. *Am. J. Dis. Child.,* 57:278, 1939.

463. Lyon, R. A., Rauh, L. W., and Stirling, J. W.: Heart Murmurs in Newborn Infants. *J. Pediat.,* 16:310, 1940.

464. McCrory, M. D., and Nash, F. W.: Hypertension in Children: A Review. *Am. J. M. Sc.,* 223:671, 1952.

465. McCue, C. M., Henningar, G. R., Davis, E., and Ray, J.: Congenital Subaortic Stenosis Caused by Fibroma of Left Ventricle. *Pediatrics,* 16:372, 1955.

466. McGoon, D. C., and Kirklin, J. W.: Pulmonic Stenosis with Intact Ventricular Septum; Treatment Utilizing Extracorporeal Circulation. *Circulation,* 17: 180, 1958.

467. McGregor, M., and Medalie, M.: Coarctation of the Aorta. *Brit. Heart J.,* 14: 531, 1952.

468. McKusick, V. A.: *Cardiovascular Sound in Health and Disease.* Baltimore, Williams & Wilkins Company, 1958.

469. McLean, D. M., Walker, S. J., and Bain, H. W.: Coxsackie B5 Virus in Association with Pericarditis and Pleurodynia. *Canad. M.A.J.,* 79:789, 1958.

470. McLean, D. M., Croft, C. C., Prince, J. T., and Heckmann, E. E.: Coxsackie and ECHO Virus Infections in Ohio during 1956. *Ohio M.J.,* 53:907, 1957.

471. MacMahon, B., McKeown, T., and Record, R. G.: The Incidence and Life Expectation of Children with Congenital Heart Disease. *Brit. Heart J.,* 15:121, 1953.

472. McMichael, J.: Dynamics of Heart Failure (Oliver-Sharpey Lectures). *Brit. M.J.,* 2:525, 578, 1952.

473. McMillan, T. M., and Bellet, S.: Auricular Flutter; Some of Its Clinical Manifestations and Its Treatment; Based on Study of 65 Cases. *Am. J. M. Sc.,* 184:33, 1932.

474. McQuiston, W. O.: Anesthetic Problems in Cardiac Surgery in Children. *Anesthesiology,* 10:590, 1949.

475. Macruz, R., Parloff, J. K., and Case, R. B.: A Method for the Electrocardiographic Recognition of Atrial Enlargement. *Circulation,* 17:882, 1958.

476. Mannheimer, E.: Phonocardiography in Children; in *Advances in Pediatrics.* Chicago, Year Book Publishers, Inc., 1955, Vol. 7, p. 171.

477. Manning, G. W., and Cropp, G. J.: The Electrocardiogram in Progressive Muscular Dystrophy. *Brit. Heart J.,* 20:416, 1958.

478. March, H. W., Gerbode, F., and Hultgren, H. N.: The Reopened Ventricular Septal Defect; A Syndrome Following Unsuccessful Closure of Interventricular Septal Defects, Particularly in Association with Infundibular Stenosis. *Circulation,* 24:250, 1961.

479. Mark, H., Jacobson, B., and Young, D.: Coexistence of Patent Ductus Arteriosus and Congenital Aortic Valvular Disease. *Circulation,* 17:359, 1958.

480. Marquis, R. M.: Ventricular Septal Defect in Early Childhood. *Brit. Heart J.,* 12: 265, 1950.

481. Idem: Longevity and the Early History of the Tetralogy of Fallot. *Brit. M.J.,* 1: 819, 1956.

482. Marquis, R. M., and Logan, A.: Congenital Aortic Stenosis and Its Surgical Treatment. *Brit. Heart J.,* 17:373, 1955.

483. Martelle, R. R., and Linde, L. M.: Cerebrovascular Accidents with Tetralogy of Fallot. *Am. J. Dis. Child.,* 101:206, 1961.

484. Massel, B. F.: ACTH and Cortisone Therapy of Rheumatic Fever and Rheumatic Carditis. *New England J. Med.,* 251:183, 221, 263, 1954.

485. Idem: Management of Rheumatic Fever: Therapy of the Acute Attack and Prevention of Recurrence. *Pediat. Clin. N. Amer.,* 5:1143, 1958.

486. Massell, B. F., Coen, W. B., and Jones, T. D.: Observations Regarding Artificially Induced Subcutaneous Nodules in Rheumatic Fever Patients. *Pediatrics,* 5:909, 1950.

487. Massell, B. F., Dow, J. W., and Jones, T. D.: Orally Administered Penicillin in Patients with Rheumatic Fever. *J.A.M.A.,* 138:1030, 1948.

488. Massell, B. F., Jhaveri, S., and Czonicer, G.: Therapy and Other Factors Influencing the Course of Rheumatic Heart Disease. (Abstr.) *Circulation,* 20:737, 1959.

489. Massell, B. F., and others: Prevention of Rheumatic Fever by Prompt Penicillin Therapy of Hemolytic Streptococcic Respiratory Infections. *J.A.M.A.,* 146: 1469, 1951.

490. Massie, E., and Walsh. T. J.: *Clinical Vectorcardiography and Electrocardiography*. Chicago, Year Book Publishers, Inc., 1960.

491. Matson, D. D., and Salam, M.: Brain Abscess in Congenital Heart Disease. *Pediatrics*, 27:772, 1961.

492. Mayer, F. E., Nadas, A. S., and Ongley, P. A.: Ebstein's Anomaly. Presentation of Ten Cases. *Circulation*, 16:1057, 1957.

493. Means, J. H.: Dyspnea. *Medicine*, 3:309, 1924.

494. Mendlowitz, M.: Clubbing and Hypertrophic Osteoarthropathy. *Medicine*, 21:269, 1942.

495. Miller, H., Uricchio, J., and Phillips, R. W.: Acute Pericarditis Associated with Infectious Mononucleosis. *New England J. Med.*, 249:136, 1953.

496. Miller, R. A., Lev, M., and Paul, M. H.: Congenital Absence of the Pulmonary Valve; The Clinical Syndrome of Tetralogy of Fallot with Pulmonary Regurgitation. *Circulation*, 26:266, 1962.

497. Mills, H., Kay, J. H., Magidson, O., Anderson, R. M., and Schiff, A.: Correction of Congenital Ventricular Septal Defect in a Patient with Previous Surgically Produced Pulmonary Artery Stenosis. *Am. J. Cardiol.*, 6:976, 1960.

498. Minhas, K., and Gasul, B. M.: Systolic Clicks: A Clinical, Phonocardiographic and Hemodynamic Evaluation. *Am. Heart J.*, 57:49, 1959.

499. Mitchell, A. M., Sackett, C. H., Hunzicker, W. J., and Levine, S. A.: The Clinical Features of Aortic Stenosis. *Am. Heart J.*, 48:684, 1954.

500. Moorhead, T. G., and Smith, E. C.: Congenital Cardiac Anomaly: Abnormal Opening between Aorta and Pulmonary Artery. *Irish J. M. Sc.*, 1923, pp. 545–9.

501. Morgan, C., and Nadas, A. S.: Chronic Atrial Tachycardia. Submitted for publication.

502. Morgan, W. L., and Bland, E. F.: Bacterial Endocarditis in the Antibiotic Era; With Special Reference to the Later Complications. *Circulation*, 19:753, 1959.

503. Morris, A. J., Chamovitz, R., Catanzaro, F. J., and Rammelkamp, C. H., Jr.: Prevention of Rheumatic Fever by Treatment of Previous Streptococcic Infections; Effect of Sulfadiazine. *J.A.M.A.*, 160:114, 1956.

504. Morrow, A. G., Braunwald, E., and Ross, J., Jr.: Left Heart Catheterization. An Appraisal of Techniques and Their Applications in Cardiovascular Diagnosis. *Arch. Int. Med.*, 105:645, 1960.

505. Morrow, A. G., Sanders, R. J., and Braunwald, E.: The Nitrous Oxide Test: An Improved Method for the Detection of Left-to-Right Shunts. *Circulation*, 17:284, 1958.

506. Morrow, A. G., Sharp, E. H., and Braunwald, E.: Congenital Aortic Stenosis: Clinical and Hemodynamic Findings, Surgical Technic, and Results of Operation. *Circulation*, 18:1091, 1958.

507. Moschcowitz, E.: Hypertension of the Pulmonary Circulation. Its Causes, Dynamics and Relation to Other Circulatory States. *Am. J.M. Sc.*, 174:388, 1927.

508. Moss, A. J., Liebling, W., and Adams, F. H.: The Flush Method for Determining Blood Pressure in Infants. II. Normal Values during the First Year of Life. *Pediatrics*, 21:950, 1958.

509. Moss, A. J., Liebling, W., Austin, W. O., and Adams, F. H.: An Evaluation of the Flush Method for Determining Blood Pressures in Infants. *Pediatrics*, 20:53, 1957.

510. Mounsey, P.: The Early Diastolic Sound of Constrictive Pericarditis. *Brit. Heart J.*, 17:143, 1955.

511. Muller, W. H., Jr.: Surgical Treatment of Transposition of Pulmonary Veins. *Ann. Surg.*, 134:683, 1951.

512. Muller, W. H., Jr., and Dammann, J. F., Jr.: The Treatment of Certain Congenital Malformations of the Heart by the Creation of Pulmonic Stenosis to Reduce Pulmonary Hypertension and Excessive Pulmonary Blood Flow. *Surg., Gynec. & Obst.*, 95:213, 1952.

513. Idem: Results Following the Creation of Pulmonary Artery Stenosis. *Ann. Surg.*, 143:816, 1956.

514. Muller, W. H., Jr., Warren, W. D., Dammann, J. F., Jr., Beckwith, J. R., and Wood, J. E., Jr.: Surgical Relief of Aortic Insufficiency by Direct Operation on the Aortic Valve. *Circulation*, 21:587, 1960.

515. Murray, G.: Closure of Defects in Cardiac Septa. *Ann. Surg.*, 128:843, 1948.

516. Mustard, W. T., and Keith, J. D.: Unpublished data.

517. Mustard, W. T., Rowe, R. D., Keith, J. D., and Sirek, A.: Coarctation of the Aorta, with Special Reference to the First Year of Life. *Ann. Surg.*, 141:429, 1955.

518. Mustard, W. T., and others: A Surgical Approach to Transposition of the Great Vessels with Extracorporeal Circuit. *Surgery*, 36:39, 1954.

519. Myers, G. B., Klein, H. A., and Stofer, B. E.: Electrocardiographic Diagnosis of Right Ventricular Hypertrophy. *Am. Heart J.*, 35:1, 1948.

520. Nadas, A. S., and Hauck, A. J.: Pediatric Aspects of Congestive Heart Failure. *Circulation*, 21:424, 1960.

521. Nadas, A. S., and Levy, J. M.: Pericarditis in Children. *Am. J. Cardiol.*, 7:109, 1961.

522. Nadas, A. S., Alimurung, M. M., and Sieracki, L. A.: Cardiac Manifestations of Friedreich's Ataxia. *New England J. Med.*, 244:239, 1951.

523. Nadas, A. S., Rudolph, A. M., and Gross, R. E.: Editorial. Pulmonary Arterial Hyptertension in Congenital Heart Disease. *Circulation*, 22:1041, 1960.

524. Nadas, A. S., Rudolph, A. M., and Hoffman, J. I. E.: Pulmonary Hypertension in Children with Systemic-Pulmonary Communications. *Circulation,* 20:744, 1960.

525. Nadas, A. S., Rudolph, A. M., and Reinhold, J. D. L.: Medical Progress: Use of Digitalis in Infants and Children; Clinical Study of Patients in Congestive Heart Failure. *New England J. Med.,* 248:98, 1953.

526. Nadas, A. S., Cogan, G., Landing, B. H., and Shwachman, H.: Studies in Pancreatic Fibrosis; Cor Pulmonale: Clinical and Pathologic Observations. *Pediatrics,* 10:319, 1952.

527. Nadas, A. S., Daeschner, C. W., Roth, A., and Blumenthal, S. L.: Paroxysmal Tachycardia in Infants and Children; Study of 41 Cases. *Pediatrics,* 9:167, 1952.

528. Nadas, A. S., Rosenbaum, H. D., Wittenborg, M. H., and Rudolph, A. M.: Tetralogy of Fallot with Unilateral Pulmonary Atresia. A Clinically Diagnosable and Surgically Significant Variant. *Circulation,* 8:328, 1953.

529. Nadas, A. S., Scott, L. P., Hauck, A. J., and Rudolph, A. M.: Spontaneous Functional Closing of Ventricular Septal Defects. *New England J. Med.,* 264: 309, 1961.

530. Neill, C., and Mounsey, P.: Auscultation in Patent Ductus Arteriosus, with a Description of Two Fistulae Simulating Patent Ductus. *Brit. Heart J.,* 20:61, 1958.

531. Neligan, G. A., Oxon, D. M., and Smith, C. A.: The Blood Pressure of Newborn Infants in Asphyxial States and in Hyaline Membrane Disease. *Pediatrics,* 26: 735, 1960.

532. Neufeld, H. N., DuShane, J. W., Wood, E. H., Kirklin, J. W., and Edwards, J. E.: Origin of Both Great Vessels from the Right Ventricle. I. Without Pulmonary Stenosis. II. With Pulmonary Stenosis. *Circulation,* 23:399, 603, 1961.

533. Neufeld, H. N., Titus, J. L., DuShane, J. W., Burchell, H. B., and Edwards, J. E.: Isolated Ventricular Septal Defect of the Persistent Common Atrioventricular Canal Type. *Circulation,* 23:685, 1961.

534. New York Heart Association, Inc.: Nomenclature and Criteria for Diagnosis of Diseases of the Heart and Blood Vessels. New York, New York Heart Association, Inc., 1953.

535. Nicholson, J. W., Burchell, H. B., and Wood, E. H.: A Method for the Continuous Recording of Evans Blue Dye Curves in Arterial Blood, and Its Application to the Diagnosis of Cardiovascular Abnormalities. *J. Lab. & Clin. Med.,* 37:353, 1951.

536. Noonan, J. A., and Nadas, A. S.: The Hypoplastic Left Heart Syndrome: An Analysis of 101 Cases. *Pediat. Clin. N. Amer.,* 5:1029, 1958.

537. Noonan, J. A., Nadas, A. S., Rudolph, A. M., and Harris, G. B.: Transposition of the Great Arteries. A Correlation of Clinical, Physiologic and Autopsy Data. *New England J. Med.,* 263:593, 637, 684, 739, 1960.

538. Ober, W. B., and Moore, T. E., Jr.: Congenital Cardiac Malformations in the Neonatal Period; An Autopsy Study. *New England J. Med.,* 253:271, 1955.

539. Ochsner, J. L., Cooley, D. A., Harris, L. C., and McNamara, D. G.: Treatment of Complete Transposition of the Great Vessels with the Blalock-Hanlon Operation. *Circulation,* 24:51, 1961.

540. Olson, R. E., Ellenbogen, E., Stern, H., and Liang, M. M. L.: An Abnormality of Cardiac Myosin Associated with Chronic Congestive Heart Failure in the Dog. (Abstr.) *J. Clin. Invest.,* 35:727, 1956.

541. Onesti, S. J., Jr., and Harned, H. S., Jr.: Absence of the Pulmonary Valve Associated with Ventricular Septal Defect. *Am. J. Cardiol.,* 2:496, 1958.

542. Ongley, P. A., Sprague, H. B., and Rappaport, M. B.: The Diastolic Murmur of Mitral Stenosis. *New England J. Med.,* 253:1049, 1955.

543. Orias, O., and Braun-Menéndez, E.: *The Heart Sounds in Normal and Pathological Conditions.* London, Oxford University Press, 1939.

544. Owen, S. G., and Wood, P.: A New Method of Determining the Degree or Absence of Mitral Obstruction: An Analysis of the Diastolic Part of Indirect Left Atrial Pressure Tracings. *Brit. Heart J.,* 17:41, 1955.

545. Owen, W. R., Thomas, W. A., Castleman, B., and Bland, E. F.: Unrecognized Emboli to the Lungs with Subsequent Cor Pulmonale. *New England J. Med.,* 249:919, 1953.

546. Paine, R., Smith, J. R., Butcher, H. R., and Howard, F.: Heart Failure and Pulmonary Edema Produced by Certain Neurologic Stimuli. *Circulation,* 5:759, 1952.

547. Palmer, H. D., and Kempf, M.: Streptococcus Viridans Bacteremia Following Extraction of Teeth; Case of Multiple Mycotic Aneurysms in Pulmonary Arteries: Report of Cases and Necropsies. *J.A.M.A.,* 113:1788, 1939.

548. Pardee, H. E. B.: Electrocardiographic Findings in Rheumatic Heart Disease. *Am. J. Med.,* 2:528, 1947.

549. Parkinson, J., and Papp, C.: Repetitive Paroxysmal Tachycardia. *Brit. Heart J.,* 9:241, 1947.

550. Patten, B. M.: The Circulatory System; Embryological; in *Growth and Development of the Child.* Part 2: Anatomy and Physiology. The White House Conference. New York, Century Company, 1933.

551. Paul, J. R., and others: *The Epidemiology of Rheumatic Fever and Some of Its Public Health Aspects.* 2nd ed. New

764   References

York, Printed for the American Heart Association by the Metropolitan Life Insurance Company, 1943.

552. Paul, M. H., and Rudolph, A. M.: Pulmonary Valve Obstruction during Cardiac Catheterization. *Circulation,* 18:53, 1958.

553. Paul, M. H., Miller, R. A., and Potts, W. J.: Long-Term Results of Aortic-Pulmonary Anastomosis for Tetralogy of Fallot: An Analysis of the First 100 Cases Eleven to Thirteen Years after Operation. *Circulation,* 23:525, 1961.

554. Paul, M. H., Rudolph, A. M., and Nadas, A. S.: Congenital Complete Atrioventricular Block: Problems of Clinical Assessment. *Circulation,* 18:183, 1958.

555. Paul, M. H., Currimbhoy, Z., Miller, R. A., and Schulman, I.: Thrombocytopenia in Cyanotic Congenital Heart Disease. (Abstr.) *Circulation,* 24:1013, 1961.

556. Paul, O., Castleman, B., and White, P. D.: Chronic Constrictive Pericarditis: Study of 53 Cases. *Am. J. M. Sc.,* 216:361, 1948.

557. Perou, M. L.: Congenital Supravalvular Aortic Stenosis. *Arch. Path.,* 71:453, 1961.

558. Perry, E. L., Burchell, H. B., and Edwards, J. E.: Congenital Communication between the Left Ventricle and the Right Atrium: Co-existing Ventricular Septal Defect and Double Tricuspid Orifice. *Proc. Staff Meet., Mayo Clin.,* 24:198, 1949.

559. Peters, J.: Edema of Acute Nephritis. *Am. J. Med.,* 14:448, 1953.

560. Place, E. H.: Heart in Diphtheria and Scarlet Fever. *New England J. Med.,* 207:864, 1932.

561. Platou, R. V.: Clinically Manifest Tuberculous Pericarditis; Report of Case with Observations on Circulatory Changes. *Am. J. Dis. Child.,* 57:1386, 1939.

562. Pleydell, M. J.: Anencephaly and Other Congenital Abnormalities: An Epidemiological Study in Northamptonshire. *Brit. M.J.,* 1:309, 1960.

563. Polani, P. E., and Campbell, M.: An Aetiological Study of Congenital Heart Disease. *Ann. Human Genetics,* 19:209, 1955.

564. Pompe, J. C.: Hypertrophie idiopathique du coeur. *Ann. d'anat. Path.,* 10:23, 1933.

565. Porter, G. H.: Sarcoid Heart Disease. *New England J. Med.,* 263:1350, 1960.

566. Potts, W. J. Smith, S., and Gibson, S.: Anastomosis of the Aorta to a Pulmonary Artery. Certain Types in Congenital Heart Disease. *J.A.M.A.,* 132:627, 1946.

567. Prinzmetal, M., and others: *The Auricular Arrhythmias.* Springfield, Ill., Charles C Thomas, 1952.

568. Prior, J. T.: Congenital Anomalies of the Mitral Valve; Two Cases Associated with Long Survival. *Am. Heart J.,* 46:649, 1953.

569. Rammelkamp, C. H., Jr.: The Lewis A. Conner Memorial Lecture. Rheumatic Heart Disease. A Challenge. *Circulation,* 17:842, 1958.

570. Rappaport, M. B., and Sprague, H. B.: Physiologic and Physical Laws That Govern Auscultation, and Their Clinical Application. *Am. Heart J.,* 21:276, 1941.

571. Idem: The Graphic Registration of the Normal Heart Sounds. *Am. Heart J.,* 23:591, 1942.

572. Idem: The Effects of Tubing Bore on Stethoscopic Efficiency. *Am. Heart J.,* 42:605, 1951.

573. Ratcliffe, J. W., Hurt, R. L., Belmonte, B., and Gerbode, F.: The Physiologic Effects of Experimental Total Pulmonary Insufficiency. *Surgery,* 41:43, 1957.

574. Rauh, L. W.: The Incidence of Organic Heart Disease in School Children. *Am. Heart J.,* 18:705, 1930.

575. Rawson, A. J., and Woske, H. M.: A Study of Etiologic Factors in So-Called Primary Pulmonary Hypertension. *Arch. Int. Med.,* 105:233, 1960.

576. Reifenstein, G. H., Levine, S. A., and Gross, R. E.: Coarctation of the Aorta; A Review of 104 Autopsied Cases of the "Adult Type," 2 Years of Age or Older. *Am. Heart J.,* 33:146, 1947.

577. Reinhold, J., Rudhe, U., and Bonham-Carter, R. E.: The Heart Sounds and the Arterial Pulse in Congenital Aortic Stenosis. *Brit. Heart J.,* 17:327, 1955.

578. Reinhold, J. D., and Nadas, A. S.: The Role of Auscultation in the Diagnosis of Congenital Heart Disease; A Phonocardiographic Study of Children. *Am. Heart J.,* 47:405, 1954.

579. Reyersbach, G., and Kuttner, A. G.: Studies on the Auriculoventricular Conduction Time of Normal Children and of Rheumatic Children without Signs of Rheumatic Activity. *Am. Heart J.,* 20:573, 1940.

580. Reynolds, J. L., Nadas, A. S., Rudolph, A. M., and Gross, R. E.: Critical Congenital Aortic Stenosis with Minimal Electrocardiographic Changes. *New England J. Med.,* 262:276, 1960.

581. Rheumatic Fever Working Party of the Medical Research Council of Great Britain and the Subcommittee of Principal Investigators of the American Council on Rheumatic Fever and Congenital Heart Disease, American Heart Association: The Treatment of Acute Rheumatic Fever in Children; A Cooperative Clinical Trial of ACTH, Cortisone and Aspirin. *Circulation,* 11:343, 1955.

582. Idem: The Evolution of Rheumatic Heart Disease in Children; Five-Year Report of a Cooperative Clinical Trial of ACTH, Cortisone, and Aspirin. *Circulation,* 22:503, 1960.

583. Rich, A. R.: A Hitherto Unrecognized Tendency to the Development of Widespread Pulmonary Vascular Obstruction in Patients with Congenital Pulmonary Stenosis (Tetralogy of Fallot). *Bull. Johns Hopkins Hosp.,* 82:389, 1948.

584. Rich, A. R., and Gregory, J. E.: Further Experimental Cardiac Lesions of Rheumatic Type Produced by Anaphylactic Hypersensitivity. *Bull. Johns Hopkins Hosp.,* 75:115, 1944.

585. Richards, M. R., Merritt, K. K., Samuels, M. H., and Langmann, A. G.: Congenital Malformation of the Cardiovascular System in a Series of 6,053 Infants. *Pediatrics,* 15:12, 1955.

586. Idem: Frequency and Significance of Cardiac Murmurs in the First Year of Life. *Pediatrics,* 15:169, 1955.

587. Riley, C. M., Freedman, A. M., and Langford, W. S.: Further Observations of Familial Dysautonomia. *Pediatrics,* 14:475, 1954.

588. Rodbard, S.: Physical Forces and the Vascular Lining. *Ann. Int. Med.,* 50:1339, 1959.

589. Roger, H.: Recherches cliniques sur la communication congénitale des deux coeurs, par inocclusion du septum interventriculaire. *Bull. Acad. Méd. de Paris,* 8:1074, 1879.

590. Rokitansky, C. F.: Die Defekte der Scheiderwände des Herzens. Quoted by J. E. Edwards.[214]

591. Root, B.: Postoperative Adrenal Insufficiency; A Review. *Current Researches in Anesth. & Analg.,* 34:78, 1955.

592. Rosenbaum, H. D., Nadas, A. S., and Neuhauser E. B. D.: Primary Myocardial Diseases in Infancy and Childhood. *Am. J. Dis. Child.,* 86:28, 1953.

593. Ross, J., Jr., Braunwald, E., and Morrow, A. G.: Transseptal Left Heart Catheterization; A New Diagnostic Method. *Progr. in Cardiovasc. Dis.,* 2:315, 1960.

594. Rossi, E.: *Herzkrankheiten im Säuglingsalter.* Stuttgart, Georg Thieme, 1954.

595. Rowe, R. D., and Uchida, I. A.: Cardiac Malformation in Mongolism. A Prospective Study of 184 Mongoloid Children. *Am. J. Med.,* 31:726, 1961.

596. Rowe, R. D., Vlad, P., and Keith, J. D.: Atypical Tetralogy of Fallot: A Noncyanotic Form with Increased Lung Vascularity. *Circulation,* 12:230, 1955.

597. Rubin, I. L., and Buchberg, A. S.: Heart in Progressive Muscular Dystrophy. *Am. Heart J.,* 43:161, 1952.

598. Rudolph, A. M.: Normal and Almost Normal Respiration in Children. Report of the Thirty-seventh Ross Conference on Pediatrics. Ross Laboratory, Columbus, Ohio, 1961, p. 65.

599. Rudolph, A. M., and Auld, P. A. M.: Physical Factors Affecting Normal and Serotonin-Constricted Pulmonary Vessels. *Am. J. Physiol.,* 198:864, 1960.

600. Rudolph, A. M., Nadas, A. S., and Borges, W. H.: Hematologic Adjustments to Cyanotic Congenital Heart Disease. *Pediatrics,* 11:454, 1953.

601. Rudolph, A. M., and Cayler, G. G.: Cardiac Catheterization in Infants and Children. *Pediat. Clin. N. Amer.,* 5:907, 1958.

602. Rudolph, A. M., Nadas, A. S., and Goodale, W. T.: Intracardiac Left-to-Right Shunt with Pulmonic Stenosis. *Am. Heart J.,* 48:808, 1954.

603. Rudolph, A. M., Mayer, F. E., Nadas, A. S., and Gross, R. E.: Patent Ductus Arteriosus. A Clinical and Hemodynamic Study of 23 Patients in the First Year of Life. *Pediatrics,* 22:892, 1958.

604. Rudolph, A. M., Paul, M. H., Sommer, L. S., and Nadas, A. S.: Effects of Tolazoline Hydrochloride (Priscoline) on Circulatory Dynamics of Patients with Pulmonary Hypertension. *Am. Heart J.,* 55:424, 1958.

605. Runco, V., Molnar, W., Meckstroth, C. V., and Ryan, J. M.: Graham Steell Murmur versus Aortic Regurgitation in Rheumatic Heart Disease: Results of Aortic Valvulography. (Abstr.) *Circulation,* 22:802, 1960.

606. Russell, D. S.: Myocarditis in Friedreich's Ataxia. *J. Path. & Bact.,* 58:739, 1946.

607. Rutstein, D. D., Nickerson, R. J., and Heald, F. P.: Seasonal Incidence of Patent Ductus Arteriosus and Maternal Rubella. *Am. J. Dis. Child.,* 84:199, 1952.

608. Sabiston, D. C., Neill, C. A., and Taussig, H. B.: The Direction of Blood Flow in Anomalous Left Coronary Artery Arising from the Pulmonary Artery. *Circulation,* 22:591, 1960.

609. Sandifort: Quoted by Brown.[102]

610. Saphir, O., Wile, S. A., and Reingold, I. M.: Myocarditis in Children. *Am. J. Dis. Child.,* 67:294, 1944.

611. Sarnoff, S. J., and Berglund, E.: Ventricular Function. I. Starling's Law of the Heart Studied by Means of Simultaneous Right and Left Ventricular Function Curves in the Dog. *Circulation,* 9:706, 1954.

612. Sasahara, A. A., Nadas, A. S., Rudolph, A. M., Wittenborg, M. H., and Gross, R. E.: Ventricular Septal Defect with Patent Ductus Arteriosus. A Clinical and Hemodynamic Study. *Circulation,* 22:254, 1960.

613. Scannell, J. G., Brewster, W. R., Jr., and Bland, E. F.: Successful Removal of a Myxoma from the Left Atrium. *New England J. Med.,* 254:601, 1956.

614. Schaefer, J. A., and Rudolph, L. A.: Corrected Transposition of Great Vessels. *Am. Heart J.,* 54:610, 1957.

615. Schiebler, G. L., Adams, P., Jr., and Anderson, R. C.: Familial Cardiomegaly in Association with the Wolff-Parkinson-White Syndrome. *Am. Heart J.,* 58:113, 1959.

616. Schiebler, G. L., and others: Congenital Corrected Transposition of the Great

Vessels: A Study of 33 Cases. *Pediatrics,* 27(5) Suppl: 849, 1961.

617. Schilder, D. P., and Harvey, W. P.: Confusion of Tricuspid Incompetence with Mitral Insufficiency—A Pitfall in the Selection of Patients for Mitral Surgery. *Am. Heart J.,* 54:352, 1957.

618. Schlomka, G.: Untersuchungen über die physiologische Unrägelmässigkeit des Herzschlages. Quoted by M. C. Joseph and L. Tenckhoff.[370]

619. Schuster, S. R., and Gross, R. E.: Surgery for Coarctation of the Aorta. A Review of 500 Cases. *J. Thor. Cardiov. Surg.,* 43:54, 1962.

620. Schwartz, S. P., and Schwedel, J. B.: Digitalis Studies on Children with Heart Disease; Effects of Digitalis on Sinus Rate of Children with Rheumatic Fever and Chronic Valvular Heart Disease. *Am. J. Dis. Child.,* 39:298, 1930.

621. Schwartz, S. P., and Weiss, M. M.: Digitalis Studies on Children with Heart Disease; Effects of Digitalis on Electrocardiograms of Children with Rheumatic Fever and Chronic Valvular Heart Disease. *Am. J. Dis. Child.,* 38: 699, 1929.

622. Schwartz, W. B., and Wallace, W. M.: Electrolyte Equilibrium during Mercurial Diuresis. *J. Clin. Invest.,* 30:1089, 1951.

623. Scott, H. W., Jr., and Sabiston, D. C., Jr.: Surgical Treatment for Congenital Aorticopulmonary Fistula. Experimental and Clinical Aspects. *J. Thoracic Surg.,* 25:26, 1953.

624. Scott, L. P., Hauck, A. J., Nadas, A. S., and Gross, R. E.: Endocardial Cushion Defect. Preoperative and Postoperative Survey. *Circulation,* 26:218, 1962.

625. Scott, R. C.: The Correlation between the Electrocardiographic Patterns of Ventricular Hypertrophy and the Anatomic Findings. *Circulation,* 21:256, 1960.

626. Scott, R. C., and others: The Syndrome of Ventricular Septal Defect with Aortic Insufficiency. *Am. J. Cardiol.,* 2:530, 1958.

627. Selzer, A.: Defect of the Ventricular Septum. *Arch. Int. Med.,* 84:798, 1949.

628. Idem: Defects of the Cardiac Septum. *J.A.M.A.,* 154:129, 1954.

629. Selzer, A., Ebnother, C. L., Packard, P., Stone, A. O., and Quinn, J. E.: Reliability of Electrocardiographic Diagnosis of Left Ventricular Hypertrophy. *Circulation,* 17:255, 1958.

630. Senning, A.: Surgical Treatment of Right Ventricular Outflow Tract Stenosis Combined with Ventricular Septal Defect and Right-Left Shunt (Fallot's Tetralogy). *Acta chir. scandinav.,* 117: 73, 1959.

631. Idem: Surgical Correction of Transposition of the Great Vessels. *Surgery,* 45: 966, 1959.

632. Idem: The Surgical Treatment of the Tetralogy of Fallot. *Schweiz. med. Wchnschr.,* 90:839, 1960.

633. Sepulveda, G., Lukas, D. S., and Steinberg, I.: Anomalous Drainage of Pulmonary Veins; Clinical, Physiologic and Angiocardiographic Features. *Am. J. Med.,* 18:883, 1955.

634. Shachnow, N., Spellman, S., and Rubin, I.: Persistent Supraventricular Tachycardia. Case Report with Review of Literature. *Circulation,* 10:232, 1954.

635. Shapiro, M. J., and Keys, A.: Prognosis of Untreated Patent Ductus Arteriosus and Results of Surgical Intervention: Clinical Series of 50 Cases and Analysis of 139 Operations. *Am. J. M. Sc.,* 206: 174, 1943.

636. Sharpey-Schafer, E. P.: Cardiac Output in Severe Anemia. *Clin. Sc.,* 5:125, 1944.

637. Shea, D. W., Kirklin, J. W., and DuShane, J. W.: Chronic Constrictive Pericarditis in Children. *Am. J. Dis. Child.,* 93: 430, 1957.

638. Shepherd, J. T., Bowers, D., and Wood, E. H.: Measurement of Cardiac Output in Man by Injection of Dye at Constant Rate into the Right Ventricle or Pulmonary Artery. *J. Appl. Physiol.,* 7: 629, 1955.

639. Shubin, H., Levinson, D. C., and Griffith, G. C.: Endocarditis Due to Coagulase-Positive Staphylococcus Pyogenes Var. Aureus. *J.A.M.A.,* 167:1218, 1958.

640. Shubin, H., Kaufman, R., Shapiro, M., and Levinson, D. C.: Cardiovascular Findings in Children with Sickle Cell Anemia. *Am. J. Cardiol.,* 6:875, 1960.

641. Sidbury, J. B., Jr., Cornblath, M., Fisher, J., and House, E.: Glycogen in Erythrocytes of Patients with Glycogen Storage Disease. *Pediatrics,* 27:103, 1961.

642. Siegel, A. C., Johnson, E. E., and Stollerman, G. H.: Controlled Studies of Streptococcal Pharyngitis in a Pediatric Population. I. Factors Related to the Attack Rate of Rheumatic Fever. *New England J. Med.,* 265:559, 1961.

643. Silverman, B. K., Nadas, A. S., Wittenborg, M. H., Goodale, W. T., and Gross, R. E.: Pulmonary Stenosis with Intact Ventricular Septum: Correlation of Clinical and Physiologic Data, with Review of Operative Results. *Am. J. Med.,* 20:53, 1956.

644. Skall-Jensen, J.: Congenital Aorticopulmonary Fistula, a Review of the Literature and Report of Two Cases. *Acta med. scandinav.,* 160:221, 1958.

645. Smith, D. E., and Matthews, M. B.: Aortic Valvular Stenosis with Coarctation of the Aorta, with Special Reference to the Development of Aortic Stenosis upon Congenital Bicuspid Valves. *Brit. Heart J.,* 17:198, 1955.

646. Smith, J. C.: Anomalous Pulmonary Veins. *Am. Heart J.,* 41:561, 1951.

647. Smith, R. D., DuShane, J. W., and Edwards, J. E.: Congenital Insufficiency of the Pulmonary Valve; Including a Case of Fetal Cardiac Failure. *Circulation,* 20:554, 1959.

648. Smith, R. M.: Blood Replacement in Tho-

racic Surgery for Children. *J.A.M.A.,* 161:1124, 1956.

649. Snellen, H. A., and Albers, F. H.: The Clinical Diagnosis of Anomalous Pulmonary Venous Drainage. *Circulation,* 6:801, 1952.

650. Sobin, S.: Experimental Creation of Cardiac Defects, in Report of the Fourteenth M. & R. Pediatric Research Conference. Columbus, Ohio, M. & R. Laboratories, 1955, p. 13.

651. Sokolow, M., and Lyon, T. P.: Ventricular Complex in Left Ventricular Hypertrophy as Obtained by Unipolar Precordial and Limb Leads. *Am. Heart. J.,* 37:161, 1949.

652. Idem: Ventricular Complex in Right Ventricular Hypertrophy as Obtained by Unipolar Precordial and Limb Leads. *Am. Heart J.,* 38:273, 1949.

653. Soloff, L. A., and Zatuchni, J.: Some Difficulties in Evaluating Functional Results after Mitral Commissurotomy. *J.A.M.A.,* 154:673, 1954.

654. Soloff, L. A., Zatuchni, J., Janton, O. H., O'Neill, T. J. E., and Glover, R. P.: Reactivation of Rheumatic Fever Following Mitral Commissurotomy. *Circulation,* 8:481, 1953.

655. Somerville, J.: Gout in Cyanotic Congenital Heart Disease. *Brit. Heart J.,* 23: 31, 1961.

656. Sones, F. M.: Cine-Cardio-Angiography. *Pediat. Clin. N. Amer.,* 5:954, 1958.

657. Soulié, P., Carlotti, J., Sicot, J. R., and Joly, F.:Etude hémodynamique du rétrécissement mitral. *Semaine d. hôp. de Paris,* 27:2627, 1951.

658. Soulié, P., Joly, F., Carlotti, J., and Sicot, J. R.: Etude comparée de l'hémodynamique dans les tétralogies et dans les trilogies de Fallot (étude de 43 cas). *Arch. mal. coeur,* 44:577, 1951.

659. Spencer, F. C., Bahnson, H. T., and Neill, C. A.: Report on the Treatment of Three Patients with Aortic Insufficiency and Ventricular Septal Defect by Plication of a Prolapsed Aortic Valve Cusp. (Abstr.) *Circulation,* 22: 816, 1960.

660. Spencer, M. P., Johnston, F. R., and Meredith, J. H.: The Origin and Interpretation of Murmurs in Coarctation of the Aorta. *Am. Heart J.,* 56: 722, 1958.

661. Sprague, H. B., and Rappaport, M. B.: The Effects of Improper Fitting of Stethoscope to Ears on Auscultatory Efficiency. *Am. Heart J.,* 43:713, 1952.

662. Stack, M. J., Rader, B., Sobol, B. J., Farber, S. J., and Eichna, L. W.: Cardiovascular Hemodynamic Functions in Complete Heart Block and the Effect of Isopropylnorepinephrine. *Circulation,* 17:526, 1958.

663. Stanton, R. E., and Fyler, D. C.: The Natural History of Pulmonary Hypertension in Children with Ventricular Septal Defects Assessed by Serial Right-

Heart Catheterization. *Pediatrics,* 27: 621, 1961.

664. Starkey, G. W. B.: Surgical Experiences in the Treatment of Congenital Mitral Stenosis and Mitral Insufficiency. *J. Thoracic Surg.,* 38:336, 1959.

665. Starling, E. H.: *The Linacre Lecture on the Law of the Heart,* Given at Cambridge. London, Longmans, Green, & Co., 1918.

666. Starr, I., Jeffers, W. A., and Meade, R. H., Jr.: The Absence of Conspicuous Increments of Venous Pressure after Severe Damage to the Right Ventricle of the Dog, with Discussion of the Relation between Clinical Congestive Failure and Heart Disease. *Am. Heart J.,* 26: 291, 1943

667. Stephenson, H. E., Jr., Reid, L. C., and Hinton, J. W.: Some Common Denominations in 1200 Cases of Cardiac Arrest. *Ann. Surg.,* 137:731, 1953.

668. Stewart, H. J., Haskell, H. S., and Evans, W. F.: The Peripheral Blood Flow and Other Observations in Coarctation of the Aorta. *Am. Heart J.,* 28:217, 1944.

669. Still, W. J. S., and Boult, E. H.: Pathogenesis of Endocardial Fibroelastosis. *Lancet,* 2:117, 1956.

670. Stoeber, E.: Weitere Untersuchungen über epidemische Myocarditis (Schwielenherz) des Säuglings. *Ztschr. f. Kinderh.,* 71:319, 592, 1952.

671. Stollerman, G. H., Johnson, E. E., and Grossman, B. J.: Streptococcal Infection in Adolescents and Adults after Prolonged Freedom from Rheumatic Fever. *Circulation,* 20:811, 1960.

672. Sujoy, B. R., Sturgis, G. P., and Massell, B. F.: Application of the Antistreptolysin-O Titer in the Evaluation of Joint Pain and in the Diagnosis of Rheumatic Fever. *New England J. Med.,* 254:95, 1956.

673. Sussman, M. L., Strauss, L., and Hodes, H. L.: Fatal Coxsackie Group B Virus Infection in the Newborn. *Am. J. Dis. Child.,* 97:483, 1959.

674. Swan, C.: Rubella in Pregnancy as an Aetiological Factor in Congenital Malformation, Stillbirth, Miscarriage, and Abortion. *J. Obst. & Gynaec., Brit. Emp.,* 56:341, 1949.

675. Swan, H., Trapnell, J. M., and Denst, J.: Congenital Mitral Stenosis and Systemic Right Ventricle with Associated Pulmonary Vascular Changes Frustrating Surgical Repair of Patent Ductus Arteriosus and Coarctation of the Aorta. *Am. Heart J.,* 38:914, 1949.

676. Swan, H. J. C., Burchell, H. B., and Wood, E. H.: Symposium on Anomalous Pulmonary Venous Connection (Drainage): Differential Diagnosis at Cardiac Catheterization of Anomalous Pulmonary Venous Drainage Related to Atrial Septal Defects or Abnormal Venous Connections. *Proc. Staff Meet., Mayo Clin.,* 28:452, 1953.

677. Swan, H. J. C., Zapata-Diaz, J., Burchell, H. B., and Wood, E. H.: Pulmonary Hypertension in Congenital Heart Disease. *Am. J. Med., 16*:12, 1954.

678. Symposium on Phonocardiography. *Am. J. Cardiol.,* 4:1, 1959.

679. Talner, N. S., Stern, A. M., and Sloan, H. E., Jr.: Congenital Mitral Insufficiency. *Circulation,* 23:339, 1961.

680. Taran, L. M.: Personal communication to the author.

681. Taran, L. M., and Szilagy, N.: The Duration of the Electrical Systole (Q-T) in Acute Rheumatic Carditis in Children. *Am. Heart J.,* 33:14, 1947.

682. Taussig, H. B.: *Congenital Malformations of the Heart.* New York, Commonwealth Fund, 1947.

683. Taussig, H. B.: *Congenital Malformations of the Heart.* Cambridge, The Commonwealth Fund, Harvard University Press, 1960, Vols. I and II.

684. Idem: Personal communication to the author.

685. Taussig, H. B., and Bing, R. J.: Complete Transposition of the Aorta and a Levoposition of the Pulmonary Artery. *Am. Heart J.,* 37:551, 1949.

686. Taylor, S. H., and Donald, K. W.: Circulatory Studies at Rest and during Exercise in Coarctation of the Aorta before and after Operation. *Brit. Heart J.,* 22:117, 1960.

687. Teare, D.: Asymmetrical Hypertrophy of the Heart in Young Adults. *Brit. Heart J.,* 20:1, 1958.

688. Tedeschi, C. G., and Stevenson, T. D., Jr.: Interstitial Myocarditis in Children. *New England J. Med.,* 244:352, 1951.

689. Therkelsen, F., and Fabricius, J.: Cor Triatriatum. *Acta chir. Scandinav.,* 119:376, 1960.

690. Therkelsen, F., Gammelgaard, P. A., and Boessen, I.: Ventricular Septal Defects in Infants Treated with Various Modifications of the Dammann-Muller Operation. *Acta chir. Scandinav.,* Suppl. 245, 1959, p. 249.

691. Thomas, C. B., France, R., and Reichsman, F.: Prophylactic Use of Sulfanilamide in Patients Susceptible to Rheumatic Fever. *J.A.M.A.,* 116:551, 1941.

692. Thomas, P., and Dejong, D.: The P Wave in the Electrocardiogram in the Diagnosis of Heart Disease. *Brit. Heart J.,* 16:241, 1954.

693. Thomas, W. A., Averill, J. H., Castleman, B., and Bland, E. F.: The Significance of Aschoff Bodies in the Left Atrial Appendage; A Comparison of 40 Biopsies Removed during Mitral Commissurotomy with Autopsy Material from 40 Patients Dying with Fulminating Rheumatic Fever. *New England J. Med.,* 249:761, 1953.

694. Thomas, W. A., Lee, K. T., McGavran, M. H., and Rabin, E. R.: Endocardial Fibroelastosis in Infants Associated with Thrombosis and Calcification of Arteries and Myocardial Infarcts. *New England J. Med.,* 255:464, 1956.

695. Thomas, W. A., Randall, R. V., Bland, E. F., and Castleman, B.: Endocardial Fibroelastosis: A Factor in Heart Disease of Obscure Etiology: A Study of 20 Autopsied Cases in Children and Adults. *New England J. Med.,* 251:327, 1954.

696. Thompson, W. P., Golden, S. E., and White, P. D.: Heart 15 to 20 Years after Severe Diphtheria. *Am. Heart J.,* 13:534, 1937.

697. Toscano-Barboza, E., and DuShane, J. W.: Ventricular Septal Defect: Correlation of Electrocardiographic and Hemodynamic Findings in 60 Proved Cases. *Am. J. Cardiol.,* 3:721, 1959.

698. Toscano-Barbosa, E., Brandenburg, R. O., and Burchell, H. B.: Electrocardiographic Studies of Cases with Intracardiac Malformations of the Atrioventricular Canal. *Proc. Staff Meet., Mayo Clin.,* 31:513, 1956.

699. Tuchman, H., and others: Superior Vena Cava Draining into Left Atrium. *Am. J. Med.,* 21:481, 1956.

700. Umansky, R., and Hauck, A. J.: Factors in the Growth of Children with Patent Ductus Arteriosus. *Pediatrics,* 30:540, 1962.

701. Van Buchem, F. S. P.: Dilatation of the Pulmonary Artery in Pulmonic Stenosis. *Circulation,* 13:719, 1956.

702. Van Buchem, F. S. P., and Eerland, L. D.: Myxoma Cordis; Diagnosis Established Preoperatively; Surgical Removal of the Tumor. *Dis. of Chest,* 31:61, 1957.

703. Van Buchem, F. S. P., Arends, A., and Schroder, E. A.: Endocardial Fibroelastosis in Adolescents and Adults. *Brit. Heart J.,* 21:229, 1959.

704. Van Epps, E. F.: Primary Pulmonary Hypertension in Brothers. *Am. J. Roentgenol.,* 78:471, 1957.

705. Van der Hauwaert, L., and Nadas, A. S.: Auscultatory Findings in Patients with a Small Ventricular Septal Defect. *Circulation,* 23:886, 1961.

706. Van Lingen, B., and others: Clinical and Cardiac Catheterization Findings Compatible with Ebstein's Anomaly of the Tricuspid Valve: A Report of Two Cases. *Am. Heart J.,* 43:77, 1952.

707. Venner, A., and Holling, H. E.: Comparison of Operation and Clinical Findings in Mitral Stenosis and Incompetence. *Brit. Heart J.,* 15:205, 1953.

708. Vince, D. J., and Keith, J. D.: The Electrocardiogram in Ventricular Septal Defect. *Circulation,* 23:225, 1961.

709. Vineberg, A., and Gialloreto, O.: Report of a Successful Operation for Stenosis of Common Pulmonary Vein (Cor Triatriatum). *Canad. M.A.J.,* 74:719, 1956.

710. Vogelpoel, L., Schrire, V., Nellen, M., and Swanepoel, A.: The Use of Amyl Nitrite in the Differentiation of Fallot's

Tetralogy and Pulmonary Stenosis with Intact Ventricular Septum. *Am. Heart J.,* 57:803, 1959.

711. Walker, G. C., and Ellis, L. B.: Quoted by Taussig.[682]

712. Wallgren, G., and Agorio, E.: Congenital Complete A-V Block in Three Siblings. *Acta paediat.,* 49:49, 1960.

713. Wannamaker, L. W., and others: Prophylaxis of Acute Rheumatic Fever by Treatment of the Preceding Streptococcal Infection with Various Amounts of Depot Penicillin. *Am. J. Med.,* 10:673, 1951.

714. Warkany, J.: Developmental Induction of Cardiovascular Anomalies, in Report of the Fourteenth M. & R. Pediatric Research Conference. Columbus, Ohio, M. & R. Laboratories, 1955, p. 9.

715. Watkins, E., and Gross, R. E.: Experiences with Surgical Repair of Atrial Septal Defects. *J. Thoracic Surg.,* 30:469, 1955.

716. Watson, D. G., and Keith, J. D.: The Q Wave in Lead V_6 in Heart Disease of Infancy and Childhood, with Special Reference to Diastolic Loading. *Am. Heart J.,* 63:629, 1962.

717. Weber, F. P.: Can the Clinical Manifestations of Congenital Heart Disease Disappear with the General Growth and Development of the Patient? *Brit. J. Child. Dis.,* 15:113, 1918.

718. Webster, B. H.: Cardiac Complications of Infectious Mononucleosis. A Review of the Literature and Report of Five Cases. *Am. J.M. Sc.,* 234:62, 1957.

719. Wegria, R., and others: Effect of Auricular Fibrillation on Coronary Blood Flow. *Am. J. Physiol.,* 160:177, 1950.

720. Weidman, W. H., and DuShane, J. W.: Some Observations Concerning Progressive Pulmonary Vascular Obstructive Disease in Children with Ventricular Septal Defect. Abstr. 106, American Pediatric Society, Seventy-first Annual meeting, Atlantic City, May 2–3, 1961, p. 104.

721. Weisenfeld, S., and Messinger, W. J.: Cardiac Involvement in Progressive Muscular Dystrophy. *Am. Heart J.,* 43:170, 1952.

722. Welch, K. J., and Kinney, T. D.: Effect of Patent Ductus Arteriosus and of Interauricular and Interventricular Septal Defects on Development of Pulmonary Vascular Lesions. *Am. J. Path.,* 24:729, 1948.

723. Wells, B.: The Assessment of Mitral Stenosis by Phonocardiography. *Brit. Heart J.,* 16:261, 1954.

724. Wenckebach, K. F.: *Die Arhythmie als Ausdruck bestimmter Funktionsstörungen des Herzens.* Leipzig, W. Engelmann, 1903.

725. Werko, L., Ek, J., Bucht, H., and Karnel, J.: Cardiac Output, Blood Pressures and Renal Dynamics in Coarctation of Aorta. Scandinav. J. Clin. & Lab. Invest., 8:193, 1956.

726. Wesselhoeft, C.: Report on Medical Progress; Communicable Diseases; Cardiovascular Disease in Diphtheria. *New England J. Med.,* 223:57, 1940.

727. White, P. D.: *Heart Disease* 3d ed. New York, Macmillan Company, 1947.

728. Idem: *Heart Disease.* 4th ed. New York, Macmillan Company, 1951.

729. Wiggers, C. J.: *Circulatory Dynamics: Physiologic Studies.* New York, Grune & Stratton, 1952.

730. Wilhelm, F., Hirsh, H. L., Hussey, H. H., and Dowling, H. F.: Treatment of Acute Bacterial Endocarditis with Penicillin. *Ann. Int. Med.,* 26:221, 1947.

731. Wilkins, R. B., Jarvis, F. J., and King, R. L.: Purulent Pericarditis Due to Hemophilus Influenzae, Type B. *Am. Heart J.,* 42:749, 1951.

732. Williams, C., and Soutter, L.: Pericardial Tamponade. Diagnosis and Treatment. *Arch. Int. Med.,* 94:571, 1954.

733. Wilson, F. N., Rosenbaum, F. F., and Johnston, F. D.: Interpretation of the Ventricular Complex of the Electrocardiogram. *Advances in Internal Medicine,* 1947, Vol. 2.

734. Wilson, M. G.: *Rheumatic Fever;* Studies of the Epidemiology, Manifestations, Diagnosis, and Treatment of the Disease during the First Three Decades. London, Commonwealth Fund, 1940.

735. Wilson, M. G., and Lim, W. N.: The Natural History of Rheumatic Heart Disease in the Third, Fourth and Fifth Decades of Life. *Circulation,* 16:700, 1957.

736. Idem: Short-Term Hormone Therapy. Its Effect in Active Rheumatic Carditis of Varying Duration. *New England J. Med.,* 260:802, 1959.

737. Wilson, R. A., and Clark, N.: Endocardial Fibroelastosis Associated with Generalized Glycogenosis. *Pediatrics,* 26:86, 1960.

738. Witham, A. C.: Double Outlet Right Ventricle; A Partial Transposition Complex. *Am. Heart J.,* 53:928, 1957.

739. Wittenborg, M. H., Neuhauser, E. B. D., and Sprunt, W. H.: Roentgenographic Findings in Congenital Tricuspid Atresia with Hypoplasia of the Right Ventricle. *Am. J. Roentgenol.,* 66:712, 1951.

740. Wolff, L., Parkinson, J., and White, P. D.: Bundle Branch Block with Short P-R Interval in Healthy Young People Prone to Paroxysmal Tachycardia. *Am. Heart J.,* 5:685, 1930.

741. Wolff, L.: *Electrocardiography: Fundamentals and Clinical Application.* 2nd ed. Philadelphia, W. B. Saunders Company, 1956.

742. Wood, E. H.: in O. Glasser: *Medical Physics.* Chicago, Year Book Publishers, Inc., 1950, Vol. 2, p. 664.

743. Idem: Symposium on Use of Indicator-Dilution Technics in the Study of the Circulation. *Circulation Research,* 10:379, 1962.

744. Wood, P.: Personal communication.

745. Idem: Congenital Heart Disease; A Review of Its Clinical Aspects in the Light of Experience Gained by Means of Modern Techniques. *Brit. M.J.,* 2:639, 1950.

746. Idem: *Diseases of the Heart and Circulation.* Philadelphia, J. B. Lippincott Company, 1950.

747. Idem: Pulmonary Hypertension. *Brit. M. Bull.,* 8:348, 1951–2.

748. Idem: *Diseases of the Heart and Circulation.* 2nd ed. London, Eyre and Spottiswoode, 1956.

749. Idem: The Eisenmenger Syndrome or Pulmonary Hypertension with Reversed Central Shunt. I and II. *Brit. M.J.,* 2: 701, 755, 1958.

750. Idem: Pulmonary Hypertension. *Mod. Concepts Cardiovasc. Dis.,* 28:513, 1959.

751. Idem: Chronic Constrictive Pericarditis. *Am. J. Cardiol.,* 7:48, 1961.

752. Wood, P., Magidson, O., and Wilson, P. A. O.: Ventricular Septal Defect, with a Note on Acyanotic Fallot's Tetralogy. *Brit. Heart J.,* 16:387, 1954.

753. Wooley, C. F., and Hosier, D. M.: Constrictive Pericarditis Due to Histoplasma Capsulatum. *New England J. Med.,* 264:1230, 1961.

754. Wright, J. L., Burchell, H. B., Kirklin, J. W., and Wood, E. H.: Congenital Displacement of the Tricuspid Valve (Ebstein's Malformation): Report of a Case with Closure of an Associated Foramen Ovale for Correction of the Right-to-Left Shunt. *Proc. Staff Meet., Mayo Clin.,* 29:278, 1954.

755. Yater, W. M., Lyon, J. A., and McNabb, P. E.: Congenital Heart Block; Review and Report of Second Case of Complete Heart Block Studied by Serial Sections through Conduction Systems. *J.A.M.A.,* 100:1831, 1933.

756. Young, M. D., and Griswold, H. E.: Situs

Inversus of the Abdominal Viscera with Levocardia; Report of 8 Cases Submitted to the Blalock-Taussig Operation. *Circulation,* 3:202, 1951.

757. Yu, P. N.: Primary Pulmonary Hypertension: Report of Six Cases and Review of Literature. *Ann. Int. Med.,* 49:1138, 1958.

758. Zeavin, I., Virtue, R. W., and Swan, H.: Cessation of Circulation in General Hypothermia. II. Anesthetic Management, *Anesthesiology,* 15:113, 1954.

759. Ziegler, R. F.: *Electrocardiographic Studies in Normal Infants and Children.* Springfield, Ill., Charles C Thomas, 1951.

760. Idem: The Genesis and Importance of the Electrocardiogram in Coarctation of the Aorta. *Circulation,* 9:371, 1954.

761. Ziegra, S. R., Kiely, B., and Morales, F.: Cardiac Catheterization in Infants with Bronchiolitis. Read at the Meeting of The Society for Pediatric Research, Swampscott, Mass., May 4, 1960.

762. Zilstra, W. G.: *A Manual of Reflection Oximetry:* And Some Other Applications of Reflection Photometry. Assen, Netherlands, Van Gorcum & Comp., 1958.

763. Zimmermann, H. A.: *Intra Vascular Catheterization.* Springfield, Ill., Charles C Thomas, 1959.

764. Zimmerman, H. A., Scott, R. W., and Becker, N. O.: Catheterization of the Left Side of the Heart in Man. *Circulation,* 1:357, 1950.

765. Zoll, P. M., Linenthal, A. J., Norman, L. R. Paul, M. H., and Gibson, W.: Treatment of Unexpected Cardiac Arrest by External Electric Stimulation of the Heart. *New England J. Med.,* 254:541, 1956.

766. Zoll, P. M., and Linenthal, A. J.: Termination of Refractory Tachycardia by External Countershock. *Circulation,* 25: 596, 1962.

APPENDIX

Tabular Data

771

Table 1. Normal Blood Pressure for Various Ages[320]

(Adapted from data in the literature)
(Figures have been rounded off to nearest decimal place)

Ages	Mean Systolic ± 2 S. D.	Mean Diastolic ± 2 S. D.
Newborn................	80 ± 16	46 ± 16
6 mos.-1 year	89 ± 29	60 ± 10*
1 year	96 ± 30	66 ± 25*
2 years................	99 ± 25	64 ± 25*
3 years................	100 ± 25	67 ± 23*
4 years................	99 ± 20	65 ± 20*
5-6 years	94 ± 14	55 ± 9
6-7 years	100 ± 15	56 ± 8
7-8 years	102 ± 15	56 ± 8
8-9 years	105 ± 16	57 ± 9
9-10 years	107 ± 16	57 ± 9
10-11 years............	111 ± 17	58 ± 10
11-12 years............	113 ± 18	59 ± 10
12-13 years............	115 ± 19	59 ± 10
13-14 years............	118 ± 19	60 ± 10

*In this study the point of muffling was taken as the diastolic pressure.

Table 2. Circulation Time by Fluorescein Method in Normal Infants and Children

Author	Distance	Number of Patients	Age	Average and Range in Seconds
Lesser et al.*	Hand to conjunctiva	55	0-5 days	10.2 (6-14)
Witzberger et al.** ..	Arm to lip	25	1-24 months	7.0 (5-9.0)
Witzberger et al.** ..	Arm to lip	51	3-13 years	11.5 (8-16)
Gasul et al.***	Arm to lip	14	4-24 months	6.5 (5-8.5)
Gasul et al.***	Arm to lip	36	3-13 years	8.5 (5-12.5)

*Am. J. Dis. Child., 83:645, 1952.
**J. Pediat., 22:726, 1943.
***J. Pediat., 34:460, 1949.

Table 3. Pattern of QRS and T Waves in Various Regions of the Heart

Surface of right ventricle, pulmonary conus	rSr', T-
Surface of right ventricle, basal (lateral wall)	rS or RS, T±
Surface of right ventricle, apical.	Rs, T+
Surface of left ventricle, basal (lateral wall)	qR or qRS, T+
Surface of left ventricle, apical	qR or qRS, T+
Cavity of right atrium	QS, T-
Cavity of right ventricle	rSr' or rS, T-
Cavity of pulmonary artery	QS, T-
Cavity of left atrium	QS, T-
Cavity of left ventricle	QS, T-
Back of the heart	Qr or QR, T-

Modified from Lepeschkin.[417]

Table 4. Rate per Minute by Electrocardiogram Interspaces between 2 QRS Complexes

5.	300	13.	115	21.	72	29.	52
6.	250	14.	107	22.	68	30.	50
7.	214	15.	100	23.	65	31.	48
8.	188	16.	 94	24.	63	32.	47
9.	167	17.	 88	25.	60	33.	45
10.	150	18.	 84	26.	58	34.	44
11.	136	19.	 79	27.	56	35.	43
12.	125	20.	 75	28.	54		

Table 5. The Mean Electrical Axis of P Wave, QRS Complex and T Wave

	P			QRS			T		
	Av.	Min.	Max.	Av.	Min.	Max.	Av.	Min.	Max.
0-24 hrs.	60	-30	90	137	75	190	77	-10	180
1 day-1 mo. . .	58	0	90	116	-5	190	37	-10	130
1-6 months . . .	56	30	90	72	35	135	44	0	90
6 mos.-1 yr. . .	55	30	75	64	30	135	39	-30	90
1-5 years	50	-30	75	63	0	110	35	-10	90
5-12 years . . .	47	-30	75	66	-15	120	38	-20	70
12-16 years. . .	54	0	90	66	-15	110	41	30	90

Modified from Ziegler.[759]

Table 6. Maximal P-R Intervals in Seconds at Different Age Levels and Varying Heart Rates

Age	Rate					
	< 71	71-90	91-110	111-130	131-150	>150
< 1 mo.			0.11	0.11	0.11	0.11
1-9 mos.			0.14	0.13	0.12	0.11
10-24 mos.			0.15	0.14	0.14	0.10
3-5 yrs.		0.16	0.16	0.16	0.13	
6-13 yrs.	0.18	0.18	0.16	0.16		

From M. M. Alimurung and B. F. Massell: The Normal P-R Interval in Infants and Children. Circulation, 13:257, 1956.

Table 7. QRS Patterns in V_1 in 521 Infants and Children[12]

Group I: 0-9 Mos. 100 Cases	Group III: 3-5 Yrs. 124 Cases
R : 2⎫ 72 (72%)⎫ 89 (89%) Rs : 70⎭ ⎬ R > S : 17 ⎭ R = S : 0 R < S : 7 rS : 4	R : 0 Rs : 13 R > S : 10 R = S : 12 R < S : 46⎫ 89 (72%)⎫ 101 (81.4%) rS : 43⎭ ⎬
Group II: 10 Mos.-2 Yrs. 98 Cases	**Group IV: 6-13 Yrs. 109 Cases**
R : 0⎫ Rs : 30⎬ 76 (77%) R > S : 46⎭ R = S : 0 R < S : 16 rS : 6	R : 0 Rs : 3 R > S : 2 R = S : 15 R < S : 42⎫ 179 (89.95%)⎫ 194 (97.5%) rS : 137⎭ ⎬

Table 8. Maximal QRS Voltage in the Chest Leads[12]

Age Group	V Lead	Q Wave					R Wave					S Wave				
		Mean	Min.	Max.	10%	90%	Mean	Min.	Max.	10%	90%	Mean	Min.	Max.	10%	90%
I	V1	0	0	0	0	0	10.3	2	22	5	17	4.95	0	23	1	12
	V2	0	0	0	0	0	15.6	5	33	9	23	10.5	0.25	28	3	19
	V4	0.18	0	2.5	0	0.5	16.7	4	36	10	24	11.3	0.25	25	5.75	17
	V5	0.6	0	3.5	0	2.5	13.1	2.5	28	7.5	23	5.74	1	15	2	10
	V6	0.83	0	3.5	0	2	9.3	0.25	24	1	16	3.12	0	11	0.5	7
II	V1	0	0	0	0	0	8.23	0.5	26	3.5	13	6.93	0.25	22	1.5	13
	V2	0	0	0	0	0	15.3	3	30	8	23	14.2	0.25	28	7	23
	V4	0.17	0	5	0	0.5	17.9	6	30	10.75	26	11.4	2	25	5	18
	V5	0.08	0	5	0	3	14.6	4	28	8	21	4	0	15	1.5	7
	V6	1.26	0	5	0	2.25	10.6	2.5	24	5	15	1.6	0	6	0.25	3.5
III	V1	0	0	0	0	0	6.5	0.5	20	2.5	11	9.8	1	25	3	17
	V2	0	0	0	0	0	12.5	3.5	25	6	19	17.3	4	33	8	27
	V4	0.12	0	3	0	0.5	18.3	5.5	37	10	28	11	1	34	5	17
	V5	1.25	0	9	0.25	3.5	18.5	7	40	11	25	3.35	0	13.5	0.75	6.25
	V6	1.28	0	8	0.25	2.5	13.7	4	28	8.25	19	1.06	0	6	0	2.5
IV	V1	0	0	0	0	0	4.9	0.5	14	2	9	10.7	1	27	4.5	18
	V2	0	0	0	0	0	9.7	2	21.5	5	14.5	19.5	6	35	11	27.5
	V4	0.13	0	2	0	0.5	18.4	3	37	11	49	10.7	0.25	24	4	19
	V5	1	0	4	0.25	2	19	5	37	13	26	2.76	0	14	0.25	6
	V6	1.04	0	4	0.25	2	13.9	4.5	33	8.5	20	0.9	0	8	0	3

Note: 10% column indicates voltage in 10 per cent of cases above the minimum, and 90% column indicates voltage in 90 per cent of cases above the minimum.

Table 9. T Wave Patterns in Leads V_1 to V_6

Lead	Group I	Group II	Group III	Group IV
V_1	± 7.0 -93.0	± 2.0 -96.0	± 2.4 -98.6	+ 3.6 ± 7.0 -89.4
V_2	+ 5.0 ±15.0 -80.0	+ 2.2 ± 5.1 -92.7	+ 9.0 ±35.4 -55.6	+42.7 ±27.2 -30.1
V_4	+52.0 ±10.0 -38.0	+75.2 ± 6.5 -18.3	+86.1 ±12.1 - 4.8	+94.0 ± 3.5 - 2.5
V_5	+93.0 ± 6.0 - 1.0	+96.0 ± 1.0 - 1.0	+99.2 ± 0.8	+100.0
V_6	+99.0 ± 1.0	+100.0	+100.0	+100.0

All figures indicate percentage incidence.
+ upright   ± diphasic   - negative

Table 10. Summary of Criteria of Left and Right Ventricular Hypertrophy

Left Ventricular Hypertrophy (in Absence of Left Bundle Branch Block)	
Limb leads	Â QRS -30° with counterclockwise loop* R in a V_L or a V_F more than 25 mm.
Chest leads	R_{V6} more than 30 mm. S_{V1} more than 25 mm. $R_{V6} + S_{V1}$ more than 50 mm. Deep q V_6 (more than 4 mm.) with tall, symmetrical T waves Intrinsicoid deflection more than 0.04 second
Strain.	Inverted T and depressed ST beyond V_4 with evidence of LVH
Right Ventricular Hypertrophy (in Absence of Right Bundle Branch Block)	
Limb leads	Â QRS more than 120° with clockwise loop R aV_R more than 5 mm.
Chest leads	$(V_{4\ r-1})$ qR pattern R - S more than 15 mm.† rsR' more than 15 mm.† Positive T in infants more than 4 days old in absence of LVH Intrinsicoid deflection more than 0.04 second
Strain.	Deeply inverted T waves and depressed ST lead V_1 to beyond V_3 with evidence of RVH

*Infants under 2 years less than +30°.
†In newborns (less than 2 months) more than 20 mm.

Table 11. Resting Oxygen Consumption

Present Study[*]			Data from the Literature[†]		
B.S.A. (M.^{2})	No.	Resting Oxygen Consumption (ml./min./M.^{2}) Mean (S.D.)	B.S.A. (M.^{2})	No.	Resting Oxygen Consumption (ml./min./M.^{2}) Mean
0.2-0.5	18		0.225-0.275	42	140
			0.275-0.325	47	150
			0.325-0.375	58	172
			0.375-0.425	81	175
			0.425-0.475	91	179
		198 (33)		319	816
0.5-1.0	38	187 (25)	0.475-1.0	620	174
1.0-1.5	50	167 (28)	1.0-1.5	174	150
1.5+	20	161 (20)	15-25 yrs.	315	138

[*]Data (from Cayler et al.) collected from The Children's Hospital Medical Center.

[†]V.A. Lee and A. Iliff: Pediatrics, 18:739, 1956; R.C. Lewis, G.M. Kinsman and A. Iliff: Am. J. Dis. Child., 53:348, 1937; W.M. Boothby, J. Berkson and H.L. Dunn: Am. J. Physiol., 116:468, 1936.

Table 12. The Significance of Oxygen Saturation Data Obtained at Cardiac Catheterization[601]
Figures Indicate Percent Saturation except in B.

A. Minimal Saturation Changes between Cardiac Chambers Indicative of Left-to-Right Shunts

Position	Minimal Saturation Increase Sets of Samples		
	1	2	3
SVC-RA	10	7	5
RA-RV	7	5	3
RV-PA	5	3	3

B. Effect of Blood Oxygen Capacity on Oxygen Content Differences

Oxygen capacity (volumes %)	10	20	30
Oxygen content at 50% saturation	5	10	15
Oxygen content at 65% saturation	6.5	13	19.5
Changes in volumes % oxygen for 15% change in oxygen saturation	1.5	3	4.5

C. Effect of Pulmonary Venous Saturation on Calculated Left-to-Right Shunts

Saturation			Left-to-Right Shunt (% of Systemic Flow)
RA	PA	PV	
		98	100%
62	80	89	200%

D. Effect of Systemic Venous Saturation on Calculated Left-to-Right Shunts

60	70	98	36%
70	80	. . . .	51%

E. Effect of Exercise on Right Atrial to Pulmonary Arterial Oxygen Saturation Differences in 5 Patients with Ventricular Left-to-Right Shunts

Right Atrial to Pulmonary Arterial Saturation Difference	
Rest	Exercise
3	16
6	13
9	24
12	27
15	30

F. Double Left-to-Right Shunt

Position	Saturation	Left-to-Right Shunt Atrial Shunt	(% of Systemic Flow) Ventricular Shunt
SVC	60		
RA	70	36%	45%
RV	77		
PV	98		

The calculations show that although the saturation increase at the first level is greater, the left-to-right shunt is smaller.

780

Table 13. Average Normal Ranges of Intracardiac and Intravascular Pressures[601]

Infants and Children		Newborn Period
Right atrium	"a" = 3-7; "v" = 2-5; m = 1-5	m = 0-3
Right ventricle.	15-30/2-5	35-65/1-5
Pulmonary artery. . . .	15-30/5-10 (m = 10-20)	35-65/20-40 (m = 25-40)
Pulmonary wedge. . . .	"a" = 3-7; "v" = 5-15; m = 5-12	
Left atrium.	"a" = 3-7; "v" = 5-15; m = 5-10	m = 1-4
Left ventricle	80-130/5-10	
Systemic artery.	90-130/60-90 (m = 70-95)	

Zero reference point--midthorax.

Table 14. Dosage Schedule for Steroid Treatment of Acute Rheumatic Fever

Period of Treatment in Days	Total Daily Dose in Mg.			
	Meticorten		Oral Cortisone	
	Over 40 lbs.	Under 40 lbs.	Over 40 lbs.	Under 40 lbs.
21	60	40	300	200
7	50	35	250	175
7	45	30	225	150
7	40	25	200	125
7	35	20	175	100
7	30	15	150	75
7	25	10	125	50
5	20	5	100	25
5	15	2.5	75	12.5
5	10		50	
6	5		25	

Table 15. Prognosis of Rheumatic Fever in 1000 Patients[63]

Initial	347 No Heart Disease			653 Heart Disease		
20 years' follow-up	4/7 without heart disease	3/7 with heart disease	10 died	1/6 without heart disease	2/6 with heart disease	3/6 died

Table 16. Practical Differential Points between Bacterial Endocarditis and Active Rheumatic Fever

	Active R.F.	B.E.
Polyarthritis.	+	0
Nodules	+	0
Chorea.	+	0
Erythema marginatum.	+	0
Pericarditis	+	0
High antistreptolysin titer	+	+
Emboli.	0	+
Spleen	0	+
Positive blood culture.	0	+

Table 17. Principal Drugs Used in Pediatric Cardiology

Drugs	Route of Administration	Dose: Initial	Maintenance	Toxicity	Indications
Anticongestives:					
Digoxin	P.O.	<2 yrs.: 0.03-0.04 mg./lb. >2 yrs.: 0.02-0.03 mg./lb.	1/4-1/3 initial dose daily	Nausea, vomiting, arrhythmias, prolonged P-R	Congestive failure, supraventricular arrhythmias
	Parenteral	75% of above	1/4 initial dose daily		
Mercuhydrin (Meralluride)	I.M.	0.1-2.0 cc.	Repeat 2-7 days	Cramps, potassium depletion, low salt syndrome, arrhythmias, acidosis, dehydration	Congestive failure, with fluid retention
Thiomerin (Mercaptomerin)	S.C. or I.V.				
Diuril (Chlorothiazide)	P.O.	0.125-0.5 Gm. 2-3 times/day	Same as initial	Potassium depletion, low salt syndrome	Congestive failure, systemic hypertension, renal edema, A-V block
Aminophylline (Theophylline ethylenediamine)	P.R. or Slow I.V. diluted in 5% D/W	3-5 mg./lb. 1-2 mg./lb.	Same as initial	Headaches, palpitation, low blood pressure	Diuretic alone or "priming" mercury, pulmonary edema, bronchospasms
Ammonium chloride	P.O.	0.5 Gm. 2-3 times/day	3-4 days before mercurial diuretic, intermittent	Gastrointestinal upset, acidosis	Supporting mercurial diuretic
Aldactone (Spironolactone)	P.O.	0.1-0.5 Gm./day	Same	Hyponatremia, potassium intoxication	Alone or with mercury for resistant edema

Table 17. Principal Drugs Used in Pediatric Cardiology (cont.)

	Route	Dose		Side effects	Indications
Antiarrhythmics:					
Quinidine sulfate	P.O.	0.1-0.4 Gm. q. 2 hr. X 8 Start with 0.1 Gm. X 8 the first day; then 0.2 Gm. the next, and so on	Effective dose q. 3-6 hours	Nausea, vomiting, tinnitus, widened QRS complexes, ventricular arrhythmia, hypotension	Ventricular arrhythmia, atrial flutter or fibrillation, paroxysmal atrial tachycardia prevention in Wolff-Parkinson-White syndrome
Quinidine gluconate	I.M.	0.1-0.5 Gm.	Effective dose q. 6-12 hours		
Procaine amide	P.O.	7 mg./lb.	0.05-0.3 Gm. q. 6 hours	Hypotension, ventricular arrhythmias	Ventricular arrhythmias
(Pronestyl)	I.M.	0.05-0.3 Gm.	Effective dose q. 6 hours		
	I.V.	0.1 Gm. slowly diluted in 5% D/W	Effective dose q. 5-10 min.		
Neostigmine (Prostigmin)	S.C.	0.05-0.5 mg.		Hyperactive gastrointestinal tract, twitching, hypotension	Paroxysmal atrial tachycardia
Isuprel (Isoproterenol)	Sublingual P.R. I.V.	2-10 mg. 3-4 times/day 5-15 mg. 3-4 times/day 4 mg./1000 ml. in constant drip until desired effect		Palpitation, precordial pain, headache, nausea, tremor	Heart block, hypotensive state
Ephedrine sulfate	P.O. and I.M. I.V.	1.7 mg./10 lb. 50 mg. (1 ml. of 5% solution) in 100 ml. in constant drip	q. 6-8 hours	See above	Heart block, hypotensive state
Antihypotensives:					
Phenylephrine hydrochloride (Neo-Synephrine)	I.V.	10 mg. (1 ml. of 1% solution) in 100 ml. in constant drip.		Bradycardia, hypertension, arrhythmias	Hypotensive state, paroxysmal atrial tachycardia
Norepinephrine (Levophed)	I.V.	4 mg./1000 ml. in constant drip until desired effect. Test dose of 1 μg./10 kg.; then adjust		See above	Hypotensive state

Table 17. Principal Drugs Used in Pediatric Cardiology (cont.)

Drugs	Route of Administration	Dose Initial	Maintenance	Toxicity	Indications
Aramine (Metaramine)	I.V.	50 mg. in 100 ml. in constant drip			Hypotension
Wyamine sulfate (Mephentermine sulfate)	I.V.	50 mg. in 100 ml. in constant drip			Hypotension
Epinephrine	I.V. I.M.	0.5 mg. (0.5 ml. of 1:1000 solution) in 100 ml. drip 0.2-0.4 mg.			Hypotension, paroxysmal atrial tachycardia
Calcium chloride	I.V. or intra-cardiac	2-4 ml. of 10% solution	Repeat q. 30-60 minutes P.R.N.	Cardiac arrest	Slow and weak cardiac action
Hypotensives: Serpasil (Reserpine)	P.O. I.M.	0.1-0.25 mg. 3-4 times/day 1-2.5 mg.	Effect in ± 1 week Effect in hours	Hypotension and brady-cardia, nasal congestion. Discontinue before surgery	Mild hypertension, chronic atrial or sinus tachycardia
Hexamethonium chloride	P.O. S.C. or I.V.	25-250 mg. with meals 0.1-1.5 mg.	2 or 3 times/day with meals 2 or 3 times/day	Postural hypotension, constipation, syncope	Severe hypotensive state
Inversine	P.O.	0.25-2.5 mg. with meals	Twice daily	As above	As above
Hydralazine (Apresoline)	P.O. I.M.	10-50 mg. 0.1 mg./lb.	4 times daily q. 4 hours	Hypotension, headaches	As above
Magnesium sulfate	I.M. I.V.	25% solution, 0.1 ml./lb. 3% solution, 0.5-100 mg./lb. in 1-hour period	Repeat q. 4-6 hours Repeat P.R.N.	Paralysis, respiratory failure, bradycardia, hypotension	As above

Table 17. Principal Drugs Used in Pediatric Cardiology (cont.)

Arfonad (Trimetaphan camphor sulfonate)	I.V.	500 mg. (10 ml.) in 1000 ml. in constant drip		As above
Miscellaneous: Morphine sulfate	S.C.	0.5-1 mg./10 lb. No more than 10 mg.	Repeat P.R.N. q. 4 hours	Central nervous system depression, respiratory failure, vomiting	Anoxic spells, congestive failure, pulmonary edema excitement
Meperidine (Demerol)	P.O. and I.M.	0.5 mg./lb.	As above	As above	As above
Nalorphine (Nalline)	I.V.	0.5-1.0 mg./30 lb.	Repeat P.R.N. in 15 minutes		Morphine poisoning
Lorfan tartrate (Levallorphan)	I.V.	0.05-1.0 mg. 50:1 ratio to morphine administered	Repeat P.R.N. in 5-minute intervals		As above

Table 18. Autopsy Findings in 26 Cases of Primary
Myocardial Disease[592]

Disease	Number of Cases
Glycogen storage disease of the heart	3
Aberrant left coronary artery.	1
Medial necrosis of the coronary arteries	2
Myocarditis	10
Endocardial fibroelastosis.	10
Total	26

Table 19. Classification of Glycogenosis[169]

Glycogen Normal		Glycogen Abnormal	
Type I	Type II	Type III	Type IV
Absent glucose-6-phosphatase	Enzyme defect unknown	Absent debrancher enzyme	Probable brancher enzyme defect
(Hepatorenal)	(Generalized)	(Limit dextrinosis)	(Cirrhotic glycogenosis)

Table 20. Physiologic Effects and Compensatory Mechanisms
in Cardiac Tamponade

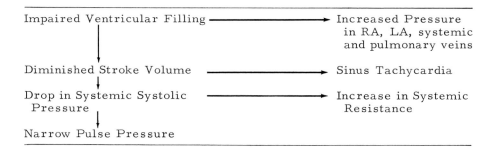

Impaired Ventricular Filling ⟶ Increased Pressure in RA, LA, systemic and pulmonary veins

Diminished Stroke Volume ⟶ Sinus Tachycardia

Drop in Systemic Systolic Pressure ⟶ Increase in Systemic Resistance

Narrow Pulse Pressure

Table 21. Hypertension in Infants and Children:
Causes and Diagnostic Aids

Etiology	Diagnostic Aids
I. Renal	
A. Acute and chronic glomerulo- nephritis Chronic nephritis secondary to anaphylactoid purpura	Clinical picture Repeated urinalyses, Addis count Concentration test, NPN Urea and creatinine clearance Renal biopsy
B. Pyelonephritis	Repeated urinalyses Repeated urine cultures plus above tests in chronic cases
C. Polycystic renal disease	Intravenous pyelograms
D. Tumors: Wilms's and neuro- blastoma	Retrograde pyelogram "Split" renal functions Exploratory laparotomy and renal biopsy
E. Ectopic kidney	
F. Hypoplastic kidney	
G. Hydronephrosis	
H. Renal artery and vein anomalies and thromboses	Above tests plus aortogram and "split" renal functions
I. Polyarteritis, disseminated lupus erythematosus	Clinical and laboratory signs of vascular disease plus renal biopsy
J. Primary arteriolar disease of the kidney	Azotemia, urine sediment abnormalities Renal biopsy or necropsy
II. Central nervous system	
A. Poliomyelitis	Clinical picture Lumbar puncture
B. Encephalitis	Above plus electroenceph- alogram
C. Rapidly expanding intracranial lesions (tumor, hemorrhage, edema)	Skull x-rays Above plus pneumoenceph- alogram or ventriculogram
III. Cardiovascular	
A. Coarctation of aorta	Femoral pulses (weak com- pared with radial) Blood pressure in legs X-ray picture (collateral, esophagogram)
B. Aortic runoffs (patent ductus arteriosus, aortic regurgi- tation, anemia, thyrotoxicosis)	Murmurs Wide pulse pressure EKG: left ventricular hypertrophy Cardiac fluoroscopy Rarely retrograde aortogram

Table 21. Hypertension in Infants and Children:
Causes and Diagnostic Aids (Cont.)

Etiology	Diagnostic Aids
IV. Endoctrine-Metabolic	
A. Secondary to cortisone or ACTH therapy	History
B. Pheochromocytoma	History, IVP Regitine-Benzodioxane tests Histamine test Urinary or blood catechol amine Urinary vanillin mandelic acid
C. Cushing's syndrome	Clinical picture 17-OH steroids
D. Congenital adrenal hyperplasia	Clinical picture 17-ketosteroid excretion
E. Primary aldosteronism	Clinical picture Low serum K
F. Porphyria	Clinical picture Urinary and fecal porphyrin excretion
V. Poisonings	
A. Lead	Clinical picture Anemia, stippled cells Cerebrospinal fluid (elevated pressure and protein) Glycosuria X-ray of long bones and skull Urine coproporphyrin (qualitative) Urine lead excretion (quantitative)
B. Mercury	Clinical picture of acrodynia Urine mercury excretion
VI. Essential	Positive family history ? Cold pressor and amytal tests

Table 22. Incidence of Major Congenital Cardiac Lesions in Maude
Abbott's 1000 Autopsied Cases of Congenital Heart Disease[1]

(In Order of Frequency)

Pulmonic stenosis with open ventricular septum	115
Patent ductus arteriosus	105
Coarctation of aorta	85
Ventricular septal defect	62
Complete transposition of the great vessels	49
Pulmonic stenosis with closed ventricular septum	35
Atrial septal defect	33
Dextrocardia	29
Cor biloculare or triloculare	27
Aortic stenosis	23
True truncus arteriosus	21
Tricuspid atresia	16
Aortic atresia	12
Aortopulmonary fenestration	10
Anomalous pulmonary venous drainage	4
Miscellaneous	374
Total	1000

Table 23. Incidence of Major Congenital Cardiac Lesions
in Paul Wood's Series[748]

Without Shunt					
General	%	Left-Sided	%	Right-Sided	%
Dextrocardia. . . .0.5		Aortic atresia. . .Rare		Ebstein's	
Familial		Aortic		anomaly of	
cardiomegaly. . .Rare		hypoplasia 0.5		tricuspid	
Friedreich's		Aortic in-		valve[*].	1.0
disease. . . . . .Rare		competence. . . . 0.5		Idiopathic di-	
Gargoylism. . . . .Rare		Aortic rings . . . .Rare		latation of	
Heart block. 1.5		Aortic stenosis . . 3.0		pulmonary	
Von Gierke's		Coarctation of		artery	1.0
disease. . . . . . .Rare		the aorta 9.0		Pulmonary	
		Cor triatriatum. .Rare		stenosis	
		Fibroelastosis . .Rare		(isolated):	
		Left coronary		Infundibular .	2.0
		artery arising		Valvular. . . .	10.0
		from pulmonary			
		artery . . . . . . .Rare			
		Mitral stenosis . .Rare			
		Right-sided			
		aortic arch			
		(isolated) . . . . .Rare			
Totals	2.0		13.0		14.0

[*]Some cases are cyanotic.

Table 23. Incidence of Major Congenital Cardiac Lesions
in Paul Wood's Series (cont.)

With Shunt			
Acyanotic Left-to-Right Shunt (Pulmonary Plethora)	%	Cyanotic Right-to-Left Shunt	%
Left ventricular enlargement:		Diminished pulmonary	
Patent ductus	13.0	blood flow:	
Aortopulmonary septal defect .	0.3	Normal or low P.A.	
Right ventricular enlargement:		pressure:	
Atrial septal defect	18.0	Left ventricular	
A.S.D. with pulmonary		enlargement:	
stenosis	2.0	Tricuspid atresia	1.5
Anomalous pulmonary venous		Anomalous drainage	
drainage (partial)		of S.V.C. or I.V.C.	
Enlargement of both ventricles:		into left atrium . . . . Rare	
Ventricular septal defect	8.0	Single ventricle with	
Ventricular septal defect with		pulmonary stenosis . . Rare	
pulmonary stenosis	1.3	Right ventricular	
Miscellaneous	3.7	enlargement:	
		Fallot's tetralogy	11.0
		Pulmonary atresia . . .	1.7
		Pulmonary stenosis	
		with reversed inter-	
		atrial shunt	3.0
		High P.A. pressure:	
		Pulmonary hypertension	
		with reversed shunt:	
		Patent ductus	2.0
		Ventricular septal	
		defect (Eisenmenger's	
		complex)	3.0
		Atrial septal defect . .	1.5
		Cor triloculare	
		biatriatum[†] . . . . . . Rare	
		Increased pulmonary	
		blood flow:	
		Transposition of great	
		vessels	1.0
		Persistent truncus . . . . Rare	
		Total anomalous pul-	
		monary venous drainage	
		into S.V.C. or R.A. . . . Rare	
		Cor biventriculare	
		triloculare . . . . Rare	
Totals	42.6		24.7

[†]Some cases may have pulmonary plethora.

Table 24. Incidence of Major Cardiac Lesions in Infants Dying in
the First Month of Life[538]

Transposition of the great vessels.	27
Interventricular septal defect.	18
Cor triloculare and cor biloculare.	12
Coarctation of aorta	11
Tetralogy of Fallot.	4
Miscellaneous	28
Total	100

Table 25. Frequency of Common Congenital Cardiac Lesions among
3786 Cases Studied at Cardiac Catheterization, Operation or Postmortem Examination in the Cardiac Division of The Children's
Hospital Medical Center, 1949-1962

Lesion	No.	%	Lesion	No.	%
Ventricular septal defect.	756	19.97	Coarctation of aorta	189	4.99
Ventricular septal defect and pulmonic stenosis	551	14.55	Transposition of great arteries	150	3.96
Patent ductus arteriosus.	466	12.31	Endocardial cushion defects.	149	3.94
			Tricuspid atresia.	47	1.24
Pulmonic stenosis	453	11.97	Miscellaneous	428	11.30
Atrial septal defect (secundum)	380	10.04			
Aortic stenosis	217	5.73	Total	3786	100

Table 26. Incidence of Various Congenital Cardiac Defects
in Keith's Series[380]

Defect	Per Cent of Total Group	Prevalence in Population, Birth-14 Years
Ventricular septal defect	22	1:4000
Patent ductus arteriosus	17	1:5500
Tetralogy of Fallot	11	1:8500
Transposition of great vessels	8	1:11,000
Atrial septal defect	7	1:13,500
Pulmonary stenosis with normal aortic root	7	1:14,500
Coarctation of aorta	6	1:16,000
Aortic and subaortic stenosis	4	1:24,000
Ventricular septal defect with pulmonary hypertension	3	1:33,000
Tricuspid atresia	3	1:35,000
Atrioventricularis communis	2	1:47,0000
Aortic atresia	2	1:39,000
Single ventricle	2	1:50,000
Total anomalous pulmonary venous drainage	2	1:55,000
Endocardial fibroelastosis	1	1:68,000
Pulmonary atresia with normal aortic root	1	1:70,000
Persistent truncus ateriosus	Less than 1	1:150,000
Ebstein's disease	Less than 1	1:210,000
Double aortic arch	Less than 1	1:250,000

Table 27. Oxygen Saturation and Oxyhemoglobin and Reduced
Hemoglobin in Normal and Cyanotic Subjects

	Normal			Cyanotic		
	O_2 Sat. %	Oxy. Hgb. gm. %	Red. Hgb. gm. %	O_2 Sat. %	Oxy. Hgb. gm. %	Red. Hgb. gm. %
Arterial blood	95	14.25	.75	75	11.25	3.75
Capillary blood (calculated)	85	12.75	2.25	65	9.75	5.25
Venous blood	75	11.25	3.75	55	8.25	6.75

Table 28. Anatomic Classification of Congenital Heart Disease

I. Communication between systemic and pulmonary circuits with
    dominantly left-to-right shunt
    A. Interatrial communications
        1. Patent foramen ovale
        2. Secundum atrial defect
        3. Endocardial cushion defect
            a. Partial
            b. Complete
    B. Interventricular communications
        1. Simple ventricular defect
            a. Small
            b. Large
        2. Complicated ventricular defect with
            a. Pulmonic stenosis
            b. Aortic regurgitation*
            c. Absent pulmonic valve
            d. Atrial defect
            e. Patent ductus arteriosus
            f. Coarctation of the aorta
        3. Single ventricle
        4. Left ventricle-right atrial shunt
    C. Communications between great vessels
        1. Patent ductus arteriosus, simple
        2. Patent ductus arteriosus complicated with
            a. Pulmonary hypertension
            b. Aortic stenosis
            c. Pulmonic stenosis
            d. Coarctation of the aorta
            e. Ventricular defect
        3. Aortopulmonary fenestrum
        4. Common truncus arteriosus
        5. Aneurysm of the sinus of Valsalva (ruptured)*
        6. Coronary arteriovenous fistula*

II. Valvar and vascular lesions with a right-to-left shunt or no
    shunt at all
    A. Coarctation of the aorta
    B. Vascular ring
    C. Aortic stenosis
        1. Supravalvar
        2. Valvar
        3. Subvalvar
        4. Muscular
    D. Aortic runoffs
        1. Fenestration of aortic leaflets
        2. Ventricular septal defect with aortic regurgitation*
        3. Bicuspid aortic valve
        4. Coronary arteriovenous fistula*
        5. Aneurysm of the sinus of valsalva*
        6. Marfan's disease

Table 28. Anatomic Classification of Congenital Heart Disease
(cont.)

    E. The hypoplastic left-heart syndrome
       1. Aortic atresia
       2. Mitral atresia
       3. Atresia of aortic arch
       4. Hypoplasia of aortic arch
    F. Mitral stenosis
    G. Mitral regurgitation
    H. Cor triatriatum
    I. Pulmonary vascular obstruction syndrome
    J. Pulmonary stenosis
       1. With intact ventricular septum
       2. With ventricular defect
    K. Pulmonary atresia with intact ventricular septum
    L. Pulmonary regurgitation
    M. Underdeveloped right ventricle with tricuspid atresia
    N. Ebstein's anomaly of tricuspid valve

III. The transpositions
    A. Complete transposition of the great arteries
    B. Partial inversion of the great arteries
       1. Taussig-Bing syndrome
       2. Double-outlet right ventricle
    C. Corrected transposition of the great arteries
       (transposition-inversion-functional correction)
    D. Complete transposition of the pulmonary veins
    E. Incomplete transposition of the pulmonary veins
    F. Transposition of venae cavae
    G. Dextrocardia
       1. Mirror image
       2. Dextroversion
    H. Levocardia

*These may be accompanied by a left-to-right shunt. See group I.

Table 29. Sudden Death in Childhood Associated with Aortic Stenosis[580]

Mortality from Sudden Death % (No. of pat. in series)	Age	Activity at Death	EKG LVH	With Strain	Symptoms
6% (67)	6 yrs.	?	+	+	Fatigue
	8 yrs.	Playing in a field	+	+	Fatigue, dyspnea, pallor
	13 yrs.	Coming home from play	+	+	Dyspnea
	14 yrs.	Bowling and basketball	+	+	? Asthma
7% (30)	6 yrs.	Died on ward awaiting operation	+	?	Fatigue, dyspnea, angina
	16 yrs.	Died on ward awaiting operation	+	?	Fatigue
4% (56)	13 yrs.	Playing Rugby football	?	?	None
	?	?	?	?	?
8% (73)	7 yrs.	Playing outdoors	+	+	Multiple syncopal spells
	15 yrs.	Walking in water 2 feet deep	+	+	One syncopal spell
	3 yrs.	Sleeping, having leg pains	-	-	One syncopal spell, fatigue
	10 yrs.	Standing watching workmen	WPW	-	Slight fatigue
	15 yrs.	Playing football	+	+	Asymptomatic
	3 mos.	Hospitalized, wheezing, gasping	+	+	?
8% (37)	?	In hospital awaiting surgery	?	?	?
	?	Walking across a schoolyard	?	?	?
	?	Walking across a beach	?	?	?
7% (15)	14 yrs.	?	?	?	Fatigue, dyspnea, angina
18% (28)	6 mos.	?	+	?	L.V. failure, age 5 mos.
	10 mos.	?	+	+	L.V. failure, age 7 mos.
	9 yrs.	?	+	+	Mild—unspecified
	11 yrs.	?	+	+	Mild—unspecified; syncope
	15 yrs.	?	+	+	Moderate—unspecified; syncope
75% (306) total					

Data drawn from seven series. Abbreviations: +, present; -, not present; LVH, left ventricular hypertrophy; ?, unknown, not reported; WPW, Wolff-Parkinson-White syndrome.

Table 30. Correlation of Postoperative Aortic Valve Gradient with
Postoperative Changes in the Electrocardiogram[414]

			Cardiographic Improvement
Gradient abolished	Valvar	2	2
	Subvalvar	4	1
Gradient diminished . . .	Valvar	3	2
	Subvalvar	0	0
Gradient unaffected. . . .	Valvar	2	0
	Subvalvar	2	0

Note that among four patients with subvalvar stenosis in whom the
gradient was abolished, only one showed significant improvement in
the electrocardiogram, whereas both patients with valvar stenosis
without residual gradient have normal tracings.

Table 31. Anatomic Lesions in 101 Patients with Hypoplastic Left
Heart Syndrome Seen at The Children's Hospital Medical Center in
Boston, 1949-1957, Inclusive[536]

	Number of Patients
Aortic valve atresia	15
With mitral atresia 2	
With mitral hypoplasia 13	
Mitral atresia	5
Mitral stenosis	4
Atresia of transverse aortic arch	6
Hypoplasia of aortic arch.	71
Total	101

Table 32. Clinical Aids in the Differentiation of the Clinical Entities Forming the Hypoplastic Left-Heart Syndrome536

Clinical Entity	Usual Length of Survival	Cyanosis	X-rays	Remarks
Aortic valve atresia . . .	Under 1 week	Moderate, generalized	Large globular heart	Sudden onset of cardiac failure and rapid, downhill course in first week of life
Mitral atresia	2-4 months	Mild, generalized	Moderate cardiac enlargement, narrow waist (occ.). Pulmonary vasculature may be diminished	X-ray somewhat atypical for group and may help in differential diagnosis
Mitral stenosis	6-24 months	Variable	Moderate cardiac enlargement, contour variable, pulmonary vasculature sometimes diminished	Paroxysmal bouts of dyspnea. Occasional typical presystolic mitral murmur
Aortic arch atresia. . .	Under 1 month	May be differential	Moderate cardiac enlargement, sometimes pulmonary plethora	Difficult to distinguish from hypoplasia. Murmurs in only half
Hypoplasia of aortic arch	Half die by 6 weeks; some survive through childhood	May be differential	Moderate cardiac enlargement, frequent pulmonary plethora	Most common form of syndrome. Relative hypertension in arms in majority

Table 33. Physiologic Classification of 50 Patients with
Transposition of the Great Arteries[536]

	No. of Patients
Group I–Intact ventricular septum.	13
Group II–With ventricular septal defect:	
A. Associated pulmonary stenosis.	11
B. Associated pulmonary vascular obstruction.	14
C. Large pulmonary blood flow with normal pulmonary resistance and no significant pulmonary stenosis . .	<u>12</u>
Total	50

Table 34. Classification of Complete Transposition
of Pulmonary Veins

	Entry	Pressure		Art. O$_2$	CE*	Survival
		PA	PV			
Without PAH* . .	Supradiaphrag-matic	N* or sl.↑	N.	85-95%	++	Likely
With PAH. . .	Infradiaphrag-matic or supra-diaphragmatic	↑↑	↑↑	20-85%	±	Unlikely

*Abbreviations: CE, cardiac enlargement; PAH, pulmonary
artery hypertension; N, normal.

Table 35. Age at Death in 42 Cases of Unilateral Anomalous
Pulmonary Venous Drainage

< 1 Year	1-20 Years	20-40 Years	40-50 Years	> 50 Years	"Adults"
6	2	6	5	9	14

From the literature.

INDEX

Page numbers in *italics* refer to illustrations.

A WAVE, in atrial pressure tracing, 160
  interpretation of, 21, *22*
abdomen, examination of, 12
abdominal pain. See *pain.*
ACTH, in rheumatic fever, 186–189
Adams-Stokes attacks, in complete heart
  block, 254
age, and blood pressure, 347, *347,* table, 773
  as factor in development of rheumatic
    fever, 173
alveolar hypoventilation, as mechanism of
  cor pulmonale, 332
Aminophylline, use with mercurial diuretics,
  322
ammonium chloride, use with mercurial diuretics, 321
amyl nitrite, effects on murmur of pulmonic
  stenosis, *619,* 621
anemia(s), as complication of tetralogy of
  Fallot, 651, *651*
  causing heart disease, 328
  in bacterial endocarditis, 218
  with pericarditis, 303
anemic heart disease, clinical picture, 329
  etiology of, 328
  physiology of, 329
  treatment, 329
aneurysm, arteriovenous. See *arteriovenous
  aneurysm.*
angiocardiography, 147
  in tetralogy of Fallot, 646
    with unilateral pulmonary atresia,
      663, *666*
  used in calculating shunts, 159
angiography, in secundum atrial defects, 379
anomalous venous drainage. See *venous
  drainage.*
anoxia, and arterial unsaturation, 353
"anoxic spells," considered in history-taking,
  4
antibiotics. See also under specific agents,
  e.g., *penicillin.*

antibiotics (*Continued*)
  in bacterial endocarditis, 221
aorta, coarctation of, 521–546
  anatomy of, 521
  associated vascular anomalies, 522
  classification of, 523
  definition, 521
  differentiation from aortic stenosis with
    congestive failure in infants, 563
  etiology of, 522
  fluoroscopic visualization, *34*
  incidence of, 521
  physiology of, 522–524, *523*
  "preductal" and "postductal," 523
  rib notching in, radiographic visualiza-
    tion, *42,* 43
  simple, 524–532
    auscultation of, 525, *526*
    catheterization studies in, 526, *529*
    clinical picture, 524–530
    complications of, 530
    course, 530
    differential diagnosis, 530
    electrocardiographic evidences of,
      525, *528*
    prognosis, 530
    radiographic evidences of, 525, *527*
    surgery in, 530
    treatment, 530–532
  with aortic stenosis, 564. See also *aortic
    stenosis.*
  with congestive failure, in infancy, 532–
    537
    auscultation of, 532
    catheterization studies in, 533,
      534
    clinical picture, 532
    course, 533, *535*
    differential diagnosis, 534–536
    electrocardiographic evidences of,
      533, *535*
    etiology, 532

801